Handbook of Transradial Interventions

The Oxford Clinical Practice Series covers an array of resources providing essential evidence-based, up-to-date information and key clinical references that will enhance the clinical knowledge of healthcare practitioners and medical students across the globe.

Handbook of Transradial Interventions

Edited by

SANJAY KUMAR CHUGH

OXFORD
UNIVERSITY PRESS

OXFORD
UNIVERSITY PRESS

Oxford University Press is a department of the University of Oxford. It furthers the University's objective of excellence in research, scholarship, and education by publishing worldwide. Oxford is a registered trade mark of Oxford University Press in the UK and in certain other countries

Published in India by
Oxford University Press
22 Workspace, 2nd Floor, 1/22 Asaf Ali Road, New Delhi 110002, India

ISBN-13 (Paperback): 978-0-19-013000-8
ISBN-10 (Paperback): 0-19-013000-8

Typeset in Minion Pro 10/13
by Newgen Knowledge Works Pvt. Ltd.
Printed and bound in India by Replika Press Pvt. Ltd.

This Book is dedicated to

My respected parents, Mrs Chand Rani Chugh and Late Shri Dharam Vir Chugh; my lovely grandchildren Dharam Veer (Jr.),
Baby Zanaiya and Baby Ayra;
my pride my joy, my son, Dr Yashasvi, and Dr Neeta my loving and courageous daughter in law;
my loving kind daughter Saumya, and Siddharth, my dearest son in law;
my wife, Dr Sunita—the love of my life:
All, God's greatest gifts to me;
and last but not the least, to All my patients.

It takes a lifetime to get there

Detailed Contents

Contributors

Sourabh Agstam, MD, DM
Advanced Cardiac Centre
Postgraduate Institute of Medical Education and Research
Chandigarh, India

Waqar Ahmed, MD
Cardiac Center, King Fahd Armed Forces Hospital
Jeddah, Saudi Arabia

Mirvat Alasnag, MD
Cardiac Center, King Fahd Armed Forces Hospital
Jeddah, Saudi Arabia

Zaid Alirhayim, MD, FACC, FSCAI
Interventional Cardiologist
King Fahad Specialist Hospital
Dammam, Saudi Arabia

Giovanni Amoroso, MD, PhD
OLVG Hospital
Amsterdam, The Netherlands

M.A. Azeez Assad, MD, DNB
Apollo Hospital
Jubilee Hills, Hyderabad, India

Hakim Benamer, MD
Ramsay Generale de Sante
Institut Cardiovasculaire Paris Sud
Massy, France

Sanjay Kumar Chugh (a.k.a Sanjay Chugh), MD, DM, FACC, FSCAI
Senior Consultant and Associate Director, Cardiology and Interventional Cardiology, Institute of Cardiac Sciences, Narayana Healthcare Superspeciality Hospital
Gurgaon, India

Sunita Chugh, MBBS, MASE
Non–invasive Cardiology, Heart and Vascular Institute
Fortis Memorial Research Institute
Gurugram, India

Yashasvi Chugh, MD
Interventional Cardiologist and Structural Heart Disease Interventionist
Baylor Scott & White Heart and Vascular Hospital
Dallas, Fortworth, Texas, USA

B. Dixit, MD, DM
Cardiology
Apollo Hospital
Hyderabad, India

Katherine Durham, MS, APN-BC
Cardiology Nurse Practitioner
Jesse Brown VA Medical Center
Chicago, USA

Daniel Feldman
Cardiology Fellow
University of Illinois at Chicago
Chicago, USA

Ganesh Paramasivan, MD, DM
Assistant Professor of Cardiology
Kasturba Medical College
Manipal Academy of Higher Education
Manipal, India

Philippe Garot, MD, FESC
Ramsay Generale de Sante
Institut Cardiovasculaire Paris Sud
Massy, France

Sudhakar George, MD, MRCP
Department of Cardiology
Royal Stoke University Hospital
UK

Tapan Ghose, MD, DNB, FACC, FSCAI
Director and Head
Department of Cardiology
Fortis Flt Lt Ranjan Dhall Hospital
New Delhi, India

Thomas Hovasse, MD
Ramsay Generale de Sante
Institut Cardiovasculaire Paris Sud
Massy, France

Shahid Karim, MD, FRCP
Consultant Cardiologist
Manchester University, NHS
Foundation Trust
Manchester, UK

Sasko Kedev, MD, PhD, FESC, FACC, FSCAI
Interventional Cardiologist
University Clinic of Cardiology
Skopje, Macedonia

Prafulla Kerkar, MD, FACC
Professor and Head
Department of Cardiology
Seth GS Medical College and KEM
Hospital
Mumbai, India

N.N. Khanna, MD, DM, FRCP, FESC, FACC, FSCAI
Senior Consultant, Interventional
Cardiology and Vascular Interventions
Indraprastha Apollo Hospitals
New Delhi, India

Dhiraj Kumar, MD, DNB, DM
Superspeciality Medical Officer
Department of Cardiology
Seth GS Medical College and KEM
Hospital
Mumbai, India

Charan Lanjewar, MD, DM, FACC, FSCAI
Associate Professor and Unit Head
Department of Cardiology
Seth GS Medical College and KEM
Hospital
Mumbai, India

Yves Louvard, MD, FSCAI
Ramsay Generale de Sante
Institut Cardiovasculaire Paris Sud
Massy, France

Mamas A. Mamas, MA, D Phil, FRCP
Professor of Interventional Cardiology
Keele University, Stoke-on-Trent
UK

Tift Mann, MD, FACC, FSCAI
Consultant Interventional
Cardiologist
North Carolina Heart and Vascular
Associates
North Carolina, USA

Saurabh Mehrotra, MD, DM
Associate Professor, Cardiology
Advanced Cardiac Centre
Postgraduate Institute of Medical
Education and Research
Chandigarh, India

Sundeep Mishra, MD, DM, FACC, FSCAI, FAPIC
Professor and Head of Cardiology
Vice Chancellor
NIIMS University
Jaipur, India

Nilavan N
Madras Medical College
Chennai, India

James Nolan, MD, FRCP
Consultant Interventional Cardiologist
Department of Cardiology
Royal Stoke University Hospital
UK

Devang S. Parikh, MD, MA
Division of Cardiology
University of Illinois at Chicago
Chicago, USA

Justin Paul Gnanaraj, MD, DM
Professor of Cardiology
Madras Medical College
Chennai, India

Shobhit Piplani, MD
Jacobi Medical Center
Albert Einstein College of Medicine
New York, USA

C. Raghu, MD, DM
Senior Consultant Interventional Cardiologist
and Head of Cardiology
Aster-Prime Hospital
Hyderabad, India

Sankaran Ramesh, MD, DM
Associate Professor
Department of Cardiology
Sri Ramachandra Medical College and Research Institute
Chennai, India

Suparna Rao, MD, DM
Registrar
Cardiology
Indraprastha Apollo Hospital
New Delhi, India

Pavankumar P. Rasalkar
Consultant Cardiology
Eden Critical Care Hospital
Chandigarh, India

Muhammad Rashid, MBBS
Keele Cardiovascular Research Group
Keele University, Stoke-on-Trent
UK

P.C. Rath, MD, DM, FACC, FSCAI, FESC
Head of Cardiology and Interventional Cardiology
Apollo Hospital
Hyderabad, India

Karim Ratib, MRCP
Department of Cardiology
Royal Stoke University Hospital
UK

Jeff Redleene
Department of Cardiology
Madras Medical College
Chennai, India
Helen Routledge
Interventional Cardiologist
Worcestershire Royal Hospital
Worcester, UK

Sanjay Sastry, MD, FRCP
Consultant Cardiologist
Manchester University, NHS Foundation Trust
Manchester, UK

Adhir Shroff, MD, MPH
Associate Professor of Medicine
Jesse Brown VA Medical Center
University of Illinois at Chicago
Chicago, USA

Mladen I. Vidovich, MD, FACC, FSCAI
Consultant Interventional Cardiologist
Division of Cardiology
University of Illinois at Chicago
Chicago, USA

Fuminobu Yoshimachi
Associate Professor
Department of Cardiology
Tokai University Hachioji Hospital
Japan

Foreword

From what initially started as a 'fringe movement' within Interventional Cardiology, transradial access has finally achieved a sense of normalcy within the field and in many cases has become the dominant form of vascular access for transcatheter cardiovascular procedures. The rapidity with which this has happened was no doubt agonizingly slow for the early pioneers in the field, but for someone like me who started training in the early 2000s, the rapidity of change has been in fact remarkable to behold. In stark contrast to when I started training, hundreds of thousands of procedures are being done worldwide transradially, and many of these are being done by operators who now view femoral access as a second and lesser alternative for access, rather than the default.

Despite the ascendancy of the transradial approach, discussions of technical best practices are still essential and hardly *passé*. In some respects, now more than ever, it is critically important to continue to assess and reassess refinements to the practice of transradial catheterization so as to continue moving our field forward. In this vein, this *Handbook of Transradial Interventions* can serve as a piloting guide for those who are unfamiliar with the techniques, as well as for seasoned veterans looking to update and expand their scope of practice. Ultimately as clinicians we are always looking for ways to better ourselves and thereby impact the care of our patients positively. Comprehensive texts like this one allow us to get much closer to this laudable goal.

Ajay J Kirtane, MD, SM
Associate Professor of Medicine at Columbia University Medical Center
Chief Academic Officer, Center for Interventional Vascular Therapy
Director, NYP/Columbia Cardiac Catheterization Laboratories

Preface

The recent European Society and the American College of Cardiology guidelines for coronary artery revascularization advocate a radial-first strategy as the default approach for percutaneous coronary interventions (PCI), regardless of clinical presentation; because of the overwhelming and irrefutable evidence of lower risk of vascular complications, bleeding and mortality, especially in acute and high risk patients, with the radial approach.

Not only has transradial access gained prime position in interventional cardiology; the paradigm has shifted further to 'forearm access', with inclusion of transulnar access, and now the latest 'distal transradial' access. This book covers it all with evidence-base and practical tips from the world leaders on the subject.

'Handbook of Transradial Interventions' which is a part of the Oxford University Press Clinical series is an exhaustive treatise that incorporates the latest topics and covers all aspects of transradial, distal radial, and transulnar interventions, from access to diagnostics and interventions including complex interventional procedures, and primary angioplasty for ST elevation myocardial infarction; along with current literature and illustrations. The book has more than 300 illustrations.

The highlights of the book are a fully illustrated chapter on practical 'tips and tricks for transradial interventions' which includes tips for transradial angioplasty in acute myocardial infarction; a separate chapter covers tips for managing complications of radial access. The chapter on complex transradial interventions is also fully illustrated and case-based.

Chapters have been added on new research and new technologies including the chapter on 'transulnar interventions' and on 'slender transradial interventions'.

For the first time, a chapter on 'appropriateness ratings for patient selection and physicians performing transradial procedures', on 'the role of

Doppler ultrasound in transradial interventions', and on 'radiation exposure and stroke risk' in transradial interventions is presented.

The 'new age' radial, the latest technique of 'distal transradial access' is discussed in a separate chapter, with illustrations.

To quote Helen Routledge, 'With constant publications and data coming through, our own "know-how" will always remain in a flux. Thus far at least, considering the overall balance of risks and benefits, the evidence most certainly favours the use of transradial access in coronary interventions. However, as in life, one must always have a back-up approach and hence to discard the trans-femoral approach totally would be foolhardy.' Hence, a chapter on management of femoral complications, including how to prevent them is included, which would be useful to default transradial operators, as femoral skills decline with fall in usage of femoral access.

This is the only book that comprehensively includes all aspects of forearm access including radial access, distal radial access, ulnar access, as well as transradial, distal trans radial, and transulnar interventions and would be an asset for junior, senior and seasoned interventional cardiologists and fellows in-training worldwide who want to learn techniques or update their skills and knowledge. It fills a much-needed void for a reference book.

We have come a long way from the days in 2002 when, after my return to India, my wife and 2 small children would stick stamps on invitations to cardiologists to attend our radial course and workshops and I would post them at the General Post Office in New Delhi, India. Radial and forearm access percutaneous coronary interventions are now popular, for their advantages to patients; but should be utilized more often, to reduce mortality risk of patients with ST elevation myocardial infarction and acute coronary syndromes. With this in mind, Chapter 10 discusses practical tips and Chapter 17 (i), (ii) present the relevant evidence for the same.

Finally, the views expressed in the chapters and permissions obtained for reproducing figures and tables in these chapters have been the sole responsibility of the respective authors.

Chief Editor
Dr Sanjay Kumar Chugh, MD Medicine, DM, Cardiology, AIIMS, New Delhi, FACC, FSCAI
Senior Consultant and Associate Director, Cardiology and Interventional Cardiology, Institute of Cardiac Sciences, Narayana Healthcare Superspeciality Hospital, Gurgaon, India

Formerly:

- Principal Consultant Escorts Heart Institute, New Delhi & FMRI, Gurgaon, India.
- Head of Department of Cardiology, Jaipur National University, IMSRC, Jaipur, Rajasthan, India.
- Fellow, Associate, Interventional Cardiology, Royal Jubilee Hospital, Victoria, BC.
- Fellow, Interventional Cardiology, St Paul's Hospital, Vancouver, UBC; & foothills Hospital, U of C, Calgary, AB.
- Clinician in Interventional Cardiology, St. George's Hospital London, UK.

Acknowledgements

I am indebted to **Dr Sunita Chugh** *for her untiring efforts; without whose help, this book would not have seen the light of day.*

I am deeply indebted to the authors of the chapters for their contributions, and to the **Consulting Editors** *for their constant help and support.*

- ***Dr Tift Mann, MD, FACC***
- ***Dr Jim Nolan, MD, FRCP***
- ***Dr Mamas Mamas, MD, FRCP***

My sincere gratitude to the **Wellness and Radial Intervention Society (WARIS)** *for its support in compiling the book, with funding to support indexing and help in launching, & promoting the book, to be able to take the technology to cardiologists worldwide.*

I acknowledge with gratitude, the whole-hearted support of

- ***Dr Naresh Trehan, Chairman, Medanta, the Medicity, Gurugram***
- ***Dr Satyajit Bose, Chief Cardiothoracic and Vascular Surgeon and Chairman,*** *The Mission Hospital, Durgapur*
- ***Dr Sandeep Bakshi,*** *Chancellor, Jaipur National University*
- ***Dr Vikram Singh Yadav, renowned Laparoscopic Surgeon***
- ***Dr Renu Yadav CEO, renowned Gynaecologist & Obstetrician, Aarvy Healthcare Superspeciality hospital, Gurugram***
  who made this book possible;

My sincere gratitude to ***all staff of Cath Labs at:***

- ***Jaipur National University Hospital, Institute for Medical Sciences and Research Centre, Jaipur, Rajasthan, India***
  (Dwarikaprasad Sharma, Ajay Singh, Ghanshyam, Geetesh Joshi, Pradeep Negi, Saurabh Dabral, Priyanka Kumari, Poonam Jangid, ChandraPrakash Garg, Noshad, and Sharif)

- **The Mission Hospital, Durgapur, WB, India**
  (Uttam Bera, Rajib Nandi, Jayanta, Abhijeet, Sangeeta, SudipKesh, Vaisakh, Sijo, Jijo)
  for helping prepare the case-illustrations and for help with collection of data.

I am grateful to -

- ***Radial Masterclass, UK; TCT, SCAI, Radial Live, and India Live*** *for promoting radials.*
- *Drs Merill Knudtson, FRCPC, FACC, Mouhieddin Traboulsi, FRCPC, FACC, JL Hansen, FRCPC, Todd Anderson, FRCPC, FACC, Michael Curtis, FRCPC, Frank Spence, FRCPC and all Staff and consultants at* **Foothills hospital, U of C, Calgary** *for angioplasty and primary angioplasty; Drs John Webb, FRCPC, FACC, Ronald Carere, FRCPC, FACC, Dr Jaap Hamburger, MD and all Staff and consultants at* **St. Paul's hospital, UBC, Vancouver, BC** *for interventional cardiology; Drs David Hilton, FRCPC, FACC, Peter Klinke, David Kinloch, FRCPC, Eric Fretz, FRCPC, and all Staff and consultants at* **Royal Jubilee hospital, Victoria, BC** *for trans-radial interventions; Dr Takashi Matsukage, MD, PhD, consultants and staff at* **Tokai University, Tokyo**, *Dr Shigero Saito, Dr Ikari; Late Dr Charles Pumphrey, MD, FRCP, Dr David E Ward, MD, FRCP, Dr Stephen Brecker, MD, FRCP, all staff and consultants at* **St. George's hospital, London, UK** *for interventional cardiology; Dr Nigel Stephens, MD, FRCP, Dr Hugh Bethell, MD, FRCP, Chris Kinsey, Ann Banfield RN, all nurses and staff of Cardiology Department at* **Northwest London Hospital, Middlesex, UK**; *Dr Ashok Seth, FRCP, Dr TS Kler MD, DM, FRCP, Dr RR Kasliwal, MD, DM, Dr Praveen Chandra, MD, DM, Dr Suman Bhandari, MD, DM, Dr Praveer Agarwal, MD, DM, Dr AK Omar, MD, Dr Sameer Srivastava, MD, DM, Dr Rajnish Sardana, MD, DM, Dr Rajneesh Kaoor, MD, DNB, Dr Aparna Jaiswal, MD, DNB, Dr Simi Minocha MD, DNB, Dr Arif Mustakeen MD, DNB, Dr Joy Chakravarti MD, Dr Ashsih Kalla, Mini SN, all residents, nurses, staff and colleagues at* **Fortis Escorts Heart Institute, New Delhi, Escorts Kalyani Heart Center and FMRI, Gurugram**; *Drs Balram Bhargava MD, DM, FRCP, FACC, VK Bahl DM, FACC, U Kaul DM, FACC*

and Consultants and staff **at CN Centre, All India Institute of Medical Sciences, New Delhi, India;** *Dr JC Ghosh MD, FRCP, Dr DC Ghosh, MD, FRCP; my friends, Dr Manas Chakravarti, Dr Pranab Basak, Dr Asutosh Ghosh MD, DM, Dr Basab Gupta, Dr Sumit Basu MD, FRCP, Consultant Cardiologist, London, Dr Siba Prasad Roy Chowdhuri Professor of Medicine at UCDavis, for their seamless help and support. And last but not the least, Special gratitude to Late Professor SC Ghosh MD, FRCP, Internal Medicine,* **Calcutta Medical College,** *for inculcating a sense of clinical judgement, the mother of all interventions.*

I am deeply indebted to our publisher, Oxford University Press, Chris Holmes, Barun Sarkar, Darshana Sarkar, Sohini Ghosh, Chandan Kumar, Amit Rai, Directors, Editors, and Staff of Oxford University Press and of Production team of Newgen Knowledge Works, Praveena A, Project Manager, Gopinath, Newgen Knowledge Works and team, who worked ceaselessly to make the book happen.

1

Overview of Transradial Access

Sanjay Kumar Chugh

Introduction

Coronary angiography was first done via the brachial artery, using the Sones technique. Subsequently, the femoral artery came to be accepted as the standard access route for coronary and other cardiac catheterization procedures. Over the past decade, the radial artery, despite its small size and other anatomical challenges, has gained popularity for access for coronary procedures, both diagnostic and interventional. Recently, distal radial access via the anatomical snuffbox has also been used as default access for transradial procedures. (Please see Chapter 26: 'Distal Radial Access for Transradial Interventions'.)

Transradial Access for Percutaneous Coronary Intervention

Radial route was first introduced by Campeau[1] for coronary angiography and by Kiemeneij and Laarman for coronary angioplasty.[2] Transradial access has since gained tremendous popularity not only because of patient comfort, with early ambulation and early discharge, but also more importantly because it has been shown to improve survival, with less bleeding and vascular complications.[3–8]

Europe, Canada, South Korea, Japan, and other parts of the world have already shifted to performing the majority of Percutaneous Coronary Intervention (PCI) transradially. Based on recent estimates provided by industry, radial access usage is over 80% in the UK and South Korea, 70% in Japan, and 40% in rest of Asia; while for Europe and USA, the figures are lower.[9]

The 2016 Report from four American College of Cardiology National Cardiovascular Data Registries on trends in U.S. cardiovascular care shows an increase in radial access for PCI from 10.9% in 2011 to 25.2% in 2014, while femoral access decreased from 88.8% to 74.5% over the same period.[10]

The National Intervention Council of India (NIC) reported in 2016 that while primary angioplasty increased by 60%, its mortality also increased by 40%. While this increase in the number of primary PCI was attributed to mushrooming of cardiac catheterization (cath) laboratory (lab) facilities in Tier 2 and 3 cities, the increased mortality was attributed to increased reporting. However, it may be relevant that most procedures were done transfemorally.[11] An NIC and wellness and radial intervention society (WARIS) questionnaire survey (2016) of 663 cardiologists in India reported that while 72% cardiologists used transradial access for coronary angiography, including those (30%) who performed elective transradial angioplasty in selected cases; only 13% were default radial-first operators (*Source:* WARIS), though a default radial-first access is recommended for coronary revascularization procedures in the recent ESC and ACC guidelines.

Randomized Studies on Transradial Interventions

A randomized comparison of percutaneous transluminal coronary angioplasty by the radial, branchial, and femoral approaches (ACCESS) trial in 1997 was the first randomized study which showed less bleeding, haematoma, and other entry site vascular complications (0% versus 2.3% versus 2%, p = 0.03) for radial versus brachial versus femoral access, while having comparable procedural success (91.7% versus 90.7% versus 90.7%, p = 0.885), procedure duration (40 min versus 39 min versus 38 min, p = 0.6), fluoroscopy times (13 min versus 12 min versus 11 min), and 1-month follow-up (6.7% versus 8.3% versus 5.3%, p = 0.6) with radial access compared to brachial or femoral access. This study, however, excluded patients with abnormal Allen's test, acute myocardial infarction (AMI), chronic total occlusion, those requiring atherectomy, and patients with haemodynamic compromise or those requiring temporary pacing or right heart catheterization. All procedures were done using right radial access (RRA), with 45° abduction of arm, wrist hyperextension. Haemostasis was achieved with occlusive tourniquets.[12]

In subsequent studies such as TEst for Myocardial infarction by Prospective Unicenter Randomization for Access sites (TEMPURA), OUTpatient Coronary Low-Profile Angioplasty Study (OUTCLAS),[8] RadIal Versus femorAL access for coronary intervention (RIVAL),[5] Trans-radial Approach (LEft versus right) aNd procedural Times during percutaneous coronary procedures (TALENT),[13] and Radial versus Femoral Randomized Investigation in ST-Elevation Acute Coronary Syndrome (RIFLE-STEACS),[6] similar results were found with less bleeding, vascular complications. RIVAL[5] and RIFLE-STEACS[6] showed significant reduction in mortality in AMI patients.

TALENT[13] (left versus right), a randomized study (n = 1467 diagnostic, n = 688 PCI), showed that left radial access (LRA) had less fluoroscopy time (149 sec) than RRA (168 sec; p = 0.0025) in diagnostic angiography only. This difference in fluoroscopy time between left and RRA was significant in the in-experienced operators and also in the elderly patients who had more tortuosities in right subclavian artery compared to left subclavian artery. (Please see Chapter 11—'Radial Access for Transradial Procedures: Right versus Left'.)

A meta-analysis of five randomized controlled trials (RCTs)[14] of 3210 patients showed that procedure failure was more with RRA compared to LRA (RR 1.65 [1.18–2.3], p = 0.003], though procedural time [weighted mean difference (WMD) = 0.99 min], fluoroscopy time (WMD = −35.79 s), contrast use (WMD = 1.7 mL), and any major complication (RR = 2) showed no significant difference between RRA and LRA. (Please see Chapter 11—'Radial Access for Transradial Procedures: Right versus Left'.)

OUTCLAS[8] was a study on outpatient PCI (n = 644). 61.5% of radial access patients versus 55% of femoral access patients, respectively, were discharged in 4–6 hours (p = 0.09), with no increase in adverse events (1.1% versus 2.6%, respectively, p = 0.2).

A Review of TRI in AMI Studies

TEMPURA[4] was the first study in ST-elevation AMI (n = 149) with reperfusion success of 96.1% versus 97.2%, p = 0.6 and in-hospital major adverse cardiac events (MACE) of 5.2% versus 8.3%, p = 0.44 for radial versus femoral access.

RIVAL,[5] a large study (n = 7021) in acute coronary syndrome (ACS) patients, including 1,958 ST-elevation (STE) AMI (STEAMI) patients showed significant survival benefit with transradial accesss in STE-AMI patients. In STEAMI patients, the mortality was 1.3% versus 3.2%, p = 0.006 with radial versus femoral access for PCI. The primary end-point [composite of death, myocardial infarction (MI), stroke, non-coronary artery bypass surgery (CABG) bleeding at 30 days] was lower with PCI using radial access compared to femoral access (3.1% versus 5.2%, p = 0.02) in the STEMI group. In a subgroup analysis, the mortality was found to be lower in large volume centres versus centres with less volume and experience (1.6% versus 3.2%). (Please see Chapter 17—'Transradial Access Site Practice and Outcomes in Patients with Acute Coronary Syndromes'.)

In RIFLE-STEACS,[6] a multicentre randomized study in STEAMI patients (n = 1001), the primary end-point (cardiac death, MI, stroke, target lesion revascularization (TLR), bleeding at 30 days) was 13.6% versus 21% with radial versus femoral access for PCI (p = 0.003), while the 30-day cardiac mortality was 5.2% versus 9.2% (p = 0.02), respectively. (Please see Chapter 17—'Transradial Access Site Practice and Outcomes in Patients with Acute Coronary Syndromes' for further details.)

Minimizing Adverse Haemorrhagic Events by TRansradial Access Site and Systemic Implementation of angioX (MATRIX) study[15] enrolled ACS patients: non-ST-elevation acute coronary syndrome (NSTEACS) (52%) and STEAMI (48%) showed 33% reduction in net adverse cardiovascular events or NACE (composite of death, MI or stroke and major [*Bleeding* Academic Research Consortium (BARC) 3 or 5] bleeding and 28% reduction in all-cause cardiovascular (CV) deaths with transradial access (TRA) compared to transfemoral access (TFA).

In a meta-analysis of 10 STEAMI randomized studies comparing TRA versus TFA (n = 3347),[16] TRA improved the survival (odds ratio (OR) 0.53), reduced major bleeding (OR 0.63), and caused fewer vascular complications (OR 0.35). Procedure time was more with TRA versus TFA (weighted mean difference = 1.76 min).

Meta-analysis of Radial Versus Femoral Access Studies

Jolly et al.[17] included 23 RCTs in their meta-analysis (n = 7020) and reported a significant reduction in major bleeding (OR 0.27–0.45,

$p < 0.001$) and death, MI, or stroke (OR 0.71, $p = 0.058$), with higher procedure failure [OR 1.29 (0.87–1.94), $p = 0.2$].

In another meta-analysis,[18] 15 RCTs and 61 observational studies were included and showed significant reduction in major bleeding with TRA (OR 0.22). Survival benefit was seen only when registry data were included. RCTs alone failed to confirm survival advantage.

Jobe and Mann[19] have suggested that all new transradial operators should start with angiograms, then sequentially graduate from PCI in type A lesions[18] to more complex types B1, B2, and C lesions; finally taking up TRA for ACS cases culminating in transradial intervention (TRI) in ST segment elevation AMI (emergent) followed by the STEMI patients with haemodynamic compromise.

Incidentally, only 2.2% operators in India use radial access as default route (in >95% cases) of their total primary PCI for acute MI (TR-PAMI) cases (*Source*: WARIS), which is a cause for concern because of the immense mortality benefit reported in RCTs.

Patient Selection for Transradial Access

- Allen's or Barbeau's test is not mandatory.
- However, because of use of transulnar access for coronary and non-coronary procedures, it is worthwhile to compress the radial artery at wrist to feel ulnar pulse simultaneously as in reverse Allen's test.
- In patients with prior forearm access, it is advisable in case of doubt to have a colour Doppler of radial and ulnar arteries to ensure that ulnar artery is not obliterated.
- All patients with a well-palpable radial pulse can undergo a radial procedure. A weak radial pulse may suggest remnant radial; also, prior use of radial for a procedure can lead to slow flow in or narrowing of radial.
- Likewise, diameter of radial artery can also be checked[20] and anomalies can be identified with pre-procedure ultrasound of arm arteries, if in doubt. (Please see Chapter 6 on 'Role of Colour Doppler Ultrasound in Transradial Interventions'.)
- Smaller radial artery lumen of the female (≤1.7 mm)[20] may present additional technical challenge of radial spasm, and crossover during PCI.[21–23]

- Compression of ipsilateral ulnar,[23] sublingual nitroglycerin,[24] slender sheaths (GSS slender), 4F diagnostic and 5F guide catheters; as well as sheathless techniques have been used in these situations.[23]
- With experience, transradial interventions can be performed in patients with haemodynamic instability.
- Transradial intervention (TRI) can be safely and effectively performed in:
  1. Patients ≥80 years
  2. Females[20–23]
  3. Obese[25]
  4. Patients with high bleeding risk or receiving anticoagulants[26–28] or GpIIb/IIIa inhibitors[29,30]
  5. After prior bypass surgery[31]
- Identification of arteries that can accommodate larger sheaths should be based upon:
  1. Preprocedural manual palpation
  2. If in doubt, colour Doppler ultrasound sizing of the artery[20] can be utilized. A radial artery of ≥2.2–2.3 mm diameter can easily accommodate a 7F sheath and guiding catheter. (For further details, please refer to Chapter 6—'Role of Colour Doppler Ultrasound in Transradial Interventions'.)

References

1. Campeau L. Percutaneous radial artery approach for coronary angiography. *Cathet Cardiovasc Diagn*. 1989;16:3–7.
2. Kiemeneij F, Laarman GJ. Percutaneous transradial artery approach for coronary stent implantation. *Cathet Cardiovasc Diagn*. 1993;30:173–8.
3. Agostoni P, Biondi-Zoccai GG, de Benedictis ML, et al. Radial vs femoral approach for percutaneous coronary diagnostics and interventional procedures: systematic overview and meta analysis of randomized trials. *J Am Coll Cardiol*. 2004;44:349–56.
4. Saito S, Tanaka S, Hiroe Y, et al. Comparative study on trans radial approach vs. trans femoral approach in primary stent implantation in patients with acute myocardial infarction: results of the test for myocardial infarction by prospective unicenter randomization for access sites (TEMPURA) trial. *Catheter Cardiovasc Interv*. 2003;59:26–33.
5. Jolly SS, Yusuf S, Cairns J, et al. RIVAL Trial Group. Radial versus femoral access for coronary angiography and intervention in patients with acute coronary

syndromes (RIVAL): a randomized, parallel group, multicentre trial. *Lancet.* 2011;377:1409–20.

6. Romagnoli E, Biondi-Zoccai G, Sciahbasi A, et al. Radial versus femoral randomized investigation in ST segment elevation acute coronary syndrome: the RIFLE-STEACS (radial versus femoral randomized investigation in ST—elevation acute coronary syndrome) study. *J Am Coll Cardiol.* 2012;60:2481–9.
7. Cooper CJ, El-Shiekh RA, Cohen DJ, et al. Effect of trans radial access on quality of life and cost of cardiac catheterization: a randomized comparison. *Am Heart J.* 1999;138:430–6.
8. Slagboom T, Kiemenej F, Laarman GJ, et al. Outpatient coronary angioplasty: feasible and safe. *Catheter Cardiovasc Interv.* 2005;64:421–7.
9. Best practices for transradial approach in diagnostic coronary angiography and intervention, pp. 5, Fig 1–7, Olivier Bertrand and Sunil Rao Eds, Wolters Kluwer publishers, 2015.
10. Masoudi FA, Ponirakis A, de Lemos JA, et al. Executive summary: trends in U.S. cardiovascular care: 2016 report from 4 ACC National Cardiovascular Data Registries. *J Am Coll Cardiol.* 2017;69:1424–6.
11. Chugh SK. Transradial interventions—from Bandwagon to movement: where we were, where we are and where we go from here. *Indian Heart J.* 2015 Nov–Dec;67(6):627–8.
12. Kiemeneij F, Laarman GJ, Odekerken D, et al. A randomized comparison of percutaneous transluminal coronary angioplasty by the radial, brachial and femoral approaches: the ACCESS study. *J Am Coll Cardiol.* 1997;29(6):1269–75.
13. Sciahbasi A, Romagnoli E, Burzotta F, et al. Trans radial approach (left vs right) and procedural times during percutaneous coronary procedures: TALENT study. *Am Heart J.* 2011;161:172–9.
14. Biondi- Zoccai G, Sciahbasi A, Bodi V, et al. Right versus left radial artery access for coronary procedures: an international collaborative systematic review and metaanalysis including 5 randomized trials and 3210 patients. *Int J Cardiol.* 2013;166:621–6.
15. Valgimigli M, Gagnor A, Calabró P, et al. MATRIX Investigators. Radial versus femoral access in patients with acute coronary syndromes undergoing invasive management: a randomised multicentre trial. *Lancet.* 2015;385(9986):2465–76. Doi: 10.1016/S0140-6736(15)60292-6
16. Joyal D, Bertrand OF, Rinfret S, et al. Metaanalysis of 10 trials on the effectiveness of radial versus femoral approach in primary percutaneous coronary intervention. *Am J Cardiol.* 2012;109:813–8.
17. Jolly SS, Amlani S, Hamon M, et al. Radial versus femoral access for coronary angiography or intervention and the impact on major bleeding and ischaemic events: a systematic review and metaanalysis of randomized trials. *Am Heart J.* 2009;157:132–40.
18. Bertrand OF, Belisle P, Joyal D, et al. Comparison of transradial and femoral approaches for percutaneous coronary interventions: a systematic review and hierarchial Bayesian meta analysis. *Am Heart J.* 2012;163:632–48.
19. Jobe RL, Mann T. Transradial consensus statement: appropriateness ratings for patient selection and physicians' performing procedures. *J Indian Med Assoc.* 2009;107(9):587–8.

20. Kumar Chugh S, Chugh S, Chugh Y, et al. Feasibility and utility of pre-procedural ultrasound imaging of the arm to facilitate transradial coronary diagnostic and interventional procedures (PRIMAFACIE-TRI). *Catheter Cardiovasc Interv.* 2013;82:64–73.
21. Pandie S, Mehta SR, Cantor WJ, et al. Radial versus femoral access for coronary angiography/intervention in women with acute coronary syndromes: insights from the RIVAL trial (Radial vs femorAL access for coronary intervention). *J Am Coll Cardiol Intv* 2015;8:505–12.
22. Chugh SK, Chugh S, Chugh Y. Towards improving transradial access in women. *J Am Coll Cardiol Intv*. 2015;8(4):638.
23. Chugh SK, Chugh Y, Chugh S. Slender transradial interventions. In: AB Mehta (Ed) *Update in Interventional Cardiology*. New Delhi: Jaypee Brothers Medical Publishers; 2017. pp. 26–36.
24. Chong AY, Lo T, George S, et al. The effect of pre-procedure sublingual nitroglycerine on radial artery diameter and Allen's test outcome – relevance to transradial catheterization. *Cardiovasc Revasc Med.* 2017.
25. Cox N, Resnic FS, Popma JJ, et al. Comparison of the risk of vascular complications associated with femoral and radial access coronary catheterization procedures in obese versus non obese patients. *Am J Cardiol.* 2004;94:1177–80.
26. Pristipino C, Pelliccia F, Granatelli A, et al. Comparison of access-related bleeding complications in women versus men undergoing percutaneous coronary catheterization using the radial versus femoral artery. *Am J Cardiol.* 2007;99:1216–21.
27. Lo TS, Buch AN, Hall IR, et al. Percutaneous left and right heart catheterization in fully anticoagulated patients utilizing the radial artery and forearm vein: a two center experience. *J Interv Cardiol.* 2006;19:258–63.
28. Hildick-Smith DJ, Walsh JT, Lowe MD, et al. Coronary angiography in the fully anticoagulated patient: the transradial route is successful and safe. *Catheter Cardiovasc Interv*. 2003;58:8–10.
29. Aguirre FV, Topol EJ, Ferguson JJ, et al. Bleeding complications with the chimeric antibody to platelet glycoprotein IIb/IIIa integrin in patients undergoing percutaneous coronary intervention. *Circulation*. 1995;91:2890–2.
30. Choussat R, Black A, Bossi I, et al. Vascular complications and clinical outcome after coronary angioplasty with platelet 2b/3a receptors blockade: comparison of transradial vs transfemoral arterial access. *Eur Heart J.* 2000;21:662–7.
31. Chugh SK. Transradial access: right or left? *Indian Heart J* 2008(Suppl A)60;1: A27–35.

2

Setting Up a Radial Programme: Equipment, Preparation, and Training

Katherine Durham, Daniel Feldman, and Adhir Shroff

Introduction

Cardiac catheterization through the radial artery has become the standard of care for many institutions, as its benefits, which include improved safety and greater patient comfort, are discovered by growing numbers of interventional cardiologists. The use of transradial access for catheterization has expanded steadily in the United States, with radial access percutaneous intervention (PCI) increasing from 1.18% in 2007 to 16.1% in 2012.[1] Most standard cardiac catheterization laboratories are capable of accommodating transradial cases with relatively simple modifications. The additional equipment, setup, and staff training required to achieve such capability will be reviewed in this chapter.

Equipment

An important concept to keep in mind when supplying equipment for a transradial lab is that conversion to transfemoral access may be necessary during any given transradial case. Therefore, equipment commonly used for transfemoral access should be readily available in all labs, even amongst 'default' radial programmes. Since there is significant overlap in much of the equipment used for transradial and transfemoral cases, this section will focus primarily on equipment needs that are *unique* to transradial access.

Patient Preparation and Table Setup

Although standard X-ray tables are used for transradial cases, patient preparation and table setup differ from that of transfemoral cases. Special equipment needed for transradial cases include an arm board, a platform for extending the wrist in a supinated position, a multi-access sterile drape, and additional radioprotective sterile drapes. Instructions detailing how this equipment is used in preparation for a case are included in the 'Patient Preparation' section.

Radial Artery Access

Depending on operator preference, two different types of needles can be used for accessing the radial artery. A bare needle is used for access via the 'anterior wall' (modified Seldinger) technique, while a catheter-sheathed needle is used for the 'posterior wall' (true Seldinger) technique (please refer to chapter on Radial Artery Puncture for details). Needles used for both techniques generally range in diameter from 19 to 22 gauge and range in length from 2 to 5 cm. The wire used to exchange the needle (or the catheter in the case of the 'posterior wall' technique) for the dilator and radial sheath is preferably a straight-tip wire with a diameter of 0.025 inches or smaller, depending on the needle size used. The radial sheath, dilator, and wire can be purchased as a packaged kit, which may contain a needle as well.

Sheaths used for transradial cases should be specifically designed for radial artery access. They are available in multiple diameters and lengths. Selection of the appropriate sheath diameters depends both on patient-specific factors, like body size, and procedure-specific factors, like anticipated equipment requirements. Importantly, multiple sheath types and sizes should be readily available in the catheterization lab in case the selected sheath must be exchanged for a different one. This may occur in the setting of ad hoc interventions, for example, in which upsizing of the sheath is necessary to accommodate larger interventional equipment. Although sheath length does not appear to impact the likelihood of radial artery spasm,[2] the risk of spasm increases in association with larger sheath diameter.[3,4] Sheath diameter is also associated with an increased risk of radial artery occlusion (RAO).[5] Thus, to minimize these risks, use of the smallest diameter sheath possible is recommended during diagnostic or planned cases. When timely intervention is vital, selecting the sheath that will easily accommodate preferred guide catheters during ST-segment elevated myocardial infarction (STEMI) cases is important and this distinction should be emphasized.[6,7]

Although a 4-French system can be adequate for diagnostic coronary angiography if an automated contrast injector is available, 5-French systems are more commonly used for diagnostic imaging. They can also accommodate for the measurement of fractional flow reserve, and experienced operators can even use 5-French systems for interventions on type-A lesions. More complicated interventions, however, require 6-French sheaths, particularly for those utilizing atherectomy devices or intravascular imaging catheters for optical coherence tomography or intravascular ultrasound. Guide catheters larger than 6-French are rarely used in transradial interventions.[6] Recently, the development of radial sheaths with thinner walls has allowed manufacturers to reduce the external diameter by one French size compared to the sheath's internal diameter. For example, a 6F Glidesheath Slender® (Terumo Interventional Systems, Somerset, New Jersey) accommodates 6-French equipment yet possesses the external diameter of nearly a traditional 5-French sheath.

Beyond using the smallest diameter sheath possible, this risk of radial artery spasm can be further minimized by using sheaths with hydrophilic coating on their external surface.[2,8,9] Pharmacologic prophylaxis against radial artery spasm can be achieved with intra-arterial administration of vasodilators following sheath insertion. Commonly used agents include non-dihydropyridine calcium channel blockers, like diltiazem or verapamil, and nitroglycerin, sometimes given in combination with each other.[6]

Another pharmacologic consideration unique to radial artery access is the administration of anticoagulants for the prevention of thrombotic RAO, even in diagnostic cases.[10] A single dose of 5,000 international units of heparin is the most commonly used agent.[6] Since specific 'cocktails' used for prevention of radial artery spasm and RAO vary based on operator preference, commonly used medications should be readily available in all labs that accommodate transradial access.

As noted in further detail, some radial operators prefer to have a portable ultrasound machine available in order to define radial artery anatomy and to guide artery cannulation in cases where radial access is challenging. For such instances, access to sterile sleeves for the ultrasound probe is necessary to maintain sterility at the access site.

Guide Wires and Diagnostic Catheters

A 0.035-inch J-tip wire is preferred as the initial guide wire in transradial cases, although wires with tighter J-curves are available and preferred by certain operators. The J-tip helps minimize the risk of entering small side branches and provides tactile feedback in case tortuosity or an obstruction is encountered. Typically, non-hydrophilic wires are used initially, although hydrophilic wires can be used for cases involving tortuous vessels or radial loops. Hydrophilic guide wires are available with three different tips: J-shaped, straight, and angled. While standard guide wires are around 150 cm in length, longer guide wires (usually 260 cm) are available for catheter exchanges in patients with anatomical challenges, such as significant subclavian or axillary tortuosity. This allows the operator to maintain wire position within the ascending aorta during catheter exchanges, which facilitates quicker and easier delivery of the next catheter.

Although most diagnostic catheters used for transfemoral cases can be used during transradial procedures, certain catheters with unique configurations have been designed specifically for right radial artery access. Two of the most common such catheters are the Jacky catheter and Tiger catheter (Optitorque™, Terumo, Somerset, New Jersey). These catheters are designed to engage both the right and the left main coronary arteries, thereby eliminating the need to exchange catheters in order to perform a complete diagnostic coronary angiogram. Successful coronary engagement using these catheters is difficult when approaching from the left upper extremity, leading most operators to preferentially use Judkins catheters in cases using left radial access.

Judkins catheters may also be necessary in right radial cases as well if adequate engagement of either coronary system is not possible with the dedicated right radial catheters.

Another major consideration regarding catheter use in transradial cases is catheter length. For radial access, it is advisable to use 110 cm catheters rather than standard 100 cm catheters.[11] The additional length may be needed to accommodate for anatomical variations like subclavian tortuosity, a long ascending aorta, or a dilated aortic root.

Interventional Equipment

Although standard guide catheter configurations used for transfemoral interventions are also used for transradial interventions, those that provide extra back-up support, such as the EBU series (Medtronic, Minneapolis, Minnesota) and the XB series (Cordis, Bridgewater, New Jersey), are often preferred for interventions on the left coronary system, particularly those performed via right radial accesses. Regardless, multiple guide catheters are available, and selection ultimately depends on operator preference. A summary of commonly used guide catheters is provided in Table 2.1.

Table 2.1 Commonly used guide catheters worldwidefor interventions on specific vessels (adapted from Bertrand 2010[6])

LAD	Left Circumflex	RCA	Left-Sided SVG	Right-Sided SVG
EBU 3.5 (27.9%)	EBU 3.5 (26.1%)	JR (70.2%)	AL (37.3%)	JR (39.6%)
JL (22.5%)	XB 3.5 (20.8%)	AR (10.2%)	JR (31%)	Multipurpose (29.2%)
XB 3.5 (18.2%)	JL (12.5%)	AL (5.8%)	LBG (19.4%)	AL (20.8%)
Other (31.4%)	Other (40.6%)	Other (13.8%)	Other (12.3%)	Other (10.4%)

LAD = left anterior descending, RCA = right circumflex artery, SVG = saphenous vein graft, EBU = Extra Backup, JL = Judkins Left, XB = Xtra Backup, JR = Judkins Right, AR = Amplatz Right, AL = Amplatz Left, LBG = Left Bypass Graft

Patient Preparation

Informed Consent and Pre-procedure Education

Attention to detail in preparation and thorough education of the patient will facilitate success with radial artery access and image acquisition for cardiac catheterization. Starting with the pre-procedure consent, explanation of the unique access risks such as radial artery spasm, bleeding, arterial dissection or perforation, and compartment syndrome, along with the discomforts that may be encountered during and after the procedure, will allow a comprehensive risk and benefit discussion. Explanation of the potential discomforts that may be encountered include temporary wrist pain when the skin is anesthetized with lidocaine and a transient burning sensation if intra-arterial calcium channel blockers are administered as an antispasmodic. Informing patients that these sensations are in the beginning of the procedure and they should not expect discomfort thereafter will provide reassurance, as pain during the procedure has been anecdotally reported to be biggest stressor for patients undergoing cardiac catheterization for the first time.

Patient anxiety and increased circulating catecholamines can increase vasomotor tone and prompt radial artery spasm.[12] Communication of any pain in the arm of access should be reinforced to the patient so that spasm, if present, can be managed immediately.[13] The need for the femoral artery access site to be available as a backup can be discussed to avoid confusion when the staff prepares both access sites for the procedure. Finally, most patients will need reinforcement of the post-procedure lifting and movement restrictions, especially if the accessed artery is of the patient's dominant arm. A conversation of the importance of these instructions will aid retention when the teaching is reinforced after the procedure.

Intravenous Access

The site of initial patient check-in and preparation varies with each institution. This is noteworthy because the department staff on this unit will need education on the optimal placement of intravenous (IV) access for the procedure to avoid interference with the sterility and equipment needed for the procedure. IV access on the opposite arm of intended radial access is ideal, and the radial artery territory on both wrists should be avoided in case of the need for access conversion to the contralateral radial artery. If IV access in the intervention arm cannot be avoided, the target site should be proximal to the wrist with preference to the level of the antecubital fossa to allow adequate space for sterile draping and placement of the post-procedure haemostasis band.[14]

Circulation Assessment

Prior to transradial cardiac catheterization, it is practical to assess for adequate circulation through patent radial and ulnar arteries. A medical history of radial artery harvest for bypass grafting, traumatic injury to the radial artery, history of Raynaud's disease, or subclavian stenosis diagnosis, along with symptoms of poor perfusion (paraesthesia, finger discolouration, and abnormal capillary refill), should prompt further investigation and assessment.[13] Pre-procedure circulation assessment varies by institution, and utilization depends on manpower, equipment, and comprehensive staff training.

One method of circulation assessment is an evolution of the Modified Allen's test that combines subsequent radial and ulnar flow isolation by manual arterial occlusion with plethysmography and pulse oximetry assessment.[15] Although its utility is controversial in the literature, this distal perfusion assessment is inexpensive, teachable, and employed by many catheterization laboratories.[16,17] Pulse oximetry is used to assess patient oxygen saturation and recorded in routine vital signs, so this equipment should be readily available in most labs. This test, anecdotally called 'The Modified Barbeau Test' (incorporating both the Barbeau and the reverse Barbeau), is performed by manual occlusion of the radial and ulnar arteries concurrently until the plethysmographic tracing is flat, with subsequent release of pressure over the radial artery allowing isolated blood flow. The process is then repeated with release of pressure over the ulnar artery to evaluate isolated ulnar patency. The plethysmography findings have previously been categorized by Barbeau et al.[15] as A, B, C, or D based on the return of a brisk waveform tracing immediately and two minutes after release of manual arterial compression. Although this method allows more precise communication of findings, an alternative method of evaluation simply classifies the result as 'normal' or 'abnormal'. A normal Modified Barbeau circulation exam would have immediate return of an oxygen plethysmography waveform after compression is released isolating the radial and ulnar arteries. An abnormal exam would be any delay in waveform return over a few seconds and can include the clinical discretion of the examiner. The pulse oximetry values of both the isolated radial and ulnar flows are additionally recorded. An example of pre-procedure charting with the Modified Barbeau assessment is: 'Right Modified Barbeau normal pre-procedure: radial saturation 98%, ulnar saturation 97%'. The mention of the right Modified Barbeau demonstrated that the procedure and planned access will be on the right wrist.

Ultrasound of the bilateral radial and ulnar arteries to determine lumen size, patency, and presence/absence of anatomical variations has been shown to be feasible and advantageous to facilitate arterial access.[18] A comprehensive understanding of the vascular anatomy before choosing an access site provides new transradial operators the confidence in sheath insertion and navigation to the aortic arch, although routine ultrasound assessment can be beneficial and utilized by experienced operators as well. Chugh et al.[18] demonstrated that colour Doppler ultrasound imaging prior to transradial catheterization decreases access site crossover and radiation times and increases procedural success rates (Figure 2.1a). A brisk radial artery flow waveform with strong peak systolic velocities obtained by duplex imaging is demonstrated in Figure 2.1b.

The final step for verifying appropriate access involves noting and recording the bilateral radial pulse grades (Figure 2.2a). Although sheath insertion is feasible with a diminished pulse, it is not a desirable site for new transradial operators. The radial pulse is characterized on a three-point scale: +1 indicates a weak pulse that may be difficult to palpate, +2 is a normal pulse that is easily palpated, and +3 indicates a bounding pulse.[13] The nursing staff may also note the radial pulse strength on the dorsal surface of the patient's hand (Figure 2.2b). This site should be assessed and recorded prior to the procedure, as the standard radial pulse assessment location will be covered by the radial haemostasis band. The extra step prior to the procedure allows adequate circulation checks and confidence that the band is not occluding the radial arterial flow.

(a) (b)

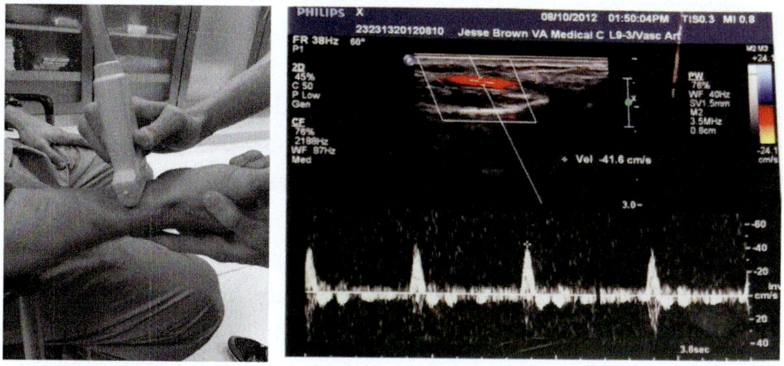

Figure 2.1 (a) An image of an ultrasound probe positioned above the right radial artery. (b) An example of duplex imaging of the radial artery, which demonstrates both a two-dimensional image of the radial artery (including colour Doppler) on the top half of the image and the velocity of blood flow in the radial artery (displayed over time) as measured by pulse wave Doppler on the bottom half of the image.

(a) (b)

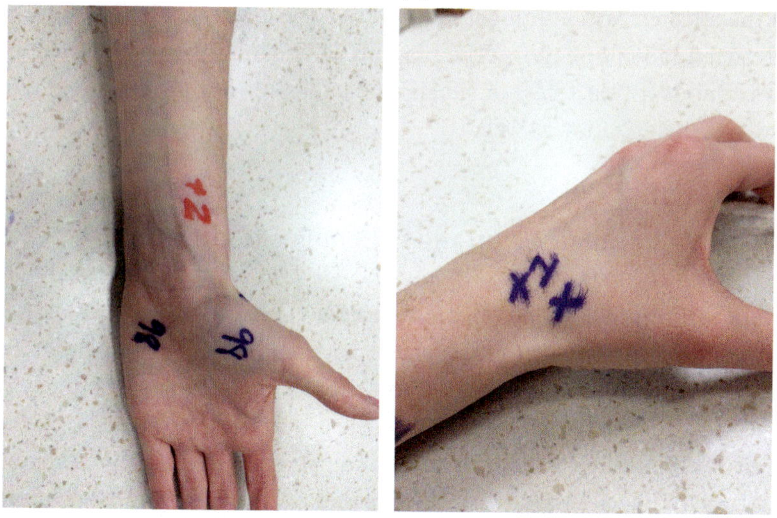

Figure 2.2 (a) An image of pulse strength written on the palmar aspect of the wrist. Isolated radial and ulnar artery oxygen plethysmography saturation values documented on the thenar and hypothenar surface on the hand, i.e. isolated radial artery saturation 98%, isolated ulnar artery saturation 98%. (b) An image of pulse strength written on the dorsal surface of the wrist.

Special Circumstances: Right Versus Left Radial Access

Although the radial artery arm of access is most objectively chosen through ultrasound evaluation,[18] the right radial artery is generally the preferred access site for radial catheterization. This preference stems from a standard laboratory setup where the operator is routinely standing on the patient's right side and does not have to reach across the patient's body with right radial artery access. The close proximity of the right arm to the operator allows a more natural position and better body mechanics during the procedure. Nevertheless, if a patient has a history of coronary artery bypass grafts with a left internal mammary artery (LIMA), left radial access is usually utilized because of the sharp angle between the subclavian axis and the internal mammary artery takeoff.[19] If left radial access is contraindicated and the patient has a LIMA bypass graft, catheters such as the Bartorelli-Cozzi catheter have been specifically developed for LIMA cannulation through the right radial artery and can be used by experienced operators. Known vascular abnormalities such as a radial loop, anomalous branching, or RAO may preclude radial access in the affected arm although loops can be traversed with techniques by advanced radial operators. The presence of a planned or established arteriovenous fistula access or subclavian stenosis is a contraindication for radial catheterization as well.

Table Setup and Patient Positioning

Table setup and patient positioning can vary and are primarily dependent on right or left radial artery access for the cardiac catheterization. For cases involving right radial access, an arm board is typically placed under the patient to allow for the appropriate positioning of the upper extremity. Although name-brand products specifically designed for transradial access are available, a standard patient transfer board can be cut, modified, and positioned for the same purpose, as demonstrated in Figure 2.3. A board is not routinely used with left transradial access because the left arm is fixed and elevated at the patient's left side or pulled slightly across his or her body in order to minimize the distance the operator must reach while standing on the patient's right side.

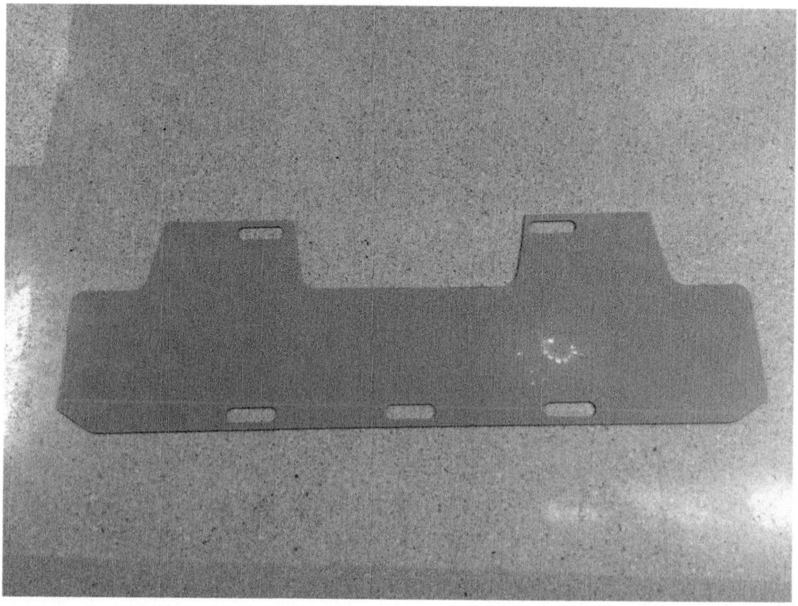

Figure 2.3 Patient transfer board cut and modified to be used as an arm positioning board.

Because the operator is reaching across the patient's body, the right arm is placed in an arm rest for a streamlined appearance and patient comfort. For patient' and operator's practicality and comfort purposes, arm positioning that is as close as possible proximal to the torso is the ideal position, in contrast to alternative positioning techniques that may require the patient's arm at a ninety-degree angle from the body. The close positioning allows the radial board to double as a work surface for equipment and wires for catheterization. Appropriate positioning for left radial access is demonstrated in Figure 2.4. For both right and left radial access, a designated platform should be used to slightly hyperextend the wrist in a flat and pronated position. An important step is ensuring the wrist is not overextended and the patient is comfortable before draping, as adjustment can be challenging when the patient is sterile and draped. Inquiring about the comfort of the shoulder should also be included, because the arm position may be difficult for patients with osteoarthritis or upper extremity mobility issues. Such positioning can be facilitated using a rolled towel or a disposable foam cradle,

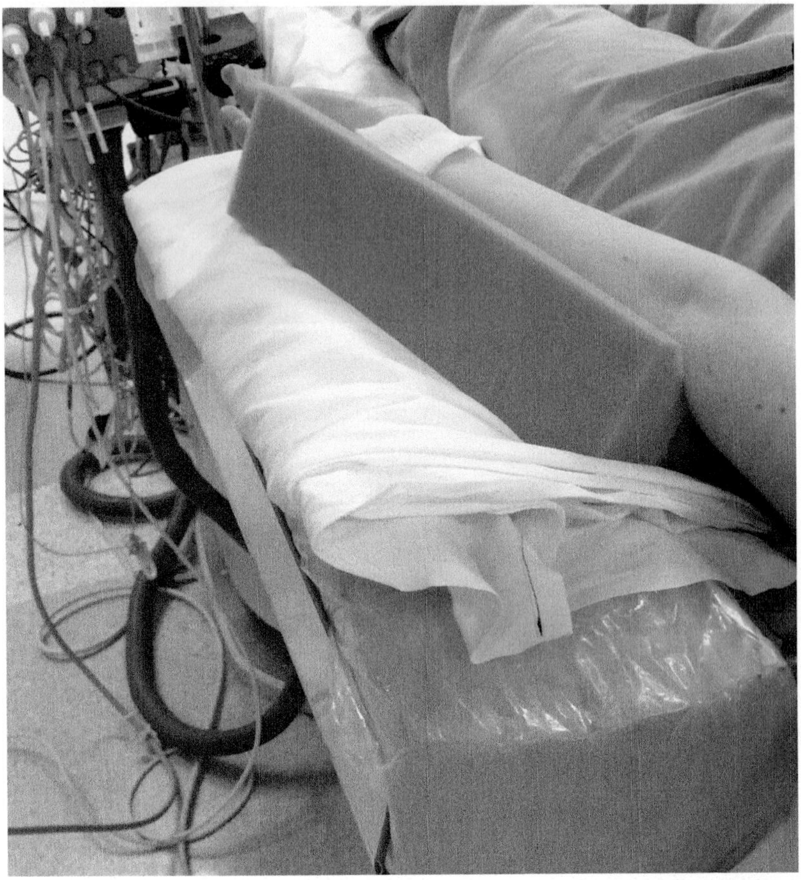

Figure 2.4 Arm positioning for left radial access.

such as the one pictured in Figure 2.5a, or failing that, a rolled towel (Figure 2.5b).

Since conversion to femoral access is always a possibility, at least one inguinal region is prepared to be used as a potential site of arterial access in addition to the wrist designated for radial access. Similar to preparation for standard femoral access, hair is removed with clippers, and all potential access sites are sterilized with a cleaning solution. The sterile field for transradial cases is typically created using a multi-access sterile drape that contains cut-outs designed to align with both wrists, the right brachial vein, and the bilateral inguinal regions (Figure 2.6).

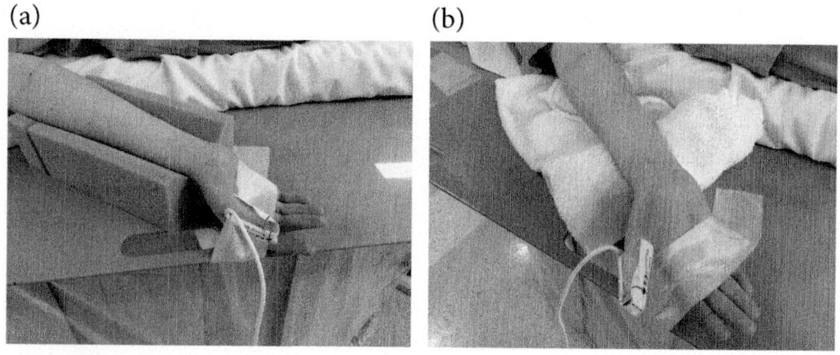

Figure 2.5 (a) Hand positioning using a foam wrist cradle. (b) Hand positioning using a rolled towel.

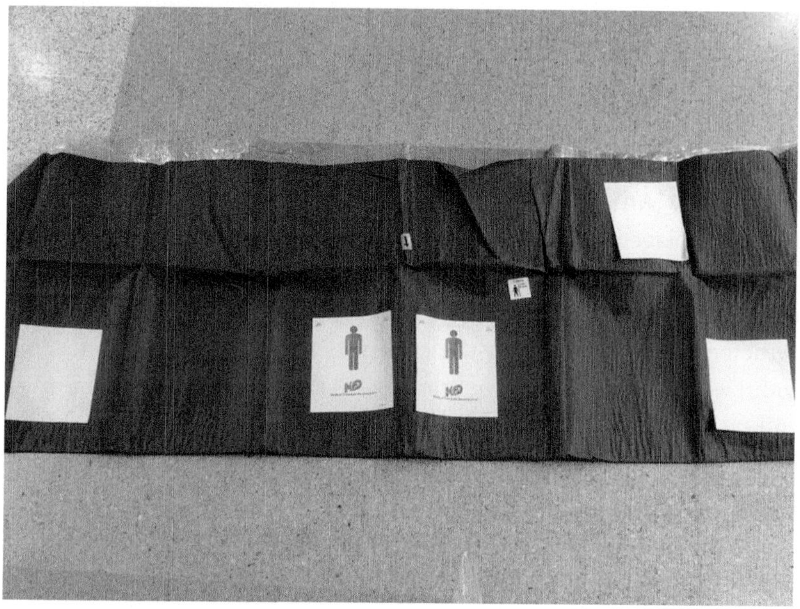

Figure 2.6 Multi-access sterile drape with cutouts that allow for exposure of the access sites for the bilateral radial arteries, right brachial vein, and bilateral femoral arteries.

The multi-access drape creates several openings for sterile preparation without a break in the draping and also facilitates rapid transition from radial access to femoral access if clinically indicated. Specific to radial access, additional radioprotective lead sterile drapes can be

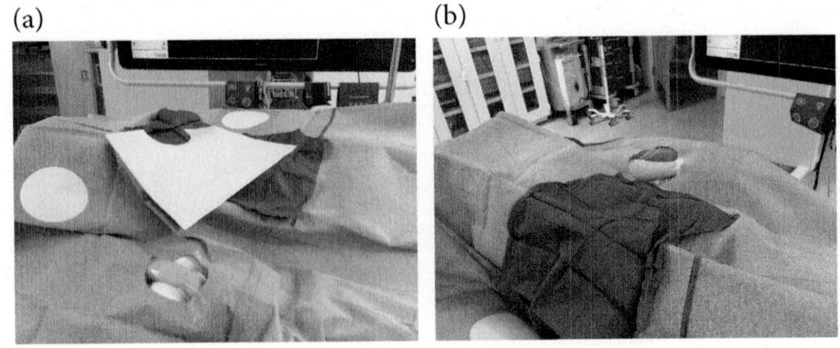

Figure 2.7 (a) A fully prepped patient for right radial access. (b) A fully prepped patient for left radial access.

placed over a patient's abdomen, pelvis, and/or right arm to minimize radiation exposure to the operator as a result of scatter.[20–22] Examples of completely draped patients ready for the start of the case are demonstrated in Figure 2.7a (right radial access) and Figure 2.7b (left radial access). After radial access is obtained, a clear occlusive dressing is usually placed over the sheath and wrist, to prevent the hydrophilic sheath from sliding out of the artery during the catheterization procedure. Planning and verbalization of the intended arm of access to the catheterization team before the patient is brought into the procedure room will ensure all setup equipment is available, and an efficient setup will result with clear interdisciplinary communication throughout the procedure.

Achieving Haemostasis

Following the conclusion of the procedure and subsequent removal of the radial sheath, haemostasis is achieved using specially designed closure bands. Multiple products are available, though each has a similar design consisting of an inflatable pad that is positioned over the access site to provide haemostatic pressure without completely occluding the vessel. Such practice, known as patent haemostasis, has been shown to reduce the risk of RAO,[23,24] thus supporting the use of closure bands in all transradial cases.

Training

Pre-procedure

The importance of thorough education for all staff who manage a transradial procedure cannot be overemphasized. Because the pre-procedure preparation starts at various sites at different institutions, the location of this training will be site specific. Although the post-procedure staff training is more extensive, interaction with the pre-procedure nurses of the projected access site from the beginning will facilitate open lines of communication and promote acceptance of the new procedure technique. The IV access considerations mentioned earlier are communicated to the preparatory staff with rationale behind ideal placement to promote understanding and retention of information. New operators may initially use more contrast dye to engage the coronary arteries and pre-procedure hydration with IV fluids can be started at this point if clinically indicated.

Post-procedure

A majority of the manpower training will be focused on the post-procedure nursing staff during the setup of a new transradial catheterization programme. Several short educational sessions will allow adequate time to cover the new information and promote retention without informational overload. Any nurse who will care for a patient post transradial catheterization should receive training, including the inpatient staff. Explanation of the radial-haemostasis band application and patent haemostasis with return demonstrations will help the staff become comfortable with the new equipment. Each catheterization lab will have a unique band deflation protocol, based on anticoagulation and provider preference, and the documentation of the schedule for band deflation should be communicated to staff prior to the first patient. Detailed instruction of the protocol for band deflation and reassurance regarding management of access site bleeding is important for patient safety. Access site bleeding can be quickly managed with reflation of the air removed from the band, which will promote haemostasis. The importance of constant reinforcement of movement and lifting restrictions to no more than five pounds for five days for patients should be communicated to staff, since many patients naturally push their weight off their wrists while transferring positions or shifting in bed. Pressure on the access site during the post-procedure recovery period can result in bleeding, haematoma formation, and longer visit times.

Other special considerations for post-procedure management are avoidance of blood pressure measurements in the ipsilateral arm of access to prevent bleeding complications. Circulation assessment of the wrist and hand following transradial catheterization is a necessary teaching point for patient safety. Circulation can be assessed by oxygen saturation and plethysmographic waveform, similar to pre-procedure assessment, and assessment of the dorsal pulse and capillary refill should also occur at frequent intervals. Because the patient has direct visualization of the arm, he or she will be able to immediately communicate any bleeding or discomforts to nursing staff for assessment and management. Ecchymosis and/or haematoma formation should be marked and documented once controlled. Patients can be discharged with a clear occlusive dressing over the access site, with a split on the wrist of access if necessary to prevent flexion. Patients should be instructed on the previously mentioned lifting restrictions, avoidance of wrist submersion in water for three days, and home site monitoring instructions. Patients can shower and remove the clear dressing in 24 hours and should keep the site open to air with no lotion or powder on the access site. Again, the most important teaching point for staff managing patients post transradial catheterization is patient safety and prevention of bleeding and continuous circulation assessments should be stressed.

Transradial Cardiac Catheterization Protocols

Developing standard protocols prior to initiating any new procedure is prudent and can communicate methods and responsibilities throughout the institution. Separate policies for radial artery access/cardiac catheterization and the radial haemostasis band removal protocol should be developed. Once interventional cardiologists and the cardiovascular team become comfortable with transradial catheterization, a protocol for same-day PCI can also be developed. Same-day PCI requires collaboration between the cardiac catheterization laboratory, pharmacy, and the short-stay unit (if applicable) for programme success. One of the benefits of radial access is decreased bleeding risks, and patients can be safely discharged around 4–5 hours after the intervention. Establishing an interdisciplinary team to develop the protocols and promote continuous communication will ease the transition to a 'radial first' catheterization programme and aid in producing optimal patient outcomes and satisfaction.

Conclusions

Most cardiac catheterization laboratories can support a transradial programme with a few specific considerations. Unique equipment includes specialized arterial sheaths, catheters specifically designed for transradial access, and haemostatic closure bands. Pharmacologic considerations include the use of spasmolytic agents to prevent radial artery spasm and anticoagulants to prevent RAO. Specialized staff training is necessary for patient preparation, lab setup, and post-procedure management. Importantly, all laboratories that utilize transradial access should be equipped and ready to convert to transfemoral access if clinically indicated.

References

1. Feldman DN, Swaminathan RV, Kaltenbach LA, et al. Adoption of radial access and comparison of outcomes to femoral access in percutaneous coronary intervention: an updated report from the national cardiovascular data registry (+). *Circulation*. 2013;127(23):2295–306.
2. Rathore S, Stables RH, Pauriah M, et al. Impact of length and hydrophilic coating of the introducer sheath on radial artery spasm during transradial coronary intervention: a randomized study. *JACC: Cardiovascular Interventions*. 1016;3(5):475–83.
3. Coppola J, Patel T, Kwan T, et al. Nitroglycerin, nitroprusside, or both, in preventing radial artery spasm during transradial artery catheterization. *The Journal of Invasive Cardiology*. 2006;18(4):155–8.
4. Goldsmit A, Kiemeneij F, Gilchrist IC, et al. Radial artery spasm associated with transradial cardiovascular procedures: results from the RAS registry. *Catheterization and Cardiovasc Interventions*. 2014;83(1):E32–6.

5. Saito S, Ikei H, Hosokawa G, et al. Influence of the ratio between radial artery inner diameter and sheath outer diameter on radial artery flow after transradial coronary intervention. *Catheterization and Cardiovascular Interventions*. 1999;46(2):173–8.
6. Bertrand OF, Rao SV, Pancholy S, et al. Transradial approach for coronary angiography and interventions: results of the first international transradial practice survey. *JACC: Cardiovascular Interventions*. 2010;3(10):1022–31.
7. Shroff A, Pancholy S, Sawlani N. Comparing radial with femoral artery access in patients with ST-segment elevation myocardial infarction: the benefits and risks. *Expert Review of Cardiovascular Therapy*. 2013;11(5):525–7.
8. Caussin C, Gharbi M, Durier C, et al. Reduction in spasm with a long hydrophylic transradial sheath. *Catheterization and Cardiovascular Interventions*. 2010;76(5): 668–72.
9. Koga S, Ikeda S, Futagawa K, et al. The use of a hydrophilic-coated catheter during transradial cardiac catheterization is associated with a low incidence of radial artery spasm. *International Journal of Cardiology*. 2004;96(2):255–8.
10. Spaulding C, Lefevre T, Funck F, et al. Left radial approach for coronary angiography: results of a prospective study. *Catheterization and Cardiovascular Diagnosis*. 1996;39(4):365–70.
11. Caputo RP, Tremmel JA, Rao S, et al. Transradial arterial access for coronary and peripheral procedures: executive summary by the Transradial Committee of the SCAI. *Catheterization and Cardiovascular Interventions*. 2011;78(6):823–39.
12. Dandekar VK, Vidovich MI, Shroff AR. Complications of transradial catheterization. *Cardiovascular Revascularization Medicine*. 2012;13(1):39–50.
13. Speiser B. Patient preparation. In: Shroff AR, editor. *Transradial Angiography and Intervention Handbook: Principles and Clinical Applications. 1. Malvern,* Pennsylvania: HMP Communications LLC; 2011.
14. Durham KA. Cardiac catheterization through the radial artery. *The American Journal of Nursing*. 2012;112(1):49–56.
15. Barbeau GR, Arsenault F, Dugas L, et al. Evaluation of the ulnopalmar arterial arches with pulse oximetry and plethysmography: comparison with the Allen's test in 1010 patients. *American Heart Journal*. 2004;147(3):489–93.
16. Bertrand OF, Carey PC, Gilchrist IC. Allen or no Allen: that is the question! *Journal of the American College of Cardiology*. 2014;63(18):1842–4.
17. Biondi-Zoccai G, Moretti C, Zuffi A, et al. Transradial access without preliminary Allen test--letter of comment on Rhyne et al. *Catheterization and Cardiovascular Interventions*. 2011;78(4):662–3; author reply 4.
18. Chugh SK, Chugh S, Chugh Y, et al. Feasibility and utility of pre-procedure ultrasound imaging of the arm to facilitate transradial coronary diagnostic and interventional procedures (PRIMAFACIE-TRI). *Catheterization and Cardiovascular Interventions*. 2013;82(1):64–73.
19. Burzotta F, Trani C, Hamon M, et al. Transradial approach for coronary angiography and interventions in patients with coronary bypass grafts: tips and tricks. *Catheterization and Cardiovascular Interventions*. 2008;72(2):263–72.
20. Iqtidar AF, Jeon C, Rothman R, et al. Reduction in operator radiation exposure during transradial catheterization and intervention using a simple lead drape. *American Heart Journal*. 2013;165(3):293–8.

21. Ertel A, Nadelson J, Shroff AR, et al. Radiation dose reduction during radial cardiac catheterization: evaluation of a dedicated radial angiography absorption shielding drape. *ISRN Cardiology*. 2012;2012:769167.
22. Lange HW, von Boetticher H. Reduction of operator radiation dose by a pelvic lead shield during cardiac catheterization by radial access: comparison with femoral access. *JACC: Cardiovascular Interventions*. 2012;5(4):445–9.
23. Cubero JM, Lombardo J, Pedrosa C, et al. Radial compression guided by mean artery pressure versus standard compression with a pneumatic device (RACOMAP). *Catheterization and Cardiovascular Interventions*. 2009;73(4):467–72.
24. Pancholy S, Coppola J, Patel T, et al. Prevention of radial artery occlusion-patent hemostasis evaluation trial (PROPHET study): a randomized comparison of traditional versus patency documented hemostasis after transradial catheterization. *Catheterization and Cardiovascular Interventions*. 2008;72(3):335–40.

3

Appropriateness Ratings for Patient Selection and Physicians Performing Transradial Procedures

Transradial Appropriateness

Tift Mann

Appropriateness of the Transradial Approach as an Access Site

The assessment of the appropriateness of the transradial approach as an access site for coronary diagnostic and interventional procedures should include an evaluation of advantages, disadvantages, and potential complications of the procedure. The benefits of transradial access have been well documented in numerous studies in the past two decades, and it is now accepted as an alternative, and sometimes preferred, approach for coronary interventional procedures.[1]

Advantages and Disadvantages

[A]The length of the transradial learning curve is directly related to previous experience and ongoing catheterization volume. However, it is generally accepted that the learning curve is in the 50–100 case range. So which physicians should learn the technique? The benefits of transradial access are greatest in patients undergoing interventional procedures. In these patients, access site bleeding complications are much lower than for the femoral approach; and morbidity, mortality, and cost are all reduced. The complication of retroperitoneal bleeding is virtually completely eliminated.[1] Thus, transradial expertise is an important asset for the interventionalist. Some practices may designate a 'radialist' in order for one operator to maintain volume and experience.

[B]In contrast to interventional procedures, diagnostic catheterizations performed from the femoral approach without anticoagulation have a very low incidence of bleeding complications. Further, with the routine use of a vascular closure device, patients may ambulate earlier and prolonged bed rest is no longer necessary.[2] Though the indications for performing *diagnostic* procedures using transradial access may appear to be less compelling; it is nevertheless important to perform diagnostic angiograms transradially in order to acquire experience with transradial catheter techniques. The expertise thus acquired helps the cardiologists in performing transradial interventions in challenging situations such as extreme obesity, peripheral vascular disease, and advanced age which benefit the most from transradial access.[1]

[C]A significant disadvantage of the transradial technique is that it involves access from a relatively small artery as well as unique skills that must be learned. These challenges[3] have been a hurdle for its adoption in the United States. Although there have been outstanding training programmes in the Far East, India, Europe, and Canada since the 1990s, it has been only in the past few years that medical centres in the United States have started to routinely offer transradial training to cardiology fellows. Thus, many cardiologists in the United States complete fellowship training with little transradial experience, and the technique must be self-taught.

Challenges

The Achilles heel of the transradial approach is radial artery occlusion. We radialists have tended to minimize this potential complication since it is virtually always clinically silent due to the dual blood supply of the hand. However, recent studies have suggested that this complication is more common than previously recognized.[4–7] A significant percentage of these occlusions will recanalize by 30 days, and hand ischaemia due to a transradial procedure is rare. However, most importantly, the artery is lost for future use.

Appropriateness Ratings of Transradial Approach

Given the issue of potential radial artery occlusion, what are the appropriateness ratings of transradial diagnostic only procedures? Generally speaking, while it is certainly appropriate to perform transradial diagnostic procedures, there probably should be a valid reason to do so. Perhaps the most important reason is simply to gain experience with transradial catheter techniques. This experience is crucial because cases with a real clinical indication for the transradial approach such as extreme obesity, peripheral vascular disease, and advanced age are often technically challenging and not straightforward.

Appropriateness Ratings and Various Coronary Syndromes

As previously noted, there are important advantages for the use of the transradial approach in interventional procedures. Appropriateness ratings for different transradial skill levels in various coronary syndromes are shown in Table 3.1. Non-interventionalists may perform the diagnostic procedure in patients with stable or unstable angina who are undergoing ad hoc procedures, particularly if there is an available interventionalist who can subsequently step in and perform the intervention. These same patients provide the non-radialist interventionalist a good opportunity to learn and gain experience with the technique.

Experienced radialists with experience prefer the technique in patients with acute coronary syndromes, especially ST elevation myocardial infarction, since a mortality benefit has been demonstrated in these patients.[8] Acute patients who present after failed thrombolytic therapy have the greatest potential benefit of the transradial approach. It is imperative, however, that the operator has sufficient experience in order to not prolong door to balloon time gaining access or performing the procedure.

Appropriateness Ratings and Previous Coronary Bypass Surgery

Appropriateness ratings for different transradial skill levels in patients with previous coronary bypass surgery are shown in Table 3.2. The catheterization of bypass grafts from the right radial artery may be difficult, and diagnostic procedures in these patients are easiest from the femoral approach and equally easy from the left radial access.

Table 3.1 Appropriateness ratings for transradial interventions by operators with different transradial skill levels in various coronary syndromes

Appropriateness Ratings for Transradial *Interventions*

	STABLE L/S	UA/ NSTEMI	STEMI/	STEMI/ TNK	STEMI/ SHOCK
NONINTERVENTIONALIST	U[1]	U[1]	I	I	I
INTERVENTIONALIST nonradialist	A	A	U[2]	U[2]	I
INTERVENTIONALIST radialist	A	A	A	A	A

Key: A = Appropriate. I = Inappropriate. U = Uncertain. U[1] = appropriate if intervention subsequently performed during same procedure by radialist. U[2] = appropriate with previous radial experience.

PCI of native vessels and right coronary bypass grafts are appropriate from the right radial approach. However, PCI of left bypass grafts and left internal mammary grafts are best performed from the left radial approach. These procedures may be technically challenging and thus carry a cautionary yellow appropriateness rating for interventionalists with limited radial experience.

Conclusion

In conclusion, with proper technique and appropriate selection of patients, transradial access is an important alternative access site for the interventionalist. A commitment to learning and maintaining the

Table 3.2 Appropriateness ratings for different transradial skill levels in patients with previous coronary bypass surgery

Appropriateness Ratings for Transradial Procedures in pts with previous CABG

	DX	PCI NATIVE	PCI SVBG	PCI IMA
NONINTERVENTIONALIST	I	I	I	I
INTERVENTIONALIST nonradialist	I	A	U[1]	U[1]
INTERVENTIONALIST radialist	I	A	A[1]	A[2]

Key: I = Inappropriate. A = Appropriate. A[1] = Appropriate but left bypass grafts best performed via left radial approach. A[2] = Appropriate but left IMA grafts best performed via left radial approach. U = Uncertain. U[1] = appropriate but may be technically challenging and should not performed early in learning curve.

technique is important as it may be easy to become discouraged during the early stages of the learning curve. Site visits to centres performing a large number of radial procedures and frequent communication with these operators to share experiences are important.

References

1. Martial H, Christian P, Carlo DM, Nolan J, Ludwig J, Tubaro M, Sabate M, Mauri-Ferre J, Huber K, Niemela K, Haude M, Wijns W, Dudek D, Fajadet J, Kiemeneij F. Consensus document on the radial approach in percutaneous cardiovascular interventions: position paper by the European Association of Percutaneous Cardiovascular Interventions and Working Groups on Acute Cardiac

Care and Thrombosis of the European Society of Cardiology. *EuroIntervention.* 2013;8:1242–51.

2. Chugh Y, Bavishi C, Faillace R, Tamis-Holland J, Mamas M, Chugh S. Safety of transradial access compared to transfemoral access with hemostatic devices (vessel plugs, suture devices & vascular clips) after percutaneous coronary. *Journal of the American College of Cardiology* 72(13 Supplement):B339.
3. Sanjay Kumar Chugh, Sunita Chugh, Yashasvi Chugh, Sunil V. Rao. Feasibility and utility of pre-procedure ultrasound imaging of the arm to facilitate transradial coronary diagnostic and interventional procedures (PRIMAFACIE-TRI). *Catheterization and Cardiovascular Interventions.* First published: 06 August 2012. 2013;82(1):64–73 https://doi.org/10.1002/ccd.24585
4. Muhammad Rashid, Chun Shing Kwok, Samir Pancholy, Sanjay Chugh, Sasko A. Kedev, Ivo Bernat, Karim Ratib, Adrian Large, Doug Fraser, James Nolan, Mamas A. Mamas. Radial artery occlusion after transradial interventions: a systematic review and meta-analysis. *Journal of the American Heart Association.* 2016 Jan;5(1):e002686. Published online 2016 Jan 25. doi: 10.1161/JAHA.115.002686
5. Pancholy S, Coppola J, Patel T, et al. Prevention of radial artery occlusion - patent hemostasis evaluation trial (PROPHET study): a randomized comparison of traditional versus patency documented hemostasis after transradial catheterization. *Catheterization and Cardiovascular Interventions.* 2008;72:335–40.
6. Cubero J, Lombardo J, Pedrosa C, et al. Radial compression guided by mean artery pressure versus standard compression with a pneumatic device (RACOMAP). *Catheterization and Cardiovascular Interventions.* 2009;73:467–72.
7. Gilchrist IC. Laissez-faire hemostasis and transradial injuries. *Catheterization and Cardiovascular Interventions.* 2009;73:473–74.
8. Andò G, Capodanno D. Radial access reduces mortality in patients with acute coronary syndromes: results from an updated trial sequential analysis of randomized trials. *JACC: Cardiovascular Interventions.* 2016;9:660–70.

4

Allen's Test and Barbeau's Test

Current Status and Relevance for Transradial Procedures

Saurabh Mehrotra, Ganesh Paramasivam, and Sundeep Mishra

Introduction

Transradial access (TRA) is emerging as the preferred access site for diagnostic and interventional procedures on the coronary tree, including primary coronary angioplasty. This can be attributed to the lower rate of vascular access site complications and bleeding with TRA as demonstrated by several studies in various clinical scenarios.[1] Additionally, patient preference, early mobilization, early hospital discharge, and a decrease in expenditure towards the treatment of access site complications have all contributed to the growing popularity of TRA.

With increasing reliance on TRA for interventions, one of the most important issue to be addressed is the consequences of radial artery occlusion post-procedurally with a reported incidence of 0.8–30%.[2] Most cases of radial artery occlusion are asymptomatic and may go undiagnosed, but the fear of ischaemic complications persist (especially in those with absence of a patent palmar arch), despite lack of evidence that radial artery occlusion leads to hand ischaemia. Most cases of hand ischaemia following TRA are due to thromboembolic occlusion of digital arteries distal to palmar arch.[3–6]

Tests for patency of palmar arch have been of interest since the introduction of TRA for coronary angiography by Campeau in 1989.[7] Allen's test (AT) (and its modification) and Barbeau's test are the two most widely used tests for patency of palmar arch. In the following sections, a brief vascular anatomy of the hand, current relevance and evidences for use of the previously provided two tests will be reviewed.

Normal Circulation of the Hand

The radial and ulnar arteries, through the superficial and deep palmar arches (SPA and DPA), provide blood supply to the hand. Branches of the common interosseous artery that originate from the ulnar artery after the radial tuberosity play a crucial role in providing blood supply to the hand (Figures 4.1 and 4.2). The ulno-palmar arches in the hand are perfused from both the ulnar and radial arteries (dual circulation). There is no static watershed point in this arrangement which ensures maintenance of perfusion when either radial or ulnar artery is compromised.[8]

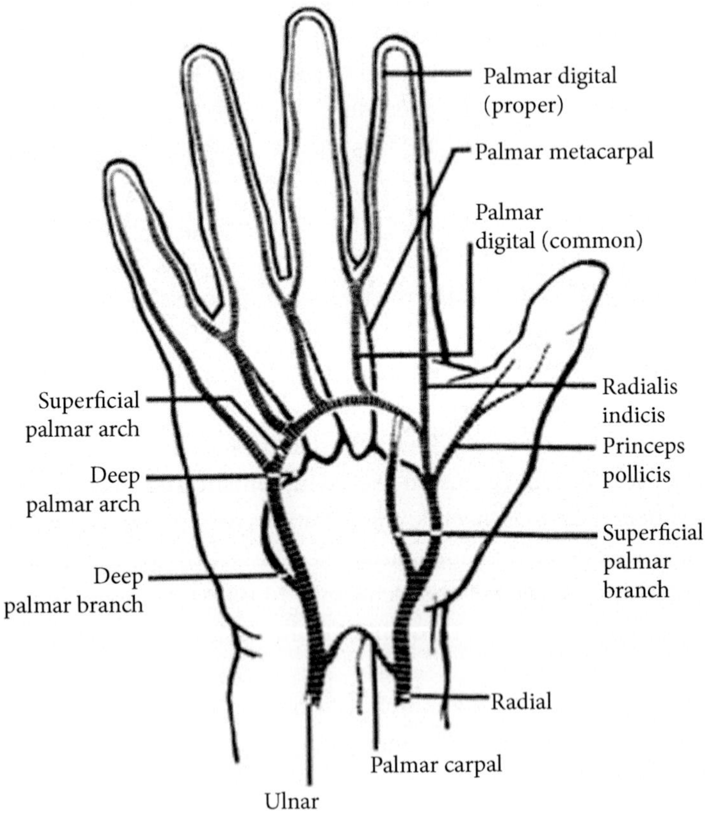

Figure 4.1 Normal circulation of hand.

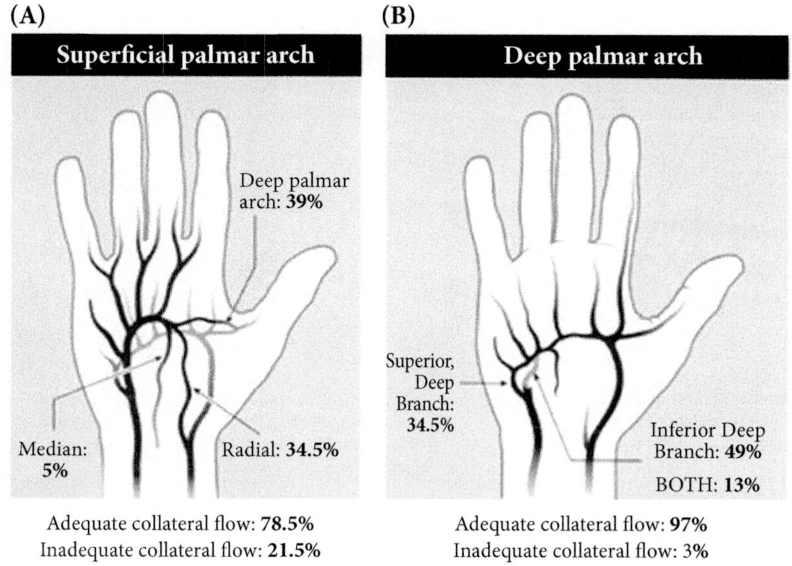

Figure 4.2 A and B Superficial and deep palmar arches of hand.

Allen's Test and Modified Allen's Test

In the original test proposed by Allen, pressure is applied to radial arteries of both the hands simultaneously after the patient tightly clenches both his fists for one minute. The examiner then compares the colour of the hands after the patient opens the fingers of both hands. Originally, AT had no time limit to assess patency of collateral circulation to the hand, seen as the return of palmar blush.[9]

In the Modified Allen's test (MAT), the patient opens and closes the hand repetitively for one minute while the examiner simultaneously occludes both the radial and ulnar arteries. The time taken for the hand to regain its colour after releasing only the ulnar artery is recorded. The test is positive indicating adequate dual circulation to the hand if the colour returns within 5–10 seconds (Figures 4.3A and 4.3B).

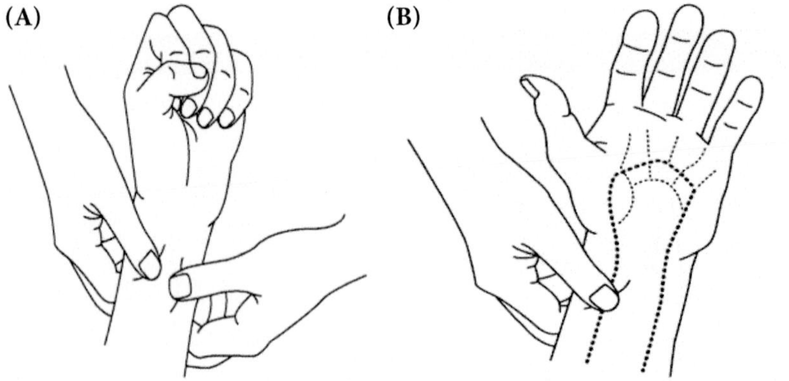

(A) Thumbs occlude radial and ulnar arteries. Pallor is produced by clenched fist.

(B) Thumb occludes radial artery while ulnar artery is released and patent. Unclenched hand returns to baseline colour because of ulnar artery and connecting arches.

Figure 4.3 A and B Modified Allen's test.[9]

Barbeau's Test

Barbeau et al. in 2004 described a more objective approach to assess the dual circulation using plethysmography instead of time to colour return.[10] In this method, a pulse oximeter is connected to the finger and the radial artery is compressed for two minutes. Depending on the adequacy of dual circulation, four different patterns can be seen on plethysmography (Figure 4.4).

Barbeau et al. studied 7,000 patients with this method. After excluding patients with a type D pattern (found in 1.5% of the patients) from undergoing TRA, no ischaemic complications were observed.[10] Barbeau's test is more objective, excludes fewer patients from undergoing TRA, and is potentially more clinically relevant than the MAT.

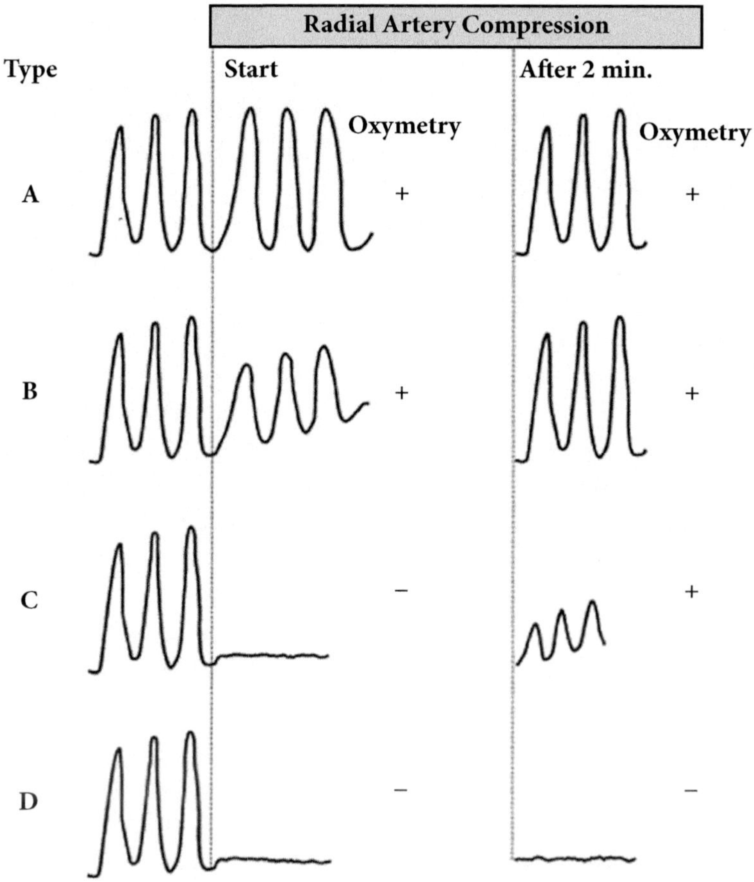

Drawing representing the 4 types of ulnopalmar arch patency findings with PL and OX, as recorded with the finger clamp applied on the thumb.

Figure 4.4 Barbeau's test. (A) No change in the waveform. (B) Diminished waveform immediately after radial artery occlusion that normalizes within 2 minutes and is associated with no change in oximetry. (C) No waveform immediately after radial artery occlusion that improves over 2 minutes and is associated with a loss of oximetry reading which also returns after 2 minutes. (D) No waveform or oximetry reading after radial artery occlusion that does not return after 2 minutes.[10]

Current Practice and Evidence

Traditionally, all patients were screened with one of these tests before being deemed fit for TRA. Patients with a negative AT and/or showing a type-D pattern on Barbeau's test were excluded from undergoing a TRA for the fear of post-procedural hand ischaemia. The incidence of lack of patency of palmar arch based on these two tests in patients undergoing cardiac catheterization is 1.5–27%.[10,11] The well-acknowledged benefits of a TRA demand an evidence-based analysis of perceived risk of hand ischaemia in such patients.

A recent international transradial practice survey found that 58% of operators used MAT and 16% used Barbeau's test, whereas 23% of operators did not perform any test prior to performing TRA-Percutaneous Coronary Intervention (PCI).[12] In a study of more than 1,000 patients undergoing coronary procedures through TRA, 25% had a negative AT but both angiography and ad hoc angioplasty was safely performed regardless of test results prior to the procedure.[13]

Among 203 patients undergoing transradial procedures, Valgimigli et al. studied the use of both the Allen's and the Barbeau's tests. Using thumb lactate levels as primary end-point and hand grip strength, ulnar frame count and thumb plethysmography as secondary end-points, this study demonstrated that these tests were of limited clinical utility as TRA was safe and feasible irrespective of tests' results.[14] Similarly, Ghuran et al. retrospectively analysed patients undergoing transradial procedure without being subjected to Allen's or Barbeau's test and suggested that pre-screening for adequacy of the dual supply of hand is not necessary.[15]

Greenwood et al. studied vascular reserve in the hand circulation. Patients with a negative AT showed a 90% reduction of blood flow to the thumb immediately after radial artery occlusion but improved to 75% reduction after 30 minutes. Simultaneously, pulse oximeter showed a 0% signal immediately following occlusion of the radial artery but rose to 64% at 30 minutes.[16]

The 'a comprehensive anatomic and functional assessment of the vasculature of the hand and relation to outcome after transradial' (ACRA) anatomy study recently evaluated the completeness of the SPA and DPA as well as their correlation with the MAT and the Barbeau test and predicting the rate of ischaemic hand complications with these non-invasive tests.[17]

Angiography was done to document vascular anatomy of the hand in 234 patients undergoing cardiac procedures through TRA. The MAT and Barbeau test were performed pre-procedurally. The function of the hand was assessed at baseline and at two years. The DPA was complete in all the patients (as demonstrated by angiography), and therefore either test was to predict its completeness. But the SPA was complete in only 54%, and both these tests were able to predict incompleteness of the SPA. With a cut-off value of >10 seconds, the sensitivity and specificity of the MAT for SPA incompleteness was 33% and 86%, respectively. In comparison, type D pattern on Barbeau test had a sensitivity of 7% and specificity of 98%, but when combined, types C and D patterns had a sensitivity and specificity of 21% and 93%, respectively, for SPA incompleteness. More importantly, an incomplete SPA was not associated with upper-extremity dysfunction ($P = 0.77$). Therefore, it was concluded that although incomplete SPA was common, the DPA always preserved blood supply to the hand. Preprocedural patency tests do not help to prevent ischaemic complications of the hand following TRA.

In a recent observational study published in 2018 by Reddy et al.,[18] they evaluated 887 hands in 445 consecutive patients prior to trans-radial angiography with Barbeau's test and reverse Barbeau's test. On initial evaluation, a 'low-risk' pattern (A or B) was seen in 780 (88%) hands and a 'high-risk' pattern (C or D) in 107 (12%) hands. When the tests were repeated 50 minutes later, 29 (27%) of high-risk hands spontaneous converted to pattern B (low-risk). This study demonstrates significant variability over short intervals suggesting that circulatory interdependence of the hand is highly dynamic, and the existing tests have poor reliability.

Based on the previously provided studies, and the observation that hand ischaemia is rare after TRA despite its widespread use in a variety of cardiovascular procedures, many experts in the field have questioned the usefulness of traditional approach of pre-screening patients before TRA.[3,17–22]

In conclusion, the use of AT, MAT, or Barbeau's (plethysmography) test is not necessary before TRA in patients undergoing cardiac catheterization. It is more important to use adequate anticoagulation and patent haemostasis techniques to avoid ischaemic complications. This will ensure that even greater number of patients undergo the safer TRA for coronary interventions while at the same time minimize complications.

References

1. Bertrand OF, Belisle P, Joyal D, Costerousse O, Rao SV, Jolly SS, et al. Comparison of transradial and femoral approaches for percutaneous coronary interventions: a systematic review and hierarchical Bayesian meta-analysis. *American Heart Journal*. 2012;163(4):632–48.
2. Wagener JF, Rao SV. Radial artery occlusion after transradial approach to cardiac catheterization. *Current Atherosclerosis Reports*. 2015;17(3):489.
3. Shah AH, Pancholy S, Shah S, Buch AN, Patel TM. Allen's test: does it have any significance in current practice? *The Journal of Invasive Cardiology*. 2015;27(5):E70–3.
4. Rademakers LM, Laarman GJ. Critical hand ischaemia after transradial cardiac catheterisation: an uncommon complication of a common procedure. *Netherlands Heart Journal*. 2012;20(9):372–5.
5. Valentine RJ, Modrall JG, Clagett GP. Hand ischemia after radial artery cannulation. *Journal of the American College of Surgeons*. 2005;201(1):18–22.
6. Lee KL, Miller JG, Laitung G. Hand ischaemia following radial artery cannulation. *Journal of Hand Surgery*. 1995;20(4):493–5.
7. Campeau L. Percutaneous radial artery approach for coronary angiography. *Catheterization and Cardiovascular Diagnosis*. 1989;16(1):3–7.
8. McGregor AD. The Allen test--an investigation of its accuracy by fluorescein angiography. *Journal of Hand Surgery*. 1987;12(1):82–5.
9. Fuhrman TM, Pippin WD, Talmage LA, Reilley TE. Evaluation of collateral circulation of the hand. *Journal of Clinical Monitoring*. 1992;8(1):28–32.
10. Barbeau GR, Arsenault F, Dugas L, Simard S, Lariviere MM. Evaluation of the ulnopalmar arterial arches with pulse oximetry and plethysmography: comparison with the Allen's test in 1010 patients. *American Heart Journal*. 2004;147(3):489–93.
11. Benit E, Vranckx P, Jaspers L, Jackmaert R, Poelmans C, Coninx R. Frequency of a positive modified Allen's test in 1,000 consecutive patients undergoing cardiac catheterization. *Catheterization and Cardiovascular Diagnosis*. 1996;38(4):352–4.
12. Bertrand OF, Rao SV, Pancholy S, Jolly SS, Rodes-Cabau J, Larose E, et al. Transradial approach for coronary angiography and interventions: results of the first international transradial practice survey. *JACC: Cardiovascular Interventions*. 2010;3(10):1022–31.
13. Maniotis C, Koutouzis M, Andreou C, Lazaris E, Tsiafoutis I, Zografos T, et al. Transradial approach for cardiac catheterization in patients with negative Allen's test. *The Journal of Invasive Cardiology*. 2015;27(9):416–20.
14. Valgimigli M, Campo G, Penzo C, Tebaldi M, Biscaglia S, Ferrari R. Transradial coronary catheterization and intervention across the whole spectrum of Allen test results. *Journal of the American College of Cardiology*. 2014;63(18):1833–41.
15. Ghuran AV, Dixon G, Holmberg S, de Belder A, Hildick-Smith D. Transradial coronary intervention without pre-screening for a dual palmar blood supply. *International Journal of Cardiology*. 2007;121(3):320–2.
16. Greenwood MJ, Della-Siega AJ, Fretz EB, Kinloch D, Klinke P, Mildenberger R, et al. Vascular communications of the hand in patients being considered for

transradial coronary angiography: is the Allen's test accurate? *Journal of the American College of Cardiology*. 2005;46(11):2013–17.

17. van Leeuwen MAH, Hollander MR, van der Heijden DJ, van de Ven PM, Opmeer KHM, Taverne YJHJ, et al. The ACRA anatomy study, a comprehensive anatomic and functional assessment of the vasculature of the hand and relation to outcome after transradial. *Circulation: Cardiovascular Interventions*. 2017;10:e005753
18. Reddy S, Pancholy PS, Pandya KP, Rai A, Patel AT, Chauhan S, et al. Variability of forearm collateral circulation: an observational study of serial hand plethysmography testing. *Cardiovascular Revascularization Medicine*. 2018; pii: S1553-8389(18)30008-3
19. Gilchrist IC. Is the Allen's test accurate for patients considered for transradial coronary angiography? *Journal of the American College of Cardiology*. 2006;48(6): 1287; author reply 8.
20. Gilchrist IC, Rao SV. De-implementing the Allen's Test. *The Journal of Invasive Cardiology*. 2015;27(5):E74.
21. Sharma R, Applegate RJ. Allen's testing prior to transradial cardiac catheterization: state of the arch. *The Journal of Invasive Cardiology*. 2015;27(9):421–2.
22. Bertrand OF, Carey PC, Gilchrist IC. Allen or no Allen: that is the question! *Journal of the American College of Cardiology*. 2014;63(18):1842–4.

5

Radial Artery Access: Puncturing the Radial Artery

Saurabh Mehrotra and Sourabh Agstam

Introduction

The transradial approach is the minimally invasive, safer, patient-friendly approach for coronary and endovascular procedures. Most expert interventionists prefer radial approach over femoral approach for coronary intervention. Radial artery approach came in limelight in 1989, when 'Lucien Campeau' published his successful series of 100 coronary angiographies performed via the left radial artery with minimal occurrence of complications.[1] Multiple randomized trials and meta-analysis comparing radial versus femoral artery access were published and American Heart Association (AHA), American College of Cardiology ACC/Society for Cardiovascular Angiography & Interventions (SCAI) guidelines now include transradial access as a class IIA recommendation.[2] However, European Society of Cardiology (ESC) guidelines 2017 includes transradial access as class I recommendation in ST Elevation Myocardial Infarction—Acute Coronary Syndrome (STEMI-ACS) for primary coronary intervention if performed by an experienced radial operator.[3]

Anatomy of Radial Artery

The brachial artery bifurcates just below the bend of the elbow into radial and ulnar artery. The radial artery traverses the lateral side of the forearm from the neck of the radius to the forepart of the styloid process in the wrist and then passes backward, around the lateral side of the carpus.

The distal portion of the artery in the forearm is superficial, being covered by the integument and the superficial and deep fascia, lying between the tendons of the brachioradialis and flexor carpi radialis over the prominence of the radius.

The flat, bony prominence of the radial artery provides ease of compression and haemostasis after sheath removal. There is no adjacent nerve structure, and hence, there is no risk of nerve injury.

Pre-procedure Testing for Dual Circulation of the Hand

In the initial few years of transradial access, all patients underwent Allen's test or Barbeau's test before access, to check for collateral circulation and to prevent hand ischaemia. Patients with abnormal Allen's test (or Barbeau's test) were initially excluded for radial approach. Controversy started when Hata et al. reported no postoperative hand ischaemia despite harvesting radial arteries for use as bypass grafts in a series of patients with abnormal collateral flow.[4] Many high-volume centres across the globe do not exclude patients on the basis of these tests. 'TransRADial coronary catheterization and intervention across the whole spectrum of Allen's test Results' (RADAR) trial showed no signs of ischaemia (based on the thumb capillary lactate level) in patients after transradial catheterization, irrespective of the Allen's test results.[5] The only absolute contraindication for transradial access is previous history of Raynaud's phenomenon. It is still controversial to regularly perform these tests before transradial approach.

Allen's test: An Allen's test is to assess collateral circulation of the hand. Both the radial and ulnar arteries are compressed simultaneously at wrist joint until the palm blanches and then release the ulnar artery. If the colour of the palm returns to normal within 10 seconds of release of the ulnar artery, there is adequate collateral circulation of palm.

Barbeau's test: The Barbeau's test is to overcome drawbacks of Allen's test. A pulse oximeter is attached on the thumb of the ipsilateral hand. A normal waveform should be observed as shown in Table 5.1. Both the radial and ulnar arteries are compressed simultaneously, and instead of observing hand colour when releasing the ulnar artery, the pulse oximetry tracing is examined. There are four responses as described later.

Table 5.1 Different responses in Barbeau's test. Type D response was considered as contraindication of radial access.[6]

	Radial artery compression			
	Start	Oximetry	After 2 minutes	Oximetry
Type A (15%)	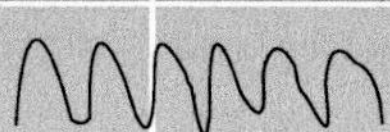	+	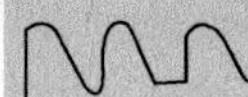	+
Type B (75%)	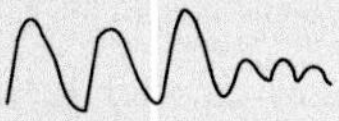	+	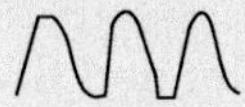	+
Type C (5%)	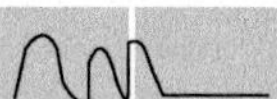	–	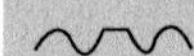	+
Type D (5%)	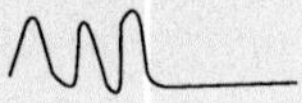	–	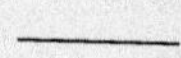	–

Radial Artery Access Technique

There are two ways to achieve radial artery access:

A. Traditional Seldinger technique or posterior wall puncture or through-and-through puncture or back-wall technique
B. Modified Seldinger technique or front wall technique or anterior wall puncture only

Most operators prefer one of two different access techniques (traditional Seldinger or modified Seldinger technique). A randomized trial comparing both the techniques reported that the through-and-through puncture technique was a reliable and faster way to achieve radial artery access with less failure rate.[6]

Stepwise Approach for Transradial Access

Step 1. Positioning of the hand for transradial access: Right or left radial artery can be used for transradial access.[7] It all depends on comfortability of the operator. Keep the patient in supine position on the angiographic table and attach arm board extension to right hand side of table. Place the patient's right arm on the board and abducted it at a 30° angle. Hyperextend the right wrist by keeping rolled towel or splint behind the wrist. Apply tape and fix fingers to arm board so that position remains stable while puncturing radial artery. In case of left radial access, place patient's left arm on a large pillow to maintain stable position. Place the forearm towards the midsection of the patient's body and strap the wrist with splint.

Step 2. Clean and drape the forearm in sterile fashion: Clean and drape the bilateral groin too as there are chances of failure of radial artery access. The site of radial artery puncture is 2 cm proximal to the radial styloid process because radial artery is most superficial in this area. *In case of poorly palpable radial artery, compress the distal radial artery at palmar crease to make proximal radial artery more superficial.*

Step 3. Premedication: Anxiety increases sympathetic activity and subsequently increases radial artery spasm. Inject 1–2 mg of midazolam and 25–50 mg fentanyl before achieving access depending on body mass index (BMI) and respiratory status. Inject 2 to 3 cc of 1% lidocaine with a 25G needle, and a wheal is raised over the puncture site.

Step 4. Radial artery puncture: The arterial puncture is performed with either a short 2.5 cm, stainless steel, 21G needle or a micropuncture intravenous (IV) catheter that consists of a fine metal needle and a 22G Teflon catheter. Feel the pulse with one hand (left hand for right hand operators) and advance the needle into radial artery at a 30° angle with other hand. In traditional Seldinger technique or back wall technique, the presence of blood in the hub of the needle of microcatheter indicates that the artery has been punctured. Advance the needle forward through the back wall of the radial artery and then, remove the fine needle and slowly withdraw small Teflon microcatheter until the appearance of brisk pulsatile flow. Advance guidewire through the microcatheter and exchange microcatheter with arterial sheath.

In modified Seldinger technique or front wall technique, advance the stainless steel needle into the front wall of radial artery. Advance the wire once blood is noticed in needle hub and it should go freely. Blood return is rarely brisk or pulsatile in this method. **Don't advance wire against resistance and rotate needle clockwise or anticlockwise until the wire can be easily advanced.** Remove the stainless steel needle and exchange it with arterial sheath. The long, smooth taper of sheath usually precludes the need for a skin nick before advancement into the vessel.

Step 5. Withdraw some blood from sheath and then flush it gently with saline to prevent air embolism. To prevent radial spasm and for maintaining vessel patency, a spasmolytic cocktail is used. Components of the cocktail commonly include nitroglycerin (100 micrograms (ug), verapamil (2.5 mg) or nicardipine or diltiazem (2.5 mg), and unfractionated heparin (UFH) (5,000 or 70 units per kilogram body weight). In our centre (PGIMER, Chandigarh), we prefer a radial cocktail consisting of 2.5 mg of diltiazem, 100 ug of nitroglycerine, and 2,500 units of UFH. Dilute the mixture with 10–20 ml of blood and inject it slowly over 1 minute to prevent patient discomfort during injection as patient feel numbness in hands.

Step 6. After the angiographic procedure, sheath should be removed meticulously. There is a concept of '**patent haemostasis**' and for which, an external band should be applied to the patient's wrist and it is inflated until haemostasis is achieved. Pulse oximetry tracing from ipsilateral thumb is seen, and air should be removed from the band until adequate anterograde flow is documented by plethysmography, while maintaining surface haemostasis.

Conclusion

Utilization and demand of radial access is increasing globally. It is safe with fewer vascular and bleeding complications when compared with femoral access. Transradial access should be accomplished using a systematic, stepwise approach. There is a steep learning curve for radial artery access, and the operator should regularly perform transradial procedures to reduce failure rate.

References

1. Campeau L. Percutaneous radial artery approach for coronary angiography. *Cathet Cardiovasc Diagn* 1989;16:3–7.
2. Levine GN, Bates ER, Blankenship JC, et al. ACC, AHA, SCAI 2011. Guideline for percutaneous coronary intervention: executive summary: a report of the

American College of Cardiology Foundation/American Heart Association Task Force on Practice Guidelines and the society for cardiovascular angiography and interventions. *Catheter Cardiovasc Interv.* 2012;79:453–95.

3. Ibanez B, James S, Agewall S, et al. 2017 ESC Guidelines for the management of acute myocardial infarction in patients presenting with ST-segment elevation. *Eur Heart J.* 2018;39:119–77.
4. Hata M, Sezai A, Niino T, et al. Radial artery harvest using the sharp scissors method for patients with pathological findings on Allen's test. *Surg Today.* 2006;36:790–92.
5. Valgimigli M, Campo G, Penzo C, et al. Trans-radial coronary catheterization and intervention across the whole spectrum of Allen's test results. *J Am Coll Cardiol.* In press.
6. Barbeau GR, Arsenault F, Dugas L, et al. Evaluation of the ulnopalmar arterial arches with pulse oximetry and plethysmography: comparison with the Allen's test in 1010 patients. *Am Heart J.* 2004;147:489–93.
7. Pancholy S, Sanghvi K, Patel T. Radial artery access technique evaluation trial: randomized comparison of Seldinger versus modified Seldinger technique for arterial access for transradial catheterization. *Catheter Cardiovasc Interv.* 2012;80:288–291.
8. Cohen MG, Rao SV. *Radial artery approach: Grossman and Baim's cardiac catheterization, angiography, and intervention.* 8 edition, Lippincot, Williams & Wilkins; 2014.

6

Role of Colour Doppler Ultrasound in Transradial Interventions

Sunita Chugh

Pre-procedure Ultrasound of Forearm Arteries (PPUAA)

Background

Challenging anatomy must be avoided to minimize the risk of complications and shorten the duration of both the procedure and radiation exposure.[1] For this reason, a systematic preliminary angiogram of the arteries of the forearm through the introducer inserted into the radial artery for 2 to 3 cm has been suggested by some authors.[2] Saito et al. (2009) described radial artery diameters using ultrasound in Japanese population and the influence of the ratio between radial artery inner diameter and sheath outer diameter on radial artery flow *after* transradial coronary intervention.[3] Chugh et al. (2013) were the first in the world to do pre-procedure ultrasound of forearm arteries (PPUAA) for sizing and color doppler assessment of radial artery *prior to* transradial interventions.[4] In the year 2002, they started with bilateral radial artery sizing in all patients planned for cardiac catheterization; subsequently, pulse wave Doppler was added to assess patency of radial and ulnar arteries; this was later followed by addition of assessment of cubital fossa to look at bifurcation of brachial artery into ulnar and radial arteries. In the year 2013, Chugh et al.[4] (2013) published their data of 2,344 patients. Other than measuring radial and ulnar artery diameters, anomalies were detected in radial artery and at cubital fossa.

Measuring Radial and Ulnar Artery Diameters Using Pre-procedure Colour Doppler Ultrasound of Forearm Arteries

Colour Doppler ultrasound has been used to measure internal diameter of arteries.

Equipment

A linear transducer with the frequency VF 10–5 MHz is required for imaging the arteries. (Figure 6.1)

Method of Measurement

Both the radial and ulnar arteries are first scanned in grey scale in transverse and longitudinal plane. With the transducer positioned longitudinally, the cursor is placed at the intima-media of anterior and posterior

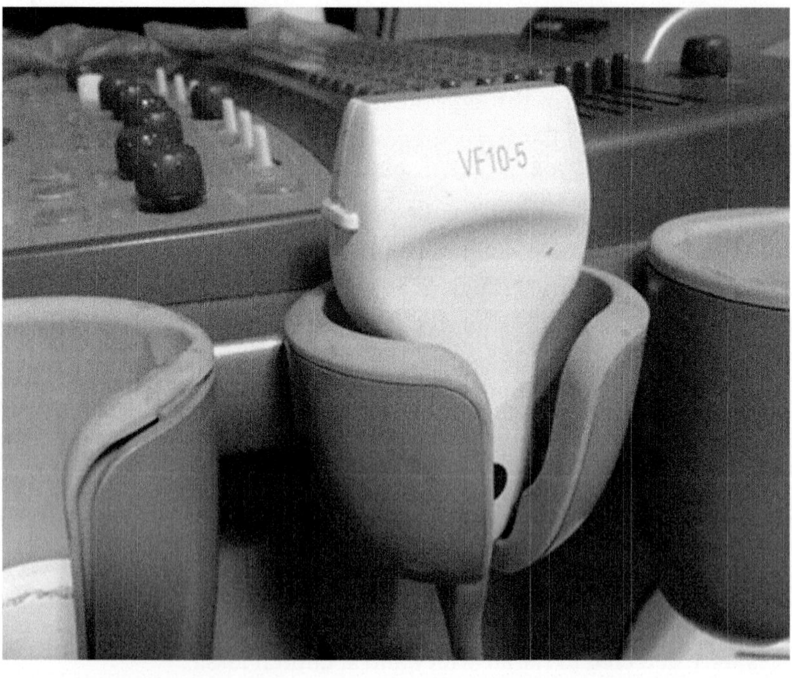

Figure 6.1 Linear probe.

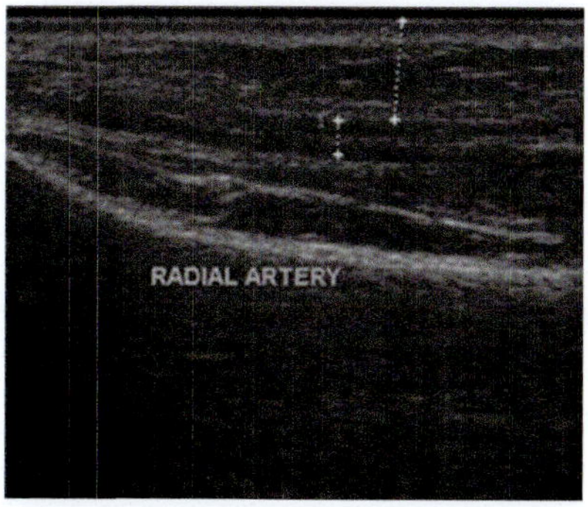

Figure 6.2a Measuring radial artery (grey scale).

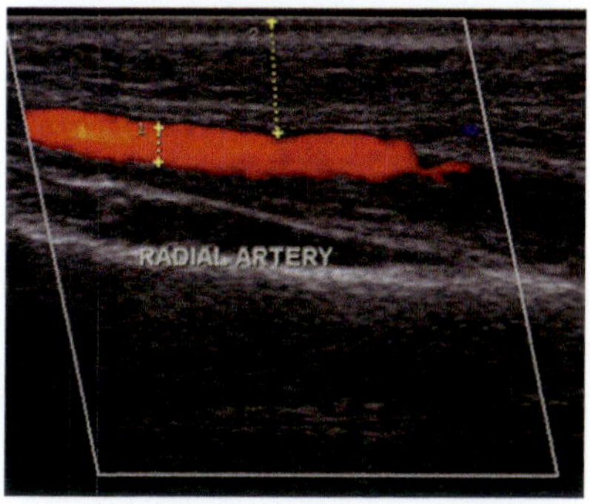

Figure 6.2b Measuring radial artery (colour Doppler).

walls to measure the inner diameter of the vessel, about 1 cm proximal to the styloid process. Next, colour Doppler imaging is performed to assess the patency of the vessel and distinguish the artery from the surrounding structures (Figures 6.2a, 6.2b, 6.3a, and 6.3b). Pulse Doppler is then done to assess the nature of the flow to rule-out monophasic flow due to high-up significant obstruction.

Radial and Ulnar Artery Diameters in the Study Population

Majority of the radial artery diameters in the Indian population that Chugh et al. (2013) studied, in National Capital Region of Delhi, were in the range of 1.8–2.1 mm (Table 6.1, Figure 6.4).

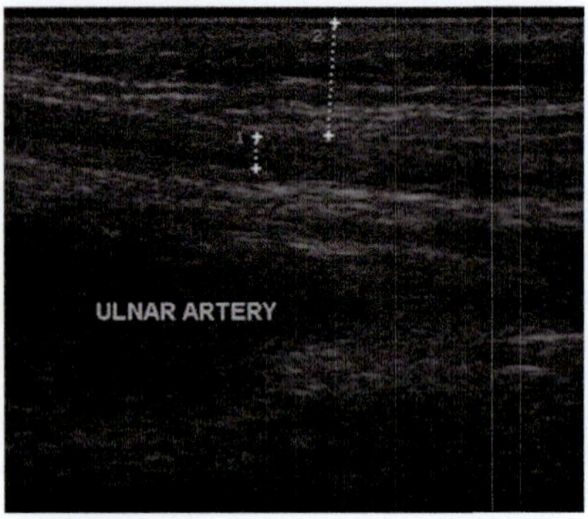

Figure 6.3a Measuring ulnar artery (grey scale).

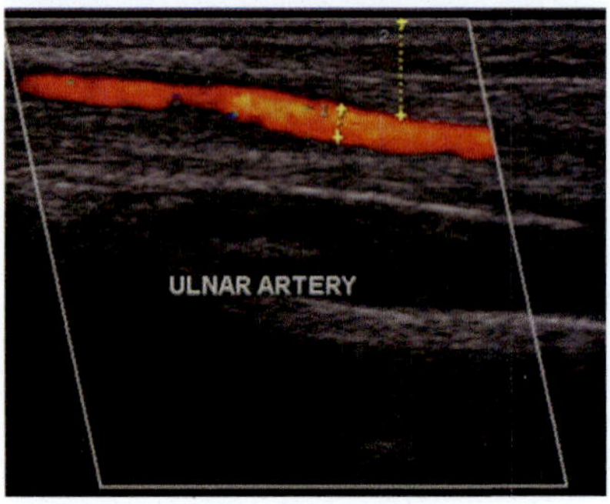

Figure 6.3b Measuring ulnar artery (colour Doppler).

Radial and Ulnar Artery Diameters in Other Ethnic Populations

There are studies on radial artery size and anatomical abnormalities in various populations.[5–7] In a South Korean cohort (n = 1191), the average radial diameter in males and female was 2.6 and 2.4 mm, respectively, and radial and brachial anomaly was found in 4.2%.[5] In another study from Europe (n = 109), the average radial diameter was 2.17 mm. There was a 10% incidence of anomaly, and left radial artery diameter (LAD) was greater than the right radial artery diameter (RAD); RAD in males was greater than that in females.[6] A study, in 100 radial artery size and

Table 6.1 Radial and ulnar artery diameters according to sex and side (n = 2,344)[4]

Size of radial and ulnar artery on the two sides	Mean diameter (mm)
Left radial artery	
Male	1.8 ± 0.29
Female	1.7 ± 0.26
Left ulnar artery	
Male	1.8 ± 0.30
Female	1.7 ± 0.3
Right radial artery	
Male	1.9 ± 1.12
Female	1.7 ± 0.29
Right ulnar artery	
Male	1.8 ± 0.30
Female	1.6 ± 0.28

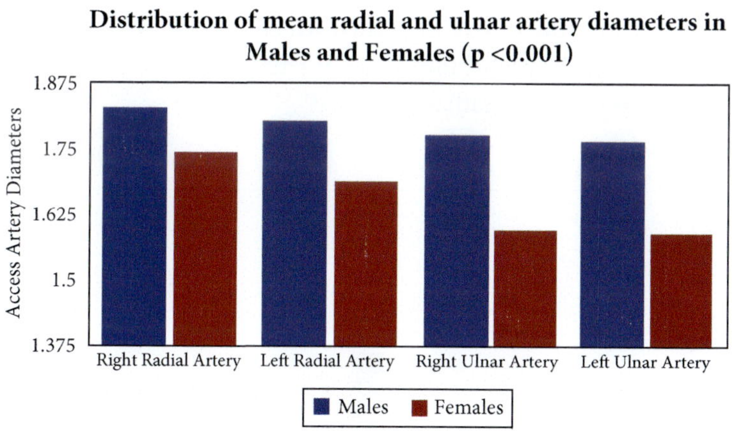

Figure 6.4 Radial and ulnar artery size according to sex and side ($n = 2,344$).[4]

age, height, weight, and body surface area of the American volunteers, found an average radial size of 2.2 mm. They found no correlation between patients; though gender variability was reported, radial artery size was found to be smaller in females.[7]

Utility of Pre-procedure Ultrasound in Measuring Diameters of Radial and Ulnar Arteries for Transradial Interventions (TRI)

Based on distribution of radial artery diameter in the population assessed by colour Doppler ultrasound, a radial sheath sizing protocol[4] was published by Chugh et al. (2013) for the first time in the world. It helps to serve as a broad outline and a guide to operators for choosing a sheath size with least mismatch to the diameter of the radial or ulnar artery to be used for access (Figure 6.5).

Sheath selection based on radial artery diameter (RAD) is also expected to minimize situations of intractable spasm requiring extreme measures such as general anesthesia to pull out unduly oversized radial sheaths from very small diameter radial arteries anecdotes of which (both published and unpublished) abound. It has the potential to prevent complications such as avulsion of radial artery which occurs because of pulling on an 8F catheter in presence of severe spasm of radial artery, first reported by Barbeau.[8–10] The likely mechanisms may have been severe radial artery to catheter size mismatch which initiates severe spasm in the radial artery. The probability of radial artery occlusion increases with bigger sheaths in smaller radial arteries.[4,11]

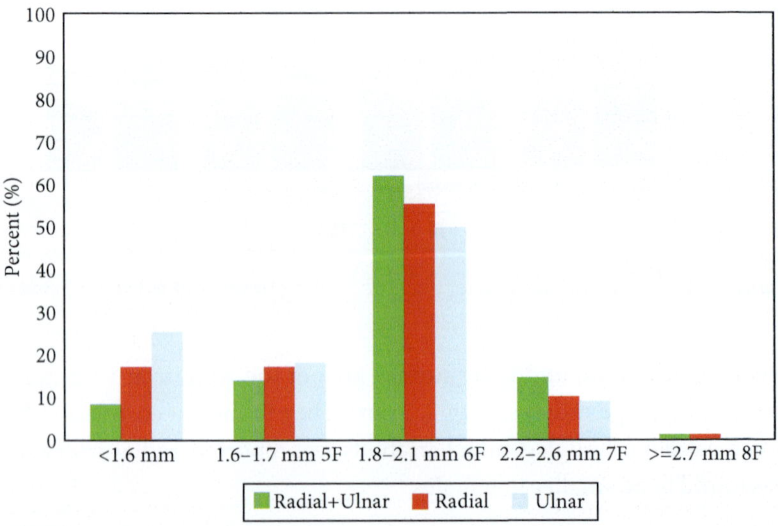

Figure 6.5 Sheath sizing protocol.[4]

A commonsense translation of French size to mm is mm x 3 = French size. Chugh et al. (2013)'s initial **sheath sizing protocol**[4] was just that:

5F Sheath would be appropriate for 5/3 = 1.7 mm Artery
6F Sheath would be appropriate for 6/3 = 2 mm Artery
7F Sheath would be appropriate for 7/3 = 2.3 mm Artery

The main concept behind this was to reduce pain and spasm by *as near* a 1:1 relation between sheath size and radial artery diameter.

With experience, larger sheath and catheter corresponding to smaller radial artery diameters up to 0.2 mm smaller for corresponding French size can be used. In smaller diameter radials, probability of radial occlusion is more, with use of a relatively bigger French radial sheath.[12] 7 F is required for Rotablation >1.75 mm burr and in some 2 stent techniques in bifurcation lesions including left main interventions. (Please see Chapter 7—'Choice of Diagnostic and Guide Catheters in Transradial Approach.)

Role of Pre-procedure Ultrasound of Arm Arteries in Detecting Anomalies of Radial Artery

As can be seen from Table 6.2, incidence of RA anomalies was 9.8%. Other than 'parallel' radial and ulnar (4.7%), and cubital loops (0.9%), intimal thickness (Figure 6.6a and 6.6b) was reported in 3.6%.[4] In two instances, where intimal thickness reported on ultrasound, it was found to be associated with severe calcification of bilateral radial and ulnar arteries

Table 6.2 Incidence of anomalies in radial artery in the study population (n = 2,344)[4]

Anomalies	Radial artery
Intimal thickness (Figure 6.2c)	3.6%
Parallel radial and ulnar (Figure 6.2a) suggesting possibility of high origin of radial from brachial or radioulnar loop or similar anomaly	4.7%
Loop seen at cubital fossa (Figure 6.2b)	0.9%
Blocked artery	0.6%

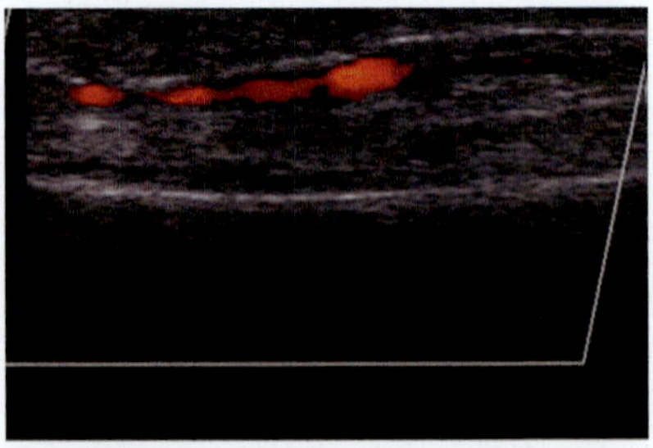

Figure 6.6a Intimal thickness.

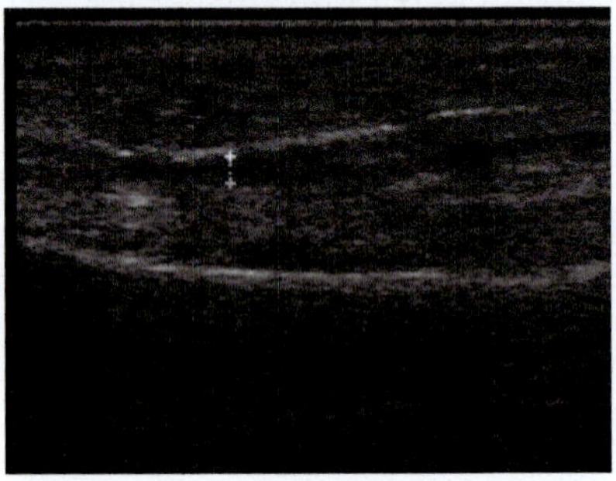

Figure 6.6b Intimal thickness.

(detected on fluoroscopy during catheterization) which led to crossover to alternate access (Figure 6.7a–c).

'Parallel' Radial and Ulnar Arteries

Wherever, on colour Doppler ultrasound, the bifurcation was not seen at the cubital fossa, the cases were grouped as 'parallel' radial and ulnar arteries, because the authors were unable to describe the various types of radial bifurcations on PPUAA. Hence, the 'parallel' group included all the types of bifurcations of radial,[1] including type-3, which with a narrow radial at bifurcation often allows a guidewire and sometimes a 4F or even 5F catheter to be advanced but not 6F; often necessitating a crossover to alternate access in cases requiring 6F angioplasty.

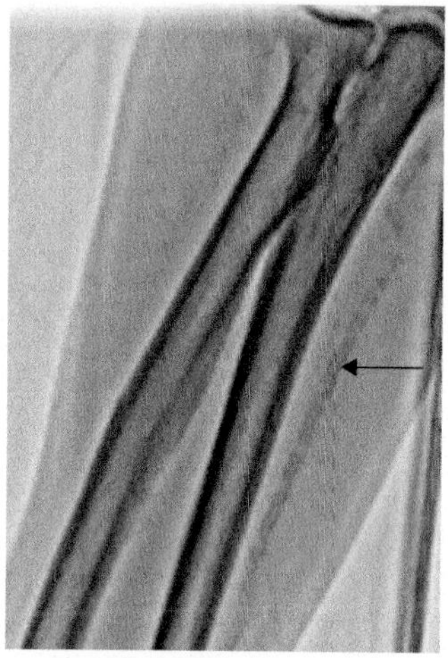

Figure 6.7a Calcific right radial and ulnar artery seen on fluoroscopy. *(Courtesy Dr Sanjay Chugh).*

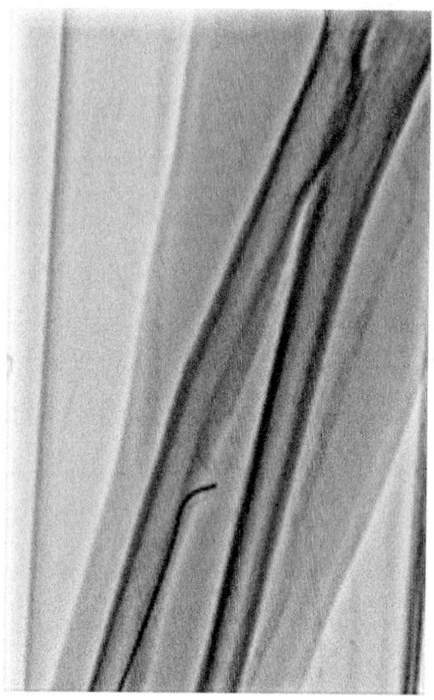

Figure 6.7b Calcific right radial and ulnar artery; angioplasty wire negotiating tortuosity in calcific right radial artery. *(Courtesy Dr Sanjay Chugh).*

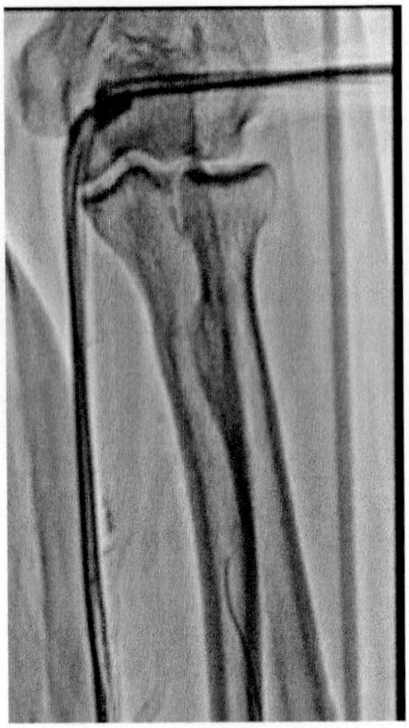

Figure 6.7c Calcific left radial and ulnar artery; angioplasty wire negotiating tortuosity in calcific left radial artery.
(Courtesy Dr Sanjay Chugh).

Role of Pre-procedure Ultrasound in Detecting Radial Artery Bifurcation Anomalies

Most remarkable is the finding of a high-up origin of radial from brachial; or in some, from the axillary artery (although not visualized on ultrasound). All high-up origins were grouped as 'parallel' radial and ulnar arteries (Figure 6.8). 'Parallel' radial and ulnar arteries were found in 4.7% (n = 2344).[4] This is an important group because in nearly 20%, the type 3 high origin of radial from brachial[1] is found, in whom the remnant radial artery is slender (Figures 6.9, 6.10a, and 6.10b), allowing a 0.038' guidewire to pass, and a 4F catheter may pass but nothing bigger can be accommodated, leading to procedure failure or crossover if ≥5F has to be used. A radio-ulnar anastomosis or cubital loop is usually present in these situations, which can often be traversed by using an angioplasty wire, to reach the brachial artery (Figure 6.11a–d). Again, although such a physical loop (Figure 6.12) was visible in only 0.9% (n = 2344), finding of 'parallel' radial and ulnar arteries included cases where a loop was not seen on colour Doppler but found on angiogram.

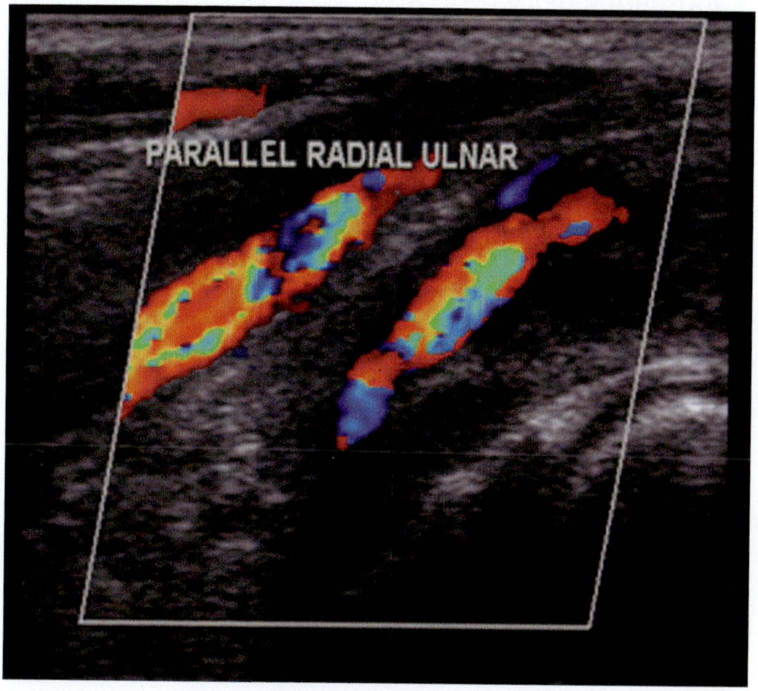

Figure 6.8 Parallel radial and ulnar artery.

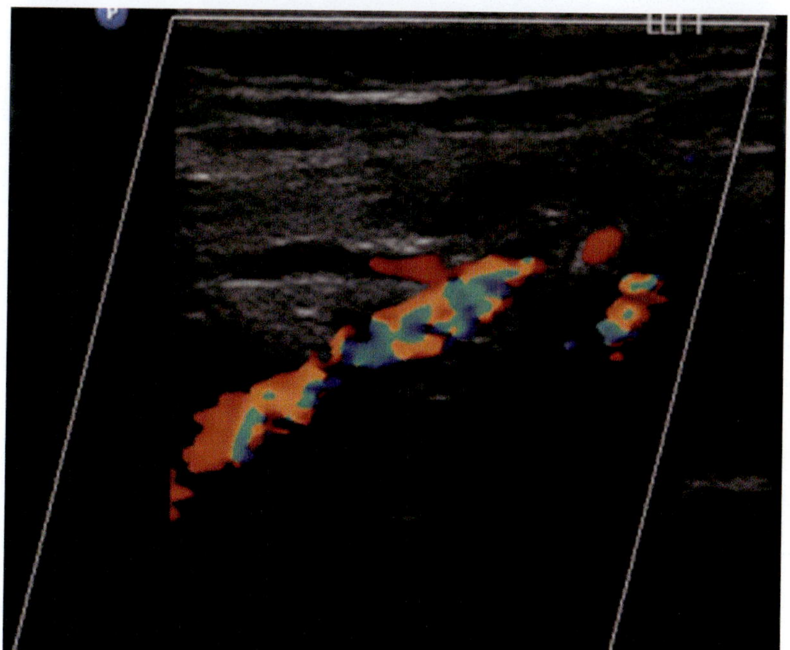
Figure 6.9 Remnant radial artery.

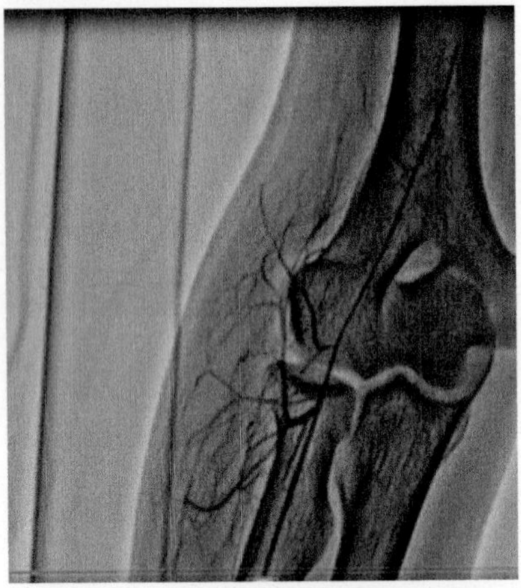

Figure 6.10a High origin type 3 radial bifurcation. (*Courtesy Dr Sanjay Chugh*).

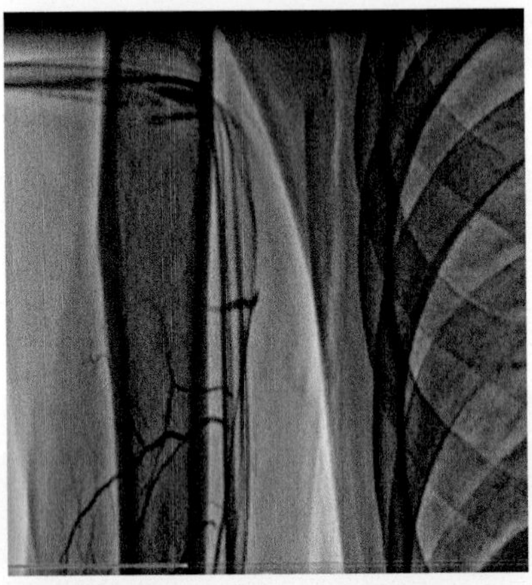

Figure 6.10b High origin type 3 radial bifurcation showing high origin of radial artery from brachial artery. (*Courtesy Dr Sanjay Chugh*).

Although PPUAA is not mandatory before transradial (TR) procedures, there is reason to believe, based on registry data,[4] and one randomized study on repeat procedures[13] that the technique would be useful in preventing procedure failure and crossovers and reducing spasm of radial artery during TR procedures.

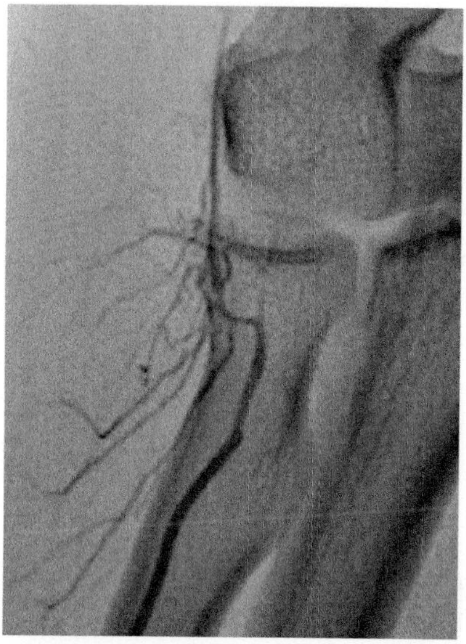

Figure 6.11a Angiogram showing a rudimentary right radial artery. (*Courtesy Dr Sanjay Chugh*).

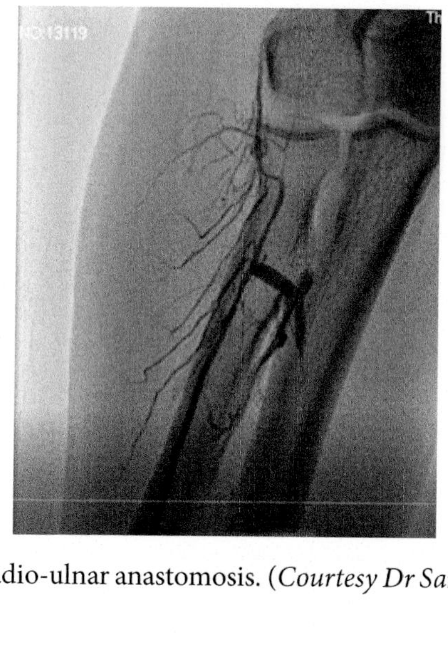

Figure 6.11b A radio-ulnar anastomosis. (*Courtesy Dr Sanjay Chugh*).

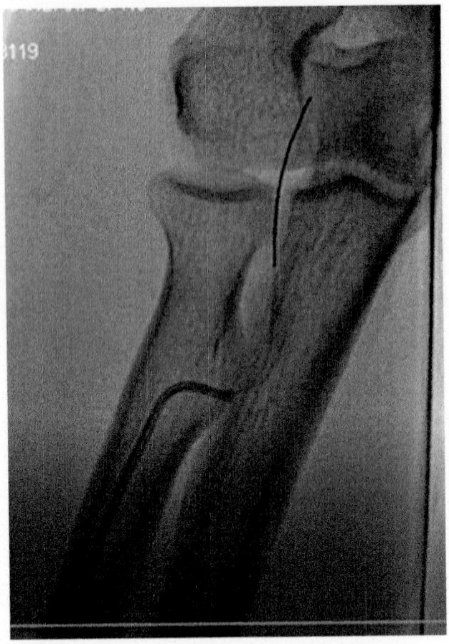

Figure 6.11c Angioplasty wire used to cross the radio-ulnar anastomosis. (*Courtesy Dr Sanjay Chugh*).

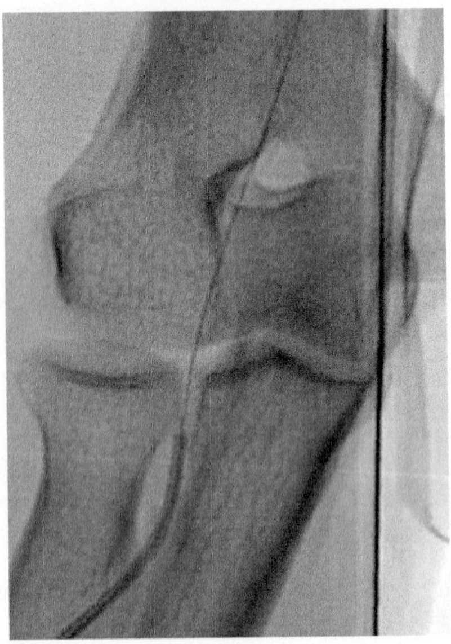

Figure 6.11d Angioplasty wire enters brachial artery via radio-ulnar anastomosis (cubital loop). (*Courtesy Dr Sanjay Chugh*).

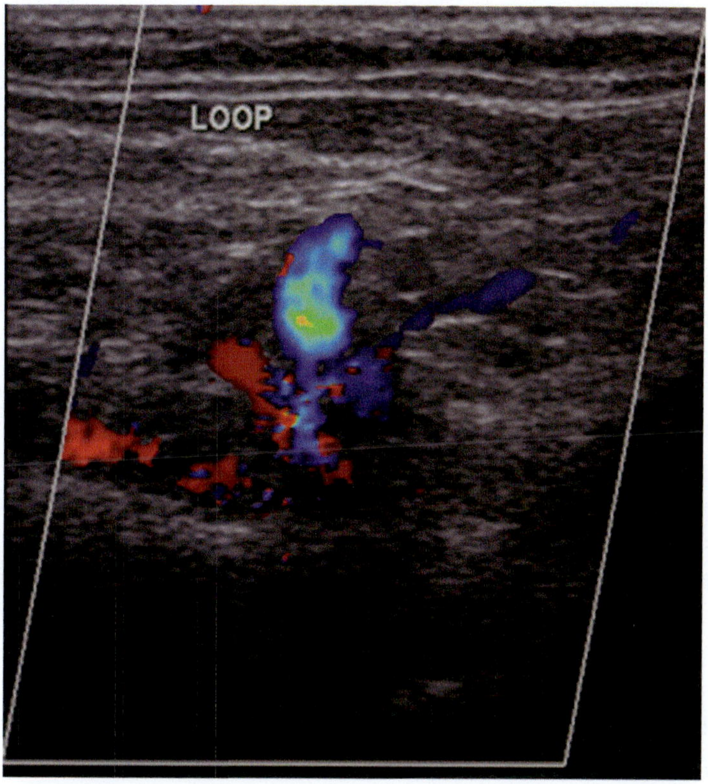

Figure 6.12 Cubital loop on colour Doppler ultrasound.

Clinical Implications of Using Pre-procedure Ultrasound of Arm Arteries for TRI

Insights from the Feasibility and Utility of Pre-procedure Ultrasound Imaging of the Arm to Facilitate Transradial Coronary Diagnostic and Interventional Procedures (PRIMAFACIE-TRI) Study

During the course of the assessment by Chugh et al. (2013) of role of colour Doppler ultrasound in their registry, they had to objectivize the assessment of spasm, in order to be able to assess the impact of pre-procedure colour Doppler on radial artery spasm (RAS) during diagnostic and interventional transradial procedures. In so doing Chugh et al. (2013) published a **grading system for RA spasm.**[4]

Grade 1: Mild Pain and Spasm not restricting catheter movement. No pause in procedure and only one dose of either or both intra-arterial Diltiazem (or Verapamil) of 5 mg and/or >0.5 mg of intravenous Midazolam.

Grade 2: Mild Pain and Spasm not restricting catheter movement. No pause in procedure and >1 dose of additional intra-arterial Diltiazem (or Verapamil) of 5 mg and/or >0.5 mg of intravenous Midazolam.

Grade 3: Moderate Pain and Spasm restricting catheter movement and necessitating a pause in procedure and >2 dose of additional intra-arterial Diltiazem (or Verapamil) >5 mg and/or >0.5 mg of intravenous Midazolam.

Grade 4: Severe Pain and Spasm disallowing any catheter movement necessitating crossover.

It helped convey severity of spasm and hence is relevant for clinical as well as research purposes to help compare impact of different pharmacologic and non-pharmacologic modalities on severity and incidence of RA spasm.

PRIMAFACIE-TRI (Feasibility and Utility of Pre-procedure Ultrasound Imaging of the Arm to Facilitate Transradial Coronary Diagnostic and Interventional Procedures),[4] a non-randomized registry of 2,344 patients showed that pre-procedure ultrasound provides useful anatomical information (Table 6.2) that reduces RA spasm, fluoroscopy time, crossover, and procedure failure (Table 6.3). The average time to do the ultrasound was 6.4 minutes, and the success rate for Coronary Angiography was 98.7% and PTCA was 97.5%.

Role of Colour Doppler Ultrasound in Repeat Transradial Procedures

Repeated coronary angiography and angioplasty procedures are required for in-stent re-stenosis and thrombosis, as well as for staged percutaneous coronary intervention (PCI) in multi-vessel coronary artery disease. Consequently, the requirement of repeat transradial interventions

Table 6.3 Procedural outcomes in the study group (n = 1872) compared to control group (n = 3441)

	Pre-Procedure Ultrasound Data Available N 2344 Selected N 1872 (CA = 1302; PCI = 570)	**Pre-Procedure Ultrasound Data Not Available (%) N 3781 Selected N 3441 (CA = 2798; PCI = 643)**	
Outcomes			
Access Artery Spasm% (_GRADE-3)	1.5	12.1	P < 0.001
Crossover (%)			
CA	1.3	4.3	P < 0.001
PCI	2.4	7.8	P < 0.001
Procedure Success (%)			
CA	98.7	92.7	P < 0.02
PCI	97.6	90.2	P < 0.01
Fluoroscopy Time (min)			
CA	3.2 ± 2.0	3.9 ± 2.5	P < 0.001
PCI	12.5 ± 5.3	24.1 ± 7.5	P < 0.001

Abbreviations: CA = coronary angiography; PCI = percutaneous coronary intervention.

(TRIs) has increased considerably. Intervention causes trauma to the artery and also affects its structure and function. Pre-procedure vascular ultrasound imaging and Doppler is an important modality that helps assess the diameter, structure, patency, and integrity of the artery after the first and before the second procedure.

The operator can decide prior to procedure whether to reuse the same vessel or choose a different vessel to avoid procedure failure and delays. Sheath size can be chosen according to vessel diameter to avoid spasm.

Elmahdy et al.[13] reported on the role of vascular ultrasound scanning in repeat transradial coronary artery intervention. The randomized study showed that pre-operative vascular ultrasound of radial artery prior to repeat transradial intervention is associated with significant reduction in vascular access time, procedure duration, RAS, and a mild increase in the radial access success rate.

TRI in Small Diameter Radial Arteries

Insights from Colour Doppler Ultrasound in Compression of Other Artery (COOA) Technique

Using colour Doppler ultrasound, we showed that with this technique, by transiently compressing the ipsilateral ulnar (≤ 5 minutes), the size of a small diameter radial artery can be increased by 12–18%, less puncture attempts were required while puncture success increased (Figures 6.13–6.15).[14] Sublingual nitroglycerin has been reported to increase the radial artery diameter.[15] The disadvantage of sublingual nitroglycerin is that it can cause drop in blood pressure in the fasting, volume-depleted, or sick patients with compromised left ventricular (LV) function and low blood pressure. On the other hand, compression of ipsilateral ulnar artery (Figure 6.16) has only local effect on the vessel compressed and has no adverse haemodynamic effects.

The increase in the access artery diameter was 16 ± 6% in arteries ≤1.5 mm at baseline (n = 374); it was 12 ± 3% ($p = 0.06$) in those (n = 390) > 1.5 mm diameter (mean = 1.8 ± 0.4 mm at baseline).

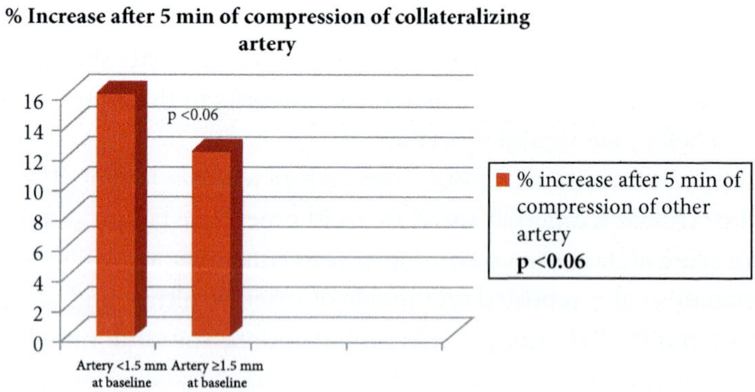

Figure 6.13 Percent increase in diameter of artery after 5-minute compression. After 5 minutes of compression of collateralizing artery, the percent increase in diameter is more in artery with baseline diameter <1.5 mm compared to ≥ 1.5 mm.

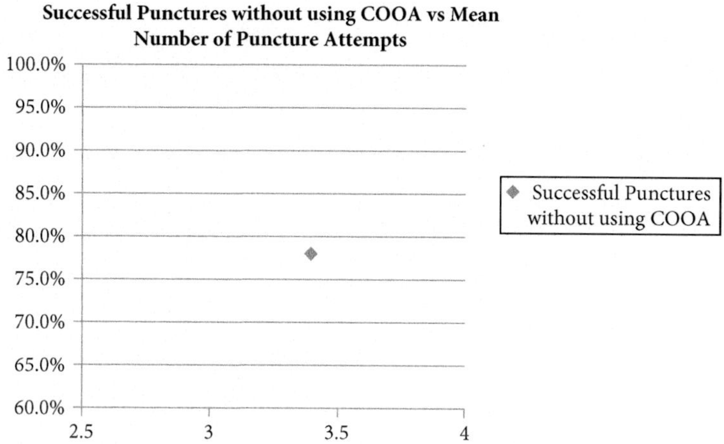

Figure 6.14 Number of puncture attempts and successful puncture without COOA.

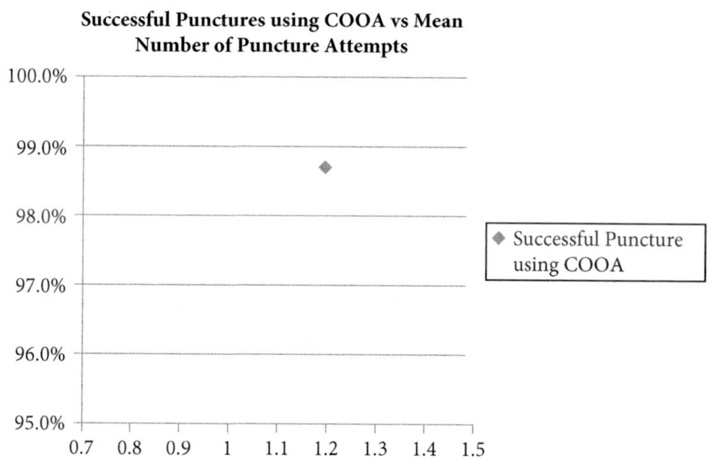

Figure 6.15 Number of puncture attempts and successful puncture with COOA.

In arteries ≤1.5 mm (mean 1.29 ± 0.21 mm): successful access occurred in 98.7% (mean puncture = 1.2) with use of compression of other artery (COOA) to enhance diameter of access artery versus 78% (mean puncture = 3.4) without COOA.[14]

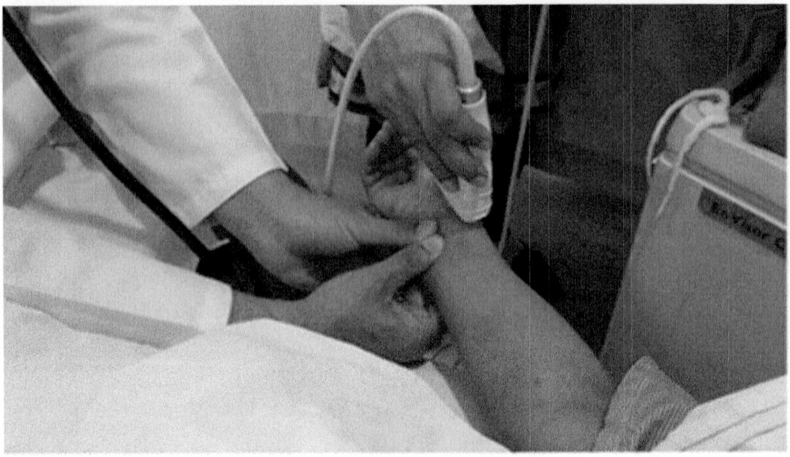

Figure 6.16 Compression of other artery.

COOA or sublingual nitroglycerin (S/L GTN) for increasing RA diameter in RA with small diameters are evolving techniques which may be used by operators prior to puncture of access artery.

Pre-procedure colour Doppler ultrasound also helps to know the size and quality of access arteries, to minimize procedure failure and complications. The above-mentioned techniques are useful, but still evolving.

Ultrasound-Guided Versus Palpation-Guided Radial Artery Puncture in Adult Population

Subsequent to publication of PRIMA FACIE TRI describing utility of PPUAA in transradial interventions by Chugh et al. in 2013, successful use of ultrasound-guidance for radial artery puncture in the cardiac catheterization laboratory was reported by Arnold Seto et al.[16] and is described below.

Radial Artery Access Through Ultrasound Trial (RAUST Trial)[16] used ultrasound-guided puncture for radial artery. Although it showed increased first pass success and efficiency of radial artery puncture with ultrasound (US) guidance, it failed to show any benefit in outcomes, including in the rate of operator-reported spasm, patient pain scores following the procedure, or bleeding complications. The first-pass success rate improved (64.8% versus 43.9%, $p < 0.0001$) and the number of attempts was reduced with US guidance [mean: 1.65 ± 1.2 versus 3.05 ± 3.4, $p < 0.0001$; median: 1 (interquartile range [IQR]: 1 to 2) versus 2 (1 to 3), $p < 0.0001$]. The time to access was reduced (88 ± 78 s versus 108 ± 112 s, $p = 0.006$; median: 64 [IQR: 45 to 94] s versus 74 [IQR: 49 to 120] s, $p = 0.01$). The study did not include the time required to prepare the US probe in the time to access and may negate the average time benefit of US guidance if performed by the operator rather than by a technician. The data should be interpreted with caution because of risk of bias. Further, ultrasound-guided radial artery puncture requires training of the operator, and availability of the ultrasound machine in the cardiac catheterization laboratory. This benefit is thus also associated with an incremental cost ($6) of sterile drapes and gel and a fixed cost for a U.S. machine that ranges from $15,000 to $25,000.[16]

A meta-analysis of seven studies[17] on the subject showed increased first pass success and significantly reduced mean attempts to success, mean time to success, and incidence of the complication of haematoma. However, none of these studies were done by cardiologists in the cardiac catheterization laboratory for transradial intervention. Most procedures were done by anesthetists and pediatricians in a largely pediatric population. Further, the number of patients in these studies was small, with concomitant risk of overestimation of treatment benefit, and there was risk of bias in all the studies. The studies also lacked consistency in the age of the patients in the study population as well as in frequency of the ultrasound probe used and experience of operators. None of the studies included difficult radial artery access such as patients with hypotension or obesity.

Another recent meta-analysis of 10 randomized controlled trials by Pacha et al.[18] showed that ultrasound-guided technique for radial artery access is associated with higher first attempt success rate of radial artery cannulation in comparison to digital palpation [OR (95% CI) 2.76 (186, 4.10); $p < 0.001$]; however, no difference was seen in overall cannulation success rate between ultrasound guided technique and digital palpation [OR (95% CI) 2.01 (1.00, 4.06); $p = 0.05$], time to cannulate [SMD (95% CI) −0.31 (−0.65, 0.04); $p = 0.30$] and mean number of attempts [MD (95% CI) −0.65 (−1.32, 0.02); $p = 0.06$]. However, because of presence of heterogeneity, results of this meta-analysis should be interpreted with caution.

The authors recommend doing pre-procedure radial artery sizing for diameter and anomalies, and radial artery puncture directly without per-operative ultrasound (USG) guidance. The investment of effort in training in ultrasound guidance is likely to be same as that required to become expert at puncturing radial arteries without USG guidance. The expertise in puncturing radial artery would then be independent of ultrasound guidance for every puncture. Since institutional practices and feasibility regarding a dedicated ultrasound machine in the catheterization laboratory may vary worldwide; the practice of puncturing the radial artery by palpation is more likely to be widely acceptable because it is not dependent on an ultrasound machine for guidance.

Role of Colour Doppler Ultrasound in Diagnosing and Managing Complications of Transradial Procedures

Colour Doppler ultrasound has been used by Chugh et al. (2015) to diagnose, assess and manage complications of transradial procedures.[19]

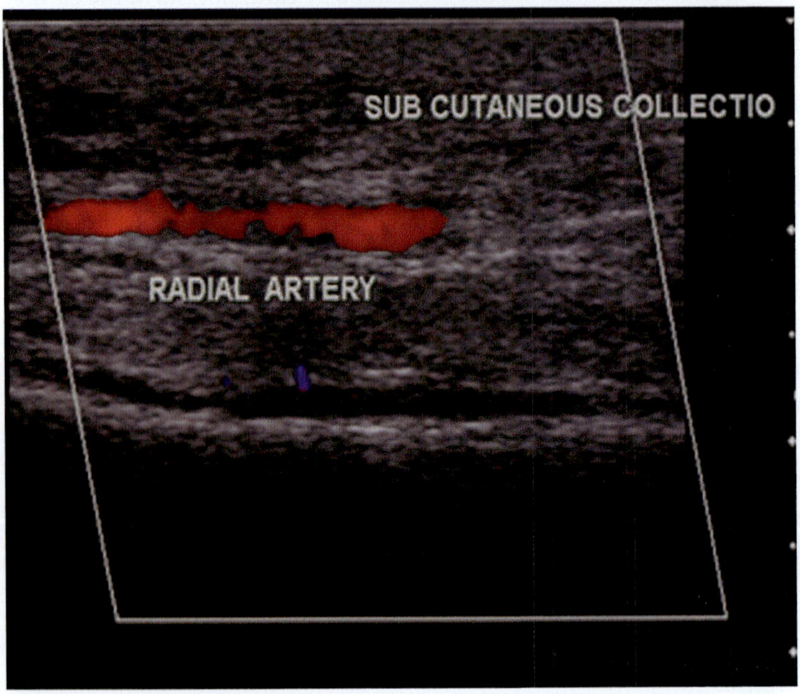

Figure 6.17 Haematoma.

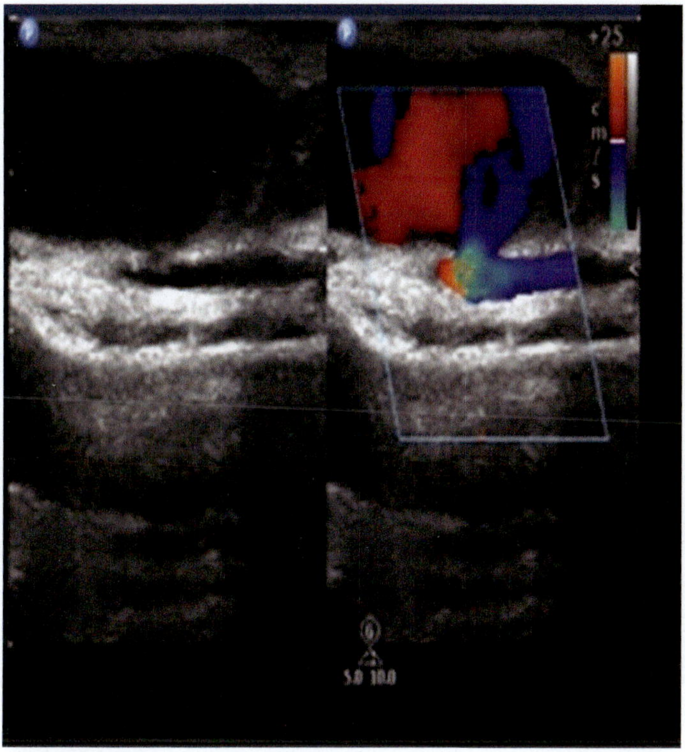

Figure 6.18 Radial pseudoaneurysm.

It has been used by Chugh et al. (2015)[19] for:

- Early detection of haematoma (Figure 6.17)
- Localization of site of active bleed
- For follow-up to confirm haemostasis, in addition
- To detect pseudo-aneurysms (Figure 6.18)
- For follow up after compression of a pseudo-aneurysm to confirm that the pseudo-aneurysm has sealed.
- It is also useful to diagnose radial artery occlusion (RAO) (Figure 6.19) post-procedure and
- For subsequent follow-up of RAO to see whether the radial artery has re-canalized at 30, 60, or 90 days.
- It also helps detect the rare development of radial arteriovenous fistula.

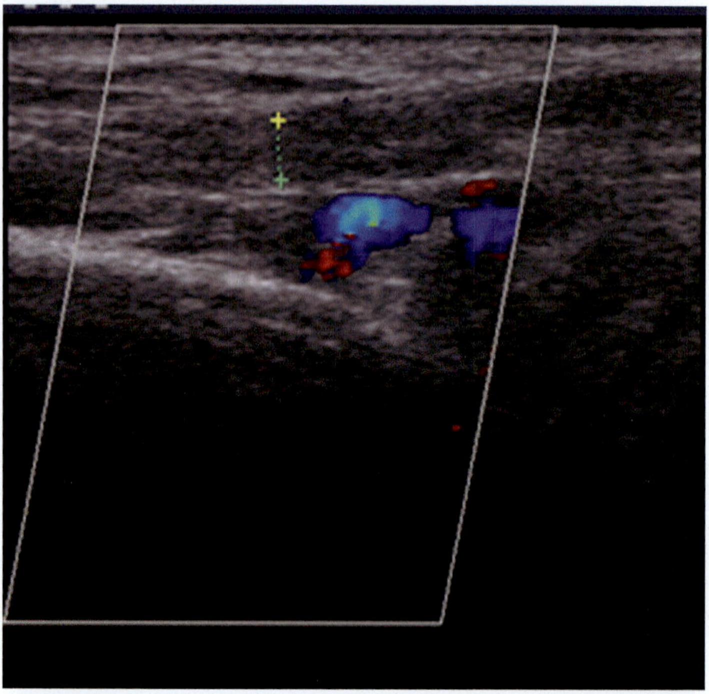

Figure 6.19 Radial artery occlusion.

References

1. Martial Hamon, Christian Pristipino, Carlo Di Mario, James Nolan, Josef Ludwig, Marco Tubaro, Manel Sabate, Josepa Mauri-Ferre, Kurt Huber, Kari Niemela, Michael Haude, William Wijns, Dariusz Dudek, Jean Fajadet, Ferdinand Kiemeneij, Geral Barbeau, Shigeru Saito, Sanjit Jolly, Yves Louvard, Tejas Patel, Sunil V Rao, Nicolaus Reifart, Philippe Gabriel, Orazio Valsecchi, Yuenjin Yang. Consensus document on the radial approach in percutaneous cardiovascular interventions: position paper by the European Association of Percutaneous Cardiovascular Interventions and Working Groups on Acute Cardiac Care and Thrombosis of the European Society of Cardiology. *EuroIntervention.* 2013;8:1242–51.
2. Lo TS, Nolan J, Fountzopoulos E, Behan M, Butler R, Hetherington SL, et al. Radial artery anomaly and its influence on transradial coronary procedural outcome. *Heart.* 2009;95(5):410.
3. Saito S, Ikei H, Hosokawa G, et al. Influence of the ratio between radial artery inner diameter and sheath outer diameter on radial artery flow after transradial coronary intervention. *Catheter Cardiovasc Interv.* 1999;46(2):173–78.

4. Kumar Chugh S, Chugh S, Chugh Y, Rao SV. Feasibility and utility of pre-procedural ultrasound imaging of the arm to facilitate transradial coronary diagnostic and interventional procedures (PRIMAFACIE-TRI). *Catheter Cardiovasc Interv*. 2013;82:64–73.
5. Byung-SuYoo, Junghan Yoon, Ji-Yean Ko, Jang-Young Kim, Seung-Hwan Lee, Sung-Oh Hwang, Kyung-Hoon Choe. Anatomical consideration of the radial artery for transradial coronary procedures: arterial diameter, branching anomaly and vessel tortuosity. *Int J Cardiol*. 2005;101(3):421–27.
6. Peruga JP, Peruga JZ, Kasprzak JD, Kręcki R, Jankowski Ł, Zając P, Plewka M. Ultrasound evaluation of forearm arteries in patients undergoing percutaneous coronary intervention via radial artery access: results of one-year follow-up. *Kardiol Pol*. 2015;73(7):502–10.
7. Velasco A, Ono C, Nugent K, Tarwater P, Kumar A. Ultrasonic evaluation of the radial artery diameter in a local population from Texas. *J Invasive Cardiol*. 2012;24(7):339–41.
8. Alkhouli M, Cohen HA, Bashir R. Radial artery avulsion – a rare complication of transradial catheterization. *Catheter Cardiovasc Interv*. 2015;85:E32–34.
9. Dieter RS, Akef A, Wolff M. Eversion endarterectomy complicating radial artery access for left heart catheterization. *Catheter Cardiovasc Interv*. 2003;58:478–80.
10. Arzamendi D, Romeo P, Gosselin G. Radial artery avulsion: a rare complication of percutaneous coronary intervention. *Revista espanola de cardiologia*. 2011;64:62.
11. Uhlemann M, Mobius-Winkler S, Mende M, et al. The Leipzig prospective vascular ultrasound registry in radial artery catheterization: impact of sheath size on vascular complications. *JACC Cardiovasc Interv*. 2012;5(1):36–43.
12. Rashid M, Kwork CS, Pancholy S, Chugh S. Radial artery occlusion after transradial intervention: a systematic review and metaanalysis. *JAHA J Am Heart Assoc*. 2016;5:e002686.
13. Elmahdy MF, Hassan M, Elquindy A. Role of vascular ultrasound scanning in repeated trans-radial coronary artery intervention (prospective randomized study). *Catheter Cardiovasc Interv*. 2017.
14. Sanjay K Chugh, Sunita Chugh, Yashasvi Chugh. Addressing the challenge of access of small radial and ulnar arteries in transradial and transulnar interventions: insights from a color Doppler study. *J Am Coll Cardiol*. 2014;64(11) Supplement: page b 240.
15. Chong AY, Lo T, George S, Ratib K, Mamas M, Nolan J. The effect of pre-procedure sublingual nitroglycerine on radial artery diameter and Allen's test outcome – relevance to transradial catheterization. *Cardiovasc Revasc Med*. 2017.
16. Seto AH, Roberts JS, Abu-Fadel MS, Czak SJ, Latif F, et al. Real time ultrasound guidance facilitates transradial access: RAUST (Radial Artery access with Ultrasound Trial). *JACC Cardiovasc Interv*. 2015;8(2):283–91. Critical care18. R93(2014).
17. Wan-Jie Gu, Hong-Tao Tie, Jing-Chen Liu, Xian-Tao Zeng. Efficacy of ultrasound-guided radial artery catheterization: a systematic review and meta-analysis of randomized controlled trials.

18. Homam Moussa Pacha, Fares Alahdab, Yasser Al-khadra, Amar Idris, Giras Rabbat, Fahed Darmoch, Mohamad Soud, Anwar Zaitoun, Amir Kaki, Sunil V Rao, Chun Shing Kwok, Mamas A Mamas, M Chadi Alraies. Ultrasound-guided versus palpation-guided radial artery catheterization in adult population: a systematic review and meta-analysis of randomized controlled trials. *YMHJ*. 2018. doi: 10.1016/j.ahj.2018.06.007
19. Sanjay Kumar Chugh, Yashasvi Chugh, Sunita Chugh. How to tackle complications in radial procedures: tips and tricks. *Indian Heart J*. 2015;67(3):275–81.

7

Choice of Diagnostic and Guide Catheters in Transradial Approach

Sankaran Ramesh, Sunita Chugh, and Sanjay Kumar Chugh

Introduction

Transradial approach (TRA) is associated with reduced access-site bleeding, greater patient comfort, early ambulation, and reduced hospital stay, and in patients with acute coronary syndromes, it is associated with reduced mortality.[1–5] TRA can, however, be very challenging. In this chapter, we discuss the choice of catheters for transradial angiography and angioplasty. For details on tips and tricks to overcome the challenges and enhance guide support, please refer to Chapter 10: 'Tips and Tricks for Transradial Interventions'.

Diagnostic Catheterization

Single-Catheter Technique

For transradial diagnostic catheterization, the authors' catheter of choice is 5F Optitorque TIG™ (TERUMO) catheter (TIG). It cannulates both left and right coronary arteries, thereby reducing the need for multiple catheter exchanges. Left ventriculography is also possible with the same catheter. The authors' practice is to use TIG as default for coronary angiography. For technique of catheter manipulation, please refer to Chapter 8: 'Technique of Engaging the Coronaries Using Transradial Access'.

There are three ways a TIG may engage the left coronary artery (LCA)[6]:

- From above level of coronary sinus in patients with narrow aortic root, as in the short-statured patients;
- At the level of LCA, in a majority with average-sized aortic roots; and
- Below level of LCA at level of base of aortic root (Figures 7.1a and 7.1b) in those with larger aortic root diameters.

In situations where TIG fails, other catheters are used.[6] A Judkins left (JL) 3.5 catheter is used in patients with a wide left main coronary artery, if the TIG catheter hooks the left circumflex artery (LCX) selectively, with poor-visualization of the left anterior descending artery (LAD). In engaging the right coronary artery (RCA) by TIG, if the conal branch is repeatedly hooked instead and the problem cannot be fixed using a Dacron angiography guidewire in the catheter to straighten the distal bend at the tip of the TIG catheter; then an Amplatz right

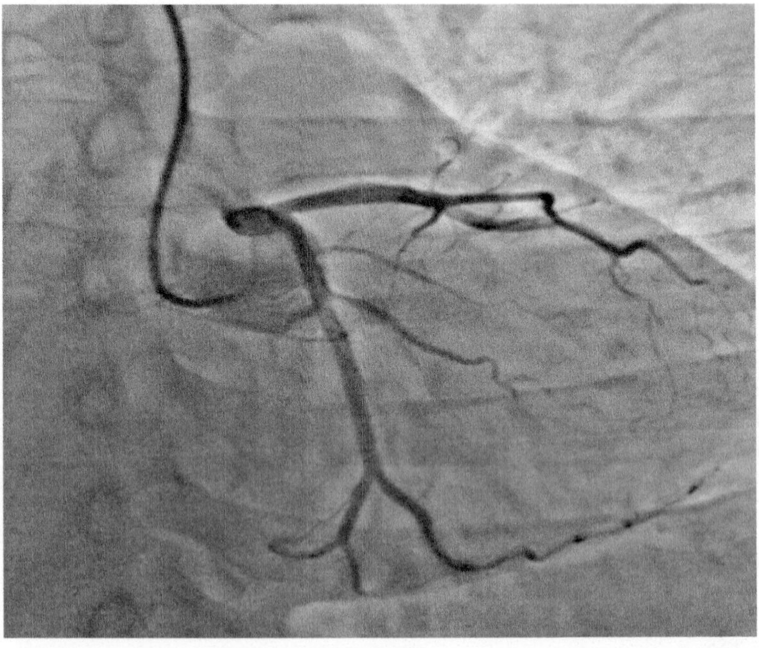

Figure 7.1a A TIG catheter pushed to the base of aortic root, tip engages the left coronary from below, in a patient with a dilated 4 cm aortic root. Right anterior oblique with caudal view.

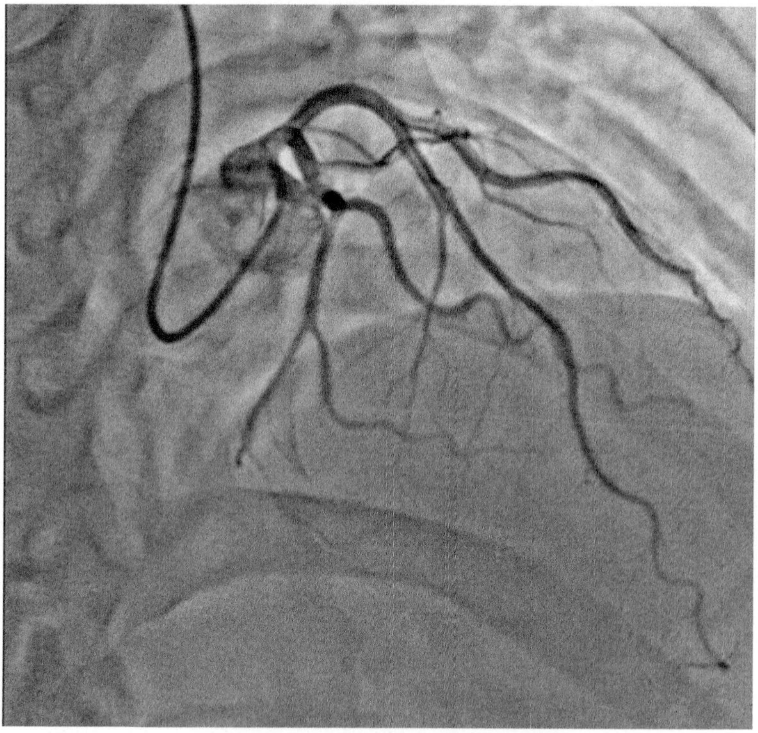

Figure 7.1b The same in antero-posterior and cranial view.

(AR) catheter may be used. In case of severe tortuosity of the subclavian artery (SCLa), it is advisable to keep an angiographic guide-wire inside the TIG catheter during its rotation to prevent the catheter from kinking. A 'big-breath' taken by the patient (the patient is asked to take a big breath and hold) helps negotiate the tortuosities. Sometimes a Glidewire® (Terumo™) is used.

Figures 7.2a–7.2h illustrate how in a 6-foot, 2-inch tall patient, a TIG catheter fell short of the coronaries because of using right distal radial access (which increases the distance to coronaries by a cm compared to standard right radial access (RRA)) and also because the patient had very tortuous right SCLa which took up additional length of catheter especially as the SCLa did not straighten up even with an angiographic guidewire in the catheter (Figure 7.2b). The TIG catheter fell short of the left coronary ostium (Figure 7.2c). To overcome the problem, the angiographic guidewire was first advanced into the catheter (Figure 7.2d); then, the wire-catheter assembly was pulled back, to straighten the tortuosity (Figure 7.2e), and

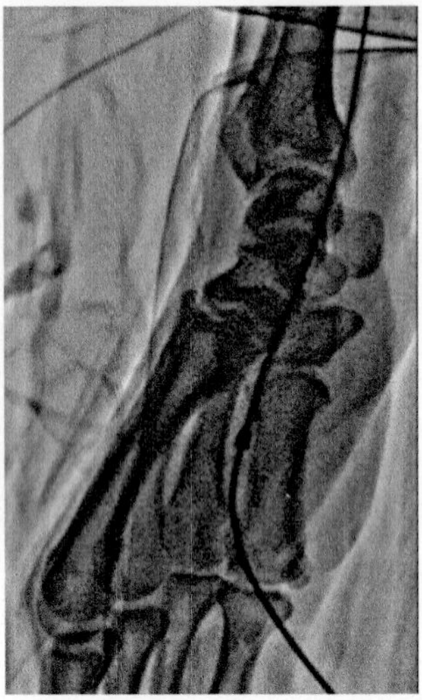

Figure 7.2a In a 6-foot, 2-inch-tall patient, distal radial access used for coronary angiogram, 5F radial sheath inserted.

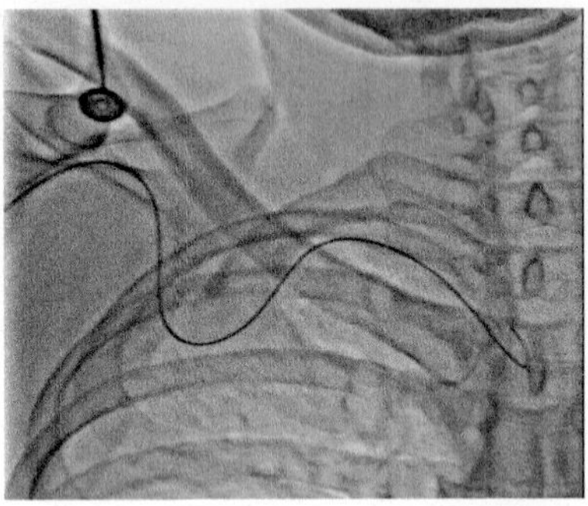

Figure 7.2b Tortuous right subclavian artery which did not straighten up with an angiographic guidewire.

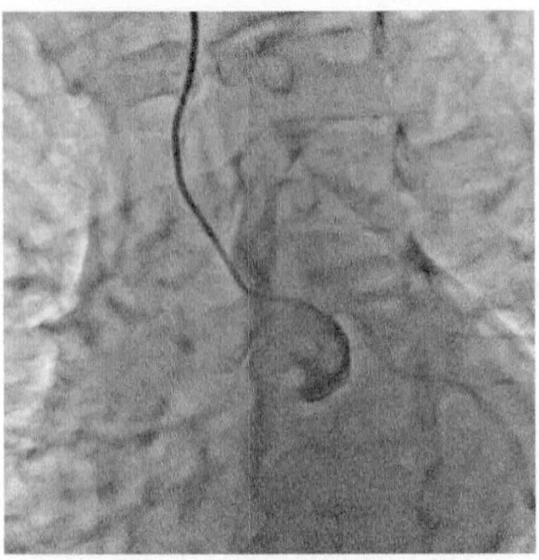

Figure 7.2c A TIG catheter fell short of the in the catheter.

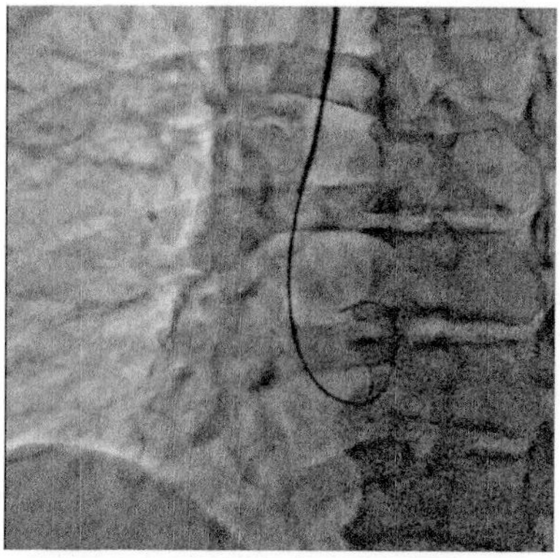

Figure 7.2d The angiographic guidewire was advanced.

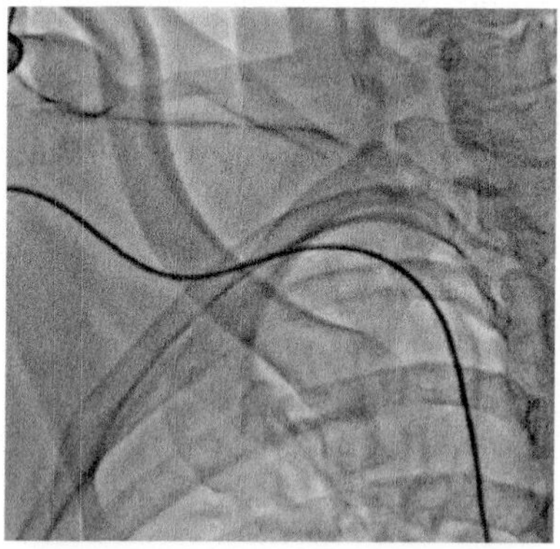

Figure 7.2e Then, the wire-catheter assembly was pulled back, to straighten the subclavian tortuosity.

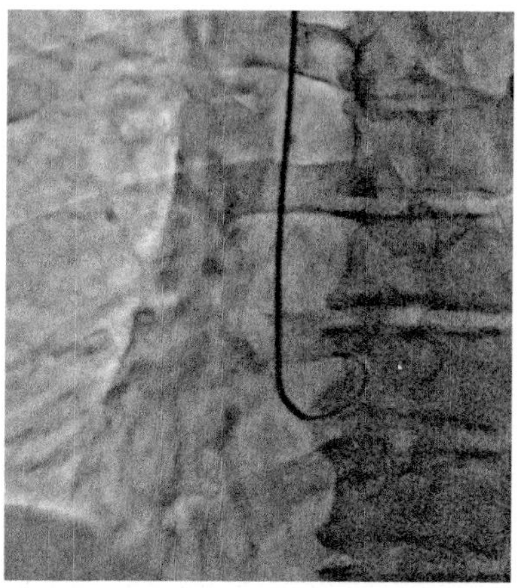

Figure 7.2f And then, the catheter was advanced again.

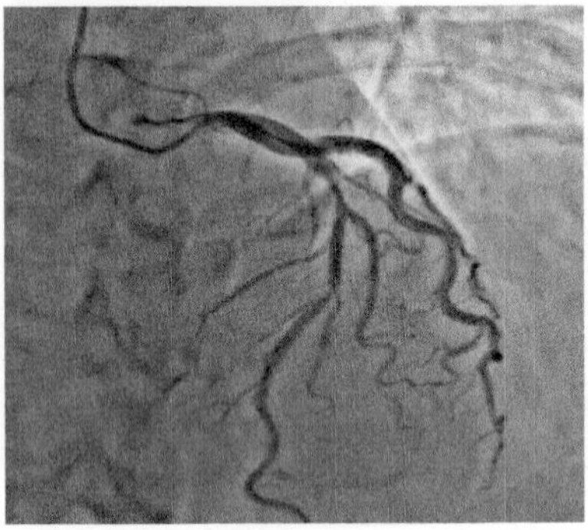

Figure 7.2g The left coronary artery could then be engaged.

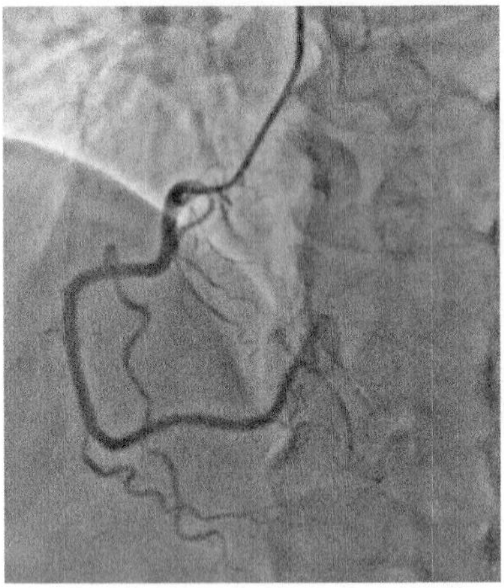

Figure 7.2h The right coronary artery was engaged using the same method.

finally, the catheter was advanced again over the wire (Figure 7.2f). The coronaries could then be engaged (Figures 7.2g and 7.2h).

In rare situations with a downward take-off of the RCA from the right coronary sinus (RCS), a multipurpose or Amplatz right curve is helpful to engage the RCA ostium.

A TIG can also be used via left radial access (LRA), though hooking the LCA through LRA may be more difficult and hence less successful than via RRA.

The various diagnostic and guide catheters (GCs) used by interventional cardiologists are shown in Tables 7.1 and 7.2.[7]

Two-Catheter Technique

Judkins right (JR) and left (JL) catheters can be used for coronary angiography, instead of a single TIG catheter. Technique of engaging the coronaries is discussed in the next chapter (Chapter 8). In case of severe subclavian tortuosity, it is advisable to keep an angiographic guidewire inside the JR catheter during its rotation to prevent the catheter from kinking. In situations where the JR selectively engages the conal branch or does not hook the RCA because of anomalous origin, then an Amplatz catheter of appropriate curve size is used. Single-catheter technique to engage both the RCA and LCA using TIG catheter reduces fluoroscopy time significantly compared to two-catheter technique using Judkins catheters.[8]

Table 7.1 Diagnostic catheter use worldwide (%) [7]

	All	U.S.	Canada-Europe	China	India	Japan
LCA						
Judkins left 3.5	44.9	37.8	49.4	25.8	15.2	26.4
Judkins left 4.0	21.6	14.6	23.1	12.9	0.0	35.6
Kimny	1.8	7.3	1.1	3.2	3.0	2.3
Multipurpose	6.2	4.9	4.3	45.2	0.0	11.5
Tiger/Tiger II	16.1	12.2	15.1	12.9	75.8	1.1
Amplatz left	2.2	1.2	2.9	0.0	0.0	1.1
Barbeau	0.2	0.0	0.3	0.0	0.0	0.0
Fajadet left	0.1	0.0	0.0	0.0	0.0	0.0
Other	7.0	22.0	3.8	0.0	6.1	21.8
RCA						
Judkins right 4.0	58.8	46.3	64.6	38.7	12.1	52.9
Kimny	1.7	7.3	1.0	3.2	3.0	2.3
Multipurpose	6.7	7.3	4.6	45.2	0.0	11.5
Tiger/Tiger II	14.9	11.0	14.4	9.7	66.7	1.1
Amplatz left	2.4	2.4	2.9	0.0	0.0	1.1
Amplatz right	2.2	3.7	2.9	0.0	0.0	0.0
Barbeau	0.5	0.0	0.8	0.0	0.0	0.0
Fajadet right	0.1	0.0	0.0	0.0	0.0	0.0
Other	12.7	22.0	8.8	3.2	18.2	31.0

(*continued*)

Table 7.1 Continued

	All	U.S.	Canada-Europe	China	India	Japan
SVG to LCA						
Judkins right	48.6	41.5	51.6	41.9	27.3	40.2
Left bypass	11.5	6.1	11.7	16.1	3.0	3.4
Amplatz left	22.6	26.8	23.4	12.9	18.2	36.8
Multipurpose	7.3	7.3	5.6	19.4	21.2	5.7
Tiger/Tiger II	3.9	6.1	3.4	9.7	6.1	0.0
Kimny	0.7	1.2	0.8	0.0	0.0	0.0
Barbeau	0.1	0.0	0.2	0.0	0.0	0.0
Fajadet	0.1	0.0	0.0	0.0	0.0	0.0
Other	5.3	11.0	3.4	0.0	24.2	13.8
SVG to RCA						
Judkins right	46.8	25.6	48.1	41.9	39.4	43.7
Right bypass	8.0	3.7	8.5	6.5	3.0	3.4
Amplatz left	12.0	7.3	10.3	25.8	18.2	34.5
Multipurpose	23.8	53.7	25.2	16.1	12.1	4.6
Tiger/Tiger II	3.1	2.4	2.9	6.5	3.0	0.0
Kimny	0.4	0.0	0.5	0.0	0.0	1.1
Barbeau	0.4	0.0	0.6	0.0	0.0	0.0
Fajadet	0.0	0.0	0.0	0.0	0.0	0.0
Other	5.6	7.3	4.0	3.2	24.2	12.6

Guide Catheters for Transradial Intervention

The average radial artery (RA) diameter is smaller than the femoral artery and has been reported to be 1.7–1.8 mm in a south Asian, Indian population and 2.2–2.6 mm in other ethnic populations.[9–12] Further, radial arteries are prone to spasm, which could lead to procedural delay and failure or crossover. Hence, to minimize RA spasm, the French size of catheters used (Table 7.3), as well as catheter manipulations should be least possible (*please see Chapter 10, Items 2, 5, and 6, Figure 10.3; and Chapter 19, Item 1*). Most transradial interventions (TRIs) can be done with 5F and 6F GCs and majority of complex percutaneous coronary interventions (PCI) (with exception of simultaneous kissing stent technique using two stents simultaneously for bifurcation lesions); rotational atherectomy (please see Chapter 14), intravascular ultrasound (IVUS), and optical coherence tomography (OCT) (*please see Chapter 16*) can be performed using 6F guiding catheters. To minimize catheter exchanges, catheter curve-size selection should be based on patient height and aortic root size on X-ray chest or echocardiogram. Catheter-shape selection is based on target vessel and take-off of the coronary artery (*please see* Chapter 10).

Optimum guide support, essential for successful completion of PCI, depends upon stability of GC engagement in the coronary when the interventional devices are advanced into the coronary artery for PCI. Guide support can be of two types: passive and active. With passive support, the GC inserted into coronary artery requires minimal manipulation; support is provided either by aortic root or opposite aortic wall and attributed to the shape of the catheter as with an Amplatz or XB guide. Active support entails operator manipulation of the catheter in some way to enhance support, such as clockwise rotation of a Judkins right catheter to deep-throat the guiding catheter for angioplasty in RCA (Figure 10.4b(v) and 10.4b(vi), Chapter 10). Guide support can be enhanced with use of a buddy wire and other techniques (*please see* Chapter 10 *for techniques and illustrations*). Active support is required more often when using 5F GC (*please see Chapter 25, 'Slender Percutaneous Coronary Interventions by Transradial Approach'*).

French Size of Guide Catheter

With 5F GCs, active support is required more often than with GC ≥ 7F in which passive support is better, while both the active and passive GC support can be derived with 6F GCs.[13] Another option for enhancing guide support is to use a guideliner,[14] which also provides additional support for PCI with 6F GC in complex tortuous, heavily calcified lesions including chronic total occlusions. With 5F catheters, it is important to be careful to de-air the catheter, as air is sucked in, because of Venturi effect, each time a balloon, stent, or wire is pulled out of the Tuohy Borst adapter. Table 7.3 shows requisite guide catheter (GC) French sizes (F) for various interventional devices for percutaneous coronary interventions.

Table 7.2 Guide catheter use worldwide (%)[7]

	All	U.S.	Canada-Europe	China	India	Japan
LAD						
Judkins left	22.5	6.3	21.6	20.7	10.0	38.4
XB 3.0	8.1	10.1	7.0	20.7	16.7	0.0
XB 3.5	18.2	26.6	18.9	13.8	6.7	5.8
Amplatz left	1.4	2.5	1.3	0.0	3.3	0.0
Tiger II	0.6	1.3	0.5	0.0	3.3	0.0
EBU 3.5	27.9	35.4	26.9	41.4	50.0	20.9
EBU 3.75	6.5	7.6	7.9	3.4	3.3	5.8
EBU 4.0	5.6	1.3	8.0	0.0	0.0	2.3
Kimny	0.8	2.5	0.8	0.0	0.0	0.0
Fajadet left	0.5	1.3	0.5	0.0	0.0	0.0
MUTA left	0.7	0.0	1.1	0.0	0.0	0.0
Other	7.1	5.1	5.4	0.0	6.7	26.7
Cx						
Judkins left	12.5	5.1	11.0	3.4	0.0	26.7
XB 3.0	6.5	6.3	4.9	13.8	13.3	1.2
XB 3.5	20.8	30.4	21.3	17.2	20.0	8.1
Amplatz left	10.8	3.8	13.0	10.3	6.7	5.8
Tiger II	0.3	0.0	0.3	0.0	3.3	0.0
EBU 3.5	26.1	26.6	25.1	48.3	43.3	25.6
EBU 3.75	6.2	15.2	6.1	3.4	6.7	7.0
EBU 4.0	8.7	2.5	11.8	0.0	3.3	3.5
Kimny	0.8	1.3	1.0	0.0	0.0	0.0
Fajadet left	0.5	2.5	0.2	3.4	0.0	0.0
MUTA left	0.4	0.0	0.7	0.0	0.0	0.0
Other	6.3	6.3	4.8	0.0	3.3	22.1
RCA						
Judkins right	70.2	69.6	70.3	93.1	80.0	48.8
Amplatz right	10.2	11.4	12.0	0.0	6.7	2.3
Amplatz left	5.8	7.6	5.4	0.0	6.7	10.5
Barbeau	1.9	1.3	2.6	3.4	0.0	0.0
Kimny	1.3	3.8	1.3	0.0	0.0	0.0
Fajadet right	0.4	0.0	0.5	0.0	0.0	0.0
MUTA right	0.2	0.0	0.3	0.0	0.0	0.0
Other	9.8	6.3	7.5	3.4	6.7	38.4

Table 7.2 Continued

	All	U.S.	Canada-Europe	China	India	Japan
Left SVG						
Left bypass graft	19.4	16.5	21.0	24.1	3.3	7.0
Amplatz left	37.3	39.2	36.6	24.1	26.7	62.8
Multipurpose	6.2	8.9	4.8	6.9	30.0	2.3
Judkins right	31.0	22.8	33.4	41.4	26.7	16.3
Barbeau	0.4	0.0	0.5	3.4	0.0	0.0
Kimny	0.7	1.3	0.8	0.0	0.0	0.0
Fajadet	0.2	0.0	0.0	0.0	0.0	0.0
Other	4.7	11.4	3.0	0.0	13.3	11.6
Right SVG						
Left bypass graft	3.5	3.8	3.1	0.0	0.0	3.5
Amplatz left	20.8	5.1	17.5	41.4	20.0	59.3
Multipurpose	29.2	65.8	30.8	13.8	26.7	4.7
Judkins right	39.6	17.7	41.8	44.8	40.0	20.9
Barbeau	0.9	0.0	1.5	0.0	0.0	0.0
Kimny	0.5	0.0	0.7	0.0	0.0	0.0
Fajadet	0.0	0.0	0.0	0.0	0.0	0.0
Other	5.5	7.6	4.6	0.0	13.3	11.6

Table 7.3 Guide catheter (GC) French size (F) for percutaneous coronary interventions

GC French size	Accomodates
5F	≤5mm Balloon; ≤4.5mm stent, IVUS from Terumo; 2.5mm cutting balloon 1.25mm Rotablator Burr (poor angiographic visualization; blood pressure has to be monitored non-invasively)
6F	All balloon, stent sizes, IVUS, OCT, Rotablation burr ≤1.5mm; Thrombosuction catheters; Spider Filter (embolic protection) for SVG intervention; Guide catheter extension (Guidezilla); Kissing balloon
7F	All of above; In addition ≥1.75mm rotablator burr; 2 stent techniques for bifurcation lesions

Abbreviations: IVUS = Intravascular ultrasound; OCT = Optical coherence tomography; SVG = Saphenous vein graft

Selection of Guide Catheter

Guide catheter selection includes the curve shape, curve size, and French size to provide stable engagement of the coronary artery with optimum GC support. GCs used are shown in Table 7.2 and Figures 7.3 and 7.4.[7] Special catheters like the Kimny can be used for both left and right coronary engagement for PCI. However, special catheters are not required, and the common femoral catheters are commonly used for transradial percutaneous coronary intervention. For TRIs of LCA, extra-backup (EBU) GC, and for RCA, the JR4 are the most popular GCs. In post-coronary bypass patients, the Amplatz-type guiding catheter for left coronary bypass vein grafts and Amplatz, JR4, or Multipurpose guiding catheter for right-sided vein grafts are commonly used. The internal mammary GC is used for left internal mammary interventions.[7] (Please see Chapter 10—'Tips and Tricks for Transradial Interventions', pages 140–141; and *Chapter 15—'Trans-Radial Interventions in Chronic Total Occlusions and Post-CABG Patients'* for further details.)

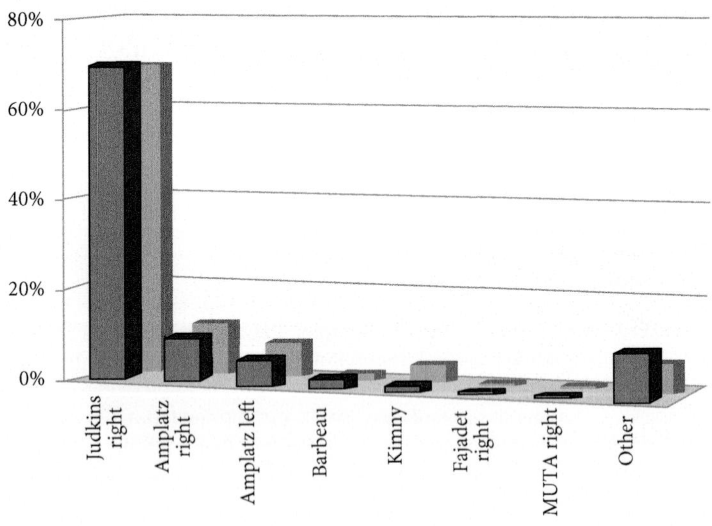

Figure 7.3 Guide catheters used for right coronary interventions [adapted from Table 4 (Bertrand et al., 2010)].[7]

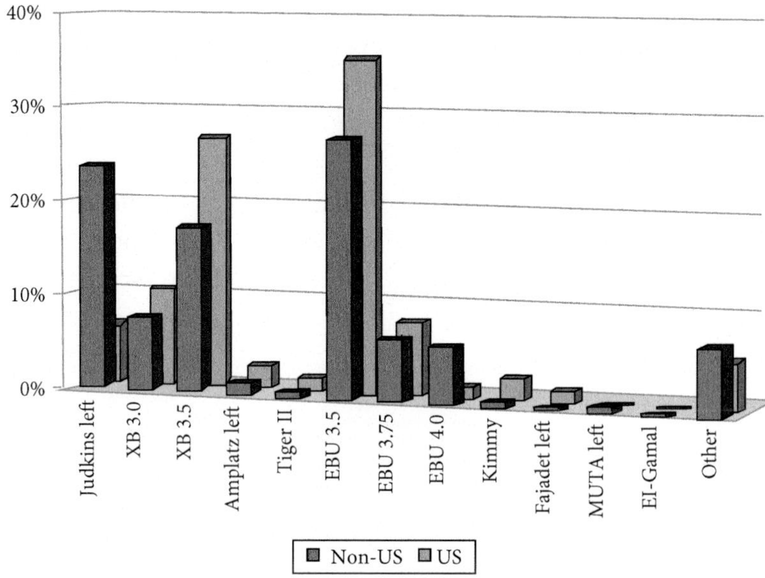

Figure 7.4 Guide catheters for left coronary interventions [adapted from Table 4 (Bertrand et al., 2010)].[7]

Guide Catheters for Left Coronary Artery

An extra-backup catheter (XB or EBU) is most commonly used by operators for PCI of the LCA (Figure 7.4). The catheter curve size used for TRI is usually 0.5F smaller than curve size used in transfemoral PCI. The extra-backup, Amplatz, and Judkins left catheter derives its support from contralateral aortic wall [Figures 7.5a and 7.6a(i)]. The Amplatz left catheter (AL1 or AL2) provides greater passive support [Figures 7.5b and 7.6a(ii)] and is preferred in chronic total occlusion (CTO), calcified lesions, and for PCI of LCX in patients with wide left main, or dilated aorta. In the latter situation, an AL2 GC may be preferred as illustrated in the case in Figure 10.9g (i–ix) in Chapter 10. The Judkins left catheter [Figures 7.5c and 7.6b(ii)] is less often preferred because it does not provide good backup support for PCI but is preferred by the authors in ostial left main stenosis or in patients with short left main and ostial disease in

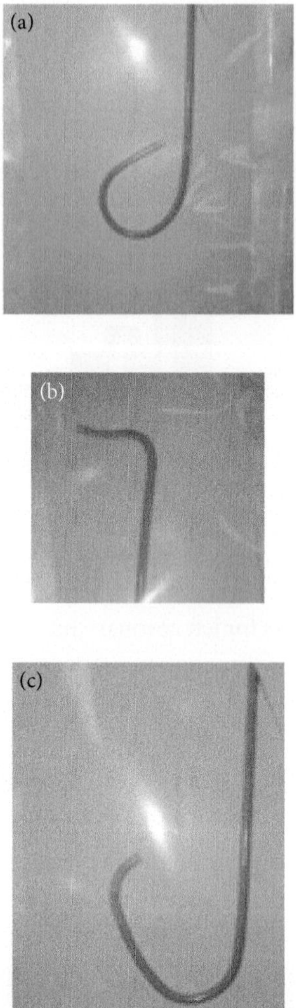

Figure 7.5 Guide catheters for left coronary artery (LCA): (a) extra-backup (XB/EBU); (b) shows Amplatz (AL) catheter; (c) shows Judkins left (JL) catheter.

LAD where it is safer (*please see Chapter 10*). A bigger curve of JL, such as a JL3.5, is sometimes preferred to enhance GC support from contralateral aortic wall for a CTO of LAD, as illustrated in Figure 10.18 (a–j) in Chapter 10.

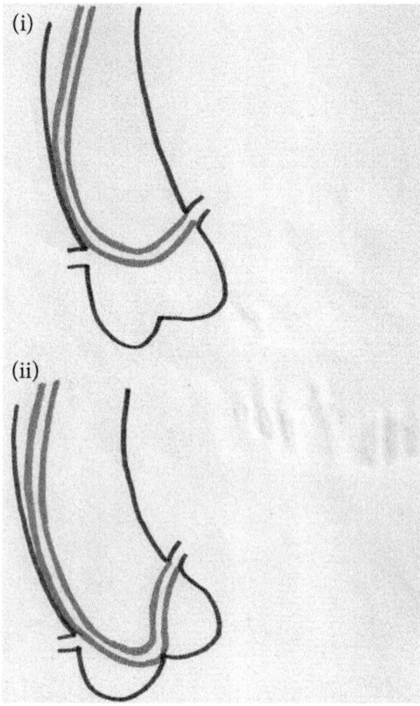

Figure 7.6a(i) XB/EBU guiding catheter engages the left coronary artery with support from contralateral aortic wall (*Sketch By: Dr Ravi Gupta*). **(ii)** Amplatz (AL) guiding catheter engages the left coronary artery with support from contralateral aortic wall and aortic valve (*Sketch By: Dr Ravi Gupta*).

Guide Catheters for Right Coronary Interventions

For most lesions in the RCA, including Shepherd's crook or tortuous right coronary; and ostial stenosis, the Judkins right catheter can be used successfully with GC manipulation for active guide support where required. For CTO of RCA or in a calcific, tortuous RCA, and in patients with dilated aorta, an Amplatz curve is preferred because of enhanced support from contralateral aortic wall with these shapes.

Figure 7.6c(i)–(iv) shows:

- The Judkins right (JR) is firmly fixed when ascending aorta is vertical [Figure 7.6c(i)].

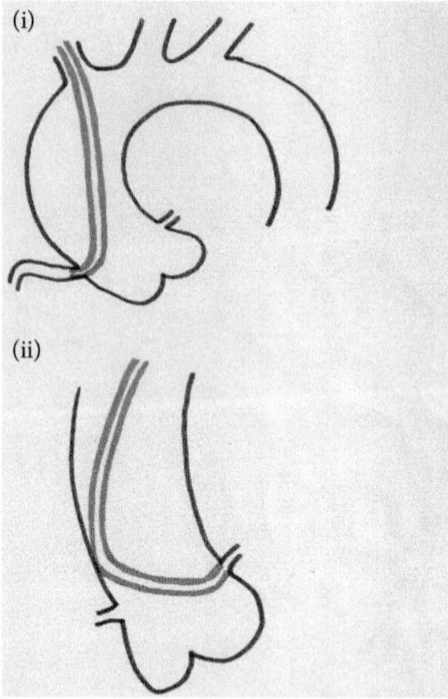

Figure 7.6b(i) Judkins right catheter engaging the right coronary artery. The Judkins right catheter is not firmly fixed when ascending aorta is horizontal (*Sketch By: Dr Ravi Gupta*). **(ii)** Judkins left (JL) catheter engaging the left coronary artery. Support from opposite aortic wall may be available with a bigger JL curve as in this illustration (*Sketch By: Dr Ravi Gupta*).

- The JR is not firmly fixed when ascending aorta is horizontal [Figure 7.6c(ii), 7.6b(i)]; in such situations for the Shepherd's crook, with up-going bend in proximal RCA, an Amplatz GC can be used if JR fails to engage the RCA. An angiography guidewire can be used inside the Amplatz catheter to get the catheter tip to point downwards. In this situation, alternatively, a JR 3.5 can be pushed-up gently while rotating it counter-clockwise (amplatzing of JR) so that the catheter sits on the coronary sinus and gets support from the opposite aortic wall, with the tip of the JR guide positioned just below the ostium of the RCA. In a Shepherd's crook, RCA, there are three options: (i) either a JR can

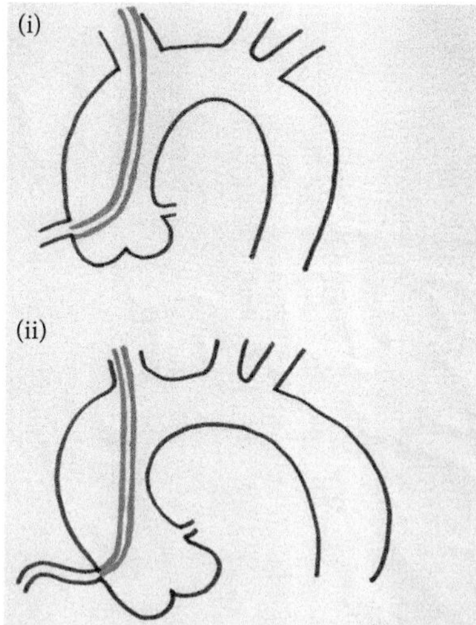

Figure 7.6c(i) Judkins right catheter is firmly fixed when ascending aorta is vertical (*Sketch By: Dr Ravi Gupta*). **(ii)** The Judkins right catheter is not firmly fixed when ascending aorta is horizontal (*Sketch By: Dr Ravi Gupta*).

be used with a soft wire such as balance middle weight, run through or Choice™ (*please see Figure 10.13(a–j), Chapter 10*) together with active manipulation for enhancing guide support; (ii) alternatively, the second option is to use an appropriate-sized Amplatz which provides passive backup support, combined with an extra-support wire for PCI. An XB right is also available for the Shepherd's crook RCA.

A TIG Optitorque diagnostic catheter from Terumo is usually successful in hooking the Shepherd's crook RCA in a horizontal aorta [Figure 7.6c (iii), Figure 7.6c (iv)].

Further, when RCA arises anteriorly or posteriorly or is anomalous, an Amplatz right [Figure 10.9d (i–xii)] Chapter 10) or left catheter is useful in engaging the RCA and provides better backup support. The latter are useful also for PCI in chronic total occlusions, calcific RCA, especially with tortuosity, as the passive support is better. Alternatively, a JR can be

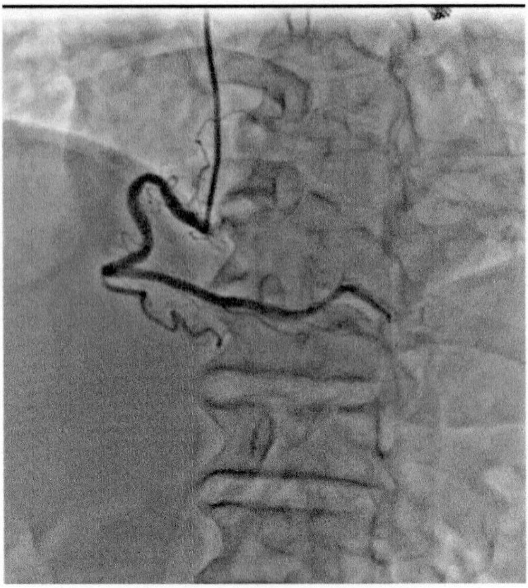

Figure 7.6c(iii) A TIG™ diagnostic catheter hooking the right coronary artery in a horizontal aorta with shepherd crook right coronary in left anterior oblique projection.

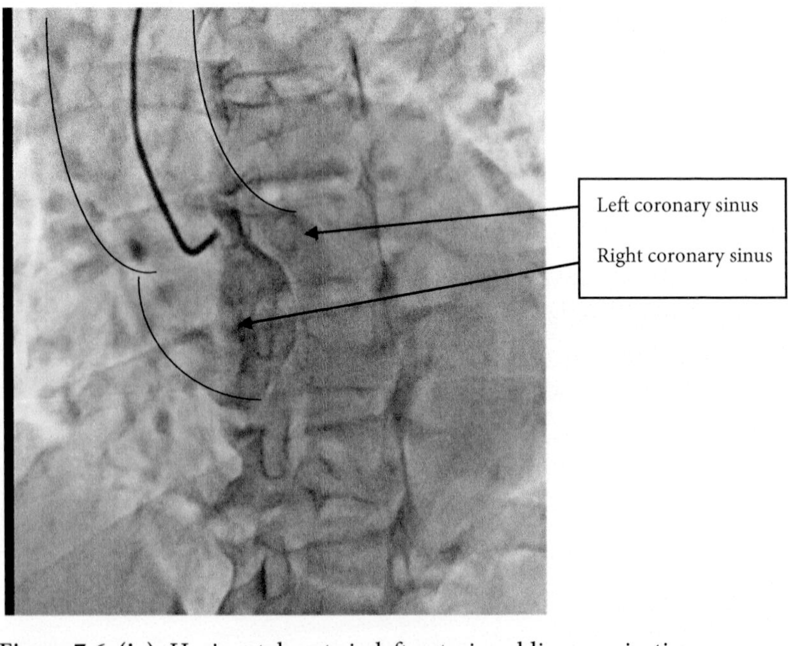

Figure 7.6c(iv) Horizontal aorta in left anterior oblique projection.

used in this situation, with active support by the operator's manipulations. An anomalous RCA from near or at left coronary sinus (LCS) can also be engaged using a TIG, multipurpose (with downward take-off) an Amplatz catheter or a JL catheter.

Special radial catheters such as Kimny, Barbeau, and Fajadet are available. The Barbeau's catheter is a modified multipurpose catheter with an additional 135° curve at the tip. The Kimny catheter can be used to cannulate both RCA and LCA and has a 45° primary curve with a secondary curve of 90°.

Engaging the Left Internal Mammary Artery Bypass Graft

Left internal mammary artery (LIMA) is best approached with left radial approach with a modified or non-modified mammary catheter (Figure 10.2e(i)–10.2e(iii), Chapter 10). The author (SKC) usually engages the LIMA in LAO view (Figures 7.7a and 7.7b). Cannulation of RIMA is usually attempted with right radial approach and is usually harder to achieve because ostium take off is at 90°.

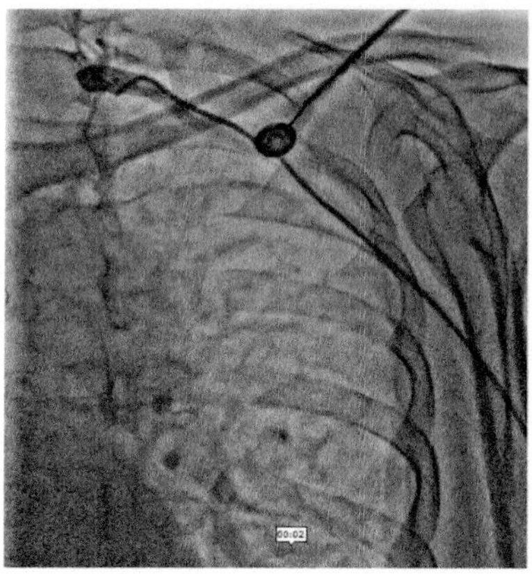

Figure 7.7a Left anterior oblique view: Non-selective contrast injection in left subclavian artery to detect origin of left internal mammary artery.

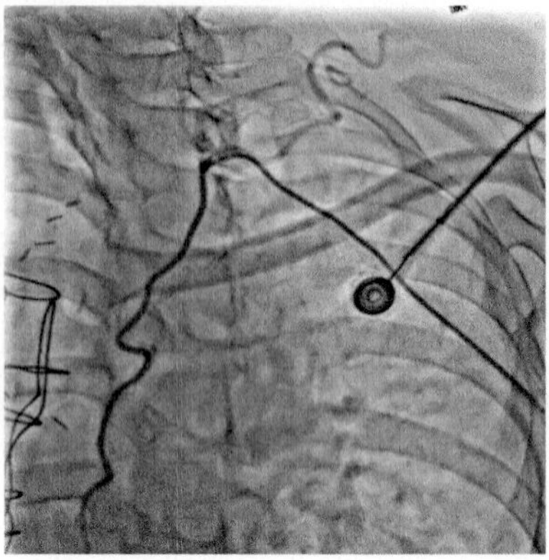

Figure 7.7b Left anterior oblique view showing a left internal mammary artery (LIMA) graft hooked by left internal mammary catheter in this view by clockwise rotation of catheter after visualizing the origin of LIMA in this view by non-selective injection into left subclavian artery, as shown in Figure 7.7a.

Chapter 10, Item 6b (viii), and Figures 10.8hy (i–xiii) illustrate the challenges and tips of hooking of coronaries and angioplasty in patients with horizontal aorta in which the anatomical position of the RCS and LCS shifts, with the LCS lying in a plane superior to the RCS. As a result, the ostium of RCA moves down to 6–7 o' clock and is often associated with an acute upward bend in RCA called Shepherd's crook. The ostium of LCA shifts up to a 12 o'clock position.

Conclusion

The majority of PCIs are performed using 6F GC, though 5F GCs remain particularly attractive because catheter-radial mismatch related to wider bore catheters increases risk of post-catheterization radial artery occlusion. Although some dedicated radial shapes have been developed, most radial operators use standard GCs commonly used for transfemoral angioplasty. It is recommended that operators should become facile with few catheters of their choice rather than try out new and fancy catheters.

Acknowledgement

We acknowledge with thanks, the help of Dr Ravi Gupta for the sketches of Figure 7.6.

References

1. Jolly SS, Cairns J, Niemela K, et al. Effect of radial versus femoral access on radiation dose and the importance of procedural volume: a substudy of the multicenter randomized RIVAL trial. *JACC: Cardiovascular Interventions*. 2013;6(3):258–66.
2. Romagnoli E, Biondi-Zoccai G, Sciahbasi A, et al. Radial versus femoral randomized investigation in ST-segment elevation acute coronary syndrome: the RIFLE-STEACS (Radial Versus Femoral Randomized Investigation in ST-Elevation Acute Coronary Syndrome) study. *Journal of the American College of Cardiology*. 2012;60(24):2481–89.
3. Bernat I, Horak D, Stasek J, et al. ST-segment elevation myocardial infarction treated by radial or femoral approach in a multicenter randomized clinical trial: the STEMI-RADIAL trial. *Journal of the American College of Cardiology*. 2014;63(10):964–72.
4. Valgimigli M, Gagnor A, Calabró P, et al. Radial versus femoral access in patients with acute coronary syndromes undergoing invasive management: a randomised multicentre trial. *The Lancet*. 2015;385(9986):2465–76.
5. András Komócsi, Dániel Aradi, Dániel Kehl, et al. Meta-analysis of randomized trials on access site selection for percutaneous coronary intervention in ST-segment elevation myocardial infarction. *Archives of Medical Science*. 2014;10(2):203–12.
6. Chugh SK, Panwar RB, Kasliwal RR, et al. Taming the tiger: a single center experience using a new catheter for transradial coronary angiography. *Catheterization and Cardiovascular Interventions*. 2006;67:788–838.
7. Bertrand OF, Rao SV, Pancholy S, et al. Transradial approach for coronary angiography and interventions: results of the first international transradial practice survey. *JACC: Cardiovascular Interventions*. 2010;3(10):1022–31.
8. Xanthopoulou I1, Stavrou K, Davlouros P, et al. Randomised comparison of JUDkins vs. tiGEr catheter in coronary angiography via the right radial artery: the JUDGE study. *EuroIntervention*. 2018;13(16):1950–58. doi: 10.4244/EIJ-D-17-00699.
9. Kumar Chugh S, Chugh S, Chugh Y, et al. Feasibility and utility of pre-procedural ultrasound imaging of the arm to facilitate transradial coronary diagnostic and interventional procedures (PRIMAFACIE-TRI). *Catheterization and Cardiovascular Interventions*. 2013;82:64–73.
10. Yoo B-S, Yoon J, Ko J-Y, et al. Anatomical consideration of the radial artery for transradial coronary procedures: arterial diameter, branching anomaly and vessel tortuosity. *International Journal of Cardiology*. 2005;101(3):421–27.
11. Peruga JP, Peruga JZ, Kasprzak JD, et al. Ultrasound evaluation of forearm arteries in patients undergoing percutaneous coronary intervention via radial artery access: results of one-year follow-up. *Kardiologia Polska*. 2015;73(7):502–10.
12. Velasco A, Ono C, Nugent K, et al. Ultrasonic evaluation of the radial artery diameter in a local population from Texas. *Journal of Invasive Cardiology*. 2012;24(7):339–41.
13. Prashant PU. *Research Reports in Clinical Cardiology*. 2014;5:213–26.
14. Efficacy and safety of the GuideLiner mother-in-child guide catheter extension in percutaneous coronary intervention.
15. Sharma D, Shah A, Osten M, et al. Efficacy and safety of the GuideLiner mother-in-child guide catheter extension in percutaneous coronary intervention. *Journal of Interventional Cardiology* 2017;30:46–55.

8
Technique of Engaging the Coronaries Using Transradial Access

Mirvat Alasnag and Waqar Ahmed

Introduction

In 1989, Lucien Campeau from the Montreal Heart Institute introduced radial artery approach for coronary angiography as a safer alternative to the brachial artery access.[1] He published a series of 100 patients, with failure in 12 patients. Diagnostic angiography was quickly followed by coronary intervention that further demonstrated the benefits of the radial approach.[2] Now the radial access is the default for coronary angiography and intervention in the majority of centres in the UK, Europe, and Asia.[3,4]

Radial Artery Access for Diagnostic Angiography

Diagnostic angiography is performed either via the right or the left radial artery. The operator's choice is to use either the standard Judkins right (JR) catheter and Judkins left (JL) catheter (Cordis Cardinal Health) or special-purpose catheters built for the radial approach. Most operators use 5F or 4F diameter catheters for diagnostic angiography.

Standard Judkins Catheters for the Diagnostic Angiography

For the left coronary artery, a JL3.5 catheter is usually preferred and a JR4 can engage the right coronary artery in almost all cases. Engaging the left coronary artery is challenging in the early learning phase. Using the femoral approach, the JL-shaped catheters engage the left coronary ostium. Via the radial approach, the operators have to learn to engage the artery from below the left coronary ostium. The JL catheter is placed in the aortic cusp over a 0.035-inch guidewire. The catheter will usually be in the non-coronary cusp. The guidewire is then withdrawn back slightly with a gentle clockwise torque. This will allow the catheter to clear the aortic valve leaflets and turn into the left coronary cusp. Subsequent further pulling up of the catheter with a continuous torque will allow the catheter to engage the left coronary ostium. If the JL3.5 catheter is unable to engage the ostium, then a JL4 for larger aortic roots, or a JL3.0 for smaller aortic roots is recommended. A Judkins Curve Left catheter can be used for a superior take off of the left coronary artery. An Amplatz 1.0 shaped catheter will engage most left coronary ostia. In larger aortic roots or unusual take-off of the left main coronary artery, an Amplatz 2.0 or guide catheters may be needed. In such cases, the XB 3 or XB 3.5 from Cordis Corporation is very helpful. Louvard et al. used the Amplatz-shaped catheters to engage both the right and the left coronary arteries in a series of 1,000 patients.[5] This serves to minimize catheter exchanges.

For the right coronary artery, the standard JR catheter is usually adequate for the majority of cases. The selection of catheters for anomalous vessels is similar to the transfemoral approach. Those range from Multipurpose to Amplatz 1.0 or 0.75.

It is imperative that wire access is maintained during all catheter exchanges, and such exchanges are performed over a 260 cm J-shaped exchange length wire or a special 210 cm wire made for the radial access (InQwire®, Merit Medical). This will avoid radial artery spasm and loss of access. In case of tortuosity of the radial or the subclavian artery system, an extra support wire like the Amplatz Super Stiff™ Guidewire (Boston Scientific) may be used. Other operators have suggested use of a hydrophilic wire such as the Glidewire® (Terumo Corporation) to smoothly negotiate the tortuosities.

Specialized Catheters

To avoid numerous catheter exchanges and to overcome the limitations of the femoral catheters, many operators use single catheters to engage the right and the left coronary arteries. Many different manufacturers market these catheters. Examples of radial-specific catheters are the Jacky Radial Catheter (Terumo Corporation), the Tiger Radial TIG Catheter (Terumo Corporation), the Ultimate 1 and 2 (Merit Medical), and the Medtronic Corporation catheters. The Medtronic catheters are four differently shaped radial catheters under the brand DxTerity TRA. All of these catheters have their own unique advantages and limitations. Chen et al. published a study comparing use of standard catheters and radial specific catheters. The endpoints included fluoroscopy time, dose-area product, total contrast volume, and total procedure time. All these parameters were found to be lower in the single catheter group (although not all were statistically significant).[6] Another published study, JUDGE study, found that Tiger-II was superior to the Judkins JL 3.5 catheter in terms of contrast volume, procedural and fluoroscopy times, spasm rate, and imaging of the right coronary artery. It was inferior in terms of imaging the left anterior descending and circumflex arteries.[7] Given the wide range of catheters, each operator should select the catheter he/she has acquired experience and comfort with use (Figures 8.1 (A–D), 8.2, 8.3, 8.4(A,B), to 8.5).

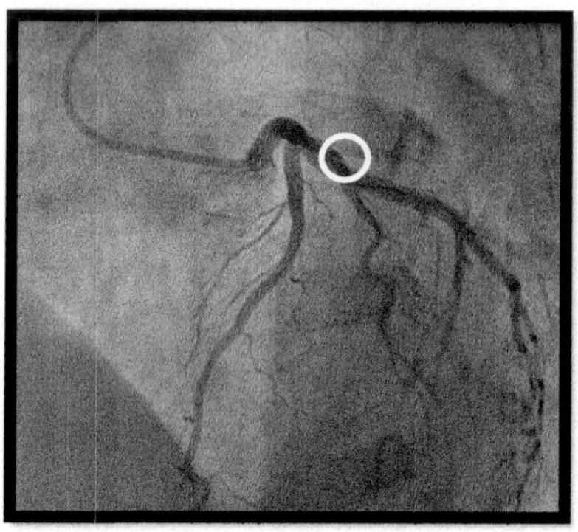

Figure 8.1A Co-axial engagement of the left main artery with a JL4 catheter (left anterior oblique cranial projection) (Figure obtained from King Fahd Armed Forces Hospital Catheterization Laboratory).

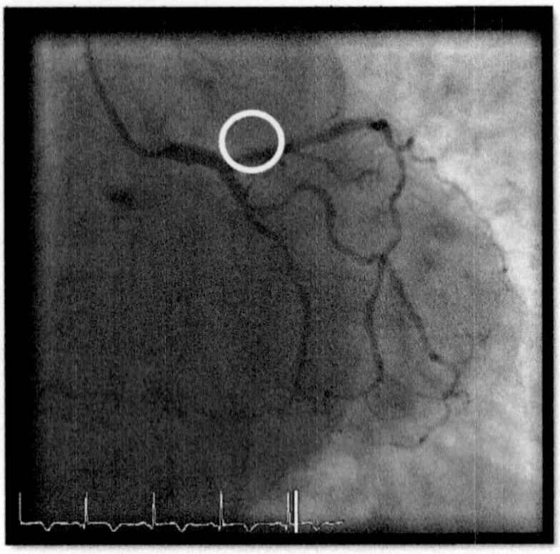

Figure 8.1B Co-axial engagement of the left main artery with a JL4 catheter (right anterior oblique caudal projection) (Figure obtained from King Fahd Armed Forces Hospital Catheterization Laboratory).

Right or Left Radial Access

When access is obtained from the right radial artery, the more to the left of the trachea, the catheter is advanced, the more likely it enters the right coronary cusp. The catheter is more likely to enter the non-coronary cusp if it is a straight descent from the ascending aorta. There are disadvantages to engage the left coronary artery from the right radial using a JL catheter. Often, a wire is retained in the catheter to straighten it. This means initial engagement is blind (no injection) and with no haemodynamic monitoring. Recently published data compared fluoroscopy time, radiation exposure, and contrast use in right versus left radial approach.[8] These studies suggested an advantage in left radial approach presumably attributed to the easier engagement of the coronary ostia using catheters that follow the natural curvature of the aorta and less tortuosity in the subclavian artery on the left side. However, the patient setup is of paramount importance in achieving a comfortable procedure for the operator in left radial cases.

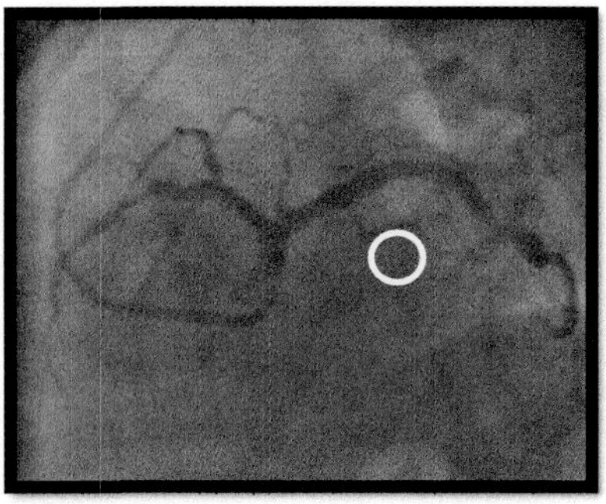

Figure 8.1C Co-axial engagement of the left main artery with a JL4 catheter (left anterior oblique caudal projection) (Figure obtained from King Fahd Armed Forces Hospital Catheterization Laboratory).

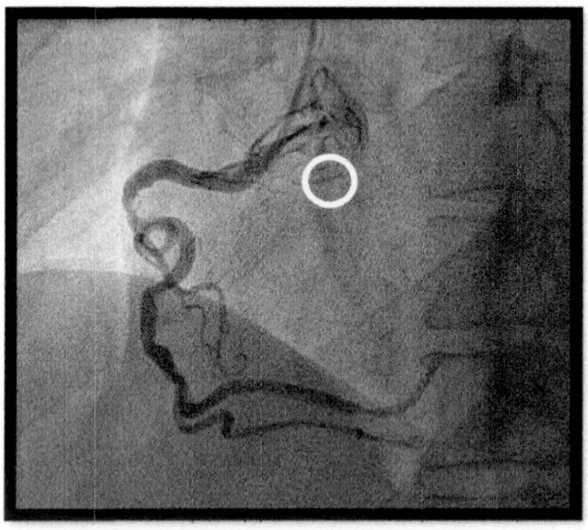

Figure 8.1D Co-axial engagement of the right coronary artery with a JR4 catheter (left anterior oblique projection) (Figure obtained from King Fahd Armed Forces Hospital Catheterization Laboratory).

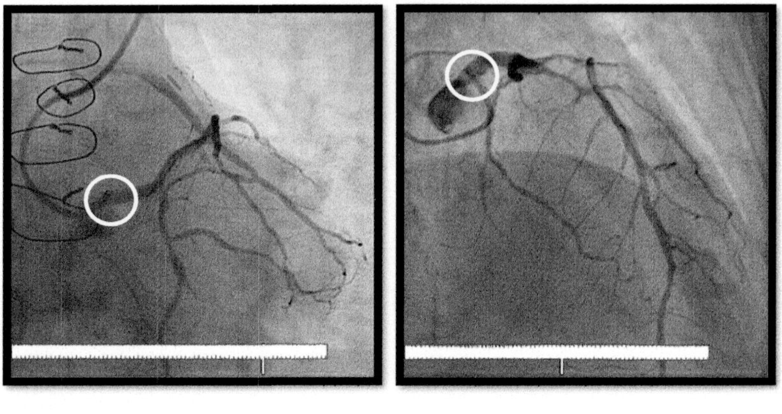

Figure 8.2 AJL4 catheter directed at the roof of the left main coronary artery (right anterior oblique caudal and cranial projections) (Figure obtained from King Fahd Armed Forces Hospital Catheterization Laboratory).

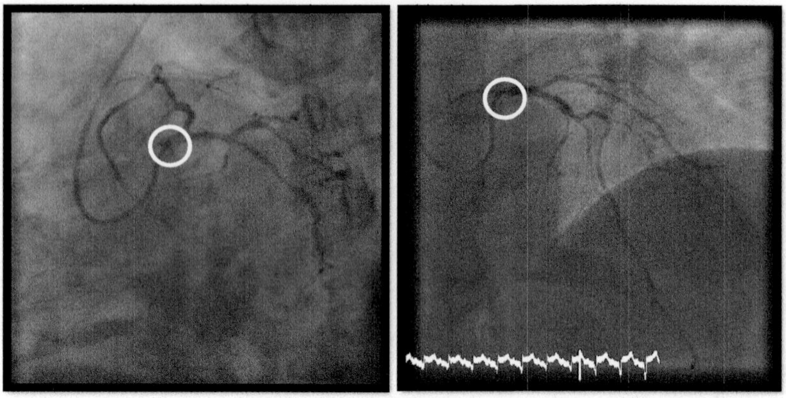

Figure 8.3 AL1 and AL2 catheters engaging the left main coronary artery (left anterior oblique caudal and right anterior oblique cranial projections) (Figure obtained from King Fahd Armed Forces Hospital Catheterization Laboratory).

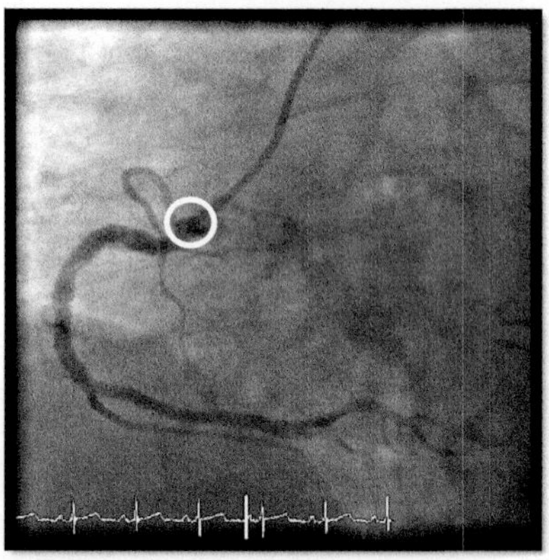

Figure 8.4A MP1 catheter engaging the right coronary artery (left anterior oblique projection) (Figure obtained from King Fahd Armed Forces Hospital Catheterization Laboratory).

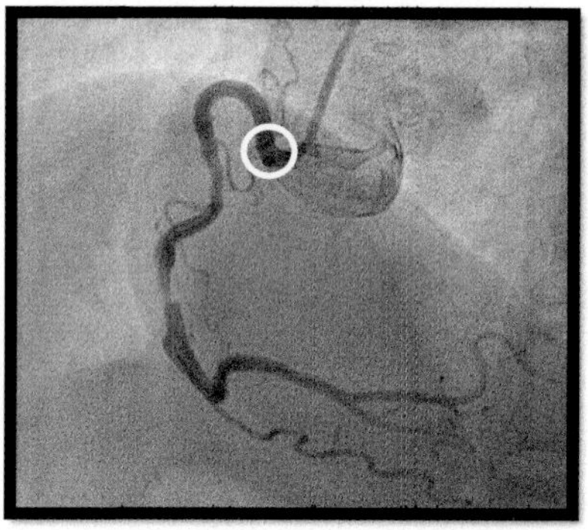

Figure 8.4B Shepherd's hook right coronary artery engaged with a JR4 catheter (left anterior oblique projection) (Figure obtained from King Fahd Armed Forces Hospital Catheterization Laboratory).

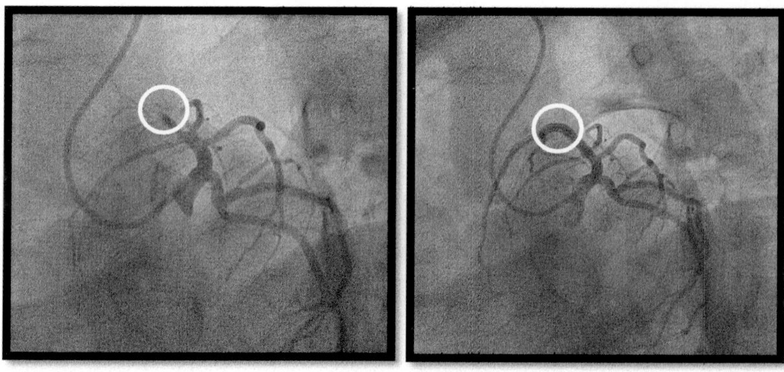

Figure 8.5 In an ST elevation MI direct engagement of the left main artery with an EBU guide catheter (pre and post intervention) (Figure obtained from King Fahd Armed Forces Hospital Catheterization Laboratory).

Selective Graft Angiography

With the development of cardiac computerized tomography (CCT), most grafts are evaluated non-invasively with CCT. For invasive evaluation, very few reports and studies evaluated the radial and femoral approaches for selective graft angiography. In the RADIAL-CABG (RADIAL Versus Femoral Access for Coronary Artery Bypass Graft Angiography), Michael et al. randomized 128 patients undergoing angiography for graft evaluation to transradial and transfemoral access. The authors concluded that there was greater radiation exposure, higher volume of contrast use, longer procedure time, and greater crossover in the transradial arm.[9] This publication was in 2013. Over the course of the past five years, no large randomized trials have examined transradial access for graft evaluation. Non-selective imaging with a pigtail and a power injector in the ascending thoracic aorta has been used previously. For selective angiography, many operators select the femoral access in order to facilitate access into the left subclavian artery and subsequently the left internal mammary artery (LIMA). Catheter selection is mostly based on operator preference and comfort. However, anatomy often dictates the choice. When using a transradial access, a universal catheter such as the Jacky, Tiger, or Ultimate catheter can be used. The advantage of a universal catheter is a single passage through the radial artery thereby potentially less time and spasm occurs during any exchange. The disadvantages of using these catheters include cost, learning curve, and more manipulation in the ascending aorta. The standard Judkins catheters are cheaper, available, and familiar to most operators. The disadvantage is more passes through the radial artery which may induce spasm and a longer procedure time. A left radial approach simplifies selective engagement of the LIMA graft and other saphenous vein grafts. Most operators, however, use the right radial artery as their default access. In such cases, often the modified mammary catheter (with a steep angle at the distal tip) is advanced into the descending thoracic aorta and then pulled back with a clockwise movement to the distal aortic arch until it reaches the ostium of the left subclavian artery. At this point, a hydrophilic 0.035 inch wire is advanced beyond the shoulder into the brachial artery for support. The catheter is then railed gently into the subclavian artery and pulled back until the LIMA is engaged. Occasionally, additional support is required and the elbow is flexed or a BP cuff is inflated to stabilize the wire and allow advancement of the catheter.[10] Regarding the catheter of choice, many resort to catheters with a long tip such as the VTK (Cook Medical, SIM1/SIM2 (Simmons catheter, Terumo Corporation), or the Bartorelli-Cozzi catheter (Modified IM catheter, Cordis Cardinal Health). Concern over long procedure time, excessive contrast use and manipulation in the arch have deterred most operators from using right radial artery for LIMA engagement (Figures 8.6(A,B) and 8.7(A,B)).

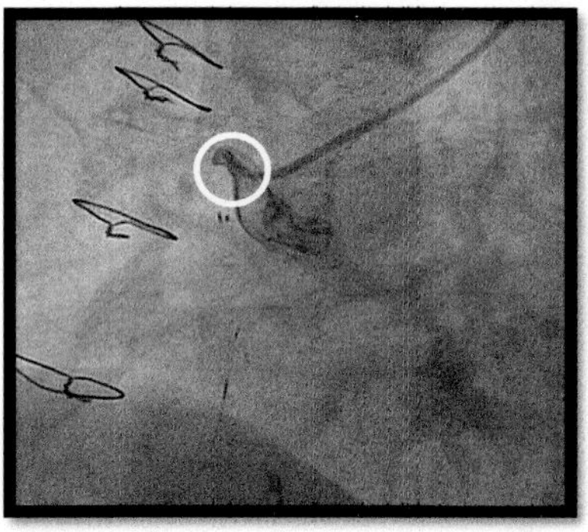

Figure 8.6A A JR4 catheter used to selectively engage a saphenous vein graft stump (left radial access) (Figure obtained from King Fahd Armed Forces Hospital Catheterization Laboratory).

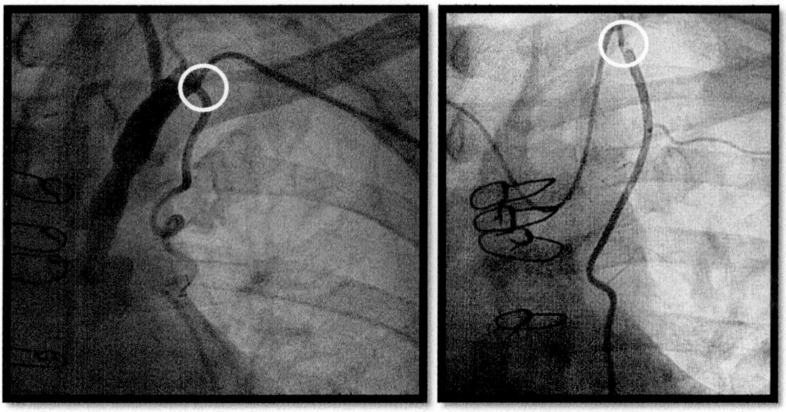

Figure 8.6B A LIMA catheter used to selectively engage a left internal mammary graft (via left and right radial access) (Figure obtained from King Fahd Armed Forces Hospital Catheterization Laboratory).

Conclusion

Selective engagement of the coronary arteries is necessary for an angiogram to be informative. If the catheters are not selectively engaged, inadequate imaging with streaming can occur. If the catheters are not coaxial, complications such as dissection can occur. Regarding interventions,

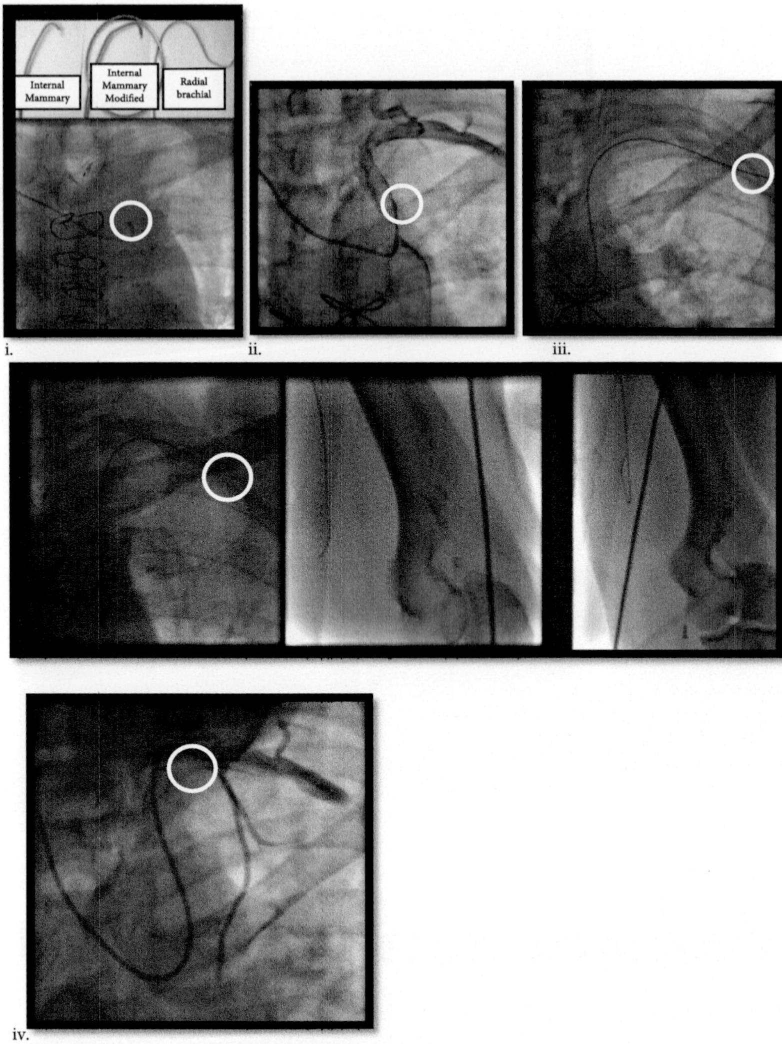

Figure 8.7A Catheters advanced from right radial access to left internal mammary artery. (Images courtesy of Patel T, et al. CCI 2012;80:316-20).

i. Advance the catheter to the distal aortic arch and pull back to the origin of the Le Subclavian Artery
ii. Inject contrast to identify the ostium of the Le Subclavian Artery
iii. Advance a hydrophilic wire into the Le Brachial Artery
iv. Advance the catheter over the wire and selectively engage the Le Internal Mammary Artery

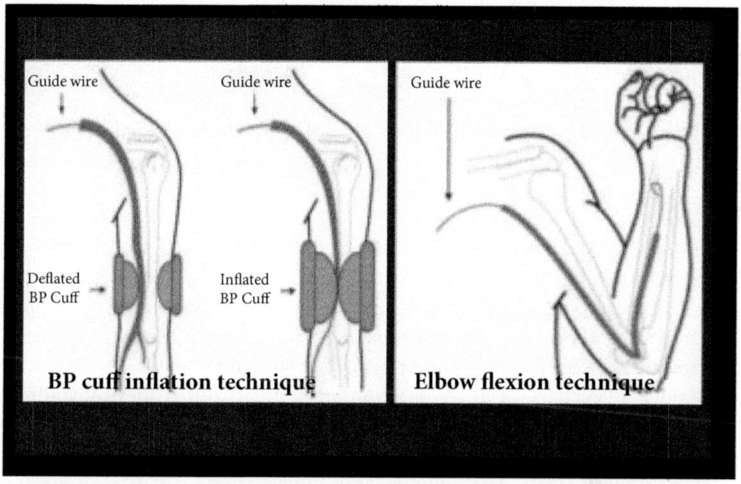

Figure 8.7B BP cuff inflation or elbow flexion techniques used to fix the wire and improve support for catheter advancement from right radial access to left internal mammary artery. (as described by Patel T, et al. CCI 2012;80:316-20).

support from the catheter of choice is mandatory. The catheter must be of appropriate shape and diameter for the planned procedure. Careful coaxial engagement is necessary for both diagnostic angiograms and interventions.

References

1. Campeau L. Percutaneous radial artery approach for coronary angiography. *Catheterization and Cardiovascular Diagnosis*.1989;16:3–7.
2. Kiemeneij F, Laarman GJ, Melker E. Transradial coronary angioplasty. *American Heart Journal*. 1995;129:1–7.
3. Bertrand OF, Rao SV, Pancholy S, Jolly SS, Rodés-Cabau L, Larose E, Costerousse O, Hamon M, Mann T. Transradial approach for coronary angiography and interventions: results of the first international transradial practice survey. *JACC: Cardiovascular Interventions*. 2010;3:1022–1031.
4. Rao SV, Ou F-S, Wang TY, Roe MT, Brindis R, Rumsfeld JR, Peterson ED. Trends in the prevalence and outcomes of radial and femoral approaches to percutaneous coronary intervention: a report from the National Cardiovascular Data Registry. *JACC: Cardiovascular Interventions*. 2008;1:379–386.

5. Louvard Y, Krol M, Pezzano M, Sheers L, Piechaud JF, Marien C, Benaim R, Lardoux H, Morice MC. Feasibility of routine transradial coronary angiography: a single operator's experience. *The Journal of Invasive Cardiology*. 1999;11:543–548.
6. Chen O, et al. Comparison of standard catheters versus radial artery specific catheter in patients who underwent coronary angiography through transradial access. *The American Journal of Cardiology*. 2016;118:357–361.
7. Xanthopoulou I, et al. Randomised comparison of JUDkins Vx tiGEr catheter in coronary angiography via the right radial artery: the JUDGE study. *EuroIntervention*. 2018.
8. Qiang F, et al. Randomized comparative study of left versus right radial approach in the setting of primary percutaneous interventions for ST-elevation myocardial infarction. *Clinical Interventions in Aging*. 2015;10:1003–1008.
9. Tesfaldet T Michael, et al. A randomized comparison of the transradial and transfemoral approaches for coronary artery bypass graft angiography and intervention: the RADIAL-CABG trial (RADIAL Versus Femoral Access for Coronary Artery Bypass Graft Angiography and Intervention). *JACC: Cardiovascular Interventions*, 2013;6(11).
10. Patel T, et al. Cannulating LIMA graft using right transradial approach: two simple and innovative techniques. *CCI* 2012;80:316–320.

9

Challenging Anatomical Variation in Radial Angiography and Angioplasty

Sudhakar George, Karim Ratib, and James Nolan

Introduction

The femoral artery has historically been the default access site for coronary angiography and interventions in many institutions across the world, although in recent years the number of procedures carried out via the radial route has increased, particularly in Europe. The first series of radial access for coronary angiography was reported by Campeau in 1989[1] and for coronary angioplasty by Kiemeneij and Laarman in 1993.[2] There are clear advantages of radial access with good-quality data demonstrating marked reductions in access site complications and bleeding. Improvement in time to ambulation has reduced costs and improved patient comfort with more patients favouring radial access. Importantly, in the subgroup of patients with acute coronary syndromes, radial access is associated with a reduction in mortality when compared to femoral procedures.[3,4] Despite the documented advantages of using radial access, the rate of uptake in some parts of the world, notably the USA, remains relatively low. Although there are several reasons for this, one important factor is the perceived long learning curve associated with transitioning to a radial approach. In this chapter, the authors describe the most frequent anatomical challenges encountered when using radial access and techniques that may be used to overcome them.

Radial Artery—The Challenges

Radial procedures can initially be more challenging due to the smaller calibre of the radial artery, its susceptibility to spasm and due to variations in anatomy en route to the coronary arteries. An angiogram of the forearm arterial tree taken following insertion of the radial sheath can be helpful in delineating the radial anatomy and highlighting potential difficulties. This is best done with a radiographic acquisition (using a stored fluoroscopy run to minimize radiation exposure) in the anteroposterior position with the arm fully externally rotated gaining maximum separation between the radius and the ulnar arteries (which helps separate out the overlying arteries). It is advised to image from the mid-radius up to the radiobrachial anastomosis, which is usually just distal to the elbow joint. Preferably vasodilators should be given first before a 50/50 mixture of contrast agent and blood (to minimize patient discomfort) is used for the angiographic acquisition.

Normal Radial Anatomy

The radial artery arises from the bifurcation of the brachial artery at the cubital fossa where it separates into the radial and ulnar arteries (Figure 9.1). The radial artery then passes down from the medial aspect of the neck of the radius to the styloid process of the anterior surface of the radius. Proximally the artery is located under the brachioradialis muscle but distally is only covered by fascia and skin and is easily compressible over the radius allowing for simple access and compression. Distal to the wrist, the branches of the radial and ulnar arteries join to form an extensive collateral network of vessels supplying the hand.

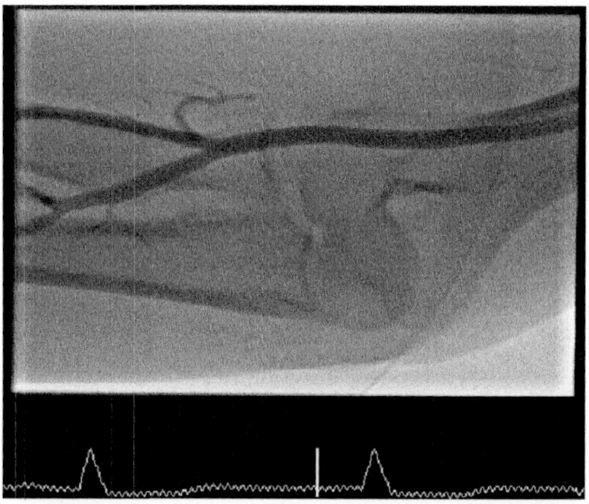

Figure 9.1 Normal radial anatomy.

Anatomical Variations of the Radial Artery

High Bifurcations

Variations in radial artery anatomy are not uncommon and have been well documented. Lo et al. analysed radial artery anatomy by angiography in a series of 1,540 consecutive patients undergoing coronary angiography or angioplasty.[5] Anatomical variations were present in 13.8% of patients. The most frequent anatomical variation was a high-bifurcating radial origin, found in 7% of their patients. Autopsy studies suggest this variation may be present in up to 14% of the population.[6] The intercondylar line of the humerus represents the proximal border of the antecubital fossa and bifurcation of the brachial artery proximal to this line is considered a 'high bifurcation'. Although high-bifurcating origins are not associated with a significantly higher rate of procedural failure, they are associated with a smaller calibre radial artery which can lead to more frequent radial spasm.[5] If difficulty is encountered, this can be overcome with use of intra-arterial vasodilators, balloon-assisted tracking (BAT), and the use of smaller calibre or hydrophilic coated diagnostic and guiding catheters. Figures 9.2 and 9.3 show a high radial bifurcation.

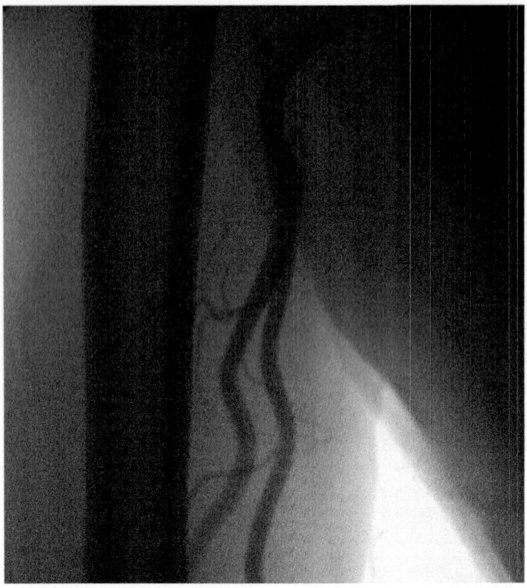

Figure 9.2 High radial artery bifurcation at level of humerus.

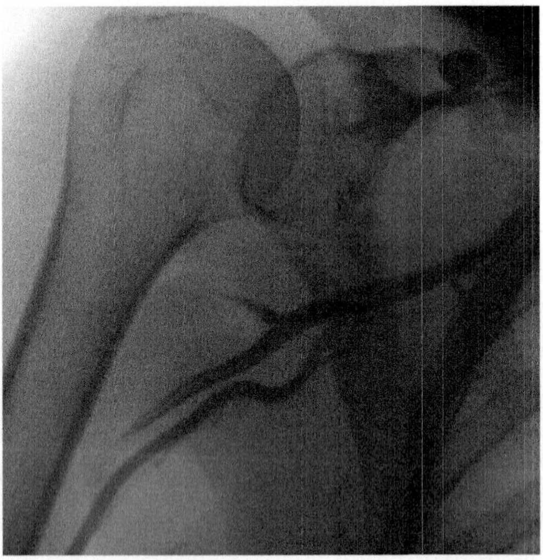

Figure 9.3 Very high radial artery bifurcation at level of axilla.

Radial Artery Tortuosity

Radial artery tortuosity can be defined as any bend but significant tortuosity usually describes a bend of greater than 90° in the vessel (Figure 9.4). The presence of significant tortuosity is associated with old age but is also more common in females and those with hypertension.[5,7] It commonly manifests as resistance to guidewire or catheter advancement. If resistance is encountered, it is imperative that an angiogram of the radial artery is taken to identify the problem. If resistance is met to passing, a standard 0.038" guidewire switching to a hydrophilic 0.032" or 0.025" guidewire will often allow passage by reducing the friction within the artery. A hydrophilic wire with a tight J-shaped tip is preferred to minimize the risk of arterial perforation when using a hydrophilic wire with little tactile feedback. An alternative option is using a standard 0.014" coronary angioplasty wire which may be simpler to torque and steer through complicated anatomy. When using smaller calibre wires, it is advised to use BAT to minimize the 'razor' effect of passing a catheter over the wire which can promote spasm.

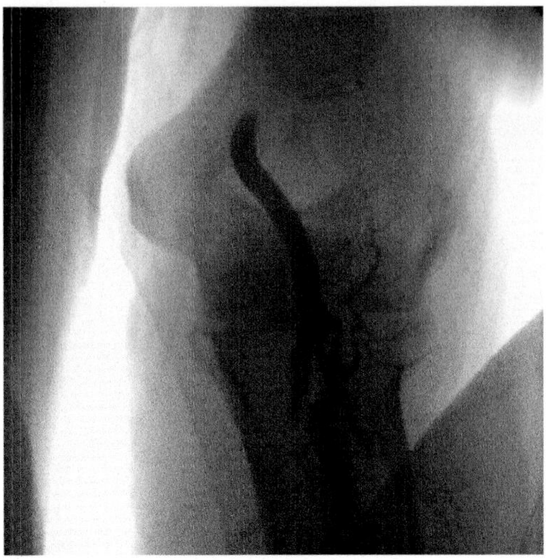

Figure 9.4 Radial artery tortuosity.

Radial Artery Loops

A radial artery loop describes a full 360° loop of the radial artery distal to the bifurcation of the brachial artery (Figure 9.5). Radial artery loops were encountered in 2.3% of the study described by Lo, and their presence was associated with a high risk of procedural failure.[5] Indeed, other groups have shown that the presence of radial loops can lead to a switch in access sites even by very experienced radial operators because of increased risk of extravasation associated with the negotiation of complex loops.[8] Again, if resistance is encountered when advancing a guidewire or catheter, a radial angiogram should be taken. Loops are difficult to navigate, and a 0.014" angioplasty wire with an appropriately shaped tip affords the best chance of success (Figure 9.6). Small loops can be straightened by using just the guidewire or after crossing with the catheter, again BAT can be helpful in negotiating a loop. Once crossed, if the loop remains, manoeuvres can be used to straighten the loop, by pulling back and torquing the wire/catheter. Straightening of loops is frequently uncomfortable for the patient and therefore it is advised to give adequate prior analgesia. Clearly any future catheter exchanges should then be carried out using an exchange length (>270 cm) guidewire. Large-diameter radial loops most frequently lead to procedural failure. The presence of a recurrent radial artery, which is frequently seen at

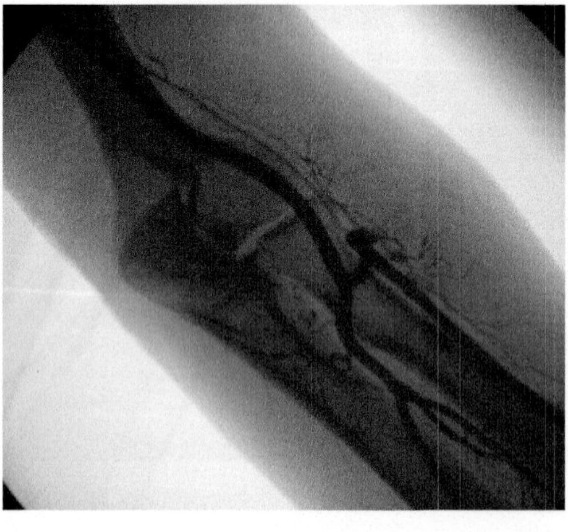

Figure 9.5 Loop in the left radial artery with aberrant radial artery from the apex of the loop.

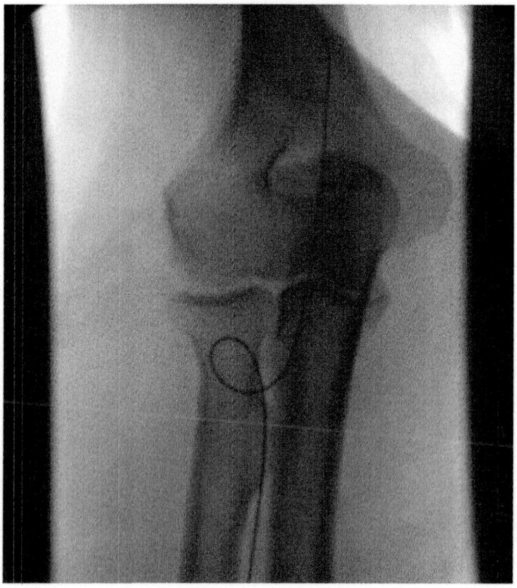

Figure 9.6 Using a wire to navigate around radial loop.

the apex of a radial loop, can be the site of perforation when wires and catheters are passed blindly up the artery through a loop and into one of these small calibre vessels.

Pre-procedural Ultrasound

Radial artery size, presence of high bifurcations, radial artery tortuosity, and radial artery loops can all be identified with the use of ultrasound scanning prior to the procedure. Some operators advocate this routinely to allow problems to be identified prior to puncture of the artery. Chugh et al. showed that pre-procedural ultrasound scanning of the arm arteries is feasible and adds just over 6 min to the total procedural time.[9] Ultrasound scanning should be performed in both upper limbs to identify the radial artery from the styloid process to the brachial artery. It is important to scan both radial arteries as radial abnormalities such as loops are often bilateral. Longitudinal views can be used to measure arterial diameter at different points along the arm. Predictably, radial artery size has been shown to have a clear association with rate of success of radial procedures[7] with small diameter of artery being associated with procedural failure.[10] Colour Doppler imaging is helpful to visualize flow and to identify the brachial artery and its bifurcation. Clearly, Doppler imaging would also identify an occluded radial artery (for example, following a previous radial artery procedure).

Radial Artery Spasm

Radial artery spasm (RAS) is frequently encountered in the presence of abnormal radial anatomy. A degree of RAS is found in around 15% of radial artery procedures[11,12] and causes patient discomfort as well as reducing the chance of procedural success. The severity of RAS can be graded on a scale developed by Chugh et al. from mild pain and spasm (grade 1) to severe pain and spasm which does not allow any catheter manipulation (grade 4).[9] Radial operators early in their learning curves may be more likely to cause RAS due to multiple attempts at puncturing the radial artery and with excessive manipulation or exchange of catheters. The first sign of RAS is often a patient complaint of pain in the forearm which should then lead to administration of adequate analgesia and vasodilators. Additionally, a forearm angiogram should be performed to delineate any abnormal anatomy and to identify any arterial perforation. A recent meta-analysis by Kwok confirmed that intra-arterial verapamil, nitroglycerine, and isosorbide mononitrate are all successful at reducing RAS.[13] The authors advocate giving one of these drugs routinely in all patients undergoing radial artery procedures, but they should certainly be administered if RAS is encountered. The patient should also be treated with an opioid-based analgesic and sedation to help control symptoms from the RAS. A repeat radial angiogram (using a small amount of contrast only) can confirm relief of the spasm. A 0.025" hydrophilic wire or 0.014" angioplasty wire can then be used to cross the affected area which will then allow for BAT of the desired catheter. Alternatively, downsizing the diagnostic or guiding catheter can allow successful completion of the procedure. Figure 9.7 shows RAS at the level of the elbow which has been relieved with intra-arterial nitroglycerine (Figure 9.8).

Balloon-Assisted Tracking

BAT is a very useful technique for negotiating a variety of difficulties including small calibre radial arteries, tortuosity (rarely needed for this), loops, and spasms.[14] The technique involves first advancing a 0.014" angioplasty wire into the aortic root. A compliant monorail balloon (for

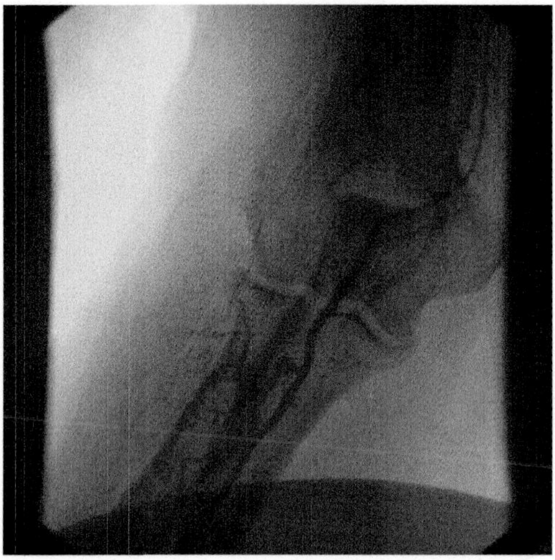

Figure 9.7 Radial artery spasm.

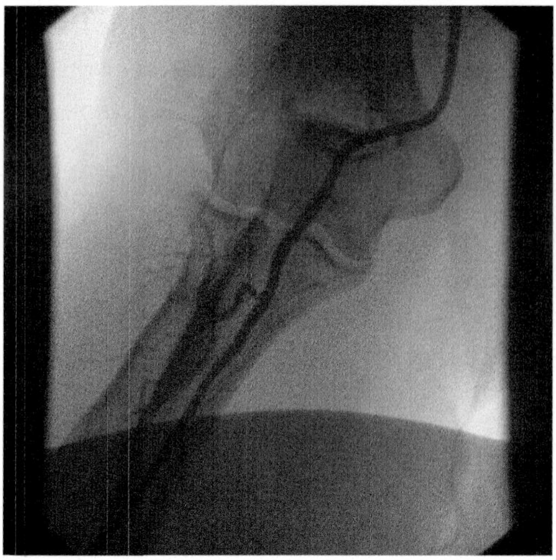

Figure 9.8 Same radial artery following intra-arterial nitrate injection.

example, 2 mm by 15 mm) is then loaded into the diagnostic or guiding catheter and advanced until the distal half protrudes from the distal end of the catheter. The balloon is then inflated to around 4–6 atmospheres. This creates a tapered, relatively soft leading edge to advance both balloon

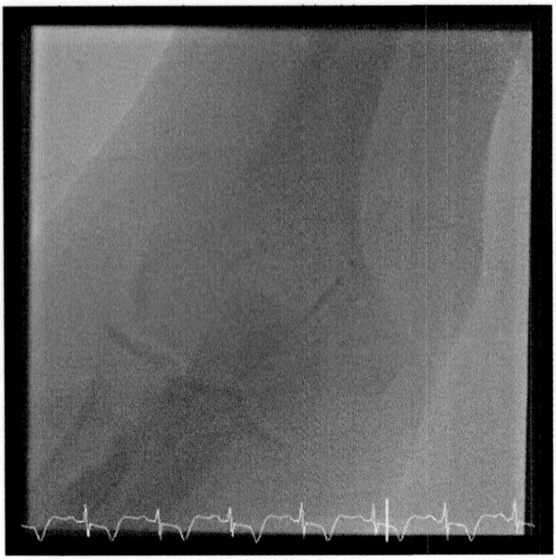

Figure 9.9 Balloon-assisted tracking of a guiding catheter through the radial artery.

and catheter over the angioplasty wire and across the area of difficulty. BAT should be carried out with care, and if any resistance is met while using the technique, caution should be advised to minimize the risk of perforation (Figure 9.9).

Radial Perforation

Radial perforation is a rare complication that is described in less than 0.5% of patients undergoing radial artery procedures.[15] The risk of radial perforation is increased by the presence of extreme radial tortuosity, loops, and spasm. Radial artery perforations can be caused by radial sheaths, guidewires, diagnostic or guiding catheters. It can also occur when exchanging from a diagnostic catheter to a larger calibre guiding catheter.

Radial artery perforation does not require the procedure to be abandoned via the radial route. Figure 9.10 demonstrates a radial artery perforation with extravasation of contrast into the tissue. BAT can be used to cross the perforation with a catheter and to perform the planned procedure. Figure 9.11 shows BAT being used to cross a radial perforation. The catheter acts to tamponade the radial perforation

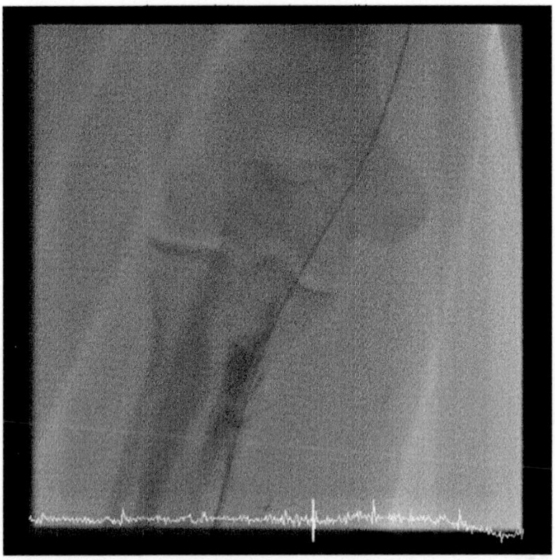

Figure 9.10 Radial artery perforation.

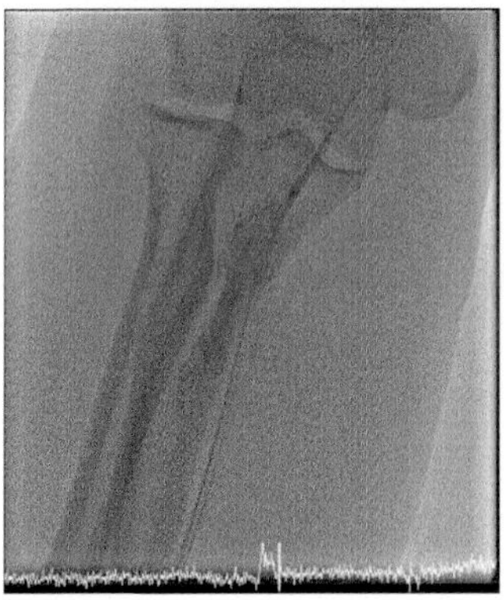

Figure 9.11 BAT allowing guiding catheter to be advanced through the area of radial perforation.

during the procedure and reduces the risk of forearm haematoma or compartment syndrome. A repeat radial angiogram at the end of the case will confirm whether active extravasation has ceased. Figure 9.12 shows that in this case, catheter tamponade has been successful at sealing the perforation.

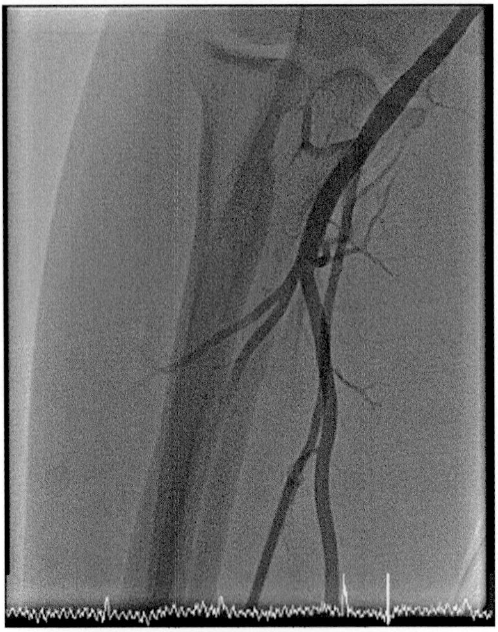

Figure 9.12 Radial angiogram after procedure completed following BAT confirming that the perforation has been sealed.

Vascular Anatomy of the Upper Arm and Shoulder

Once the guidewire has been successfully advanced through the radial artery, the operator then has to contend with the anatomical variations present in the upper arm and shoulder. The following topics will discuss the normal anatomy in this region followed by some of the common variations that can make coronary artery cannulation challenging.

Normal Anatomy of Upper Arm and Shoulder

The aortic arch gives off the innominate artery on the right which bifurcates into the right subclavian artery and the right common carotid

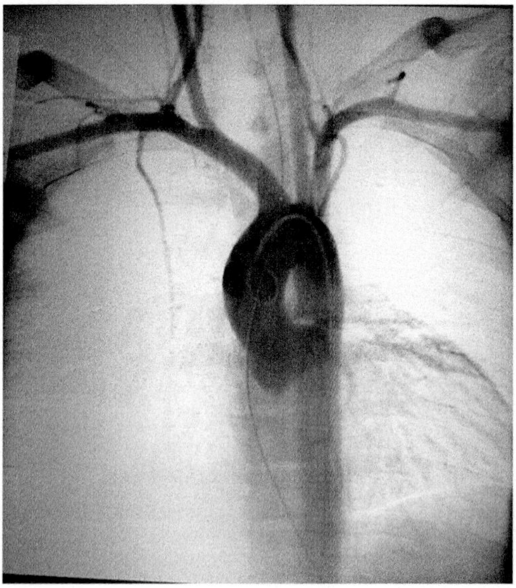

Figure 9.13 Normal aortic arch and great vessels. Copyright: http://www.meddean.luc.edu/lumen/meded/radio/curriculum/Vascular/Vessels_thorax_f.htm

artery. From its origin, the subclavian artery travels laterally between the scalene muscles and becomes the axillary artery at the lateral border of the first rib. The axillary artery passes into the upper arm where it becomes the brachial artery at the lower margin of teres major. On the left, the subclavian artery arises directly from the aortic arch before travelling laterally and becoming the axillary artery and then brachial artery (Figure 9.13).

Anatomical Variations of Upper Arm and Shoulder

Tortuosity

As at the level of the subclavian artery, tortuosity can be characterized as minor or significant (>90° bend). Tortuosity at the subclavian-innominate junction on the right can present as difficulty in advancing the guidewire (Figure 9.14). Deep inspiration by the patient can be helpful in straightening the vessel and can facilitate advancement of

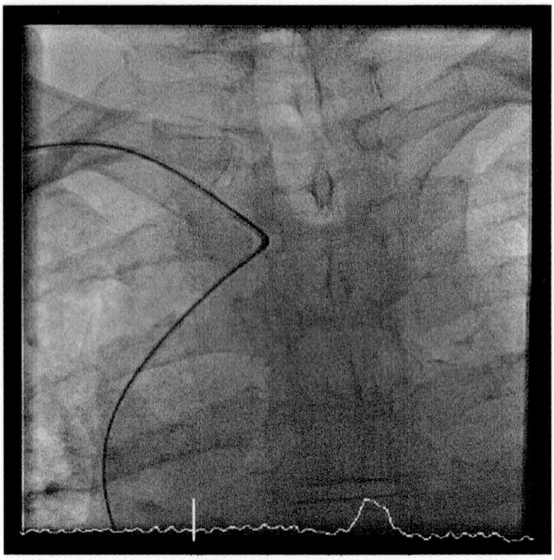

Figure 9.14 Tortuosity of the right subclavian artery.

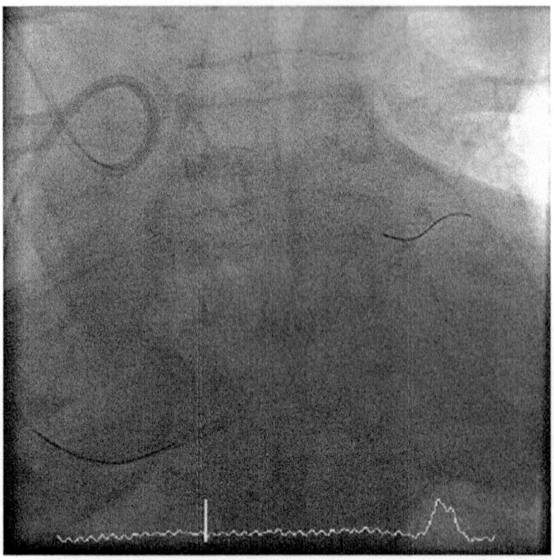

Figure 9.15 PCI taking place with right subclavian tortuosity.

the guidewire. If this is unsuccessful, an angiogram delineating the anatomy may be helpful. Again, switching to a 0.025" hydrophilic J-tipped wire or a 0.014" angioplasty wire and/or using BAT can also be helpful (Figure 9.15).

Loops

Loops encountered in the subclavian-innominate area should be treated in the same way as those in the radial artery. Loops can be traversed using hydrophilic J-tipped wires or appropriately shaped 0.014" angioplasty wires. Advancing a diagnostic or guiding catheter over the wire followed by gentle manipulation can help to straighten the loop and make coronary artery cannulation less challenging. If the operator experiences difficulty in advancing diagnostic or guiding catheters over the wire, then again, BAT can be used to good effect. Catheter manipulation within the ascending aorta may be facilitated by the use of supportive guide wires (Figure 9.16).

Atherosclerotic Disease

Occasionally stenotic lesions of the subclavian or innominate vessels are seen. These initially present as difficulty in advancing the guidewire or catheter and can be confirmed with coronary angiography. Depending on the degree of severity of the lesion, they may be crossed with a normal guidewire or with a 0.014" angioplasty wire. If the stenosis is not

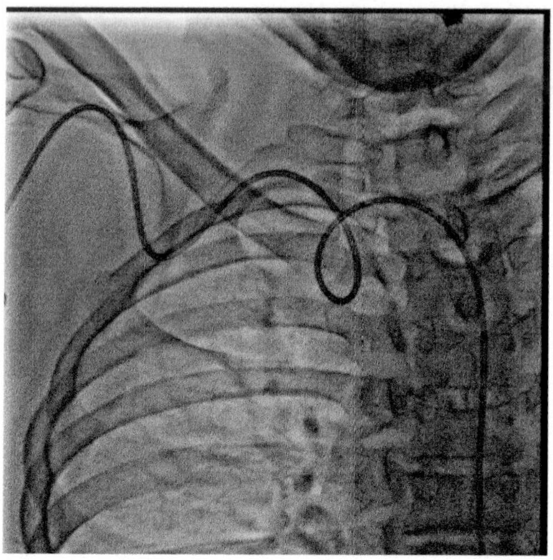

Figure 9.16 Loop in the subclavian and brachiocephalic artery.
Copyright: http://www.angiologist.com/vascular-intervention/radial-artery-access-for-renal-interventions/

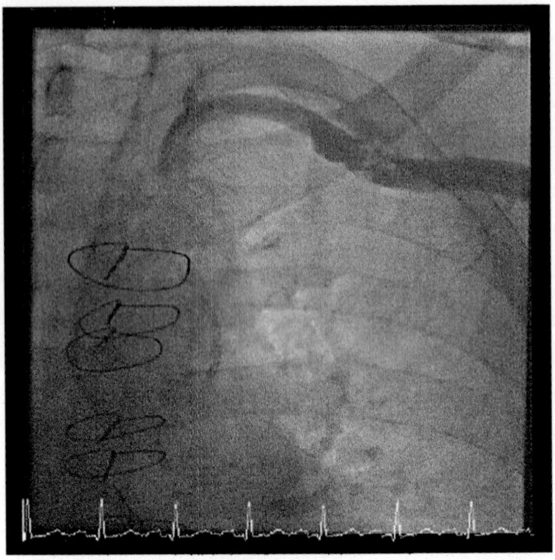

Figure 9.17 Stenosis in a left subclavian artery.

particularly significant, the coronary procedure should be performed as planned. If the stenosis obstructs delivery of equipment, then it can be treated with balloon angioplasty alone or followed by stenting if the operator is appropriately trained. Atherosclerosis of the radial artery itself is rarely seen. Figure 9.17 shows an angiogram of a left subclavian artery stenosis in a patient who had previously undergone coronary artery bypass grafting with vein grafts and a left internal mammary artery graft. Although a wire from the left radial artery passed easily into the aortic root, catheter advancement was not possible. Angiography confirmed a tight left subclavian artery stenosis. Figure 9.18 demonstrates balloon dilatation of the subclavian artery stenosis using a multi-purpose catheter and a non-compliant 6 mm balloon. This allowed the easy passage of catheters to the aortic root.

Congenital Abnormalities

Aortic Arch

The most commonly seen pattern of aortic arch gives rise to three great vessels: innominate artery, left common carotid artery, and left subclavian artery. This pattern is seen in around 70% of patients.[16] Anatomical variations of this pattern are seen and can make navigation of the guidewire

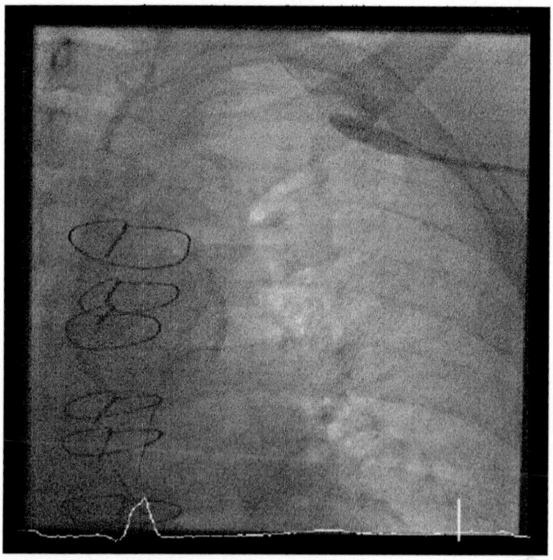

Figure 9.18 Balloon dilatation of a left subclavian artery stenosis.

into the aortic root more difficult. The next most common variation in aortic arch anatomy is where the innominate and left common carotid arteries share a common origin. This occurs in around 13% of the population. Another variant which occurs in around 9% of the population occurs when the left common carotid artery originates from the innominate artery.[16] These variations (seen in Figures 9.19, 9.20, and 9.21), though relatively frequent, cause no procedural difficulty and so are often not detected by the operator.

Aberrant Right Subclavian Artery

An aberrant right subclavian artery (also known as arteria lusoria) has an estimated incidence of 0.5–2%. Instead of originating from the innominate artery, an aberrant right subclavian artery originates directly from the aortic arch distal to the left subclavian artery. In 80% of cases, it then passes behind the oesophagus to make its way to the right upper limb. In the remaining cases, it passes either between the oesophagus and trachea (15%) or in front of the trachea (5%).

As can be seen from Figures 9.22 and 9.23, a wire travelling along an aberrant right subclavian artery is biased towards entering the descending rather than ascending aorta. Deep inspiration from the patient

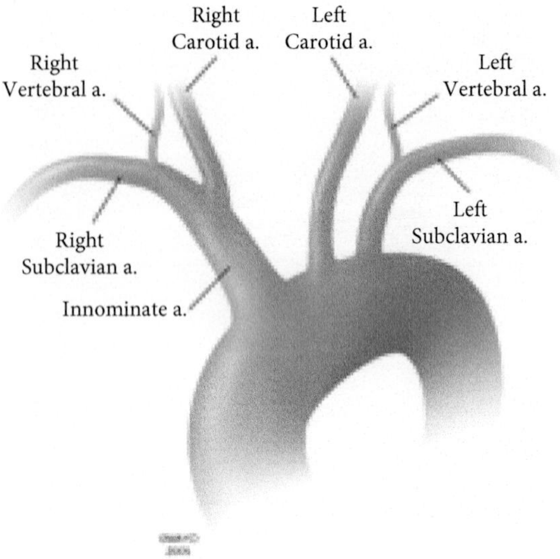

Figure 9.19 Most common form of aortic arch.[16] Copyright: *AJNR Am J Neuroradiol.*

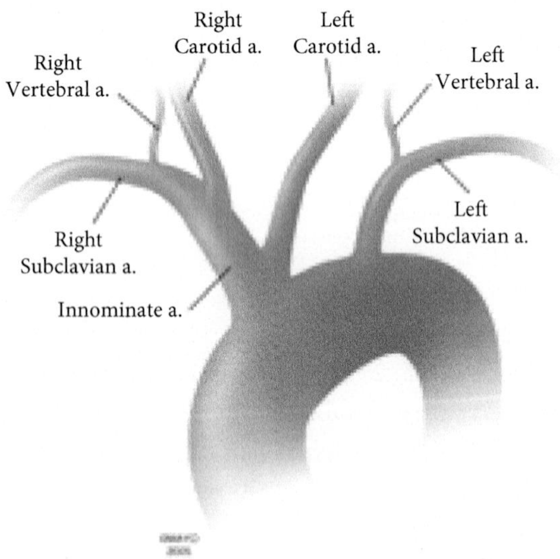

Figure 9.20 Second most common aortic arch pattern with common origin of the innominate and left common carotid arteries.[16] Copyright: *AJNR Am J Neuroradiol.*

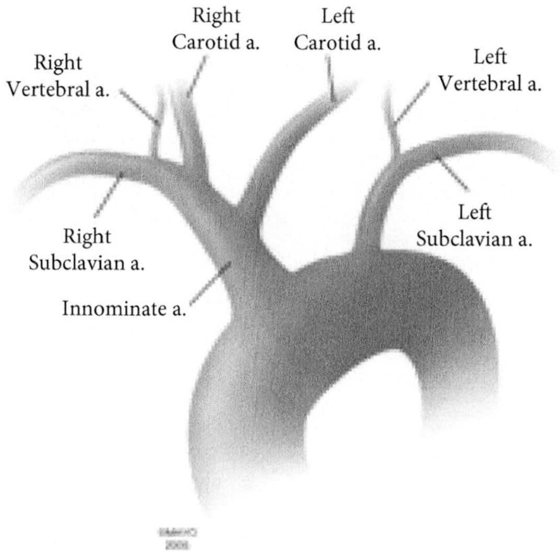

Figure 9.21 Left common carotid artery originates from innominate artery.
Copyright: *AJNR Am J Neuroradiol.*

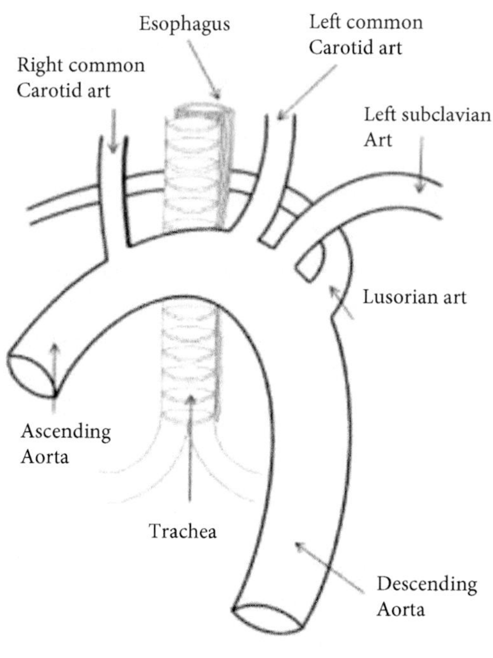

Figure 9.22 Schematic of aberrant right subclavian artery (Lusoria artery)[17].
Copyright: *American Journal of Gastroenterology* (*Am J Gastroenterol.* 2000 Jun;95(6):1411–6).

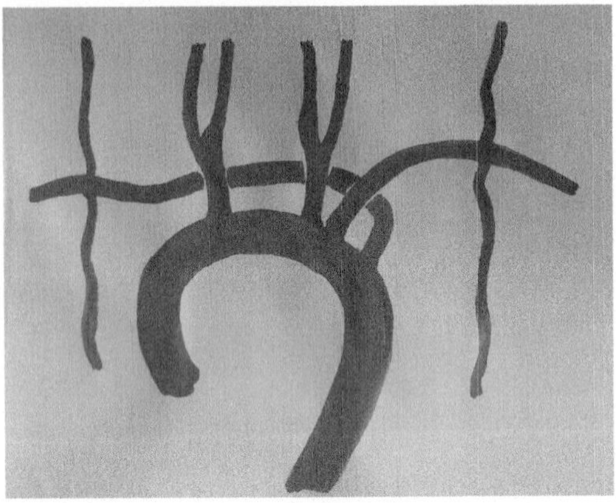

Figure 9.23 Angiogram showing aberrant right subclavian artery.
[Copyright: Kopp R, Wizgall I, Kreuzer E, et al. Surgical and endovascular treatment of symptomatic aberrant right subclavian artery (arteria lusoria). *Vascular*. 2007 Mar–Apr;15(2):84–91].

can be helpful in attempting to manipulate the wire into the ascending aorta. If this is unsuccessful, then directing a diagnostic catheter (for example a Judkins right) can facilitate correct passage of the wire: Working in the left anterior oblique (LAO) projection the wire is passed into the descending aorta. This can then be slowly withdrawn and the catheter turned towards the direction of the ascending aorta (towards the left of the screen in the LAO projection), the wire is then advanced when in the correct position. This is a challenging anatomical situation. Even when access is gained to the ascending aorta, difficulty in controlling catheter manipulation is universal, and only the most experienced operators can overcome this problem. When an inexperienced radial operator encounters an aberrant subclavian artery, switching to a different access site can be the best option if a highly experienced operator is not available to assist.

Right Aortic Arch

Right aortic arch is a rare variation found in <0.1% of the population, according to a review of the literature.[18] The most common form has an aberrant left subclavian artery with the vessels coming off in the order: left common carotid artery, right common carotid artery, right subclavian

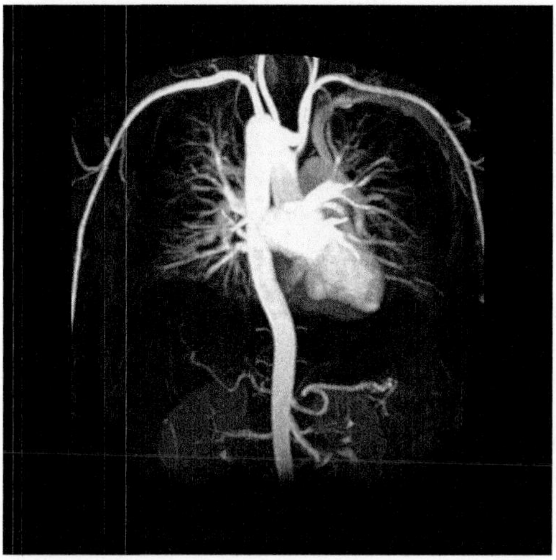

Figure 9.24 Right aortic arch. (Image courtesy: Dr Maxime St-Amant, Radiopaedia.org, rID: 20698).

artery, and left subclavian artery. Again, if difficulty is encountered when advancing the guidewire, an angiogram will help to clarify the anatomy and make successful navigation more likely. If such a rare anomaly is suspected, a CT of the aorta will accurately delineate the anatomy and guide selection of the most appropriate access site (Figure 9.24).

Conclusion

Coronary intervention via the radial route presents a unique set of challenges to operators. An understanding of the basic vascular anatomy from the heart to the radial puncture site and knowledge of some simple techniques can help to increase the likelihood of a successful outcome.

References

1. Campeau L. Percutaneous radial artery approach for coronary angiography. *Cathet Cardiovasc Diagn*. 1989;16:3–7.
2. Kiemeneij F, Laarman GJ. Percutaneous transradial artery approach for coronary stent implantation. *Cathet Cardiovasc Diagn*. 1993;30:173–178.

3. Mamas MA, Ratib K, Routledge H, Neyses L, Fraser DG, de Belder M, Ludman PF, Nolan J, British Cardiovascular Intervention Society and the National Institute for Cardiovascular Outcomes Research. Influence of arterial access site selection on outcomes in primary percutaneous coronary intervention: are the results of randomized trials achievable in clinical practice? *JACC Cardiovasc Interv*. 2013;6:698–706.
4. Mamas MA, Nolan J, de Belder MA, Zaman A, Kinnaird T, Curzen N, Kwok CS, Buchan I, Ludman P, Kontopantelis E, British Cardiovascular Intervention Society (BCIS) and the National Institute for Clinical Outcomes Research (NICOR). Changes in arterial access site and association with mortality in the United Kingdom: observations from a national percutaneous coronary intervention database. *Circulation*. 2016;133:1655–1667.
5. Lo TS, Nolan J, Fountzopoulos E, Behan M, Butler R, Hetherington SL, Vijayalakshmi K, Rajagopal R, Fraser D, Zaman A, Hildick-Smith D. Radial artery anomaly and its influence on transradial coronary procedural outcome. *Heart Br Card Soc*. 2009;95:410–415.
6. Rodríguez-Niedenführ M, Vázquez T, Nearn L, Ferreira B, Parkin I, Sañudo JR. Variations of the arterial pattern in the upper limb revisited: a morphological and statistical study, with a review of the literature. *J Anat*. 2001;199:547–566.
7. Dehghani P, Mohammad A, Bajaj R, Hong T, Suen CM, Sharieff W, Chisholm RJ, Kutryk MJB, Fam NP, Cheema AN. Mechanism and predictors of failed transradial approach for percutaneous coronary interventions. *JACC Cardiovasc Interv*. 2009;2:1057–1064.
8. Louvard Y, Lefèvre T. Loops and transradial approach in coronary diagnosis and intervention. *Catheter Cardiovasc Interv Off J Soc Card Angiogr Interv*. 2000;51:250–252.
9. Chugh SK, Chugh S, Chugh Y, Rao SV. Feasibility and utility of pre-procedure ultrasound imaging of the arm to facilitate transradial coronary diagnostic and interventional procedures (PRIMAFACIE-TRI). *Catheter Cardiovasc Interv Off J Soc Card Angiogr Interv*. 2013;82:64–73.
10. Guédès A, Dangoisse V, Gabriel L, Jamart J, Chenu P, Marchandise B, Schroeder E. Low rate of conversion to transfemoral approach when attempting both radial arteries for coronary angiography and percutaneous coronary intervention: a study of 1,826 consecutive procedures. *J Invasive Cardiol*. 2010;22:391–397.
11. Kiemeneij F, Vajifdar BU, Eccleshall SC, Laarman G, Slagboom T, van der Wieken R. Evaluation of a spasmolytic cocktail to prevent radial artery spasm during coronary procedures. *Catheter Cardiovasc Interv Off J Soc Card Angiogr Interv*. 2003;58:281–284.
12. Ruiz-Salmerón RJ, Mora R, Vélez-Gimón M, Ortiz J, Fernández C, Vidal B, Masotti M, Betriu A. [Radial artery spasm in transradial cardiac catheterization. Assessment of factors related to its occurrence, and of its consequences during follow-up]. *Rev Esp Cardiol*. 2005;58:504–511.
13. Kwok CS, Rashid M, Fraser D, Nolan J, Mamas M. Intra-arterial vasodilators to prevent radial artery spasm: a systematic review and pooled analysis of clinical studies. *Cardiovasc Revascularization Med Mol Interv*. 2015;16:484–490.
14. Patel T, Shah S, Pancholy S. Balloon-assisted tracking of a guide catheter through difficult radial anatomy: a technical report. *Catheter Cardiovasc Interv Off J Soc Card Angiogr Interv*. 2013;81:E215–E218.

15. Patel T, Shah S, Sanghavi K, Pancholy S. Management of radial and brachial artery perforations during transradial procedures--a practical approach. *J Invasive Cardiol.* 2009;21:544–547.
16. Layton KF, Kallmes DF, Cloft HJ, Lindell EP, Cox VS. Bovine aortic arch variant in humans: clarification of a common misnomer. *AJNR Am J Neuroradiol.* 2006;27:1541–1542.
17. Janssen M, Baggen MG, Veen HF, Smout AJ, Bekkers JA, Jonkman JG, Ouwendijk RJ. Dysphagia lusoria: clinical aspects, manometric findings, diagnosis, and therapy. *Am J Gastroenterol.* 2000;95:1411–1416.
18. Cinà CS, Althani H, Pasenau J, Abouzahr L. Kommerell's diverticulum and right-sided aortic arch: a cohort study and review of the literature. *J Vasc Surg.* 2004;39:131–139.

10

Tips and Tricks for Transradial Interventions

Yashasvi Chugh, Sunita Chugh, and Sanjay Kumar Chugh

Introduction

Transradial access (TRA) has evolved as a popular successful alternative to femoral route,[1,2] with its benefits of reduced major bleeding and vascular complications, lower costs and patient comfort with early mobilization.[3–8] However, TRA has a steep learning curve,[9] with challenges in radial access,[10] which include radial artery spasm, anatomical arterial and aortic anomalies,[11–13] that often lead to increase in procedural and fluoroscopy times as well as radiation exposure, besides procedure failure and crossover.[1–3,6,7]

Reasons for transradial procedure failure are as follows:

- Access failure: 52.6% of all procedure failures,[14] are because of inability to successfully puncture or wire the radial artery; while 38% of failures.[15] relate to radial artery spasm.
- Inability to advance guide catheters to the ascending aorta is reported as reason of failure of transradial (TR) percutaneous coronary intervention (PCI) in 51% of patients[16] because of radial spasm or anatomical abnormalities in the radial artery ranging from small diameter radial artery (SDRA) to loops, brachial and subclavian tortuosities and aortic anomalies. Small diameter of radial artery increased failure [odds ratio (OR) 2.6, 95% confidence interval (CI) 1.4–5.0; $p = 0.003$] and similarly a difficult access resulted in a greater risk of failure (OR 2.5, 95% CI 1.3–4.9; $p = 0.006$).[14]
- Short stature (OR: 0.97; 95% CI: 0.95–0.99, $p = 0.02$) essentially because of smaller diameter radial arteries[16] and

- Old age (≥75 years) (OR: 3.86; 95% CI: 2.33–6.40, $p = 0.0006$) are also recognized as independent predictors of failure.[16] In the elderly, this is because of tortuous and diseased arteries.

Overcoming the Potential Challenges in Transradial Procedures

Radial Access: Puncture

Failure to puncture or wire the radial artery is reported in 52.6%; of failures[14] but was found to be less than 1% when combined with pre-procedure ultrasound of arm arteries (PPUAA).[17]

Patient Preparation for Radial Access

- The contralateral arm should have a venous cannula and a maintenance drip should be on flow appropriate to the left ventricular function and clinical status of the patient. This is important because patients are fasting and liable to drop blood pressure. Also, because there is no femoral venous access, the arm cannula helps ensure an adequate, patent venous access for administering emergency medicines and intravenous fluids. A non-invasive blood pressure cuff for monitoring blood pressure should be on the contralateral arm and be set on auto-mode, as per clinical requirement of the case. Blood pressure reading from the radial sheath is unreliable because of spasm in radial artery. In these situations, a non-invasive blood pressure (NIBP) cuff provides blood pressure recording, till a catheter reaches the central aorta.[18]
- For anxious patients, intravenous injection of Midazolam in small doses (0.5 mg) up to total of 2 mg is beneficial to allay anxiety and reduce risk of spasm. Since pain leads to more anxiety and spasm, injection of Fentanyl injected slowly intravenously in small doses of 12.5 mcg and repeated as required up to 50 mcg relieves pain and should be used in patients at the earliest hint of pain. It is important to be cautious when using these medications in patients with sleep apnea and chronic obstructive airway disease, who tend to desaturate rapidly with sedation.[18]

- Injection of Verapamil or Diltiazem[19] alone or in combination with nitroglycerine and/or Nicorandil[20] should be readily available, diluted for intra-arterial use; usually 3–5 mg of Diltiazem or Verapamil and 50–100 mcg of nitroglycerine are used intra-arterially.[20] The authors sometimes use Nicorandil in doses of 2.5 mg intrarterially.[21]
- To minimize spasm in radial artery, the usual practice of the authors is to administer 3–5 mg of Diltiazem or Verapamil intra-arterially after introduction of sheath, at end of procedure, before sheath removal, as well as after every catheter exchange.
- The authors administer injection heparin, 70 U/Kg, or 5,000 units for an average 70 kg patient for diagnostic catheterization. For PCI, heparin is administered in dose of 70–100 IU/Kg body weight[22]; additional doses are repeated according to activated clotting time (ACT), with aim to maintain ACT at 250–300 seconds during procedure.
- Injection atropine should be kept ready for intravenous use, because vagal reactions can occur.

Radial Artery Puncture

The site of puncture (Figure 10.1) should be 2 cm proximal to the styloid process because beyond this point the artery usually has a bend and can lead to access failure.

Anatomical snuffbox has also been used to access the distal radial artery (DRA) on the dorsum of the hand (Figure 10.1a). The boundaries of the snuffbox are shown in the illustration. It is important to direct the needle in the direction of the radial artery at the wrist. Hand position is important (Figure 10.1b); the patient's hand muscles must be relaxed for successful puncture. Prior sedation often helps in relaxing the patient's hand in anxious patients (Please refer to the chapter on 'Distal Transradial Access' for further details).

Puncture can be done using a bare metal micro-puncture needle or a sheathed needle.

- Using a Bare Metal Needle [From Cook® or Cordis (Figures 10.1c and 10.1d)]: The puncture is done to anterior wall of the artery using

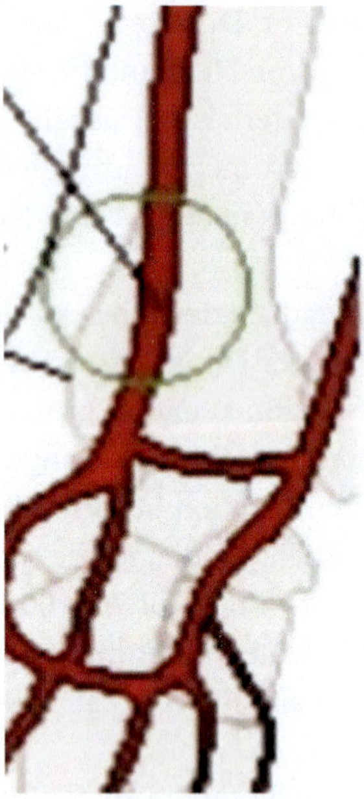

Figure 10.1 Ideal site for puncture on radial artery: 2 cm proximal to styloid process.

a bare metal 'micro-puncture needle' (Figure 10.1e) and a radial sheath using seldinger technique, similar to that used for femoral access.

- Puncture can also be done using a Terumo™ sheathed needle (Figures 10.1f(i) and 10.1.6bf(ii)) or a 20G Jelco venous canula, using transfixion technique in which the radial artery is punctured through both anterior and posterior walls. After a speck of blood appears in the hub of the needle (Figure 10.1g), the needle is pushed beyond the posterior wall, following which, the stillete is removed. The cannula is then slowly withdrawn till the latter is intraluminal with the artery and the blood then gushes out of the cannula. At this point, the 0.018" sheath wire is introduced into the cannula. Following this, the cannula is removed and a sheath is threaded over the sheath wire. Small diameter radial arteries often do not spurt when the cannula is intraluminal with the artery during withdrawal

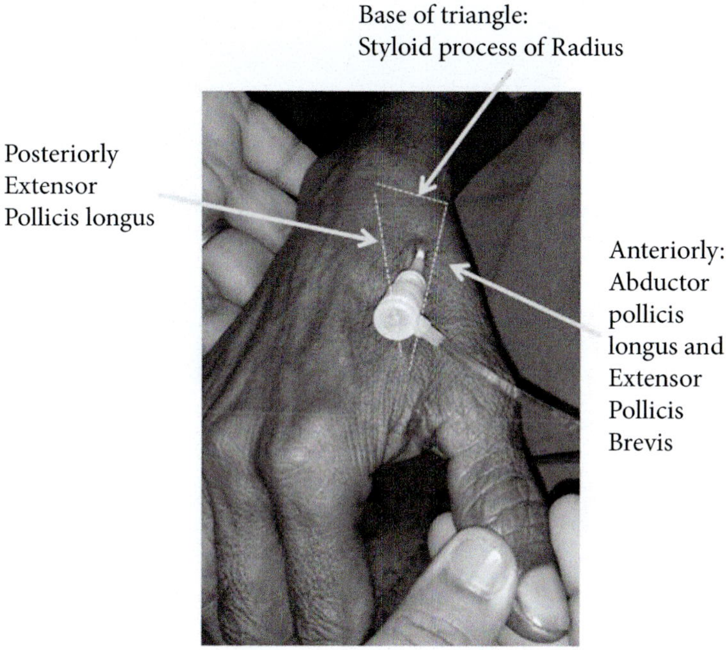

Figure 10.1a Anatomical landmarks for anatomical snuffbox: Posteriorly: Extensor Pollicis longus; Anteriorly: Abductor Pollicis longus and Extensor Pollicis Brevis; Base of triangle: Styloid process of Radius. Radial sheath is inserted in radial artery which traverses the floor of the snuffbox.

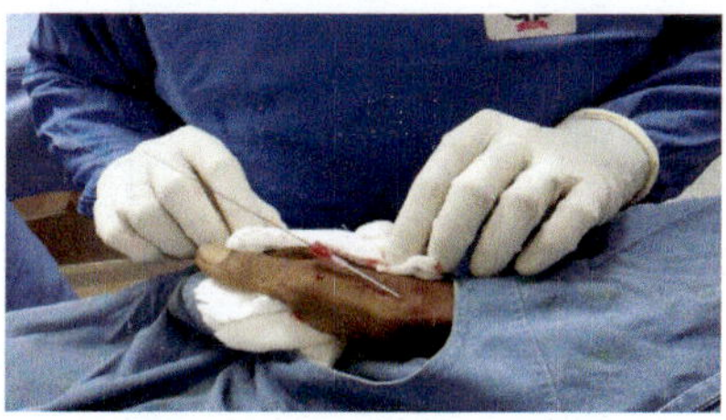

Figure 10.1b Hand position for distal radial access in anatomical snuffbox. Patient's palm is placed on a sterile towel roll so that the forearm is in 30° pronation and extended backwards by 15°. This allows the snuffbox to open up and the radial artery in the snuffbox to be felt. This can then be punctured with the needle at 20° angle to the dorsum of hand. Note the direction of puncture is downwards and parallel to inner border of first metatarsal bone. Hand position is very crucial for successful puncture of distal radial artery in anatomical snuffbox.

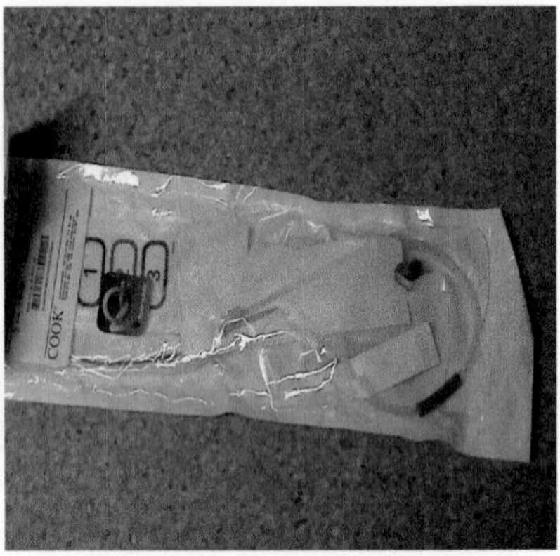

Figure 10.1c Cook® Sheath.

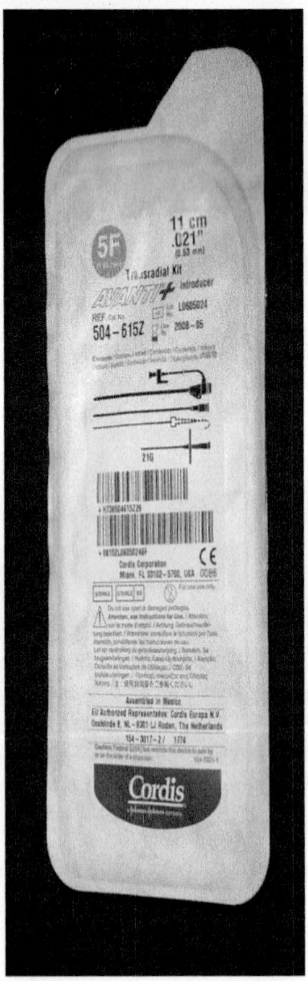

Figure 10.1d Cordis™ Sheath.

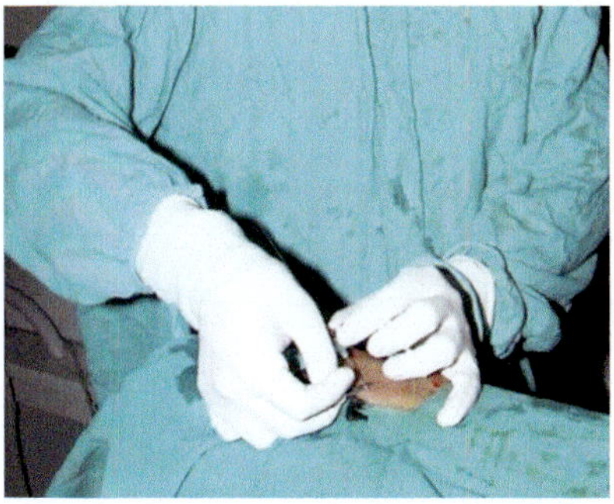

Figure 10.1e Puncture technique using a bare metal micro-puncture needle (Cook®).

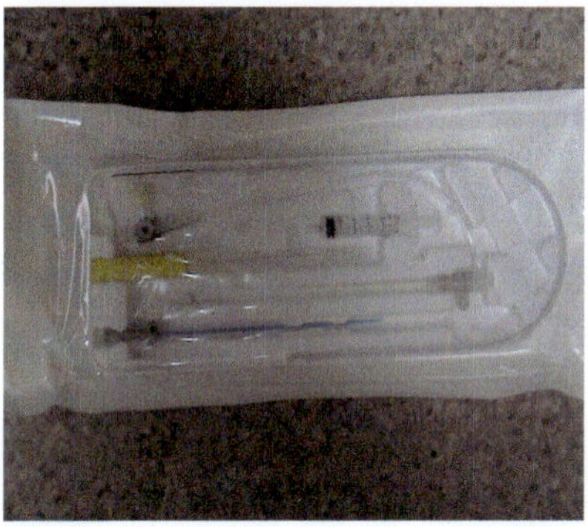

Figure 10.1f(i) Terumo™ Sheath kits.

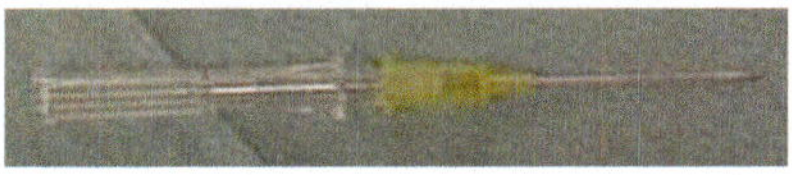

Figure 10.1f(ii) Terumo™ needle with sheath.

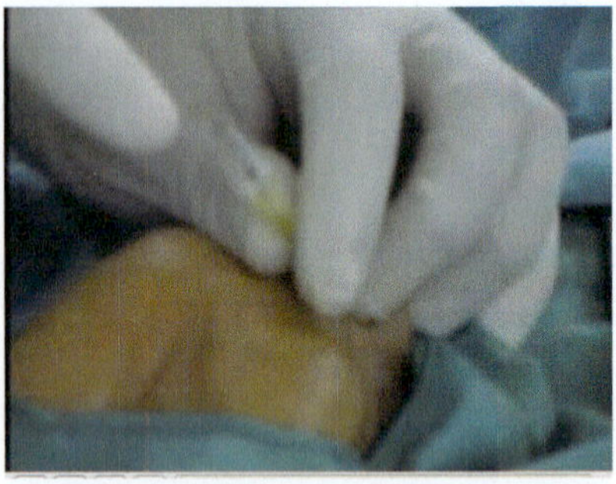

Figure 10.1g A sheathed Terumo needle is used to puncture the radial artery 2 cm proximal to styloid process of radius. As the needle is advanced and punctures the radial artery, a speck of blood appears in the hub of the needle. (Not shown in picture) After this, the needle is advanced further to puncture the posterior wall of the radial artery. Thereafter, the stilette is withdrawn, leaving the cannula in.

of the cannula as described above. A trick is to introduce the 0.018" sheath wire in the cannula as soon as a thin column of blood fills up the cannula up to the hub. Then if the wire does not progress into the artery (Figure 10.1h(i)), gentle withdrawal of the cannula with gentle repeated attempts to push the wire forward often allows the wire to traverse into the artery (Figure 10.1h(ii)).

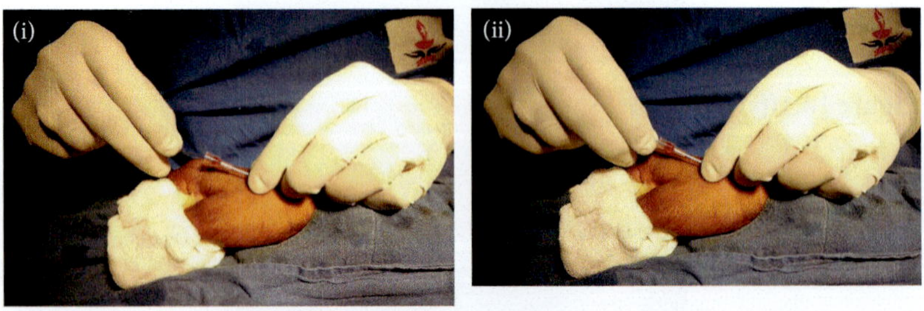

Figure 10.1h(i,ii) Trick of accessing a small diameter radial artery (SDRA): The radial artery is punctured using a 20G Gelco™ venous cannula. The cannula is the slowly rotated and pulled back gently. A 0.018" sheath wire is then introduced into it as soon as a thin column of blood fills up the cannula up to the hub (Figure 10.8a). Then, if the wire does not progress into the artery, gentle withdrawal of the cannula with attempts to push the wire forward often allows the wire to traverse into the artery (Figure 10.8b). These figures illustrate the technique in puncture of a small distal radial artery in the anatomical snuffbox. The same technique can be used for standard radial access in small distal radial artery.

Right or Left, Which Radial Artery to Use?

Comparative data of right radial artery versus left radial artery is presented in the chapter on '*Transradial interventions: right or left*'. The practical approach and tips are presented here.

- Most operators prefer to use right radial artery as default. Failure to engage the coronary arteries because of anatomical variations has been reported in 10% patients using right radial access; which was successfully completed via the left radial artery (LRA).[14]
- The left radial artery is best punctured from the left side of the patient, with the arm of patient abducted to 90° (Figure 10.2a). After access is obtained, the procedure then continues from the right side of the patient (Figure 10.2b).

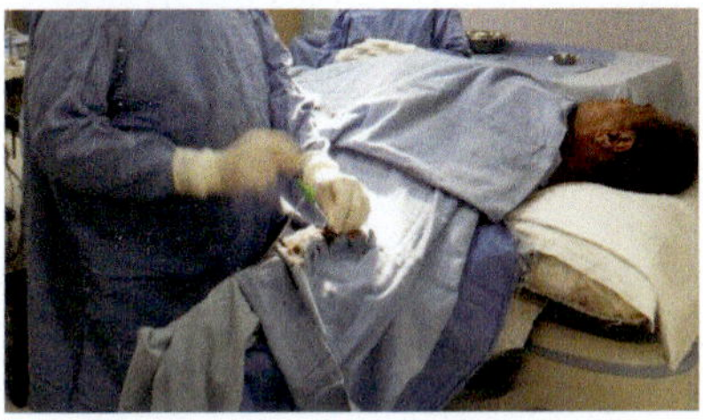

Figure 10.2a Cath-lab arrangements for left RA/UA puncture. Puncture is done from left of patient with patient arm abducted to 90°.

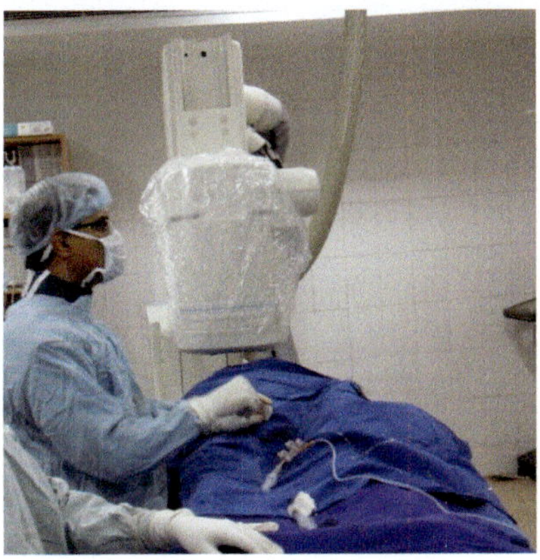

Figure 10.2b Rest of the catheterization procedure is then done from the right of the patient.

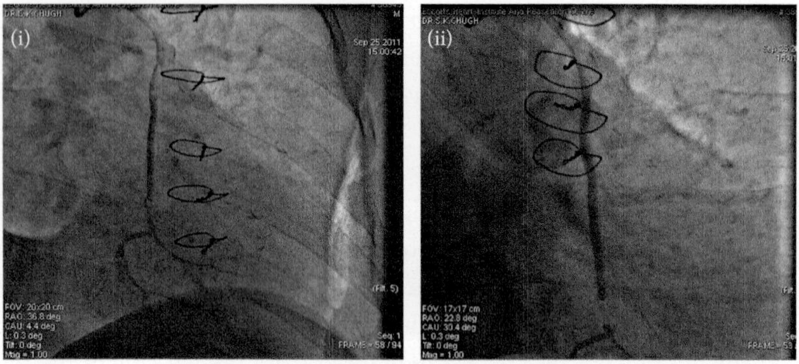

Figure 10.2c(i) and (ii) Saphenous vein graft to second obtuse marginal (OM2) has a critical stenosis with filling defect at the site of anastomosis.

- The authors prefer the left radial access in post-coronary artery bypass graft (post-CABG) patients because hooking saphenous vein grafts (SVGs) and also left internal mammary artery (LIMA) is easier from the left side. Hooking of the LIMA from right radial access leads to failure in 26.7% cases.[14] SVGs can be engaged from left radial artery using an Amplatz right [Figure 10.2c (i–ix)]. Other catheters that may be used are TIG™, left coronary bypass, multipurpose and Amplatz left [Figure 10.2d(i–viii)].

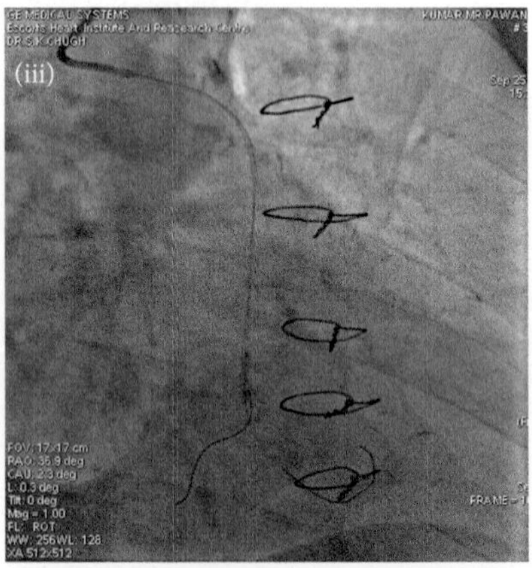

Figure 10.2c(iii) Two BMW wires one in each branch of the second obtuse marginal inserted via the saphenous vein graft. A 6F AR2 guide used, 2 × 8 mm balloon used to pre-dilate the lesion.

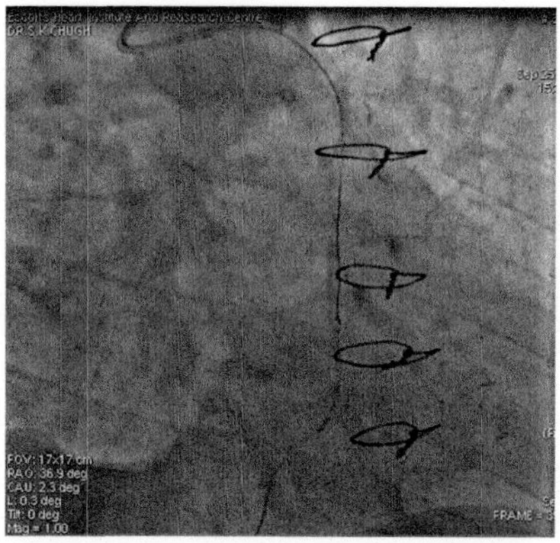

Figure 10.2c(iv) Stent in position from SVG to the bigger (lower) branch of second obtuse marginal.

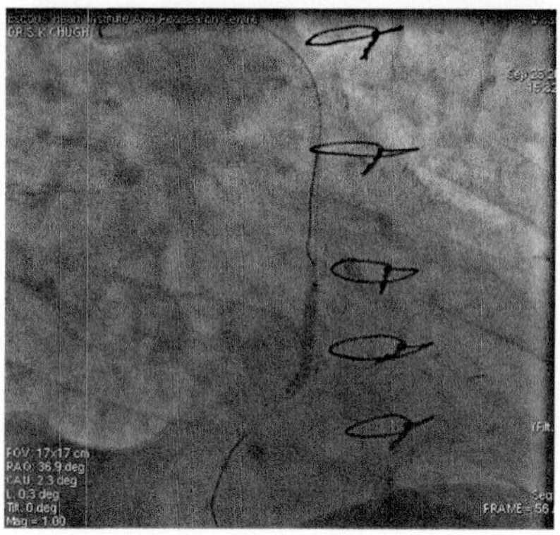

Figure 10.2c(v) 2.5 × 18 mm stent deployed at nominal pressure.

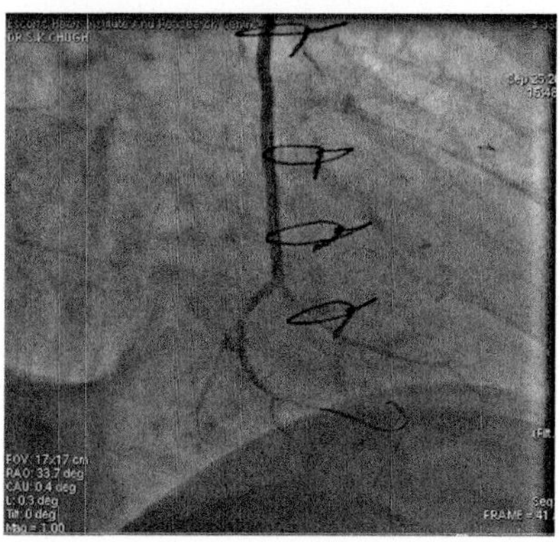

Figure 10.2c(vi) Post-deployment dissection noted at distal edge of stent.

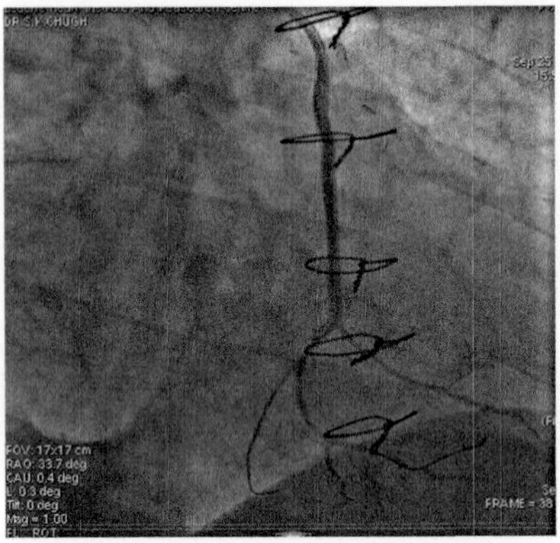

Figure 10.2c(vii) Second stent positioned distal to the first stent.

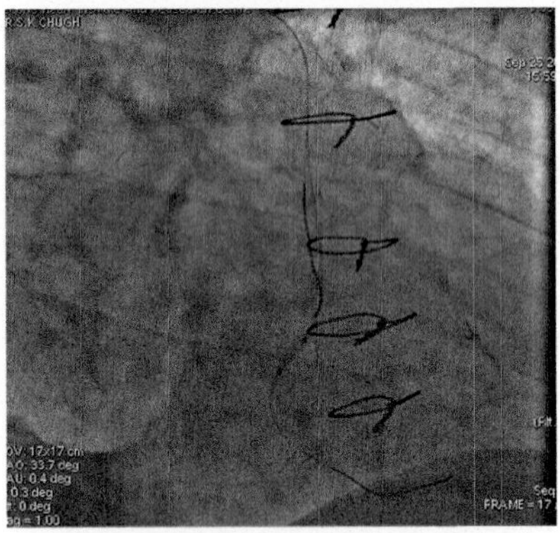

Figure 10.2c(viii) Second stent deployed in overlap with first stent.

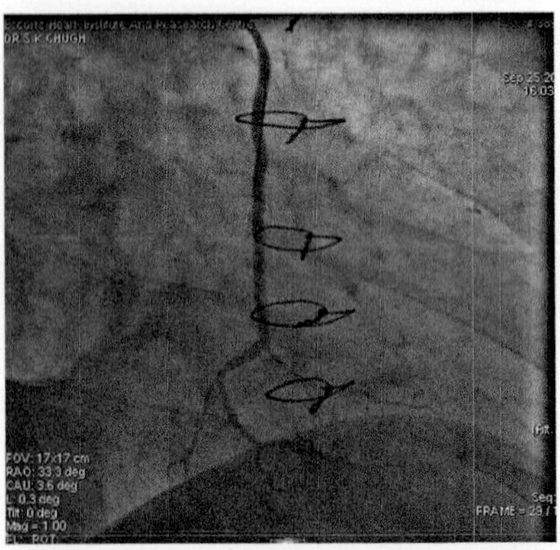

Figure 10.2c(ix) Final angiogram showing TIMI 3 flow.

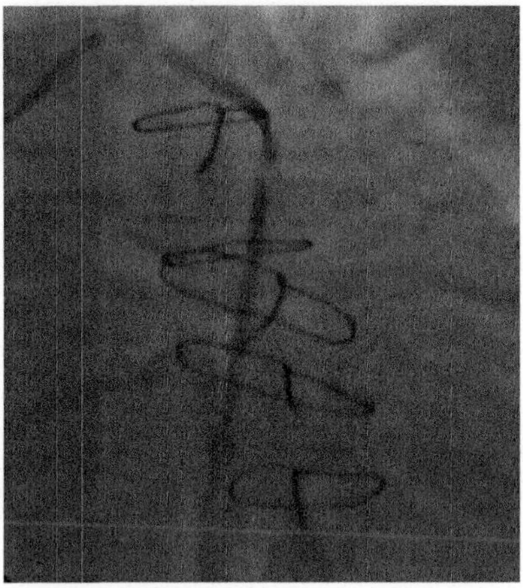

Figure 10.2d(i) AL1 guide catheter (GC) used to hook a 15-year-old, degenerated saphenous vein graft (SVG) to second obtuse marginal (OM2) with a critical, over 95% stenosis in the body of the SVG in a 70-year-old, post-bypass patient.

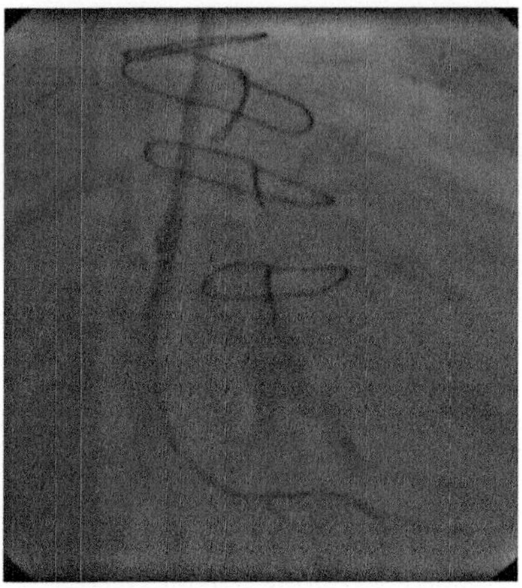

Figure 10.2d(ii) BMW wire used to cross the lesion. A spider filter inserted in the distal part of the vein graft.

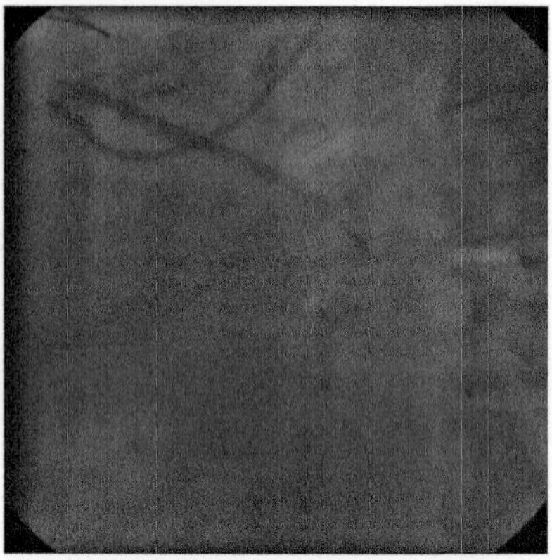

Figure 10.2d(iii) Spider filter is deployed.

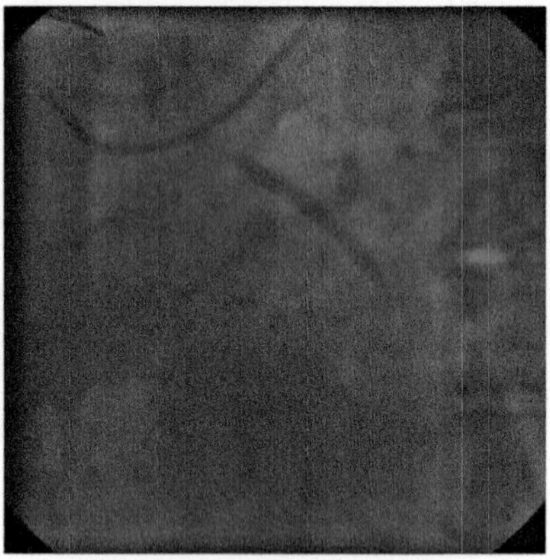

Figure 10.2d(iv) 2.75 × 23 mm stent deployed at the lesion.

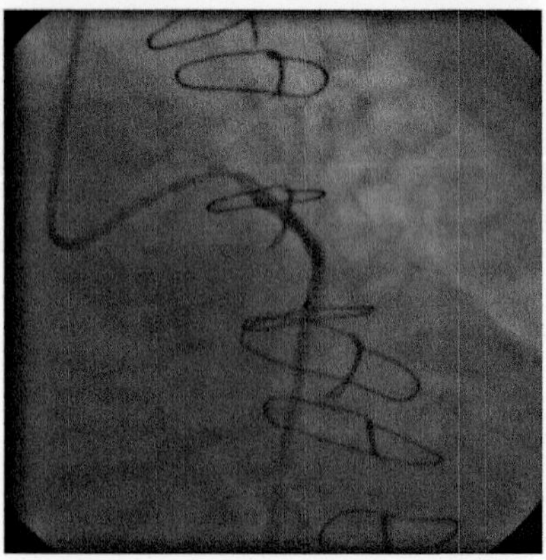

Figure 10.2d(v) Angiogram shows TIMI 3 flow in the vessel.

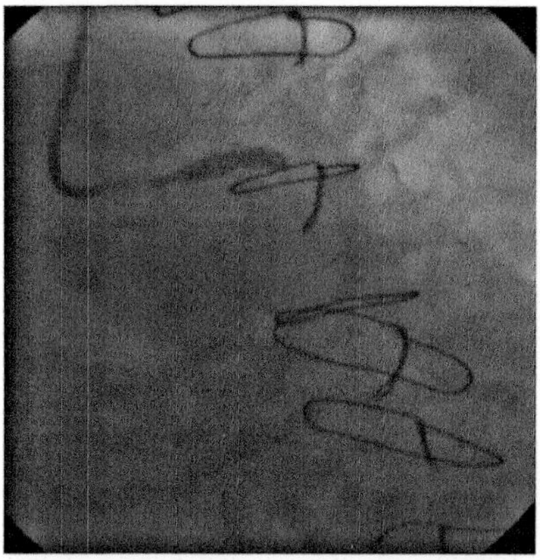

Figure 10.2d(vi) Stent is post-dilated with 3-mm balloon.

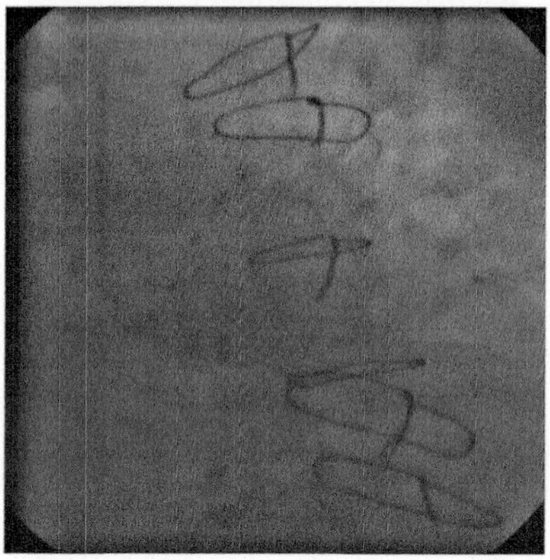

Figure 10.2d(vii) Filter is recaptured and being withdrawn into the guide.

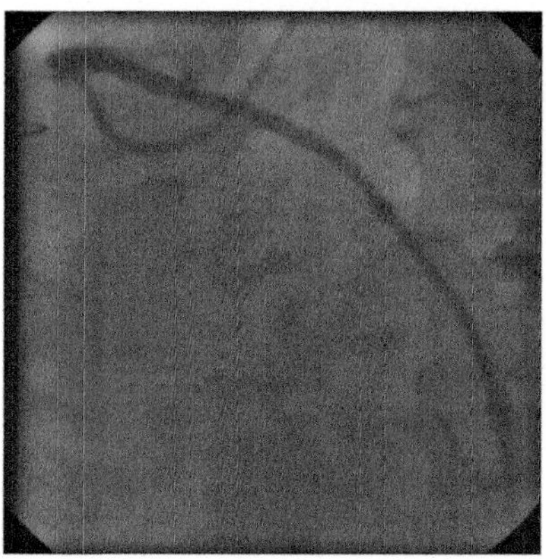

Figure 10.2d(viii) Final angiogram shows TIMI 3 flow.

A LIMA guide catheter (GC) is used for LIMA interventions or interventions in the native artery distal to LIMA anastomosis [Figure 10.2e(i–iii)].

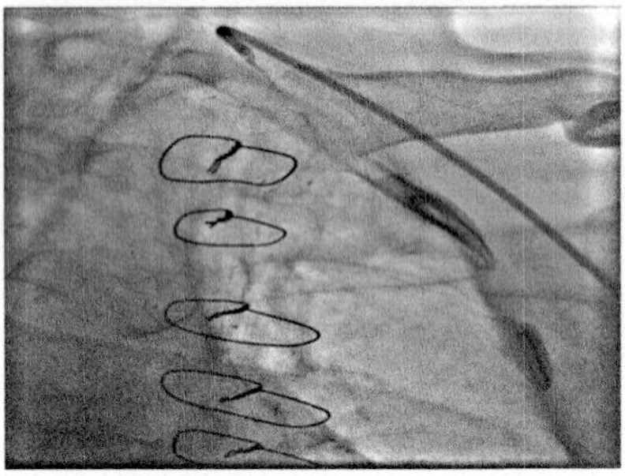

Figure 10.2e(i) A 6F left internal mammary artery (LIMA) guiding catheter used through left radial access to engage the LIMA.

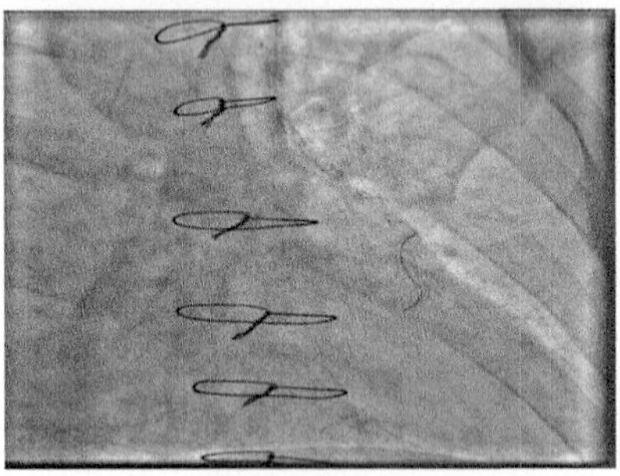

Figure 10.2e(ii) A wire crosses the lesion at anastomosis of LIMA graft to the left anterior descending artery (LAD).

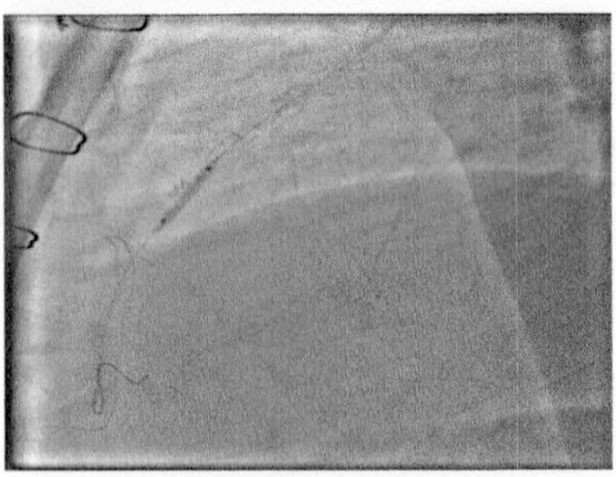

Figure 10.2e(iii) Stent deployed at the lesion.

- Although radial artery (RA) of any diameter can be used for radial access; as per modification of the authors' sheath sizing protocol (Figure 10.3), 5F sheath and catheters are used for radial artery diameter (RAD) more than or equal to 1.6 mm, 6F is used for RAD more than or equal to 1.7 mm and 7F for RAD more than or equal to 2.0 mm. For percutaneous coronary interventions (PCIs), the authors prefer 6F.[17] The reason for such selection of sheath French size based on RAD is that accommodating for a 20% increase in diameter of radial artery with use of intra-arterial vasodilators as above, the sheath: artery ratio is close to 1:1, and was found to minimize overstretch of the artery and hence reduce spasm, pain and difficulty in manipulation of catheters as occurs with grade 3 spasm[17] (*see below for spasm grades*). Hence, radial arteries with diameter 0.2 mm less than that mentioned in the protocol (Figure 10.3) have been used by the authors successfully for corresponding French size sheath.

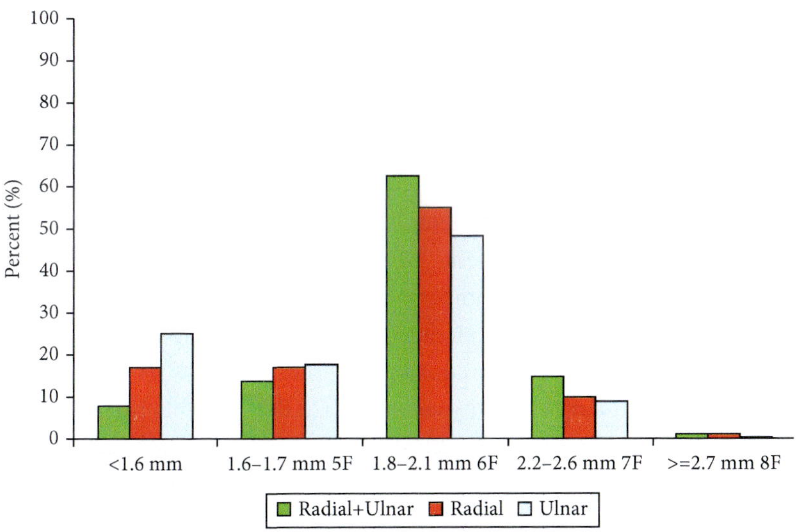

Figure 10.3 Sheath sizing protocol (Chugh et al.[17]).

- The authors use alternate access for small diameter radial arteries if the attempt to puncture them fails. To minimize risk of failure, if the artery feels small or if RA is less than1.3 mm, the authors prefer to start the case with either ulnar artery (UA) on the right or left radial or ulnar, whichever is bigger. The authors' default access artery is the right radial artery (RRA) because it is easier to puncture and comfortable for operator. Performing a procedure on left arm from right side of patient requires bending which strains the back of the operator. Hence, RA is preferred over UA, also because of a more superficial location, lack of adjacent nerves and easier haemostasis.

- Again if a loop, with accessory radial artery or a narrow radial artery arising from high up brachial or axillary artery is encountered on the right (Type-3 bifurcation[1]), crossover to alternate access may be required; which, for the authors', is to left radial artery; although there is a 2% chance of bi-laterality of the same abnormality. Such loops or high origin of radial artery from brachial or axillary artery can be predicted by PPUAA[17]; although PPUAA is not routinely practiced because of logistical difficulties relating to cost and availability of the procedure for the purpose in most hospitals and hence neither there is consensus for PPUAA at present nor it is mandatory. However, PPUAA is a useful option (*for details, please see Chapter 6 on Role of Doppler Ultrasound in Transradial Interventions*).
- **Left radial access is preferred over right radial access** in the following cases:
  - Occluded or small diameter RRA
  - Failed right radial access
  - Known anomaly in right arm artery suggested by PPUAA
  - Chronic total occlusion, or a tortuous, calcific or Shepherd's crook right coronary artery requiring complex PCI
  - Post-coronary artery bypass graft (CABG) patients: where bypass grafts need to be engaged
  - Deformity or scar of right arm/forearm making puncture difficult
  - Severe tortuosity of right subclavian artery
- In the following situations, **ulnar access was preferred over radial access:**
  - In presence of bilateral small, diseased or calcific radial arteries or
  - Anatomical abnormalities detected on ultrasound such as presence of a loop or accessory radial artery,
  - A high origin of radial from axillary artery or from the brachial artery proximal to the antecubital fossa. In the latter, type 3

bifurcation, the radial artery is narrow, allowing a guidewire to cross but it is often difficult to take 5F or 6F catheters through it.

Access Artery Spasm

Spasm of radial artery (RA) is one of the most common reasons for crossover or procedure failure in transradial interventions (TRIs).[15] Once RA spasm (RAS) develops, it makes catheter manipulation difficult, leading to procedural delays, discomfort to patients and procedure failure. A RAS grading given below is useful to quantify the problem in an individual and helps correlate severity of spasm with precipitating factors. (Please see Chapter 19, 'Complications of Transradial Access: Management and Prevention').

Arterial Spasm Grades (Chugh et al.[17])

- **Grade-4:** Severe pain and spasm disallowing any catheter movement necessitating crossover.
- **Grade-3:** Moderate pain and spasm restricting catheter movement and necessitating a pause in procedure and more than two additional doses of 5 mg intra-arterial Diltiazem or Verapamil, and/or 1 mg of intravenous Midazolam.
- **Grade-2:** Mild pain and spasm not restricting catheter movement; no pause in procedure but more than one additional dose of 5 mg intra-arterial Diltiazem (or Verapamil) and/or 0.5 mg of intravenous Midazolam.
- **Grade-1:** Mild pain and spasm not restricting catheter movement; no pause in procedure and only one additional dose of either or both 5 mg intra-arterial Diltiazem (or Verapamil) and/or 0.5 mg of intravenous Midazolam.

Preventing and Managing RA Spasm

- RAS can be prevented by using arterial sheaths with a sheath to artery diameter of as near possible to less than 1.1 which reduces radial artery stretch.[23] Ideal sheath to RA diameter is less than :1.1.
- Though consensus is lacking, a PPUAA[17] measures arterial diameters which can be a rough guide to selecting the nearest compatible

sheath size that would be expected to cause the least sheath; artery mismatch, based on the radial or ulnar artery diameter as illustrated in this sheath sizing protocol (Figure 10.3).[17]

- Pre-procedure ultrasound of arm arteries also helps identify anatomical abnormalities in the arm arteries, which has been reported to reduce patient discomfort, as well as procedure and fluoroscopy times even in patients undergoing second procedure.[24]
- Intra-arterial administration of Verapamil or Diltiazem, alone or in combination with Nitroglycerine after sheath insertion, after every catheter exchange and before sheath removal helps to prevent and manage RA spasm.
- Catheter manipulations, stiff catheters and multiple catheter exchanges contribute to RA spasm.[18] These should be avoided by thoughtful planning of appropriate choice of catheter size and shape to minimize manipulation or exchange of catheters.
- A sheathless technique has been described to minimize stretch of radial artery because the outer diameter of a radial sheath is 2F larger than its internal diameter. In the sheathless technique, a catheter is introduced directly and advanced into the radial artery without a sheath[25–27] with reported procedural success rate of 95% and radial artery occlusion rate of 2.5%. There are difficulties, however, with sheathless guiding, in exchanging catheters and also injecting spasmolytics, should radial artery spasm occur. The former can be overcome with the Cordis Railway Sheathless system™'; while the latter can be surmounted by injecting the spasmolytic into the brachial artery via the GC, when the same is being exchanged. This is also a useful technique for TRI in small diameter radial arteries.

Small Diameter Radial Arteries

- No definition of 'small diameter radial arteries' exists in literature. Our definition of SDRA is a radial artery with diameter less than or equal to1.7 mm. The reason for using 1.7 mm cut-off is that compared to patients with radial artery diameter less than or equal to 1.7 mm, in patients with more than 1.7 mm, crossovers (procedure failure) and access artery occlusions were 3.9% versus 0.9% and 2.8% versus 0.8%, respectively ($p < 0.0001$).[28]

- Female sex, low body mass index, and short stature are associated with SDRA[16]
- With compression of the ulnar artery, the diameter of a radial artery can be enhanced (Figure 10.3a(i–ii) and 10.3b).[30] The diameter of 1.1–1.6 mm arteries can be enhanced; though the percentage increase in diameter is variable and difficult to predict. The technique also enhances puncture success, including first pass success and reduction in number of punctures required to gain access.[29]

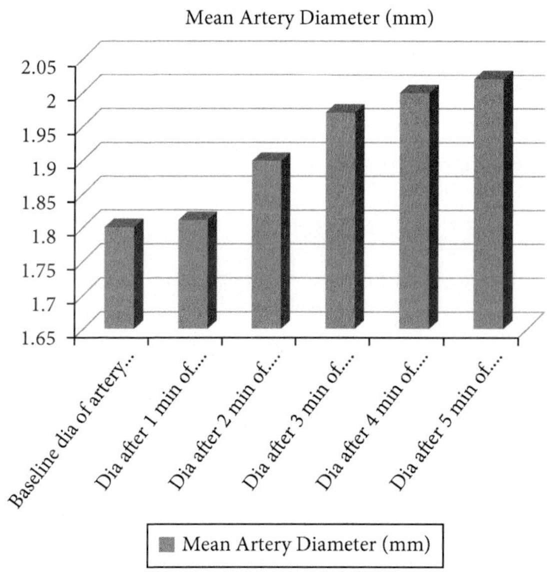

Figure 10.3a(i) Per minute enhancement in the mean diameter (MD) of the radial artery (RA) over 5 minutes of compression of the ipsilateral ulnar artery for radial artery mean diameter (RAMD) of 1.65 mm at baseline. (*Compression of the other artery (COOA) Technique*[23]).

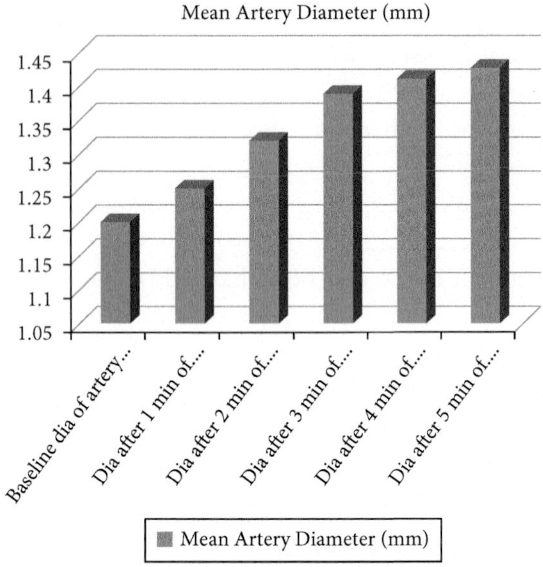

Figure 10.3a(ii) Per minute enhancement in the mean diameter (MD) of the radial artery (RA) over 5 minutes of compression of the ipsilateral ulnar artery for radial artery mean diameter (RAMD) of 1.05 mm at baseline. (*Compression of the other artery (COOA) Technique*[23]).

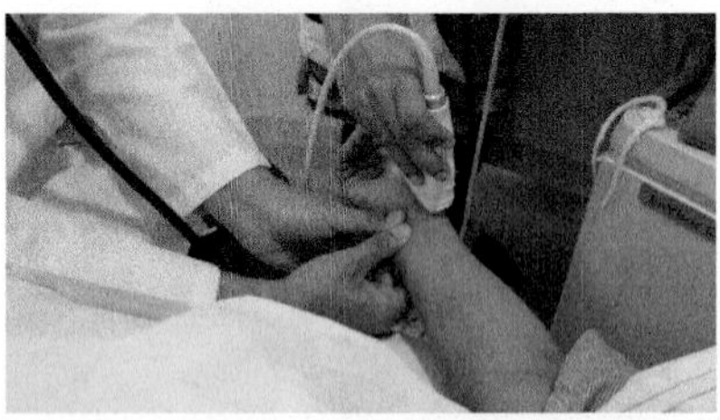

Figure 10.3b Technique of compression of the ipsilateral ulnar artery[23] with simultaneous study of increase in the size of radial artery diameter in real-time with colour Doppler ultrasound using a linear probe.

- For the first time in the world outside of Japan, transradial angioplasty through 4French guiding catheters was done by the author (SKC) and Dr Takashi Matsukage in India at Radial Live 2013. Angioplasty to a right coronary artery was done (Figure 10.4a). Miniature catheters, balloons and wires are manufactured and commercially available in Japan; kissing balloon through 5French guiding catheter (Figure 10.4b) and trifurcation kissing balloon through 6French guiding catheter is possible (Figure 10.4b(i)).

- The Glidesheath slender® (GSS™, Terumo) which gives a 5F lumen in 4F sheath can be used safely and successfully with 5F guiding catheters for complex PCI in patients with SDRA using conventional wires, balloons and stents; with exclusion of bifurcation lesions having large side-branch (requiring kissing balloon angioplasty or 2 stent strategy) and calcific lesions requiring rotablation. RA spasm and crossovers did not occur in the 9 patients reported.[30]

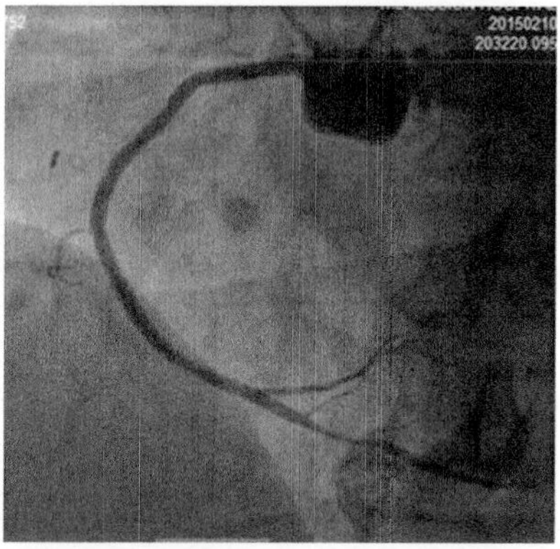

Figure 10.4a 4F angioplasty of right coronary artery: final result after successful transradial angioplasty.

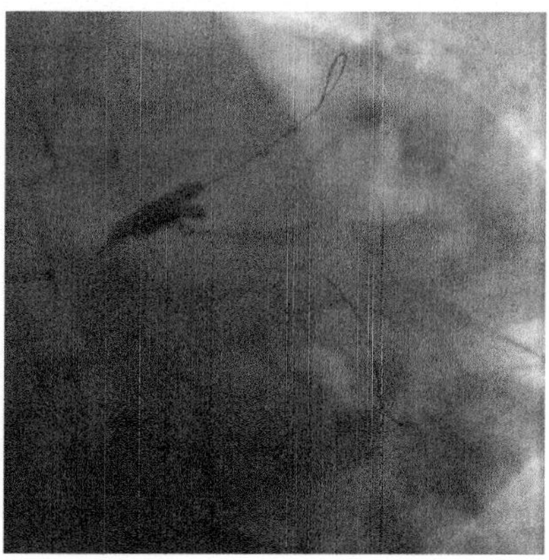

Figure 10.4b Kissing balloon through 5 French guiding catheter. (*Courtesy Dr Takashi Matsukage, Tokyo, Japan*).

- 5F guiding catheter lacks support (please see illustrative case figures 10.4b(ia);10.4b(ii–vii)) which can be overcome by 'deep intubation' of the guiding catheter into the right coronary artery, always over a balloon or stent (Figure 10.4b(iii) & 10.4b(v)). A GuideLiner® cannot be used with 5F guiding catheter; though a Heartrail® 4F guiding catheter (Terumo) can be used through it, in 'mother and child' technique to deliver a stent into the lesion in tortuous and calcific coronary arteries (see Chapter 25 on 'Slender Percutaneous Coronary Interventions by Transradial Approach').

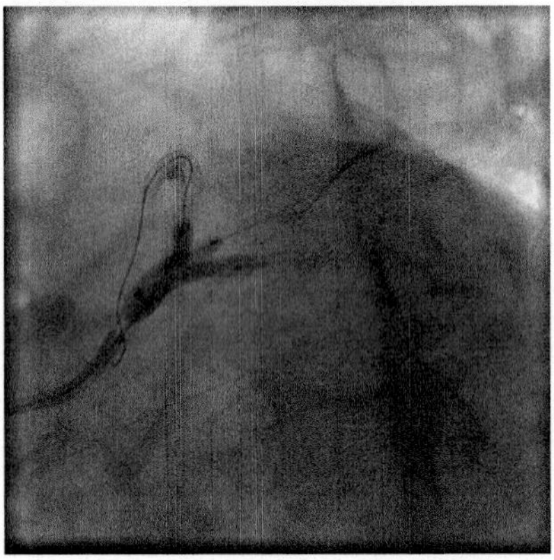

Figure 10.4b(i) Trifurcation kissing balloon through 6 French guiding catheter.

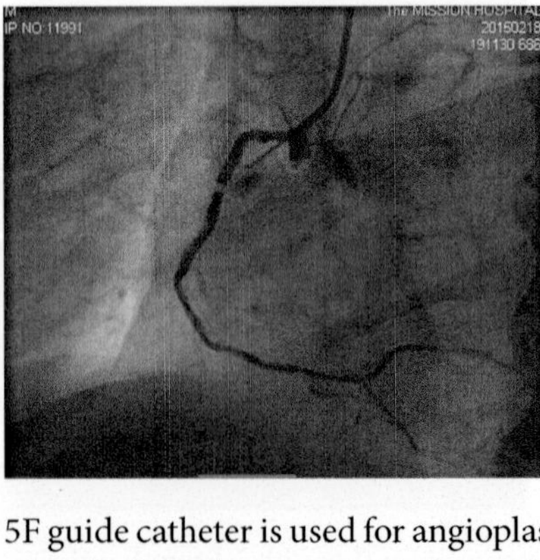

Figure 10.4b(ia) A 5F guide catheter is used for angioplasty of a critical stenosis in mid- heavily calcific right coronary with ostial disease. A 6F caused damping of pressures. Note distal diffuse disease.

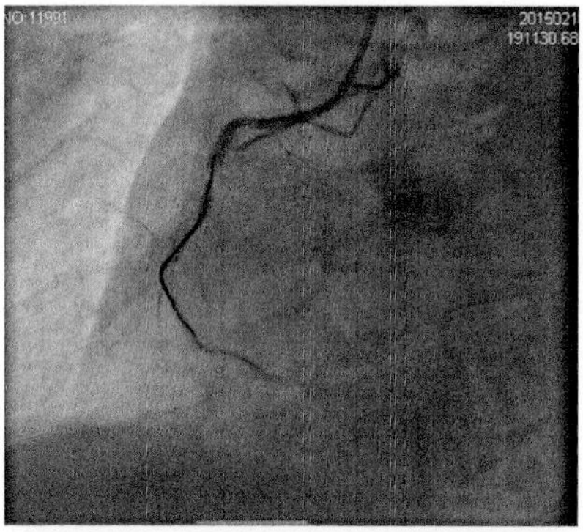

Figure 10.4b(ii) Two BMW wires reach distal right coronary artery.

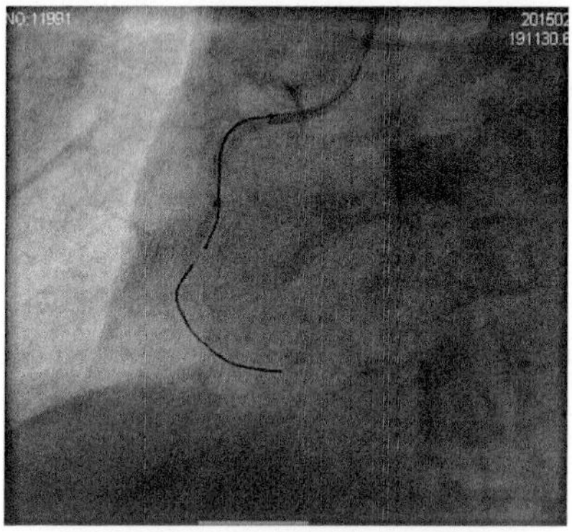

Figure 10.4b(iii) The 5F JR guide is deeply intubated over the balloon for active support to get the balloon down to the lesion.

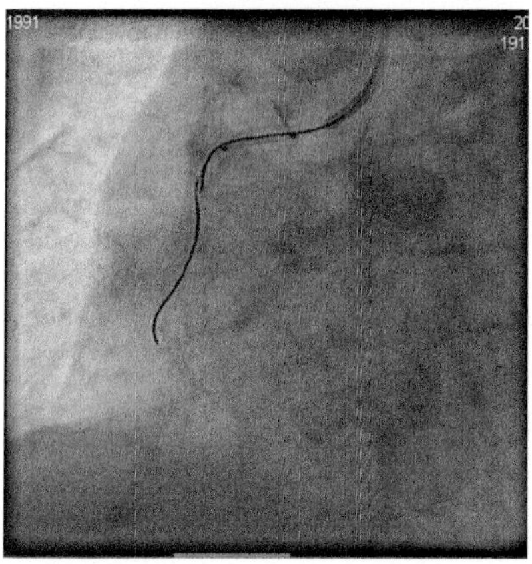

Figure 10.4b(iv) The stent does not track beyond the ostium of the heavily calcific right coronary artery (RCA).

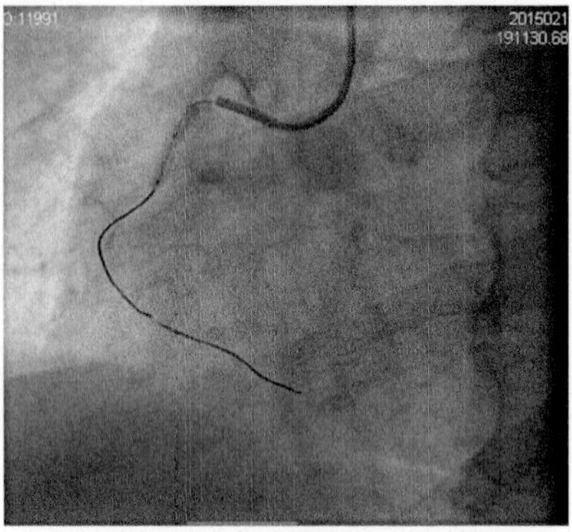

Figure 10.4b(v) The 5F guide catheter being deep throated over the balloon for active guide support in this heavily calcific right coronary artery with ostial disease to get the stent down to the lesion. Rotablation and GuideLiner were not feasible with 5F guide catheter.

- 5F guiding catheter has poorer visualization by angiography, because of reduced lumen of the catheter. Hence pre-dilatation allows better visualization of distal vessel during stent placement.
- It is important to be mindful of air being sucked in through the Tuohy-Borst adapter, while removing balloon from the guiding catheter.

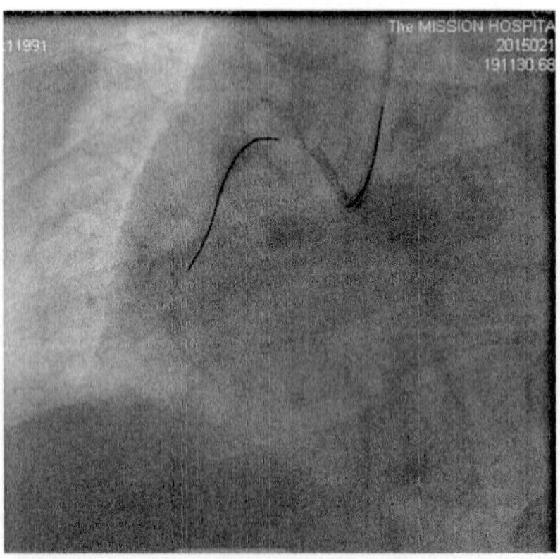

Figure 10.4b(vi) The 5F guide catheter being deep throated over the stent for active guide support in this heavily calcific right coronary artery with ostial disease to get the stent down to the lesion.

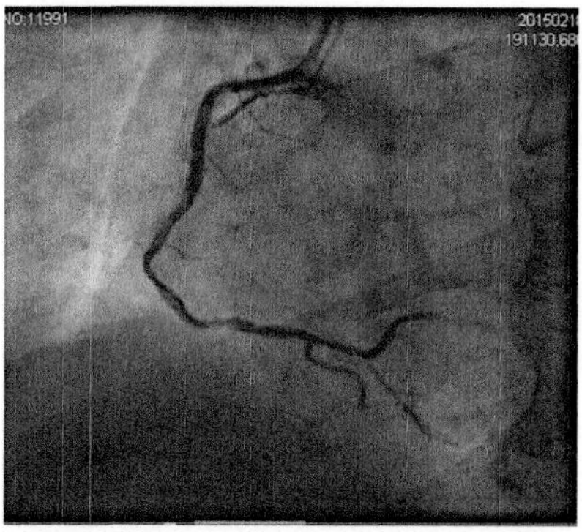

Figure 10.4b(vii) Angiogram after successful stent deployment at culprit lesion shows TIMI-3 flow.

- Rotablation can be done through 5F guiding catheter; but suffers from poor visualization and blood pressure cannot be recorded invasively during the procedure. Hence non-invasive blood pressure recording has to be used. Hence this is not ideal and not recommended.

Slender and sheathless techniques are described separately in Chapter 25 (Slender Percutaneous Coronary Interventions by Transradial Approach).

Radial Artery Anomalies

Abnormalities in forearm arteries such as cubital loops or tortuosities lead to failure in interventions through the radial approach.[14,16,31] Although such loops may be traversed successfully with a 0.014" angioplasty guidewire, it could lead to procedural delays with prolonged fluoroscopy time and radiation exposure to both patient and operator, besides causing grade 3–4 spasms which could lead to procedure failure or necessitate crossover to alternative access. For these reasons and also because the negotiation of such anomalies is fraught with risk of complications such as vessel rupture and extravasation, the European Society of Cardiology, in its consensus document[1] recommends that challenging anatomy must be avoided to minimize the risk of complications and shorten the duration of both procedure and radiation exposure. For this reason, a systematic preliminary angiogram of the arteries of the forearm through the introducer inserted into the radial artery for 2–3 cm has been suggested by some authors.[1,32] However, if abnormal anatomy is found on the preliminary angiogram of the radial artery and the operator decides not to negotiate the same for advancing the catheter up to the coronary arteries, this would lead to a crossover to alternate access. On the other hand, a Pre-Procedure colour Doppler Ultrasound of the Arm Arteries (PPUAA)[17] (see below) is preferable, because, by giving prior information on arterial anomalies of arm arteries (please see Table 10.1), it allows such choice of access to be made even before the radial artery is punctured, thus preventing a crossover to alternate access. However, the use of PPUAA is optional and at the discretion of the operator, based on local logistics and feasibility of performing PPUAA,[17] which varies between centers worldwide.

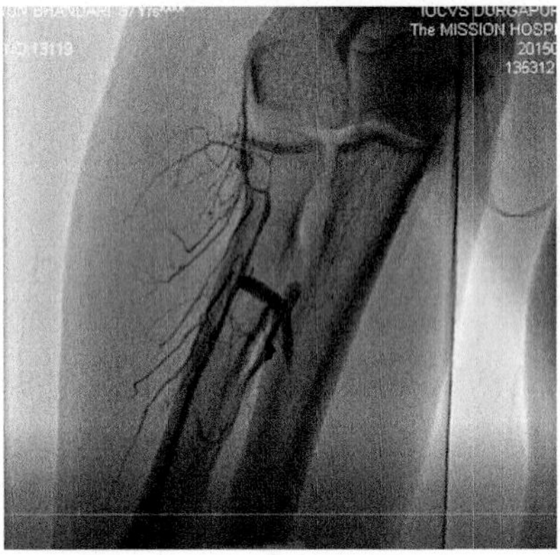

Figure 10.4c(i) Contrast injection in right radial artery shows a cubital loop and high origin rudimentary radial artery (Type 3).[1]

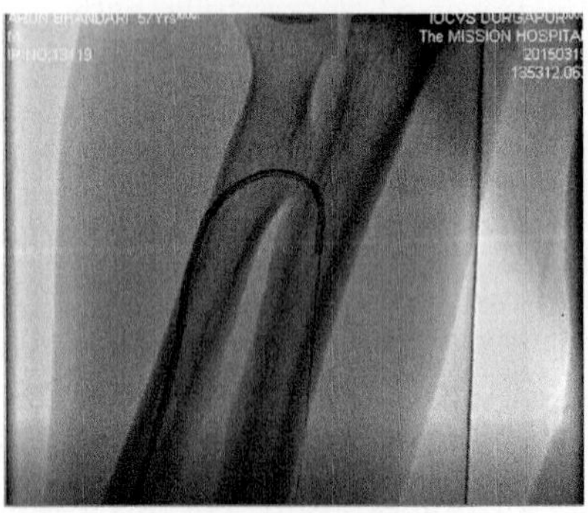

Figure 10.4c(ii) Injection of contrast through right radial artery shows a complex radio-ulnar anastomosis (loop) at 90° to right radial artery.

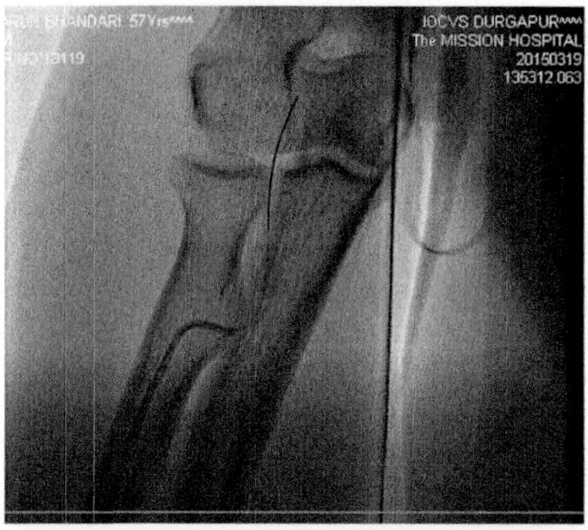

Figure 10.4c(iii) Negotiating wire and catheter across loop.

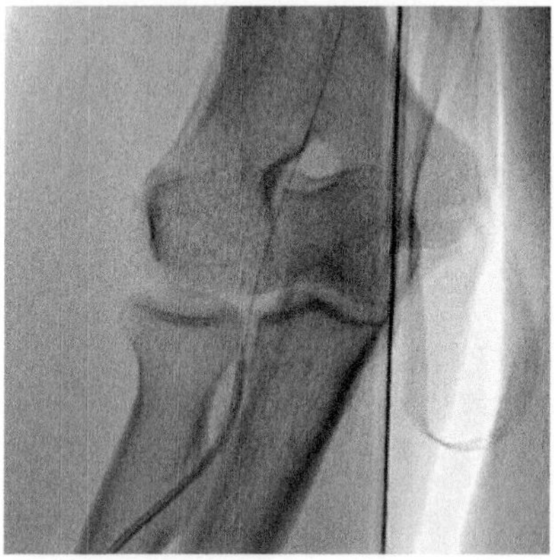

Figure 10.4c(iv) Catheter is withdrawn and angioplasty wire is manipulated upwards across the loop into the brachial artery.

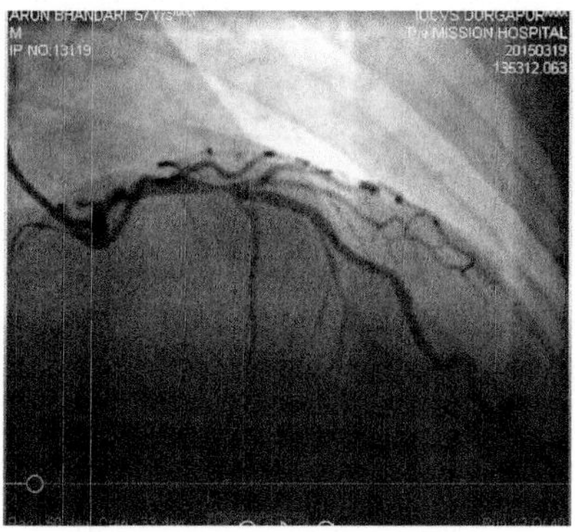

Figure 10.4c(v) The angiogram reveals the culprit vessel; left anterior descending artery (LAD) has a critical 90% stenosis in mid LAD.

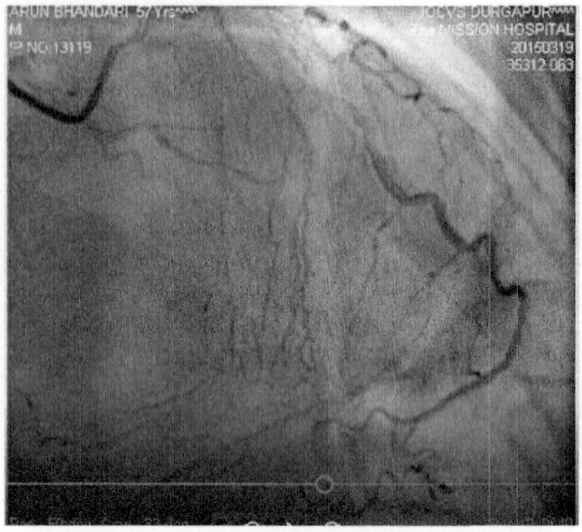

Figure 10.4c(vi) Angiogram showing collaterals to right coronary artery from the culprit vessel, left anterior descending artery (LAD).

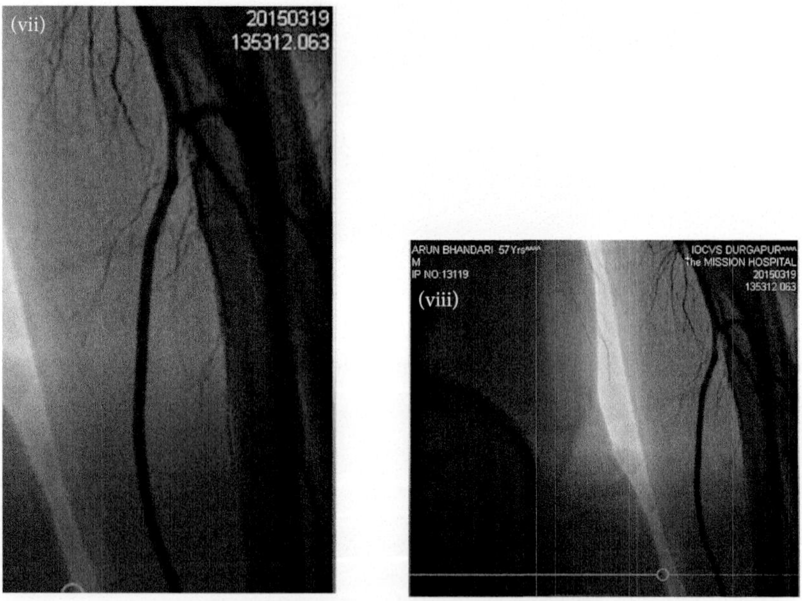

Figure 10.4c(vii–viii) Access through the left radial artery: a high origin of radial from brachial artery.

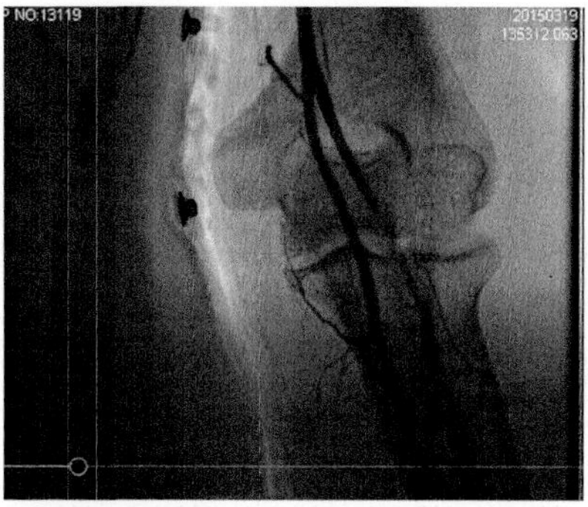

Figure 10.4c(ix) A 6F JL3.0 guiding catheter engages the left coronary artery. Lesion in left anterior descending artery (LAD) is crossed with a BMW wire. Second BMW wire is in first diagonal branch (D1).

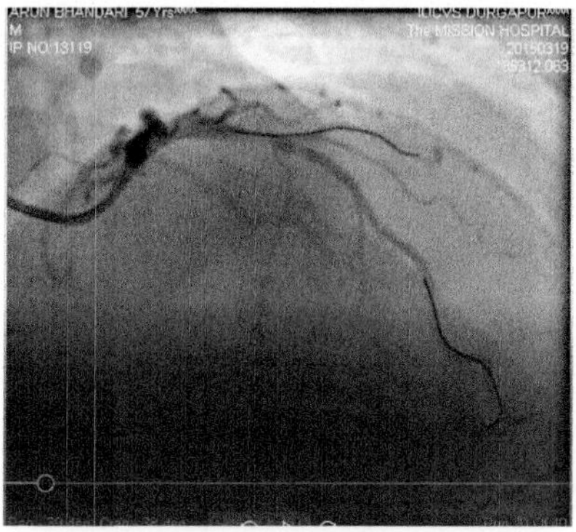

Figure 10.4c(x) Stent deployed at LAD lesion.

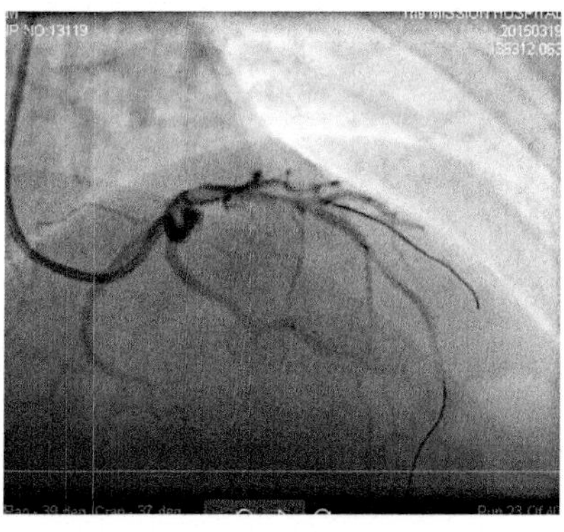

Figure 10.4c(xi) Angiogram after stent deployment.

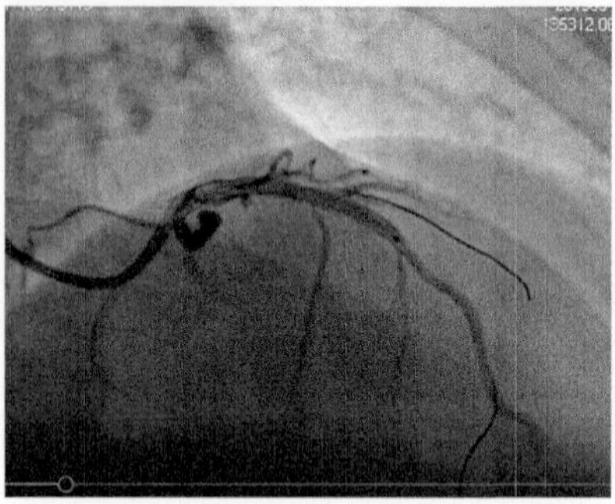

Figure 10.4c(xii) Post-dilatation of stent after wires in LAD and D1 were exchanged.

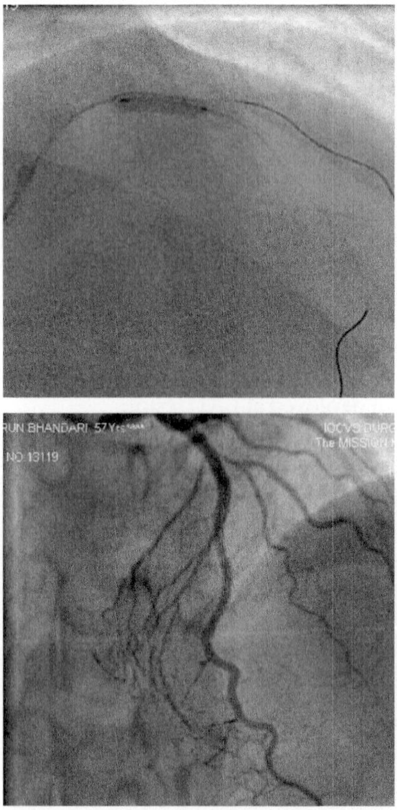

Figure 10.4c(xiii) Final result, TIMI 3 flow.

Table 10.1 Radial Arterial Anomalies Noted on Pre-procedure Ultrasound of Arm Arteries[17]

Anomalies	Radial Artery
Intimal thickness	3.6%
Parallel Radial and Ulnar suggesting possibility of high origin of radial from Brachial or Radioulnar loop or similar anomaly	4.7%
Loop seen at Cubital Fossa	0.9%
Blocked artery	0.6%

- The authors describe a case of acute ST elevation anterior myocardial infarction in a 65-year-old male, who was taken up for primary angioplasty via right radial access. A cubital loop on the right side was traversed using an angioplasty wire [Figure 10.4c(i–iv)]. and a 5F TIG™ catheter was then advanced over it to complete the diagnostic angiogram The angiogram revealed an occluded right coronary artery collateralized from the culprit left anterior descending artery (LAD) which had a mid 90% stenosis [Figure 10.4c(v–vi)]. In order to avoid the risk of trauma and extravasation at the site of cubital loop while advancing a 6F guiding catheter for angioplasty through the cubital loop, the authors decided to access the left radial artery which also was incidentally found to have a high origin from brachial artery [Figure 104c(viii–xi)]. The angioplasty was completed successfully [Figure 10.4c(xi–xiii)] via left radial access.
- There are data from the authors' registry that the failure can be successfully minimized to under 1% with the use of pre-procedure colour Doppler of the arm arteries[17] to identify these anomalies prior to procedure. Having done that, if a loop (Figure 10.5a) is detected on the right side pre-procedurally, an ipsilateral ulnar access can be electively chosen instead of right radial access; or alternatively, a contralateral radial or ulnar access may be chosen. The choice can be made before the patient is taken up for procedure in the catheterization laboratory.
- Cubital loops can be traversed using an angioplasty wire and then the diagnostic catheter tracks over it and a guide catheter tracks on the

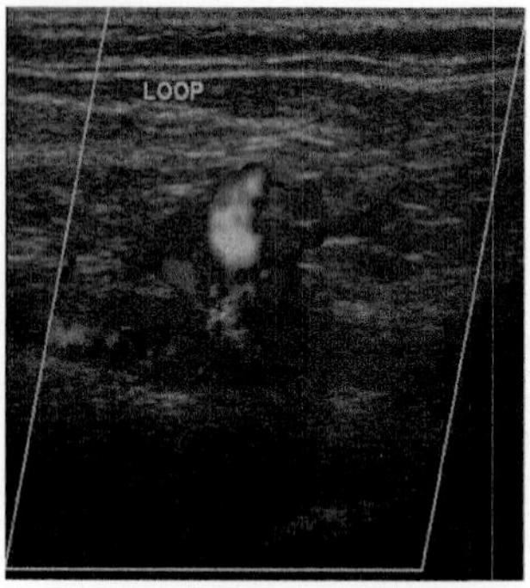

Figure 10.5a Cubital loop on colour Doppler ultrasound. (*Courtesy Dr Sunita Chugh* FMRI, Gurugram, India).

angioplasty wire with a deflated balloon, which can then be utilized for the angioplasty as illustrated in Figures 10.5b to 10.5h

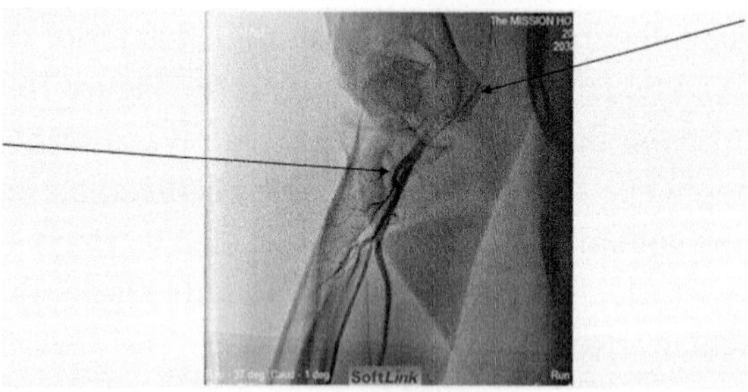

Figure 10.5b A test injection of contrast shows a type-3 high origin of radial from brachial artery with radio-ulnar anastomosis (cubital loop) and a rudimentary radial artery[1] where the wire had tracked.

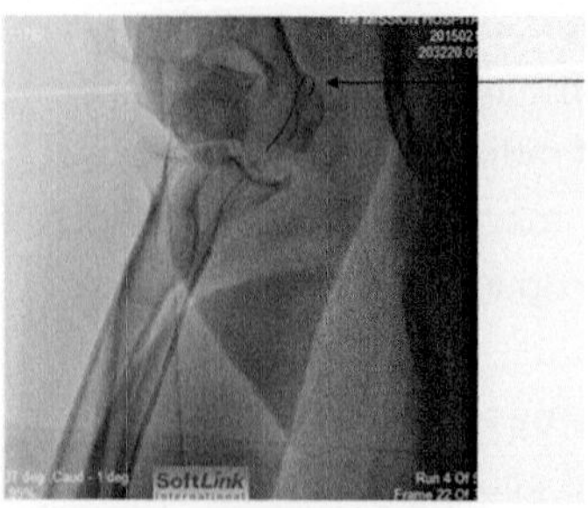

Figure 10.5c An angioplasty (balance middle weight) wire is used to cross the loop into brachial artery.

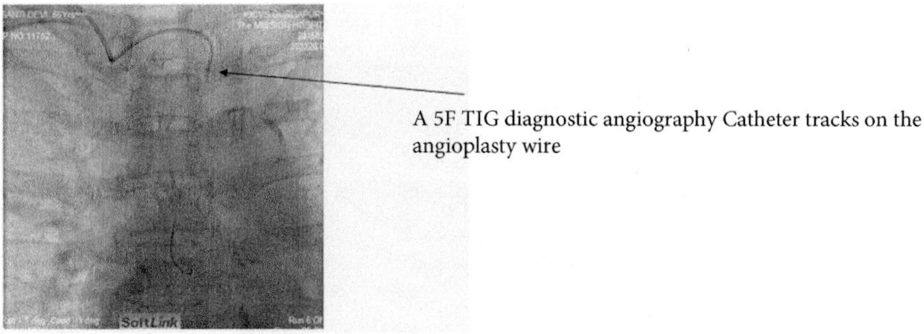

Figure 10.5d A TIG™ catheter then tracks over the angioplasty wire crossing subclavian tortuosity.

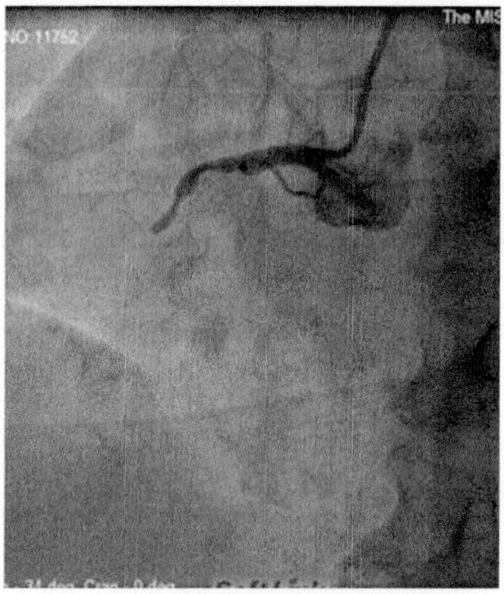

Figure 10.5e The TIG™ catheter hooks the right coronary artery which shows total occlusion.

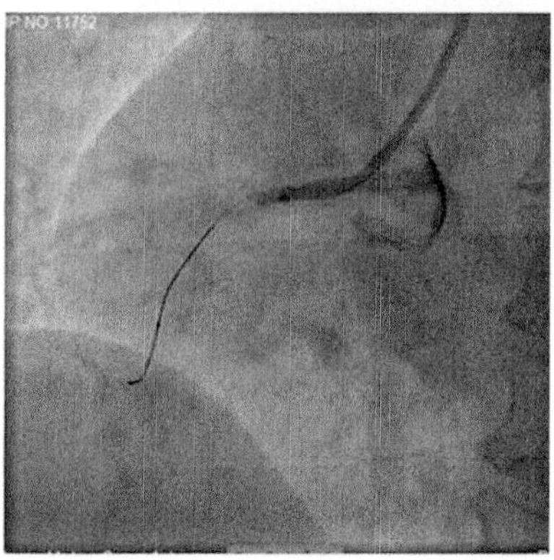

Figure 10.5f The TIG™ catheter is exchanged for a JR 3.5 Guiding catheter over a 0.035", 360 cm J tip Dacron woven angiographic guidewire. The occluded Shepherd's crook right coronary artery is being crossed using a 1.5-mm balloon over it to enhance support.

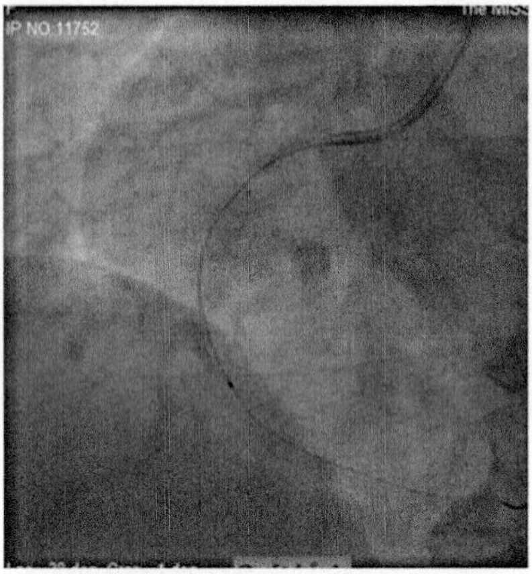

Figure 10.5g After crossing the occlusion, an Export thrombosuction catheter in use to remove thrombus to visualize the distal vessel for choosing appropriate stent size after pre-dilatation with the 1.5 mm angioplasty balloon used to support the wire to cross the occlusion failed to show distal vessel.

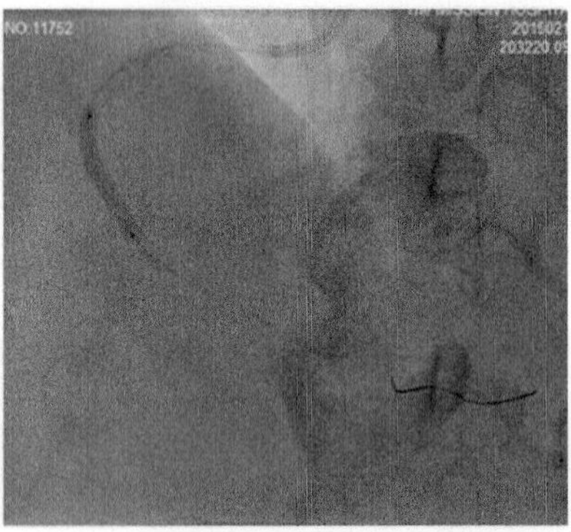

2 stents deployed, post-dilatation in progress

Figure 10.5h Two stents deployed successfully.

- With the described fallacies of Allen's and Barbeau's tests,[33] it stands to reason to perform a pre-procedure Doppler[34] to detect an upstream obstruction in the radial artery or an occlusion of radial or ulnar artery.
- However if the same is not feasible, then contrast injections may be done after gaining radial access, to look for a stenosis upstream in radial artery.[1,32]

- Contrast injections can be more painful in upper limb arteries; hence, it is preferable to dilute non-ionic contrast to minimize patient discomfort.
- A 0.014" angioplasty wire can be used to successfully negotiate acute bends [Figure 10.5h(i–ii)] or tortuosities in the radial artery [Figure 10.5h(iii–v)] and a stenosis with spasm in radial artery at bifurcation of brachial artery [Figure 10.5h(vi–viii)].

Technique of pre-procedure ultrasound of the arm arteries (PPUAA)[17] and ultrasound guided puncture is described separately in the Chapter on *Role of pre-procedure ultrasound of arm arteries.*

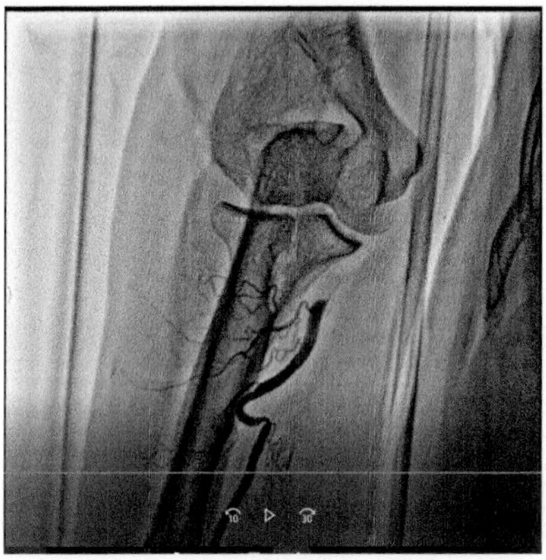

Figure 10.5h(i) Acute bend in radial artery.

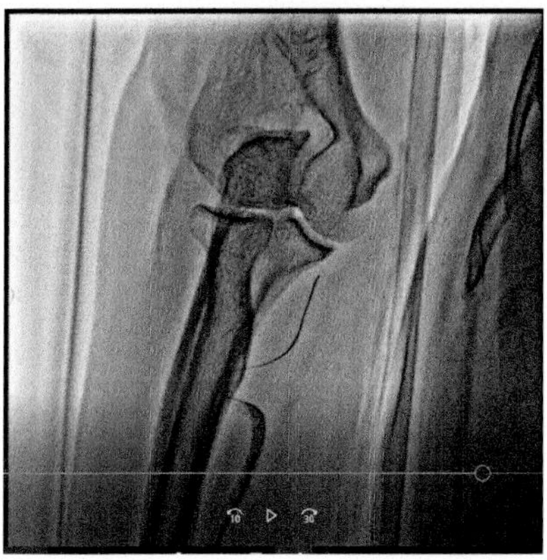

Figure 10.5h(ii) Angioplasty wire to cross acute bend in radial artery.

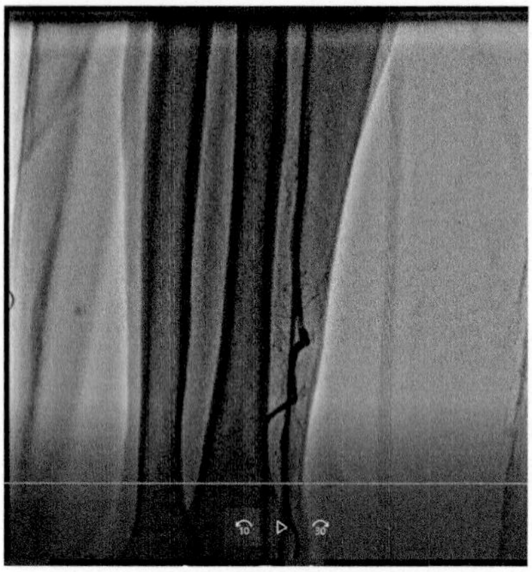

Figure 10.5h(iii) Tortuous radial artery with spasm crossed by angioplasty wire.

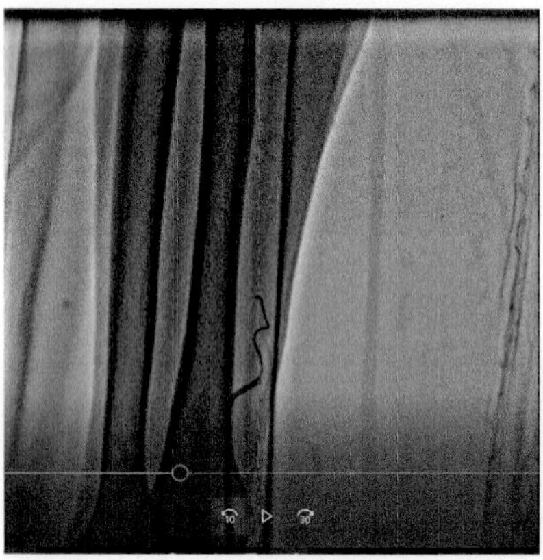

Figure 10.5h(iv) Angioplasty wire crosses the segment of tortuosity and spasm in radial artery.

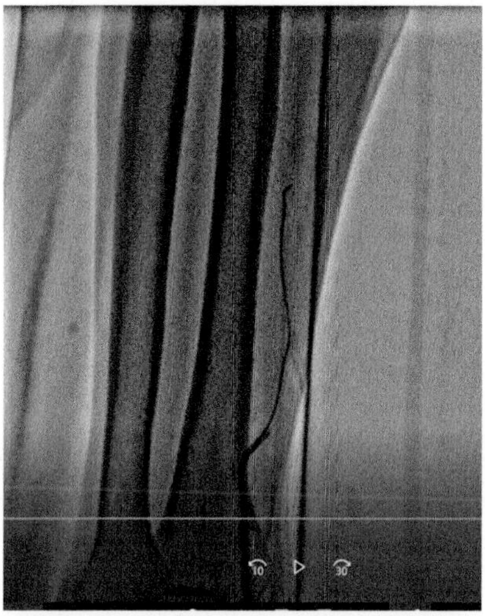

Figure 10.5h(v) Angioplasty wire crossed the segment of tortuosity and spasm in radial artery.

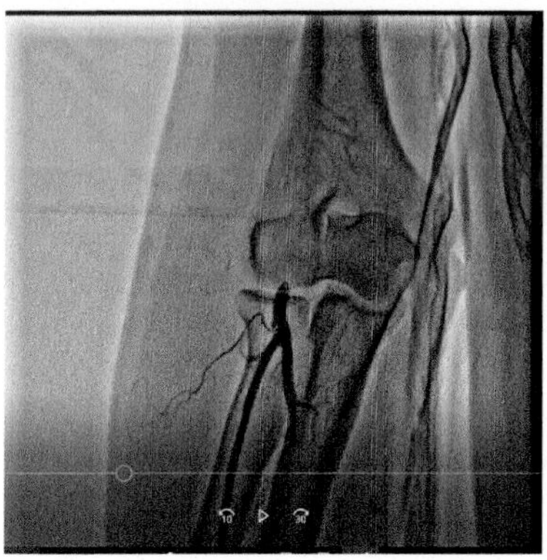

Figure 10.5h(vi) A stenosis and spasm at origin of the radial at bifurcation of brachial artery.

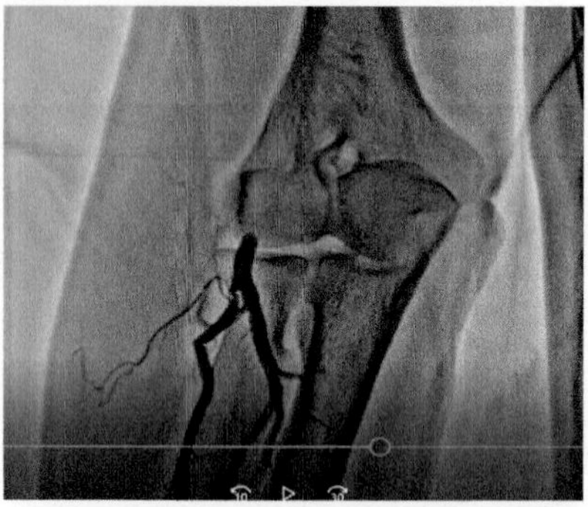

Figure 10.5h(vii) Stenosis and spasm at origin of the radial artery is visualized with contrast injection in left anterior oblique projection.

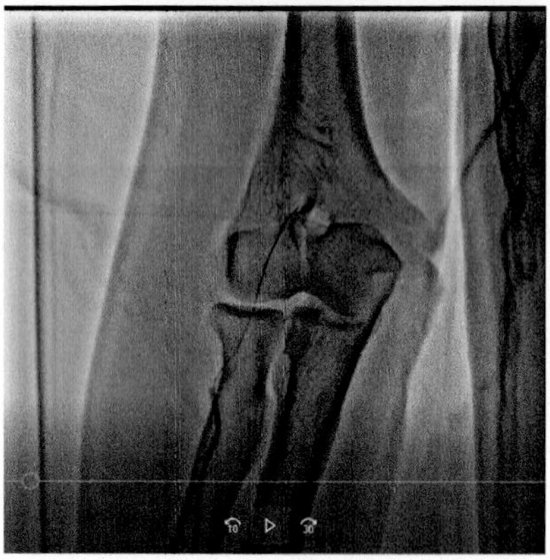

Figure 10.5h(viii) Stenosis and spasm at origin of the radial artery was crossed using an angioplasty wire.

Traversing the Subclavian Artery

- *Proceeding from the subclavian artery to the aorta*: In crossing the subclavian tortuosities [Figure 10.5i(i–iii)], asking the patient to take a deep breath enables the guidewire to flip into the ascending aorta. Big breath of the patient also helps if the angiographic guidewire tracks into descending aorta [Figure 10.5i(iv)]. The angiographic guidewire alone or with catheter is withdrawn from the descending aorta while the patient takes a big breath; the assembly or guidewire flips into ascending aorta [Figure 10.5i(v–vii)].

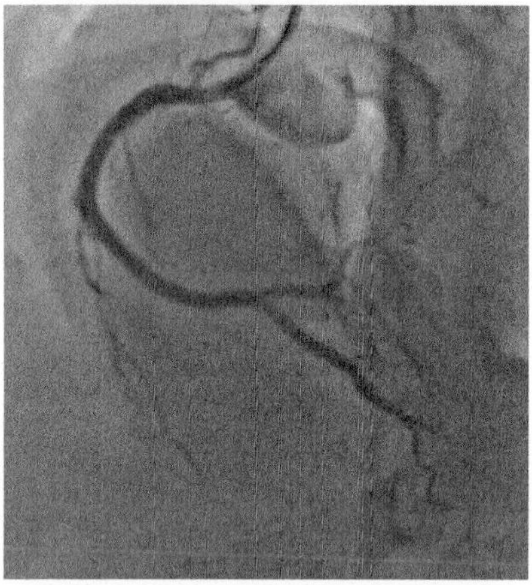

Figure 10.5i Final TIMI 3 flow.

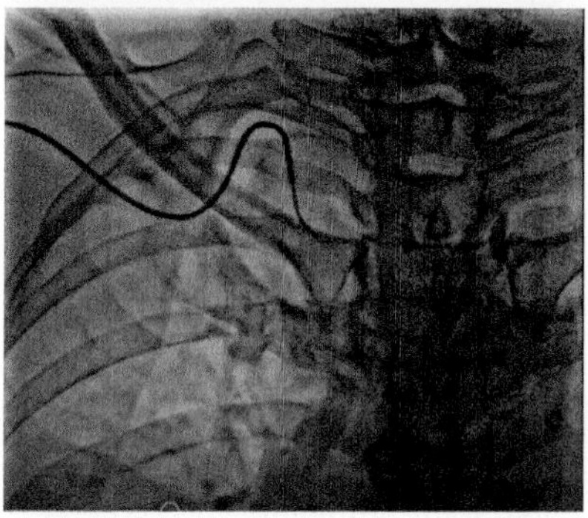

Figure 10.5i(i) Angiographic guidewire crossing the subclavian tortuosity.

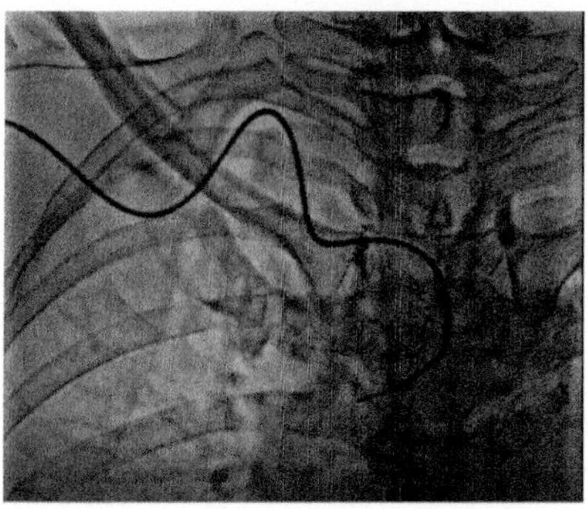

Figure 10.5i(ii) Asking the patient to take a deep breath enables the guidewire and catheter to flip into the ascending aorta.

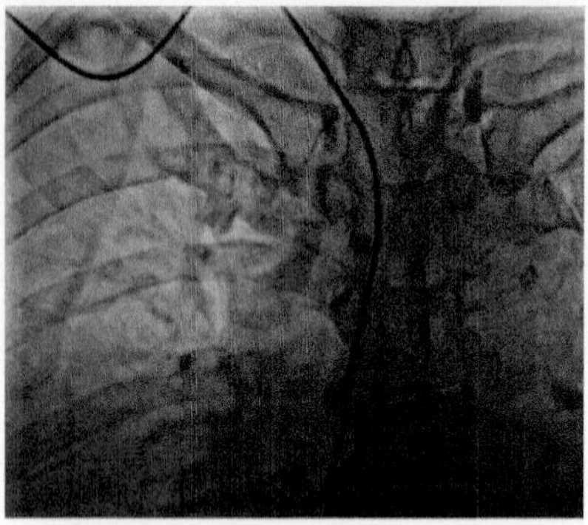

Figure 10.5i(iii) Gentle advancement of guidewire brings the catheter down further in ascending aorta.

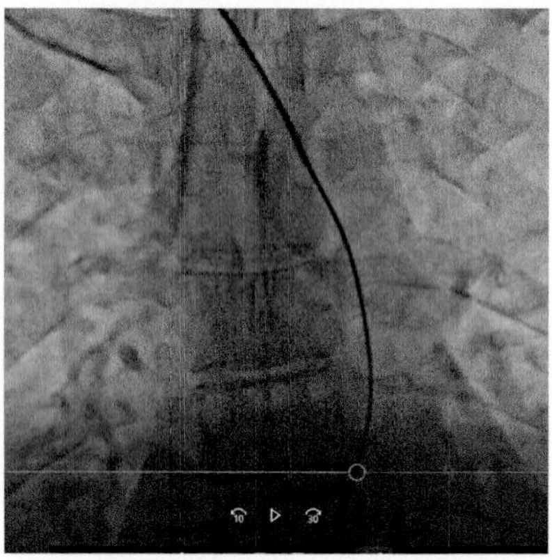

Figure 10.5i(iv) Angiographic guidewire and catheter track into descending aorta.

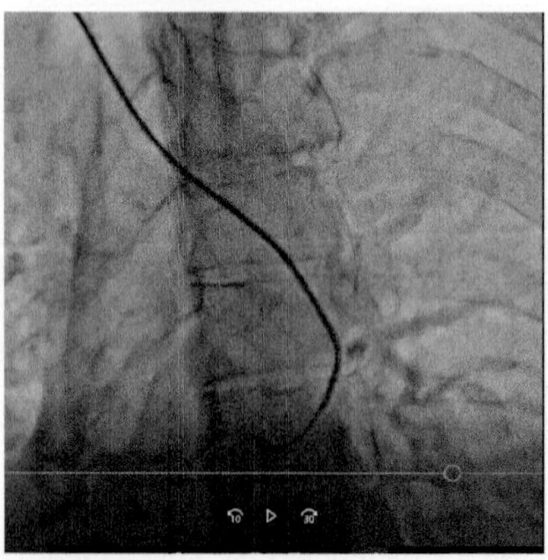

Figure 10.5i(v) The angiographic guidewire and catheter assembly is withdrawn from the descending aorta while the patient takes a big breath.

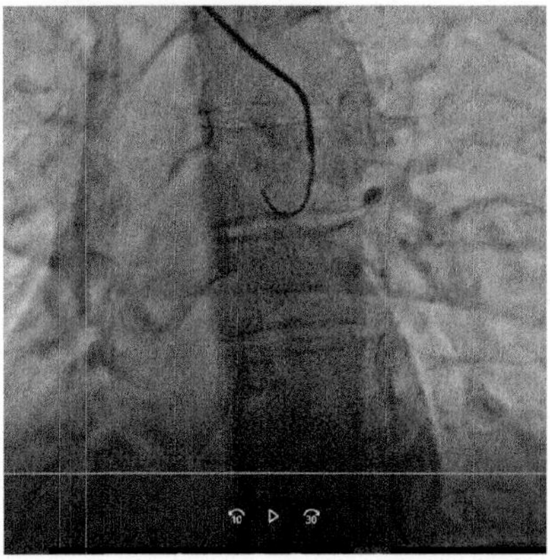

Figure 10.5i(vi) The assembly flips into ascending aorta.

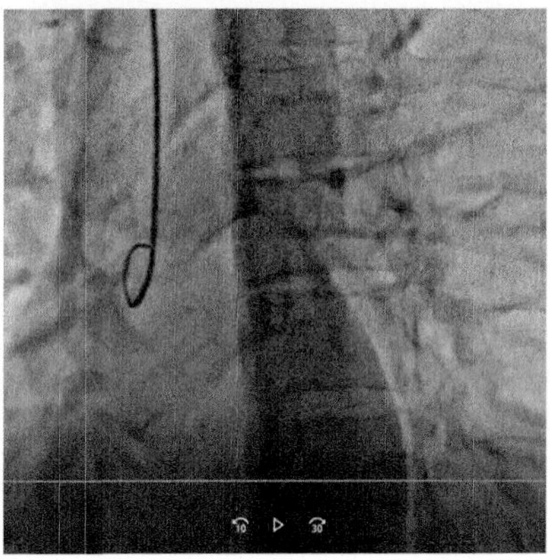

Figure 10.5i(vii) Wire being withdrawn from the catheter before engaging the coronary artery.

- Tortuosity is found more commonly in the right compared to the left subclavian artery (1:9.5).[35] A 0.035" Terumo Glidewire® helps negotiate the subclavian/brachiocephalic tortuosities. A big breath by the patient is often additionally very helpful in traversing the tortuosity [Figure 10.5j(i–iii)].

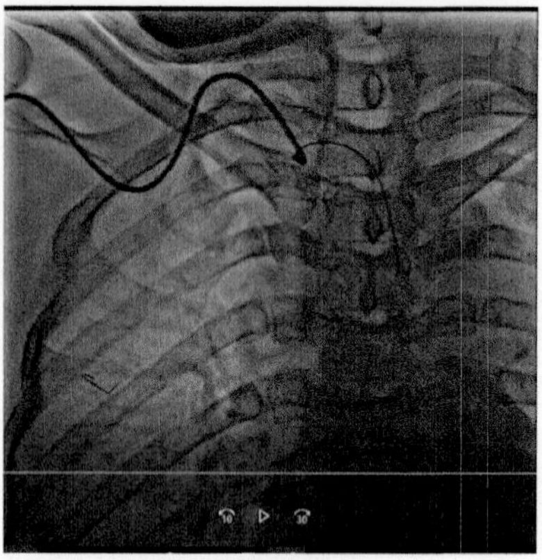

Figure 10.5j(i) Tortuosity in right subclavian artery being crossed using a 0.035-inch Terumo Glidewire®.

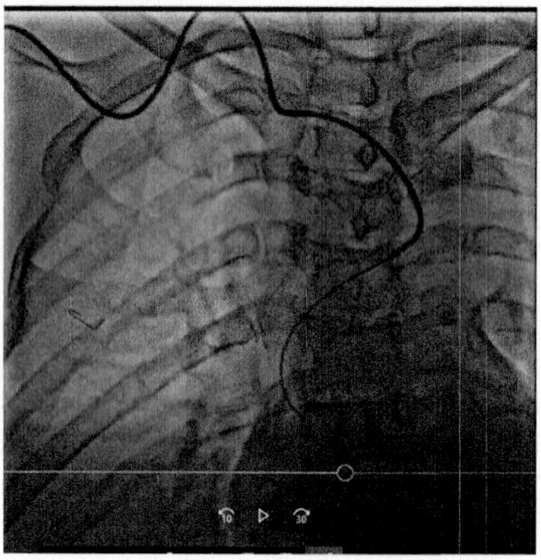

Figure 10.5j(ii) With the help of big breath, the catheter and wire reach the ascending aorta.

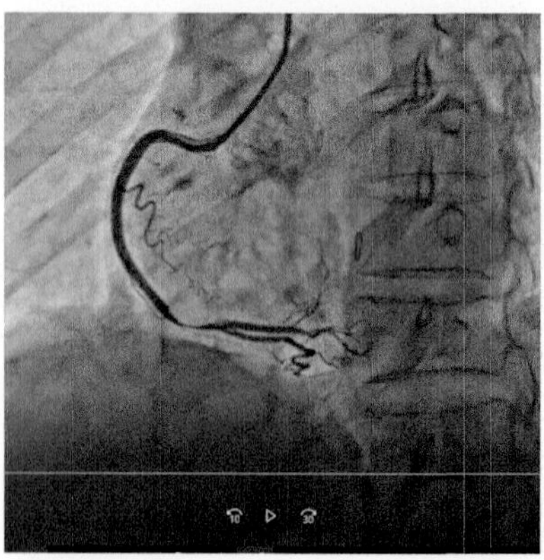

Figure 10.5j(iii) The right coronary artery is engaged, which shows the critical distal culprit lesion.

A left-sided approach is preferred in the elderly (>75 years) due to a lower incidence of tortuosity on this side.[18] Again, strokes, though rare, are more common in the elderly; it may be related to more catheter manipulations in presence of severe tortuosity of right subclavian artery. In a propensity match analysis, left radial access (LRA) was associated with a significant decrease in in-hospital stroke (OR: 0.52, 95% CI: 0.37–0.82; p = 0.005)[36] (please see Chapter 11).

- An angioplasty wire like BMW or Runthrough wire can also be used to traverse tortuous subclavian arteries [Figure 10.5k(i–ii)] sometimes, with a 360° loop in subclavian, or when a terumo glidewire fails to negotiate the tortous subclavian artery. Asking the patient to take a big breath along with manipulation of the diagnostic catheter facilitates movement of the wire and catheter down from tortuous subclavian artery to the ascending aorta [Figure 10.5k(iii–iv)]. Stiff guidewires such as Amplatz, on the other hand, can cause concertina and increase resistance to passage of a catheter.

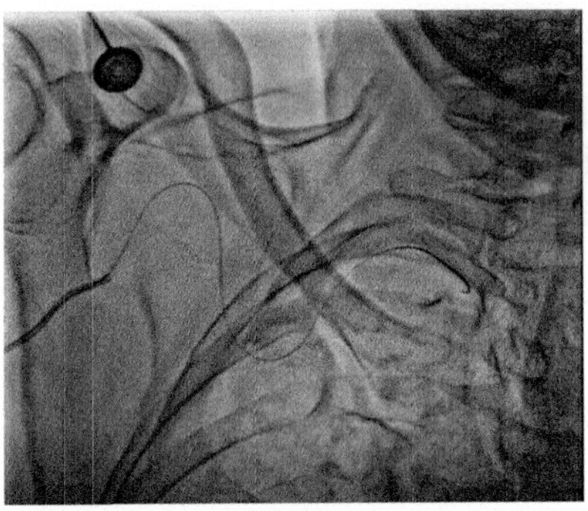

Figure 10.5k(i) Angioplasty wire used to cross subclavian tortuosity.

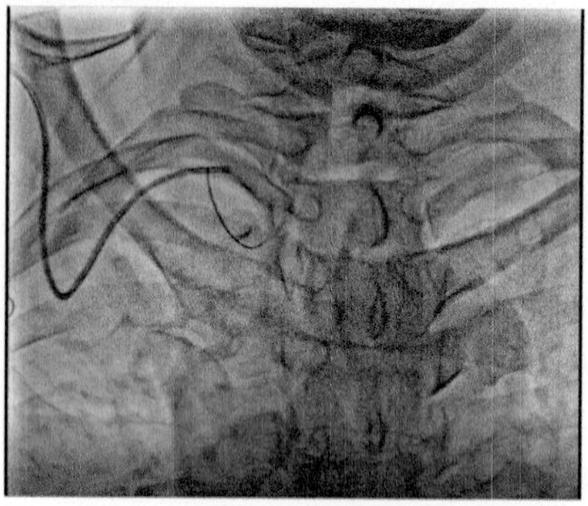

Figure 10.5k(ii) The diagnostic catheter tracks over the angioplasty wire.

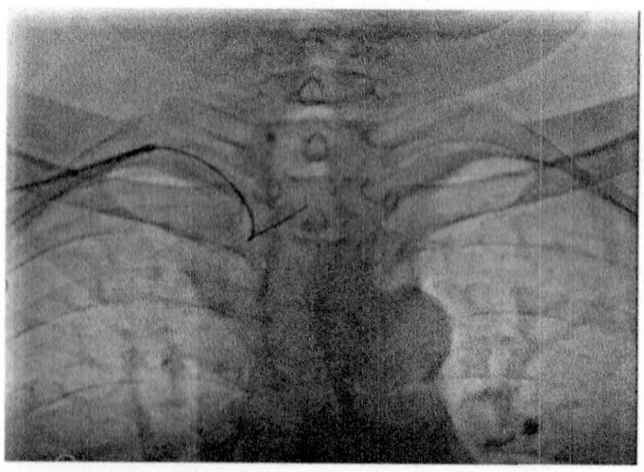

Figure 10.5k(iii) A big breath is used to flip the wire from the subclavian artery towards the brachiocephalic artery.

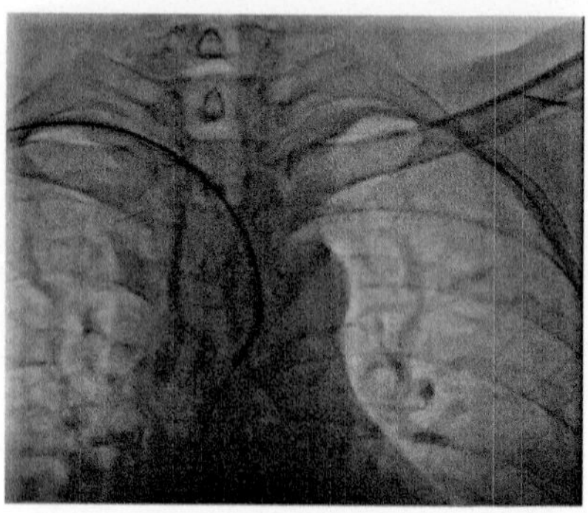

Figure 10.5k(iv) Catheter descends on angioplasty wire to ascending aorta.

- To save time, as in an acute myocardial infarction setting, when taking a guiding catheter over an angioplasty wire, the authors recommend tracking it on a deflated angioplasty balloon to minimize the razor effect of the edge of the guiding catheter (Figure 10.5l). The same wire and balloon could then be used for angioplasty after engaging the coronary artery. The authors do not use an inflated balloon at the tip of the guiding catheter as described in balloon assisted tracking (BAT), because of serious concerns[37] regarding risk of extravasation and post-procedure radial occlusion.

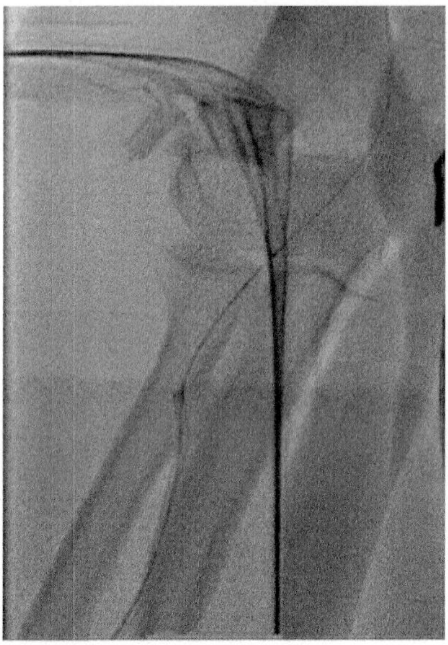

Figure 10.5l Taking a guide catheter over an angioplasty wire. The guide tracks on a deflated angioplasty balloon.

- A subclavian or brachiocephalic artery, though patent, may appear blocked as flow may not be seen with a retrograde test injection done through a catheter traversing a tortuous subclavian artery (Figure 10.6a). A test injection of contrast through the catheter in right anterior oblique view showed a part of the right brachiocephalic artery leading to the arch of aorta (Figure 10.6a(i)). A 0.0014" angioplasty wire enters the descending aorta (Figure 10.6b) and is deflected on from the aortic knuckle (Figure 10.6b(i)) to reach the ascending aorta (Figure 10.6b(ii)). The same was used to cross the occlusion in right coronary artery (RCA) (Figure 10.6c), after engaging the RCA with a JR4, 6F guide catheter which tracked over the angioplasty wire with a deflated balloon. Export™ thrombosuction was done (Figure 10.6d). Following thrombosuction (Figure 10.6e) and stenting of the culprit lesion, Figure 10.6f shows final TIMI-3 flow in RCA, and a right anterior oblique view showed that the right subclavian artery was actually patent (Figure 10.6f(i)).

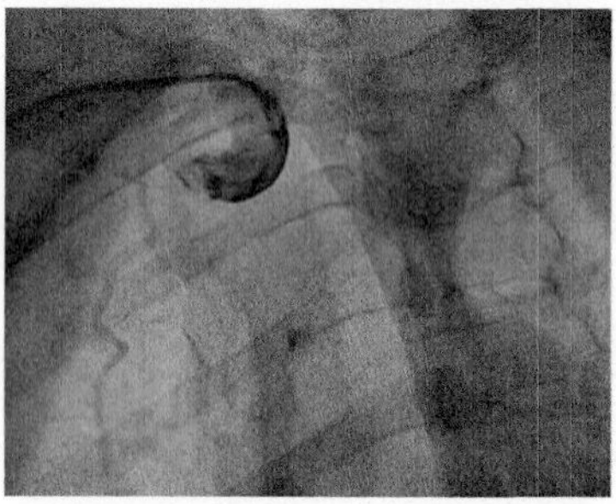

Figure 10.6a Subclavian artery appears blocked with a test injection done through a catheter traversing a tortuous subclavian artery.

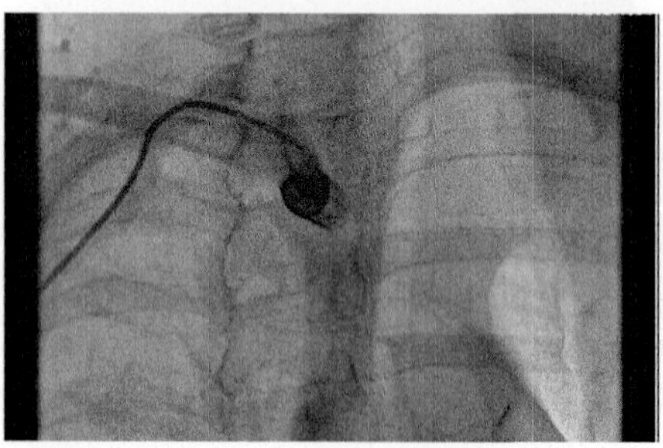

Figure 10.6a(i) A test injection of contrast through the catheter in right anterior oblique view showed a part of the right brachiocephalic artery leading to the arch of aorta.

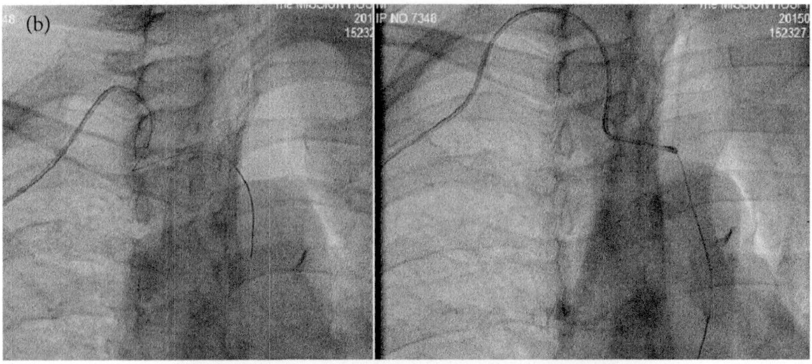

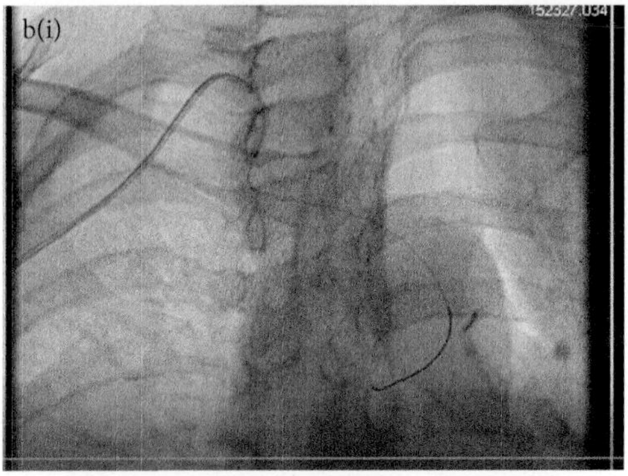

Figure 10.6b, 10.6b(i) and 10.6b(ii) A 0.0014" angioplasty wire was used to enter the ascending aorta.

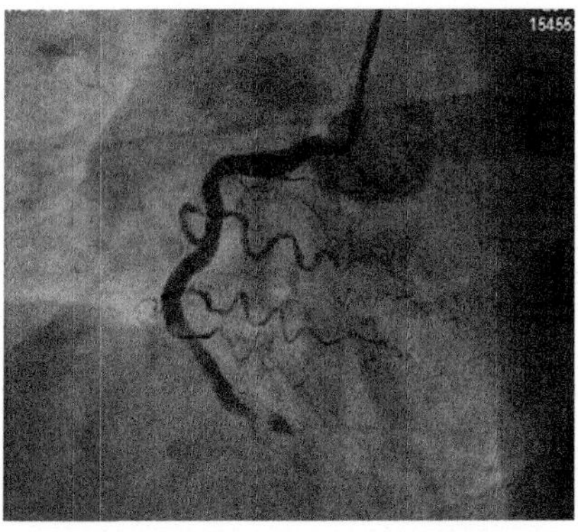

Figure 10.6c Occlusion in right coronary artery (RCA). A JR4, 6F guide catheter used to engage the RCA. Same angioplasty wire is used to cross the lesion.

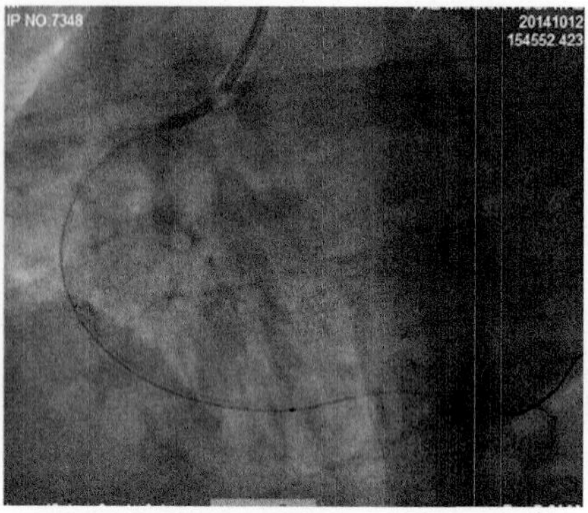

Figure 10.6d Export thrombosuction.

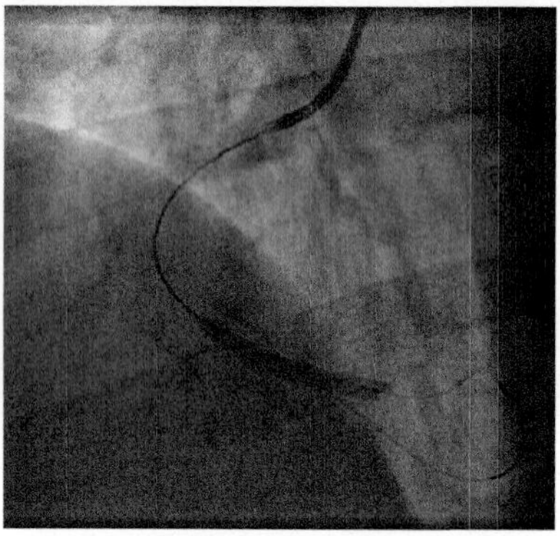

Figure 10.6e Post-thrombosuction stent deployment.

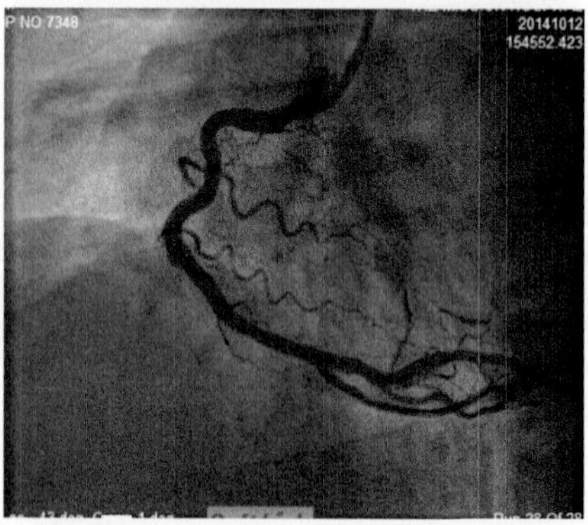

Figure 10.6f Final TIMI 3 flow in right coronary artery (RCA) after stenting of the culprit lesion.

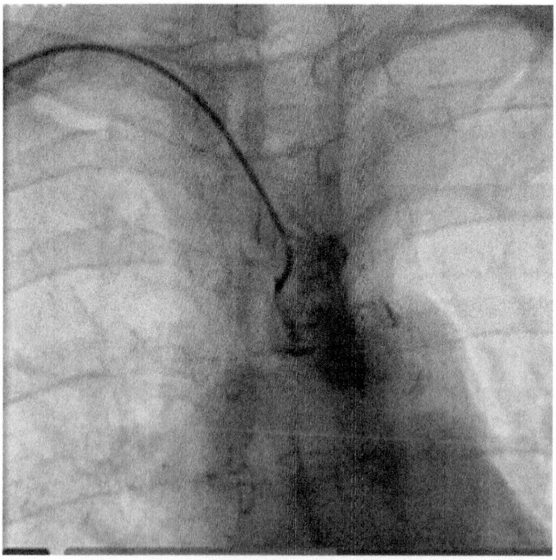

Figure 10.6f(i) Contrast injection through catheter in right anterior oblique view shows retrograde contrast flow into brachiocephalic.

- Retro-oesophageal right subclavian artery (RORSA): Sometimes, the wire and catheter tracks from the right brachiocephalic artery directly to descending aorta. In these situations, the usual big breath fails to bring the wire and catheter into ascending aorta. Depending on site of origin of subclavian artery in a RORSA, a test injection of contrast through the catheter may help visualize the arch of aorta (Figure 10.7) or descending aorta (Figure 10.7a). A 0.035" or 0.038" Terumo Glidewire® can be deflected off the aortic knuckle (Figure 10.7b) into ascending aorta. The catheter then tracks over it and the angiogram is completed (Figure 10.7c-i). A JL 3.0 (Figure 10.8a, 10.8b(i–viii)) or XB3.0 [Figure 10.8c (i–vii)] guide catheter may be preferred to engage the left coronary artery in patients with RORSA for PCI to left circumflex artery (LCX). Figure 10.8c(i) and Figure 10.8c(ii) are images of left coronary artery performed using a TIG diagnostic catheter showing an occluded LCx as the culprit in a patient with acute myocardial infarction.

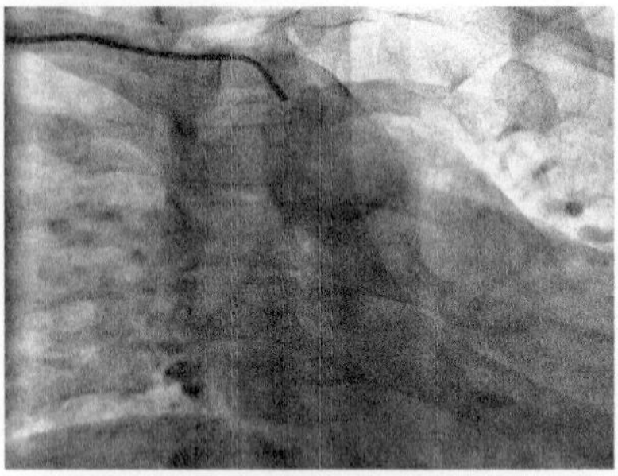

Figure 10.7 Injection of contrast through the catheter to visualize the origin of retro-oesophageal right subdavian artery from the arch of aorta.

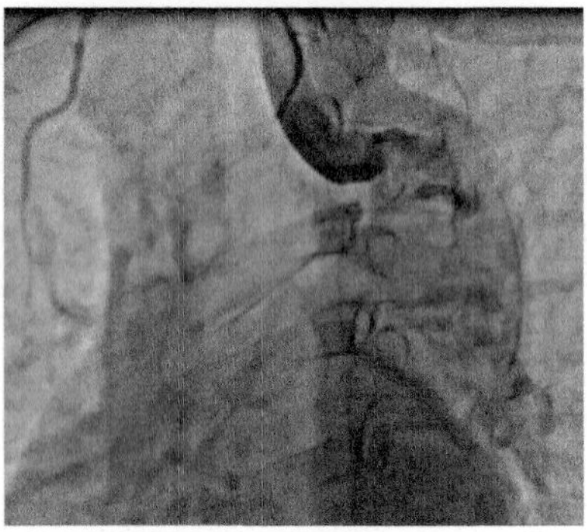

Figure 10.7a Injection of contrast through the catheter to visualize the origin of retro-oesophageal right subclavian artery from descending aorta.

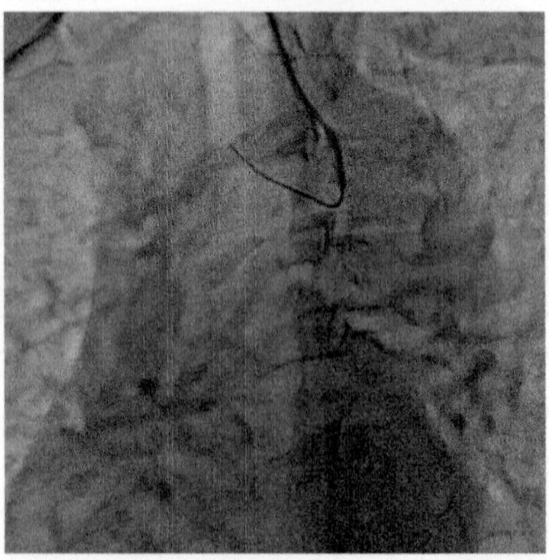

Figure 10.7b Terumo Glidewire® being deflected of the aortic knuckle tortuous ascending aorta.

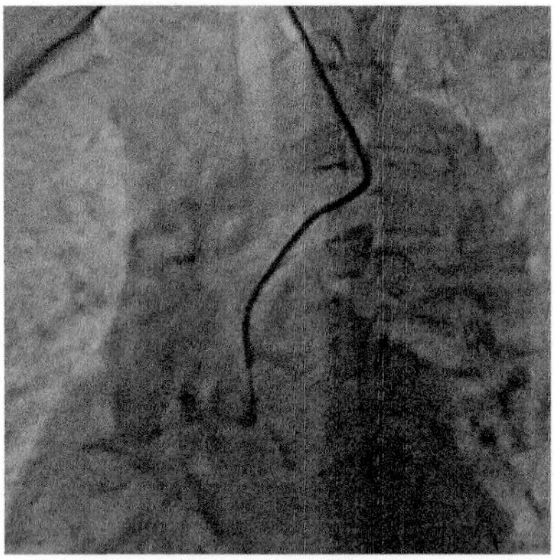

Figure 10.7c Catheter tracks on it.

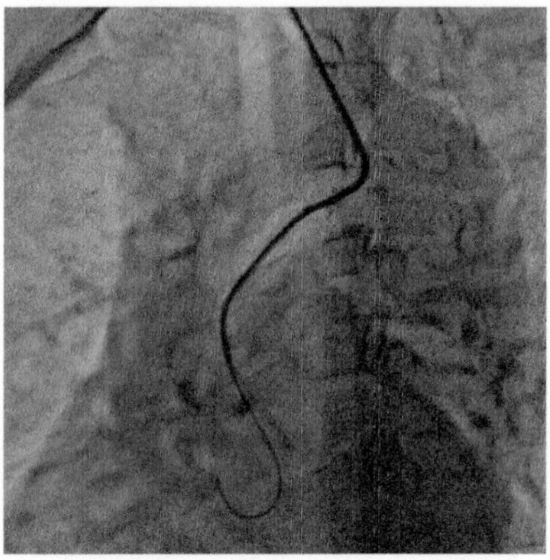

Figure 10.7d Catheter tracks further into ascending aorta.

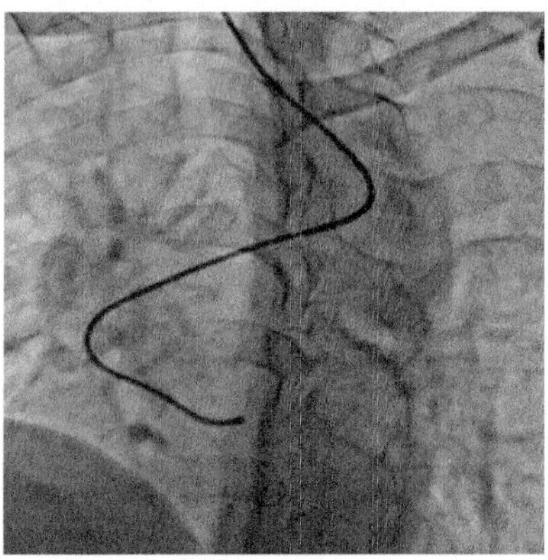

Figure 10.7e Catheter in ascending aorta.

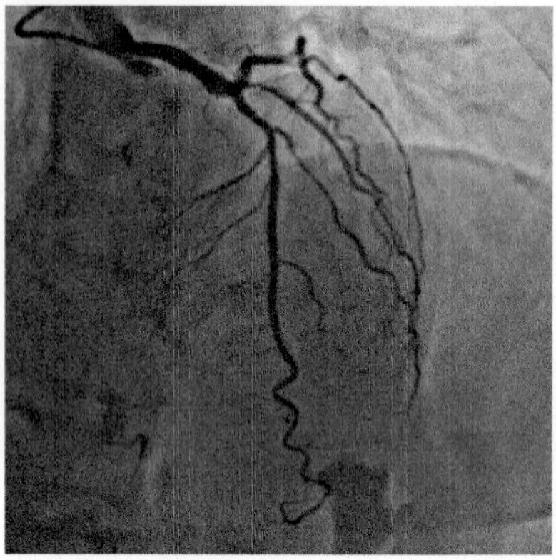

Figure 10.7f Judkins Left 3.5 diagnostic catheter engages the left coronary artery.

(g)

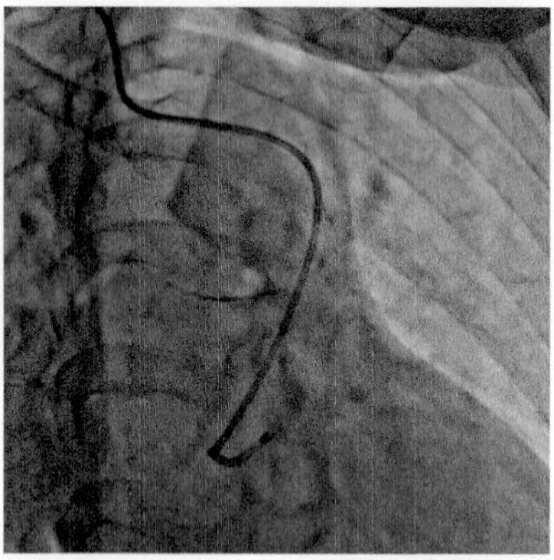

(h)

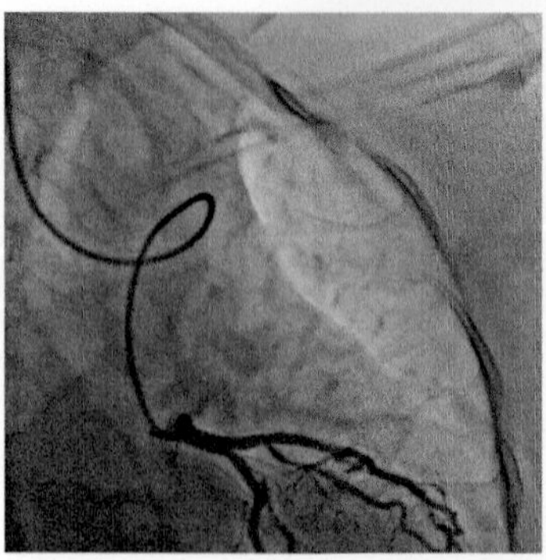

(i)

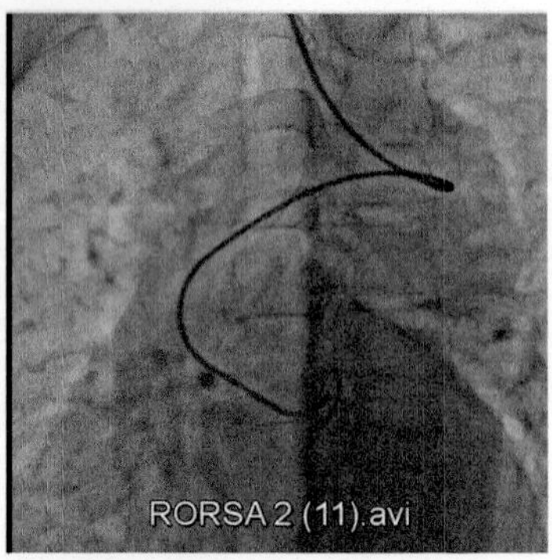

Figures 10.7g–i Show shape of left coronary catheter in various views.

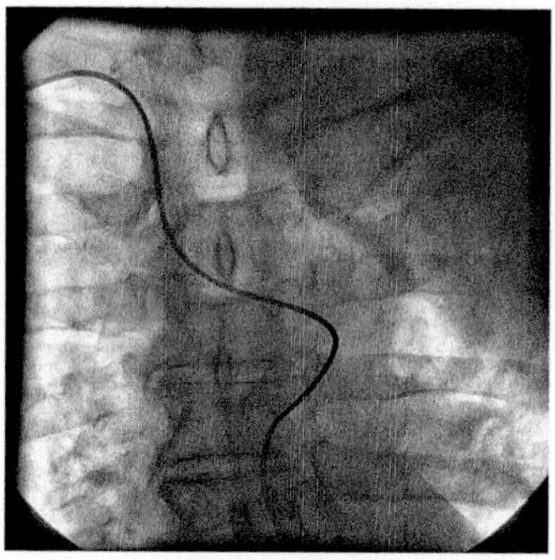

Figure 10.8a Catheter appearance in a retro-oesophageal right subclavian artery as seen during an angiogram.

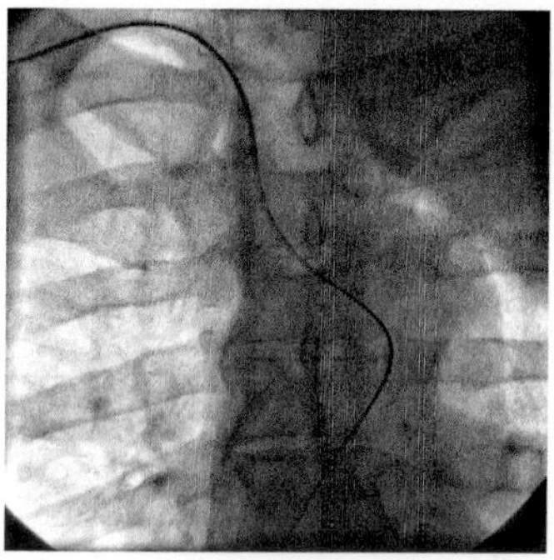

Figure 10.8b(i) Shows a 6F JL 3.0 guide catheter traversing the retro-oesophageal right subclavian artery into the ascending aorta.

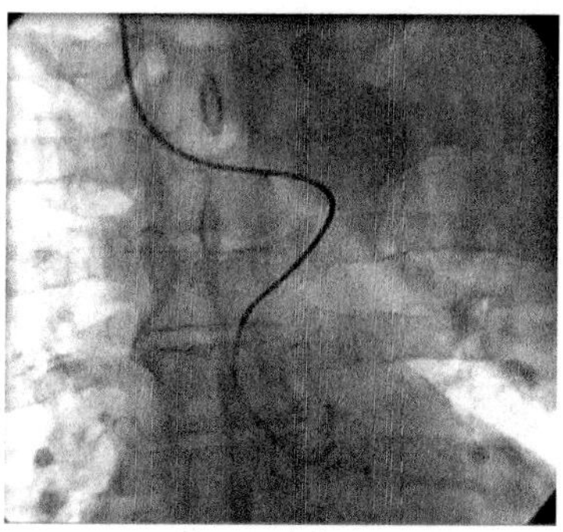

Figure 10.8b(ii) The 6F, Judkins Left (JL) 3.0 guiding catheter engages the left coronary artery.

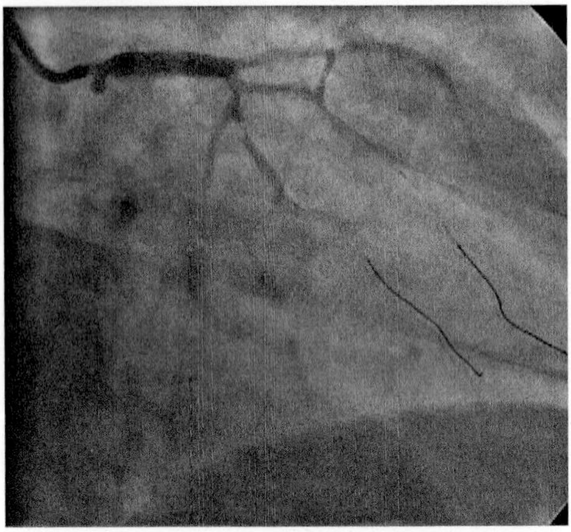

Figure 10.8b(iii) Second balanced middle weight (BMW) wire inserted in first obtuse marginal branch to enhance guide support.

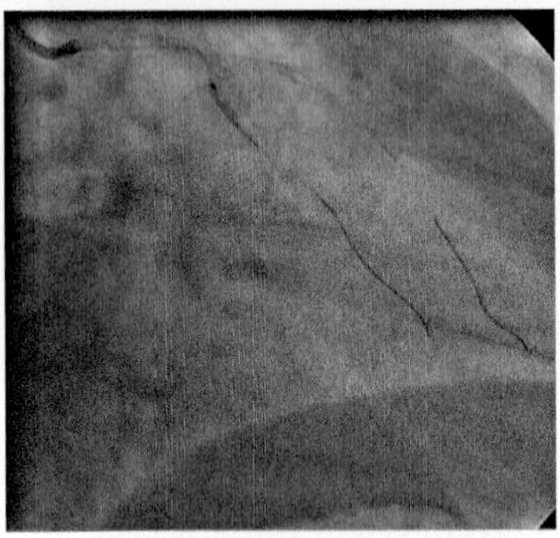

Figure 10.8b(iv) Pre-dilataion balloon in position at lesion in second obtuse marginal branch (OM2).

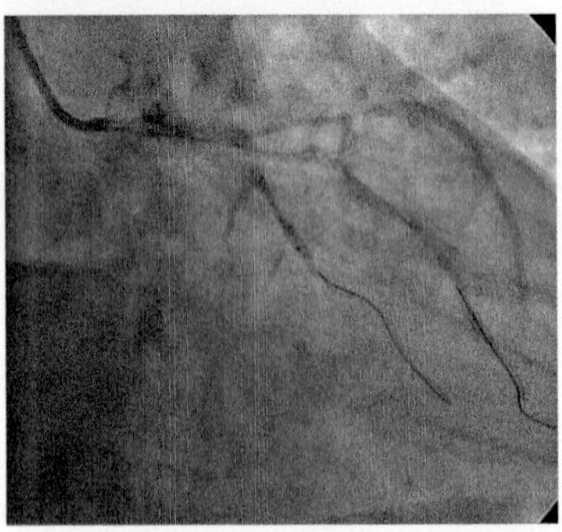

Figure 10.8b(v) Lesion predilated.

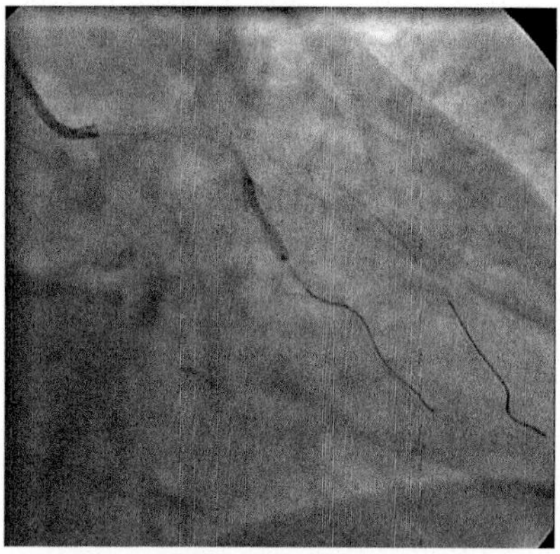

Figure 10.8b(vi) Stent in position at lesion in second obtuse marginal branch (OM2).

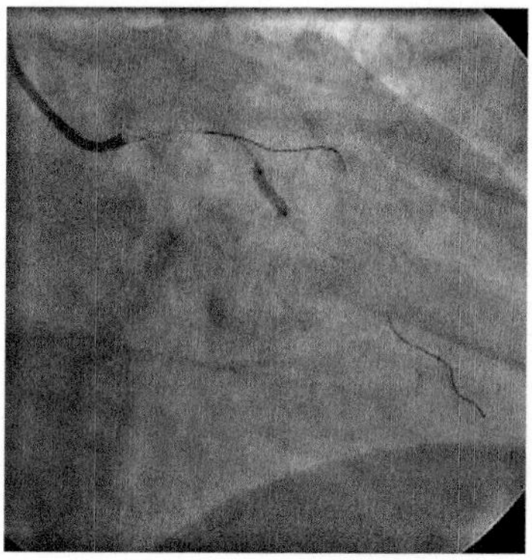

Figure 10.8b(vii) Post-dilatation of stent.

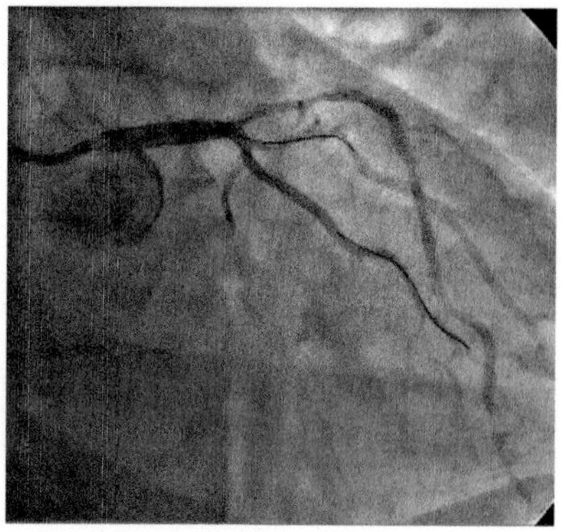

Figure 10.8b(viii) Final.

Figure 10.8b(i–viii) Case of angioplasty to second obtuse marginal branch (OM2) of left circumflex artery in a patient with retro- oesophageal right subclavian artery (RORSA). A 6F, Judkins Left (JL) 3.0 guiding catheter used to hook the left coronary artery. Second balance middle weight (BMW) wire inserted in first obtuse marginal branch to enhance guide support.

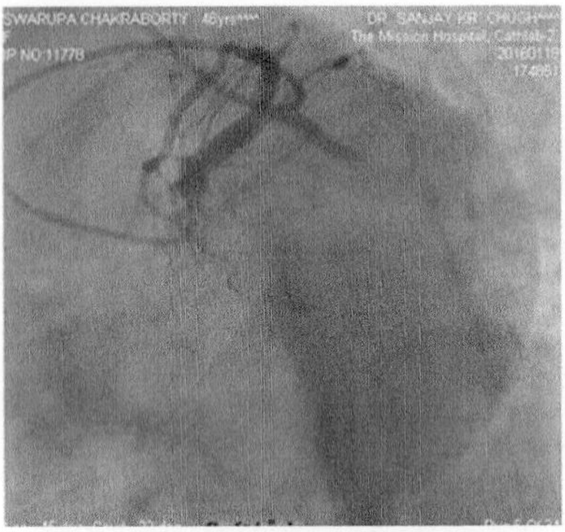

Figure 10.8c(i) Shape of TIG™ catheter in retro-oesophageal right subclavian artery in left anterior oblique with caudal view; note the occluded culprit vessel LCX in a patient with acute myocardial infarction taken up for primary angioplasty.

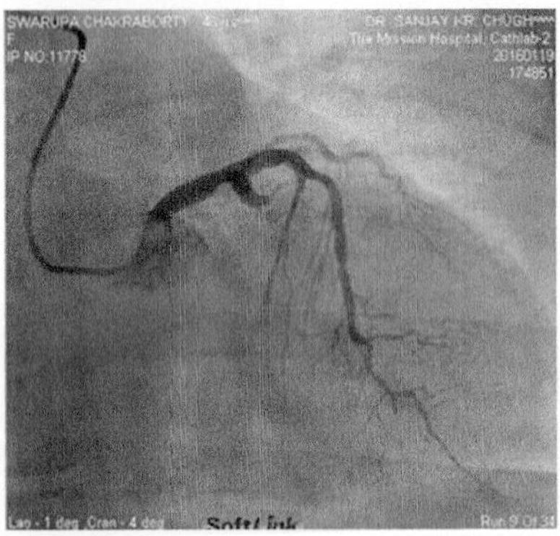

Figure 10.8c(ii) Shape of TIG™ catheter in retro-oesophageal right subclavian artery in anteroposterior cranial view.

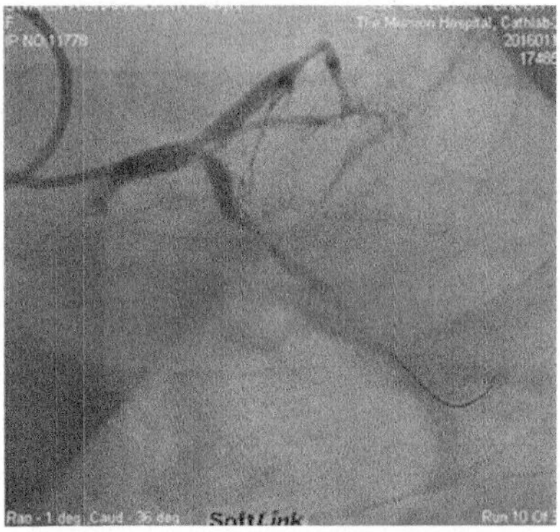

Figure 10.8c(iii) A balance middle weight (BMW) wire across the occluded left circumflex artery (LCX) for primary angioplasty.

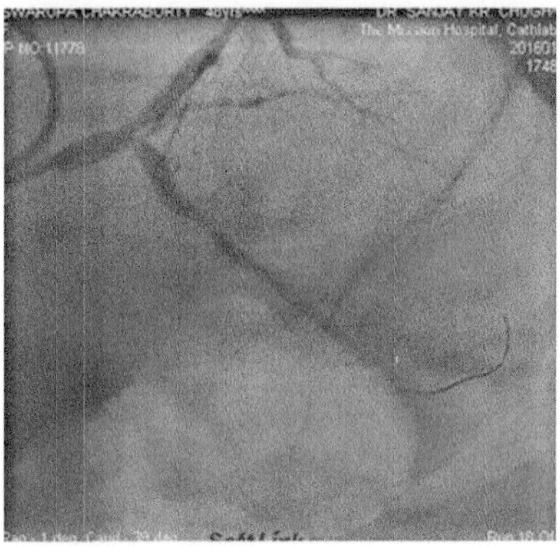

Figure 10.8c(iv) Balloon pre-dilatation.

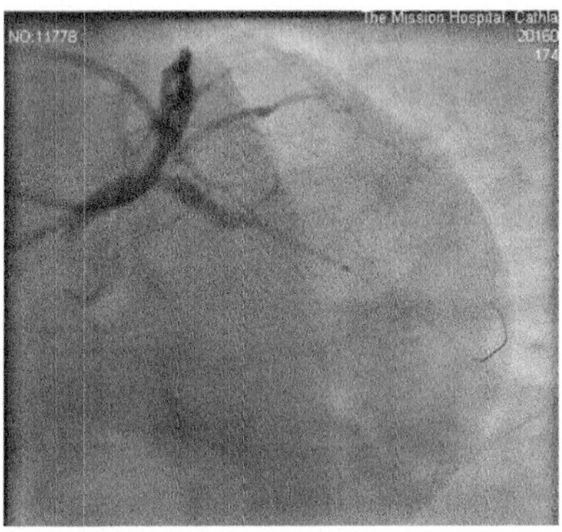

Figure 10.8c(v) Stent in position for implantation.

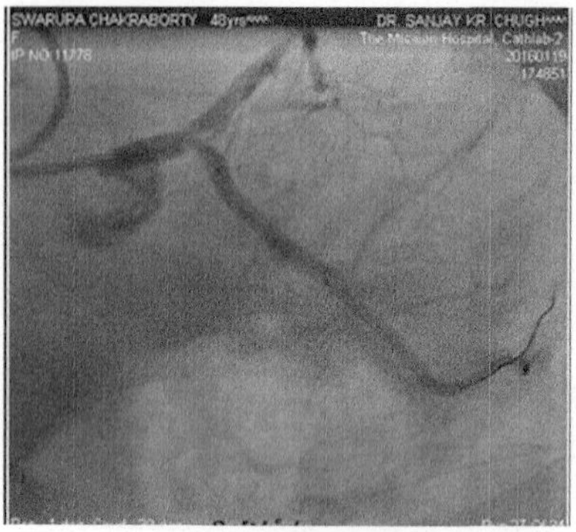

Figure 10.8c(vi) Post-stent.

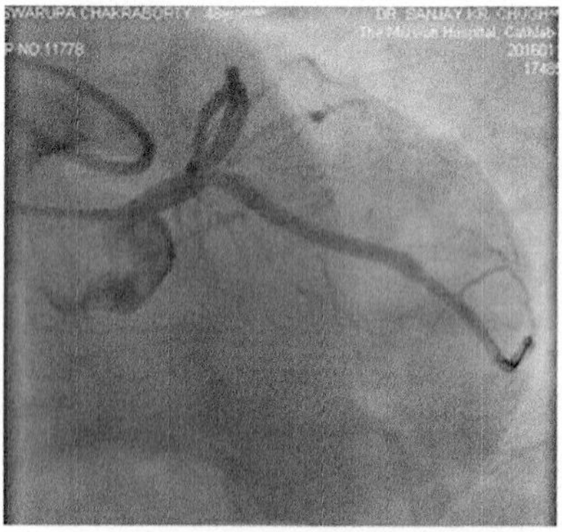

Figure 10.8c(vii) Final angiogram showing TIMI 3 flow.

- For RCA, in patients with RORSA, a JR3.5 is commonly successful in engaging it.

Some operators avoid going through a RORSA by converting to left radial access for angioplasty once a RORSA is identified during diagnostic coronary angiography from the right radial artery.

Engaging the Coronaries: Selection of Diagnostic and Guiding Catheters

Choice of Catheter for Diagnostic Coronary Angiograms

- For right radial access, a TIG™ catheter is preferred and was reported to be the most popular diagnostic catheter used by operators in

India (Table 10.2).[38] If right coronary artery (RCA) cannot be hooked with TIG™, then JR or AR is used. If TIG™ selectively engages the left circumflex artery (LCX), as in a wide left main coronary artery, then a JL 3.5 diagnostic catheter is used for engaging the left anterior descending artery (LAD).[39]

- Catheter curve size selection can be done on the basis of height of patient (bigger curves for taller patients) and aortic root assessed on skiagram of chest and/or echocardiogram.[18,40]
- For left radial access, Judkins left (JL) and right (JR) catheters are preferred. TIG™ may also be used. A smaller curve of JL catheter fits better when using left radial access compared to curve size required from right radial access.[18,40]
- As in patients with RORSA, distal origin of brachiocephalic from aortic arch or severe tortuosities in the brachiocephalic or subclavian arteries also affect catheter curve size. As described above, smaller curve of JL or extra back up (XB™) often fits better in these situations.[18,40]
- Choice of shape and size of catheter curve for left coronary artery[18,40] also depends on take-off of coronary artery and abnormality of aortic root such as in horizontal aorta or unfolding of aorta.

Choice of Guiding Catheter

- In the worldwide practice survey, EBU3.5 was found to be the most commonly used catheter for left coronary artery (Table 10.2).[38] For interventions in left anterior descending artery (LAD), a JL or EBU or

Table 10.2 Choice of Guiding Catheters[40]

Guiding Catheter	Vessel
JL/XB/EBU	Left Anterior Descending Artery
XB/AL/JL/EBU	Left Circumflex Artery
JR/AR/AL	Right Coronary Artery
AR/AL/MPA2	Saphenous Vein Graft
IMA	Left Internal Mammary Artery

Judkins Right (JR), Judkins Left (JL), Extra Back up (EBU), Amplatz Left (AL), Amplatz Right (AR), Back-up (XB), Internal Mammary Artery (IMA)

XB is preferred. For LCX, again, an XB, EBU, JL or AL may be used. An XB or EBU are most commonly used.[18]

- Choice of GC curve size, as for choice of diagnostic catheter (please see above), is based on height of patients (bigger curves for taller patients), and aortic root which can be assessed on echocardiogram.[18]
- The shape and curve size of left coronary guiding catheter, depends not only on whether LAD or LCX is to be tackled, it also depends on the take-off of the coronary artery as described above for diagnostic catheters. An Amplatz or extra-backup is preferred for a higher take-off of left coronary artery.
- As in patients with RORSA, in patients who have a distal origin of brachiocephalic from aortic arch or severe tortuosities in the brachiocephalic or subclavian arteries, a smaller curve of JL, EBU or XB fits better in these situations. In a patient with RORSA, usually a JR hooks the RCA. In an anomalous RCA with RORSA, an AR2 guide catheter may be required to hook the RCA [Figure 10.8d(i–xi)].

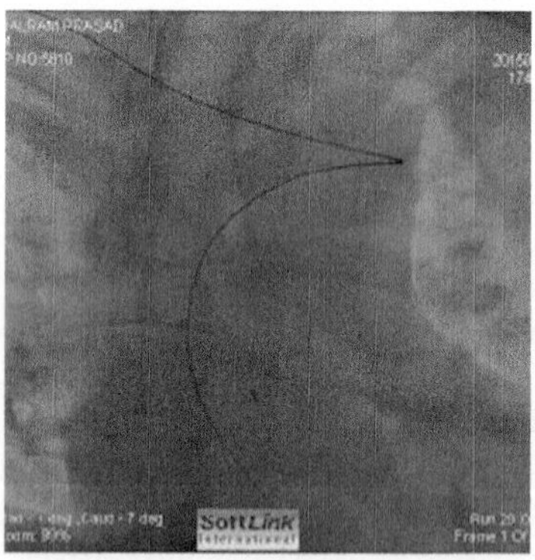

Figure 10.8d(i) Shape of guidewire in retro-oesophageal right subclavian artery seen in left anterior oblique view.

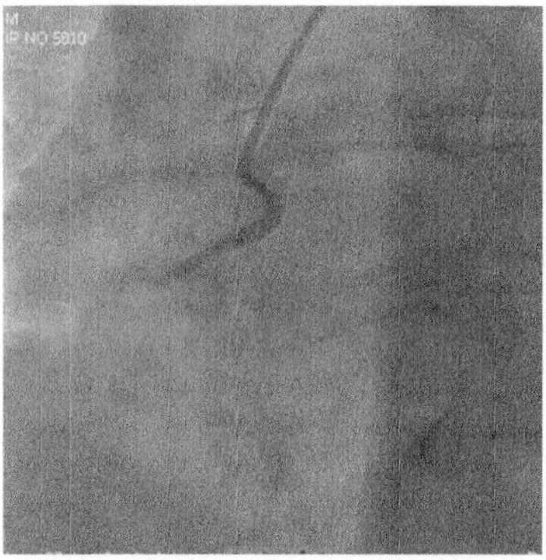

Figure 10.8d(ii) An Amplatz Right (AR)2 guide catheter hooks the anomalous right coronary artery.

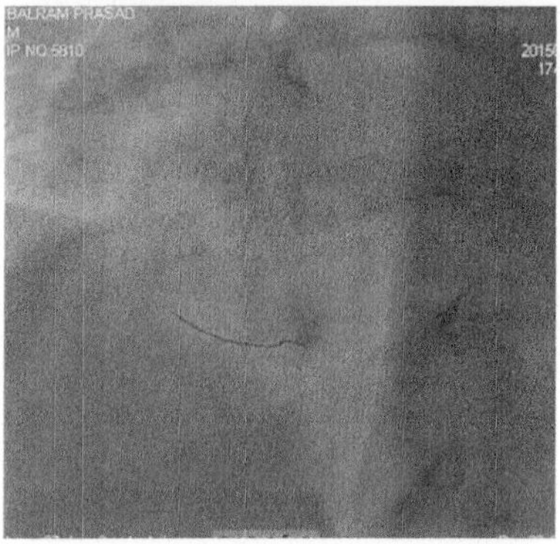

Figure 10.8d(iii) A balance middle weight (BMW) wire in right coronary artery.

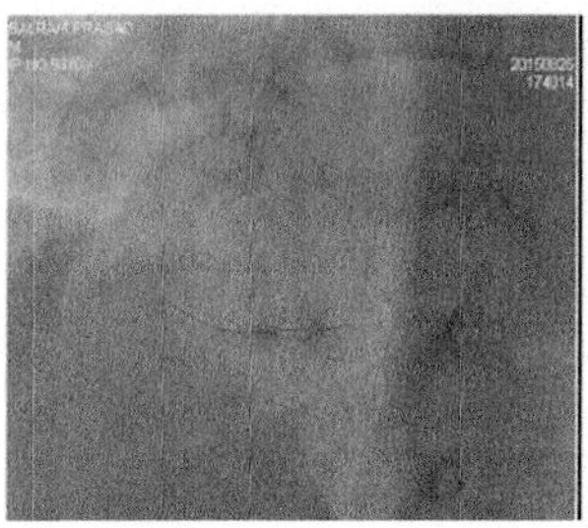

Figure 10.8d(iv) A balance middle weight (BMW) wire crosses thrombotic occlusion in distal right coronary artery.

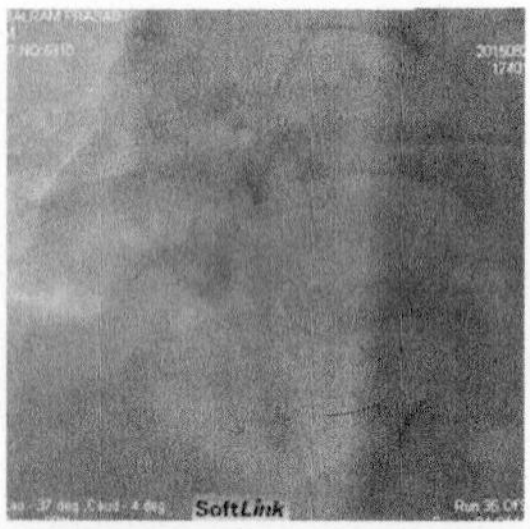

Figure 10.8d(v) Export thrombosuction being done.

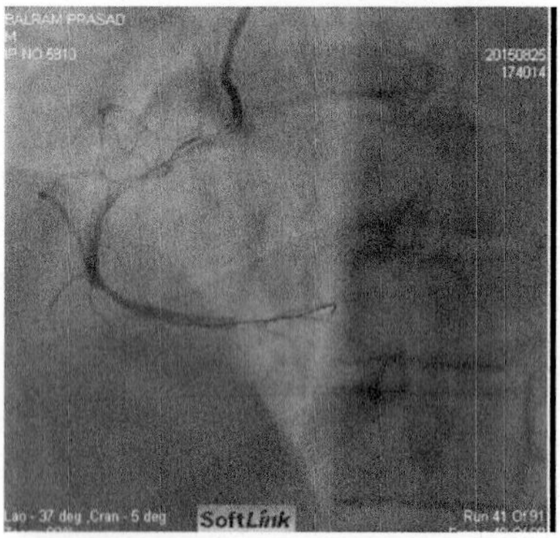

Figure 10.8d(vi) Post thrombosuction.

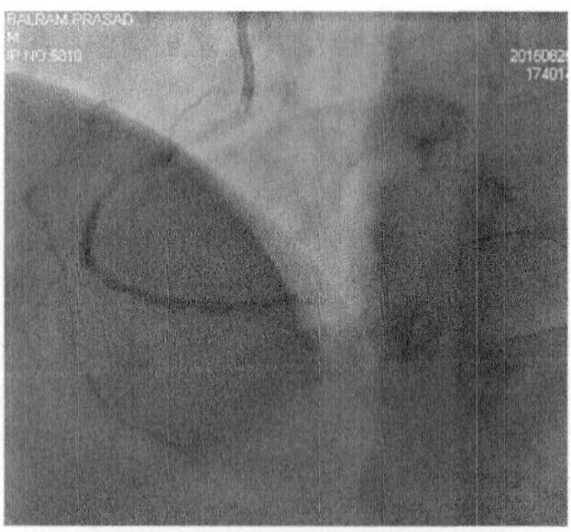

Figure 10.8d(vii) Distal stent being positioned.

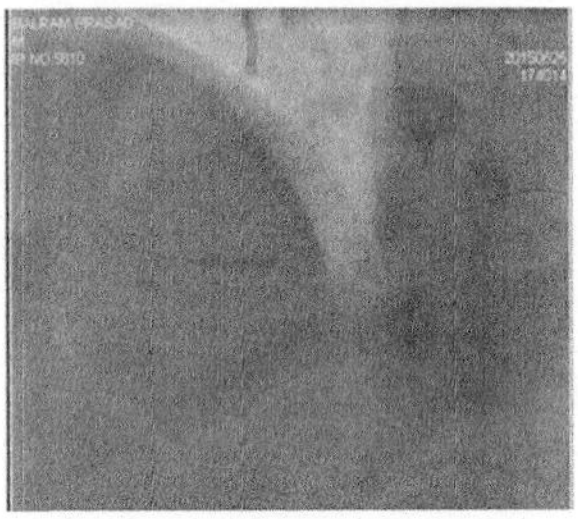

Figure 10.8d(viii) Distal right coronary artery (RCA) stent being deployed.

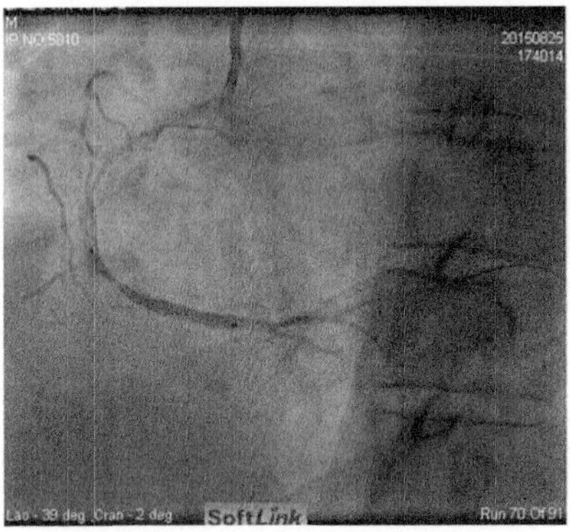

Figure 10.8d(ix) Second stent being positioned to cover the mid-right coronary lesion, in overlap with the distal stent.

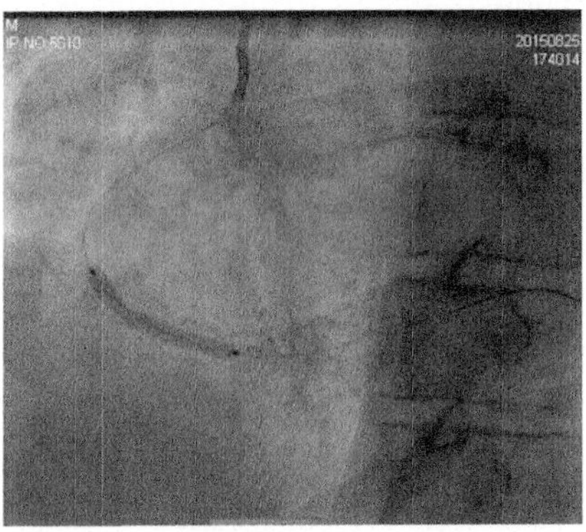

Figure 10.8d(x) Mid right coronary artery (RCA) stent being deployed.

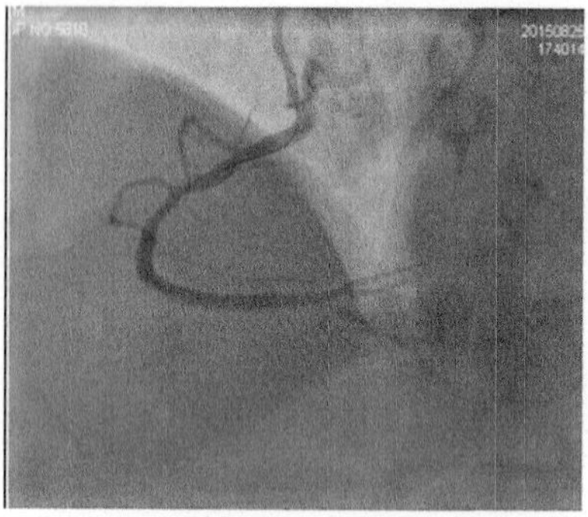

Figure 10.8d(xi) Final result, after post-dilatation of stent.

- Non-JL shapes such as Amplatz left (AL) or XB are preferred for a long left main coronary artery [Figure 10.8hx(i–vii)] or in patients with tortuous, angulated, distal or calcific lesions in LAD or LCX. The AL or XB/EBU guide tip reaches up to the ostium of the LCX, thus making the deliverability of angioplasty wire, balloon or stent easier in patients with acute angulation at origin of LCX [Figure 10.8e(i–viii)] or with hairpin bends in LCX [Figure 10.8f(i–x)]. An example of use of AL2 for good guide support in a patient with severe aortic regurgitation and dilated aortic root for percutaneous coronary intervention (PCI) to LCX and OM2 for ischaemic mitral regurgitation is shown in Figure 10.8g (i–ix) *(please see legends to Figure 10.8g(i–ix) for details of the case*). Again, a JL gives little support in an up-going left coronary artery, so non-JL shapes are used in such situations.

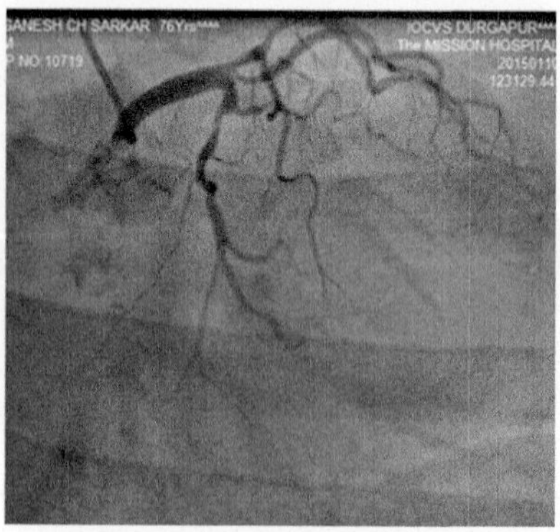

Figure 10.8e(i) Example of long left main artery with an acute angled hairpin bend at origin of left circumflex artery (LCX) with a 95% stenosis in proximal LCX.

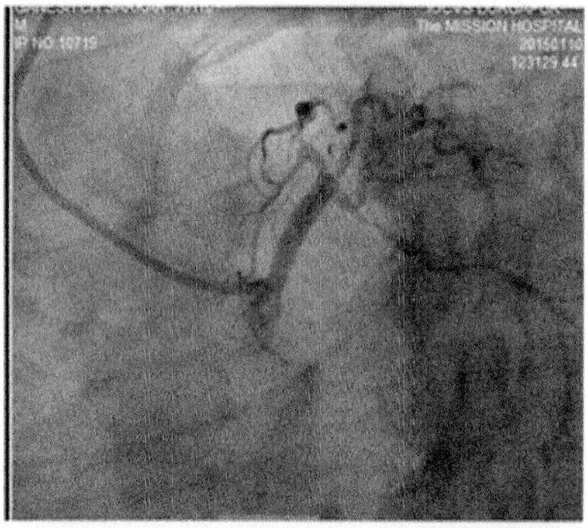

Figure 10.8e(ii) Left coronary angiogram showing long left main artery with an acute angled hairpin bend at origin of left circumflex artery (LCX) with a 95% stenosis in proximal LCX in left anterior oblique caudal view.

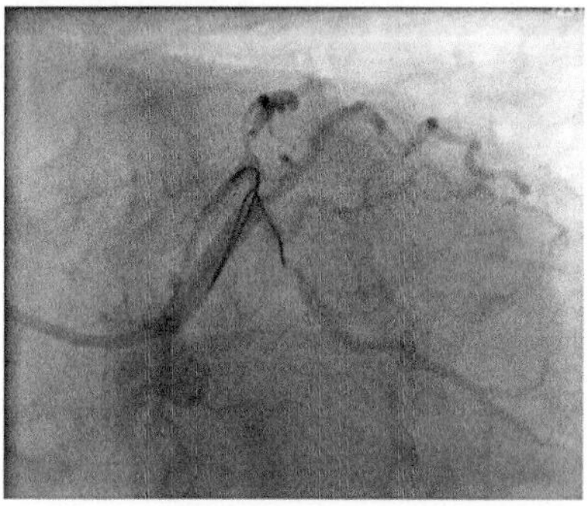

Figure 10.8e(iii) The balance middle weight (BMW) wire in LCX does not progress beyond the lesion because the 6F Judkins Left (JL)3.0 guide does not provide any support. A second BMW wire is inserted in left anterior descending artery (LAD) to enhance support.

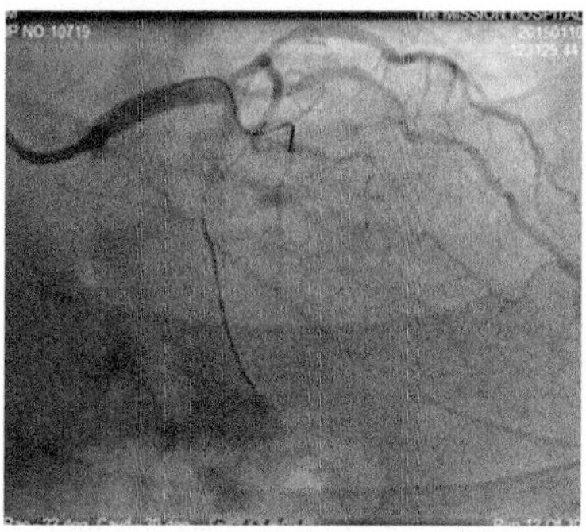

Figure 10.8e(iv) Guide catheter changed to XB3.0 enables the lesion to be crossed. Second wire in OM 1.

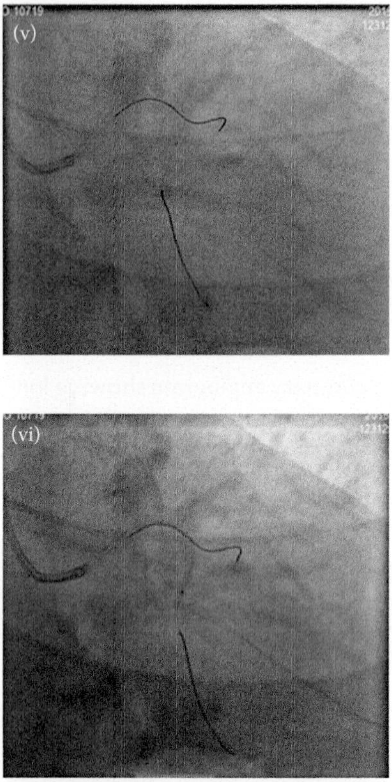

Figure 10.8e(v,vi) Lesion predilated with a 1.5-mm balloon. Subsequently a 2.0-mm balloon was also used for re-dilation.

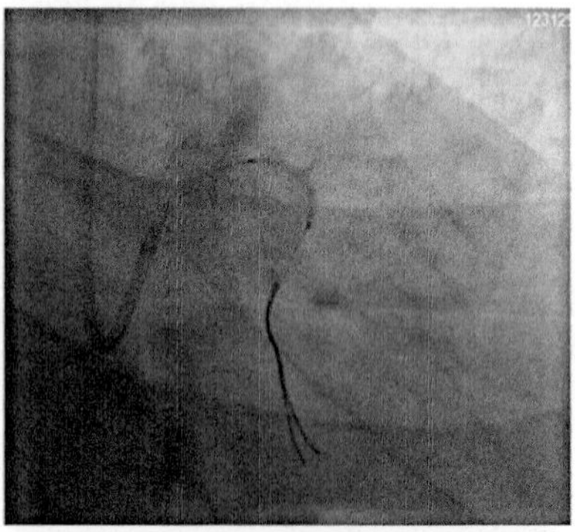

Figure 10.8e(vii) Second balance middle weight (BMW) wire is now down the main left circumflex artery (LCX) to enhance guide support. The 2.5 mm × 15 mm stent does not negotiate the hairpin bend at origin of LCX.

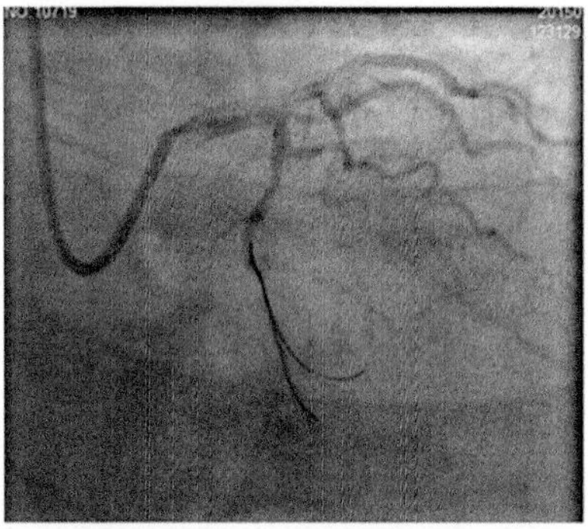

Figure 10.8e(viii) The guide tip is pushed up, in power position, its tip now closer to the ostium of the LCX, which increases the power to push the stent across the hairpin bend at LCX origin, and deliver the stent successfully into the lesion.

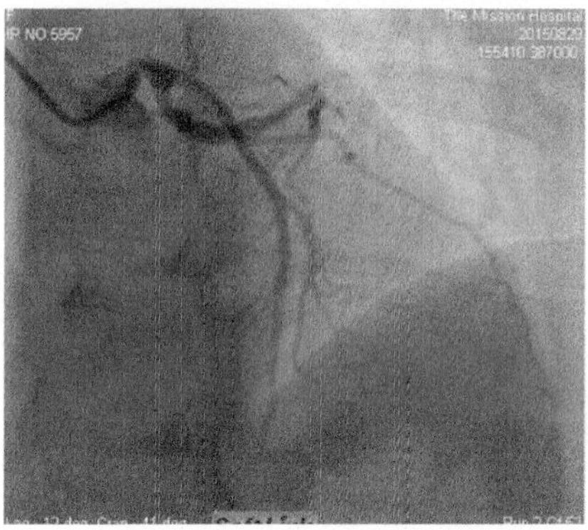

Figure 10.8f(i) Hairpin bend at LCX origin and at origin of OM2.

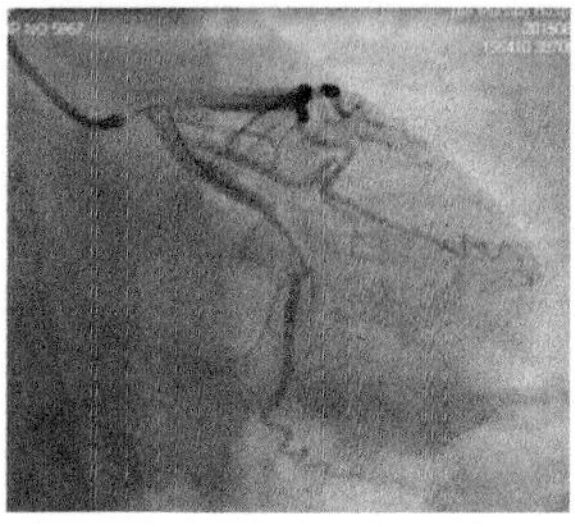

Figure 10.8f(ii) With JL guiding catheter, the BMW wire does not advance into LCX because of first hairpin bend at LCX ostium.

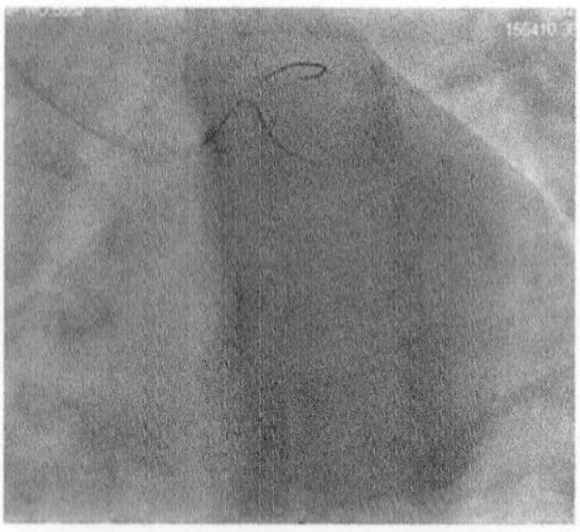

Figure 10.8f(iii) Even after a second (buddy)wire is inserted in left anterior descending artery to enhance support; the JL guide, support is inadequate for wire advancement in LCX because of the hairpin bend at LCX ostium.

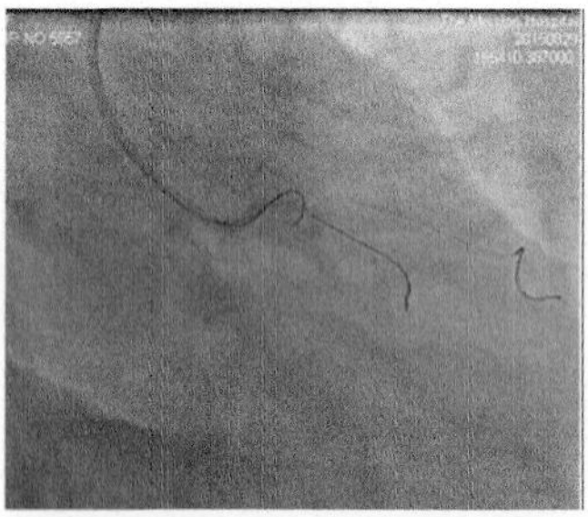

Figure 10.8f(iv) Even with 2 additional BMW wires (in LAD and OM1), guide support with JL is poor and the BMW wire in use for the LCX cannot be advanced because of the hairpin bend at LCX ostium.

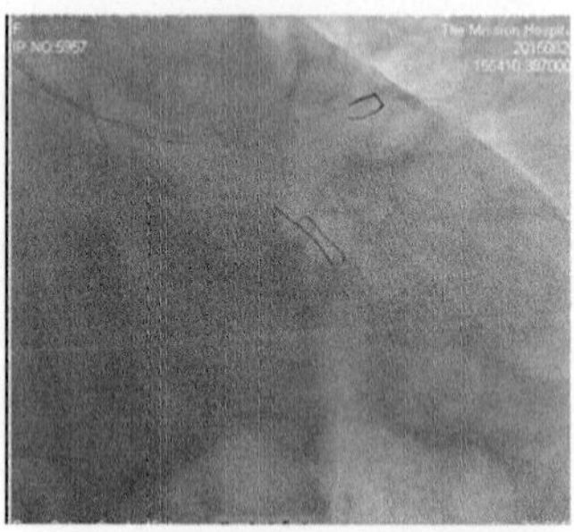

Figure 10.8f(v) Change of guide to XB 3 is rewarding as with a BMW wire in LAD for additional support, a BMW wire can now be advanced successfully in the LCX.

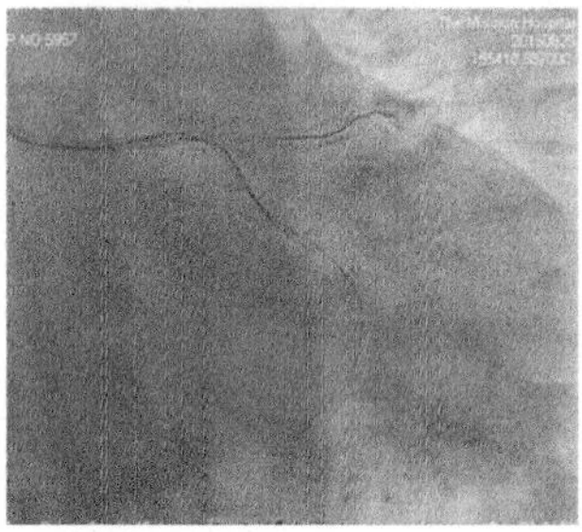

Figure 10.8f(vi) A Whisper wire easily negotiated the second bend in proximal OM2. Since the tip of the BMW wire which was first advanced in the LCX was damaged, it could not be advanced into the OM2 but helped straighten the first hairpin bend at the origin of the LCX.

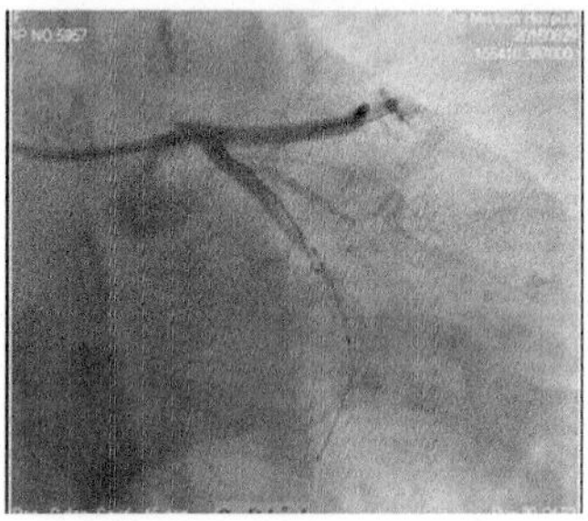

Figure 10.8f(vii) A 2.5 × 18 mm, Xience V® stent (Abbott Vascular) is positioned on the LCX-OM2 junction without difficulty. The second wire in the LCX helped straighten the first bend.

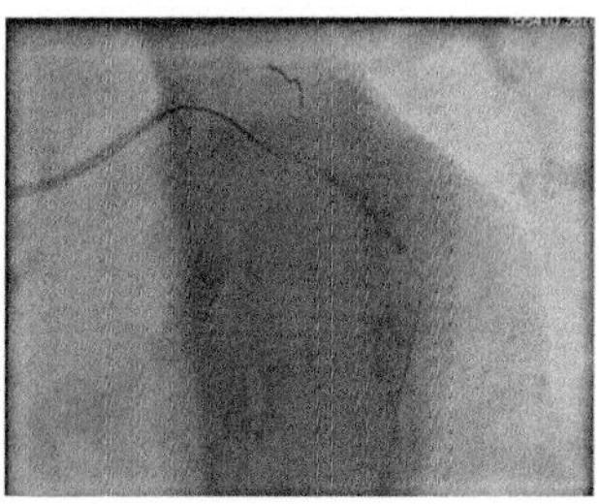

Figure10.8f(viii) Stent being deployed.

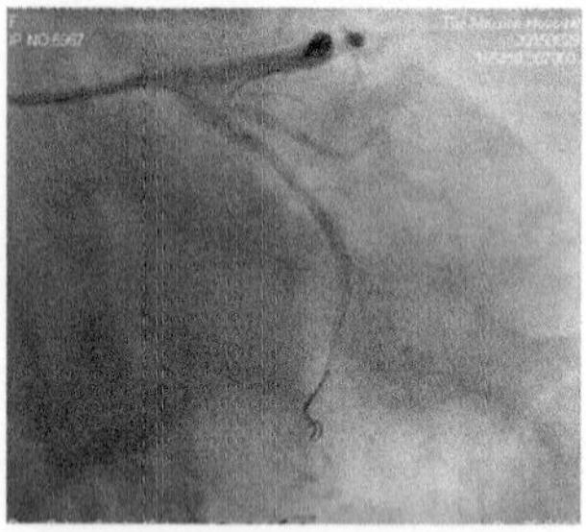

Figure 10.8f(ix) Second Xience V® 3 × 23 mm stent being deployed in overlap.

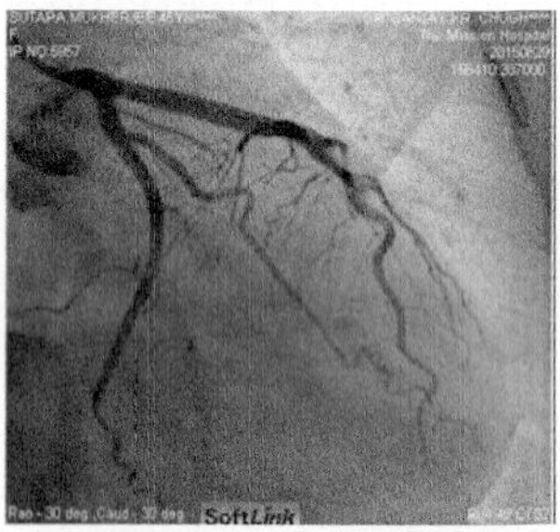

Figure 10.8f(x) Final result, TIMI 3 flow, successful PCI.

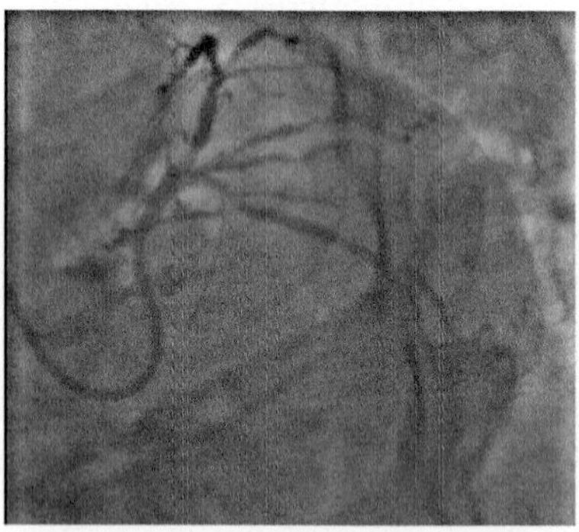

Figure 10.8g(i) AL2 guide used for PCI to culprit vessel LCX-OM2 in a post-bypass case of acute coronary syndrome with ischemic severe mitral regurgitation with heart failure, and moderately severe aortic regurgitation with dilated aortic root. Note the proximal lesion in the left circumflex artery and the distal lesion in second obtuse marginal (OM2) at bifurcation (Medina 0, 1, 0).

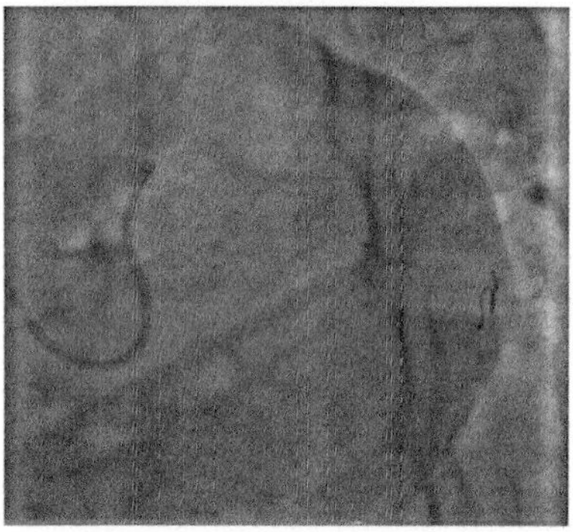

Figure 10.8g(ii) Distal lesion in OM2 at bifurcation is pre-dilated with a 2-mm balloon.

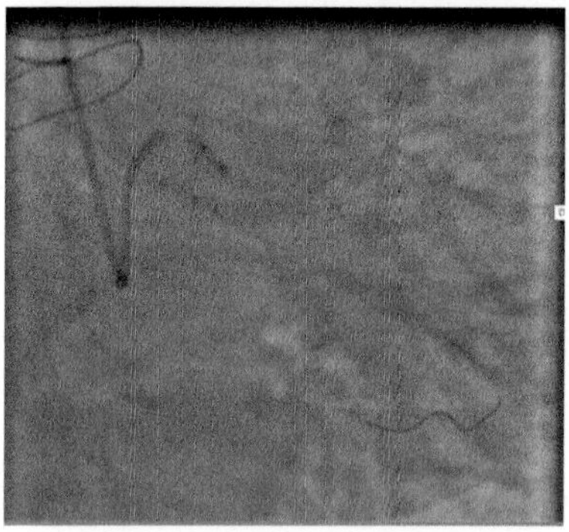

Figure 10.8g(iii) Proximal lesion in LCX pre-dilated with 2.5 × 8 mm balloon.

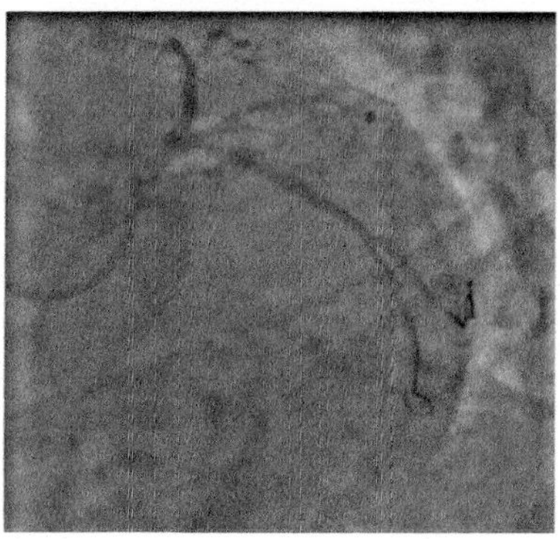

Figure 10.8g(iv) 2.5 × 23 mm Xience V® stent being positioned in OM2 across the bifurcation.

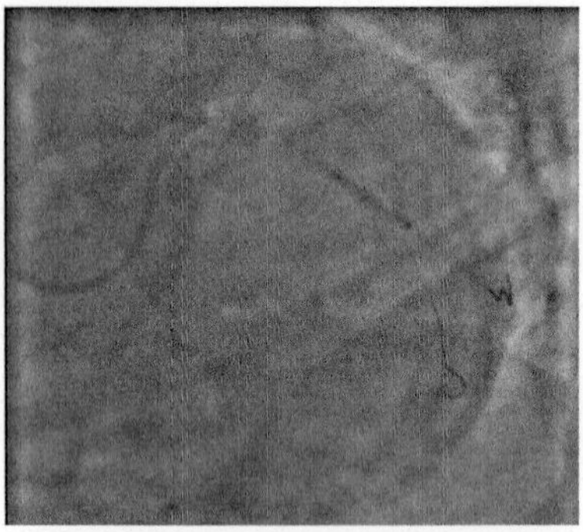

Figure 10.8g(v) 2.5 × 23 mm Xience V® stent being deployed in OM2.

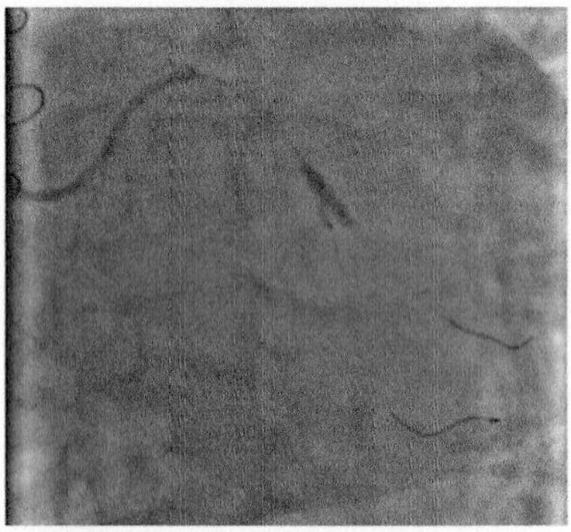

Figure 10.8g(vi) Kissing balloon in progress at OM2 bifurcation through 6F guiding catheter [Maverick™ balloons (Boston Scientific)].

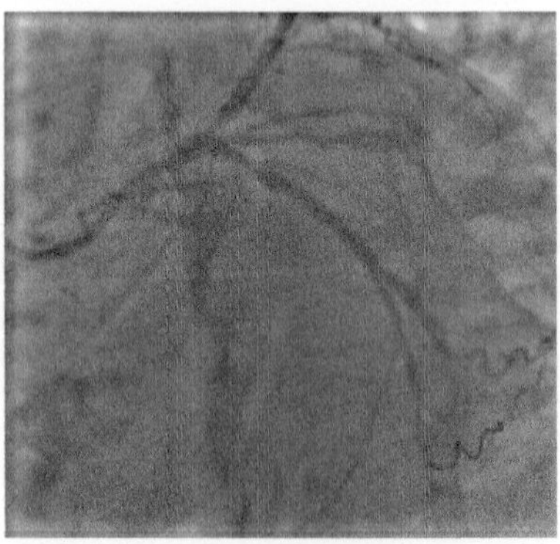

Figure 10.8g(vii) Proximal stent being positioned.

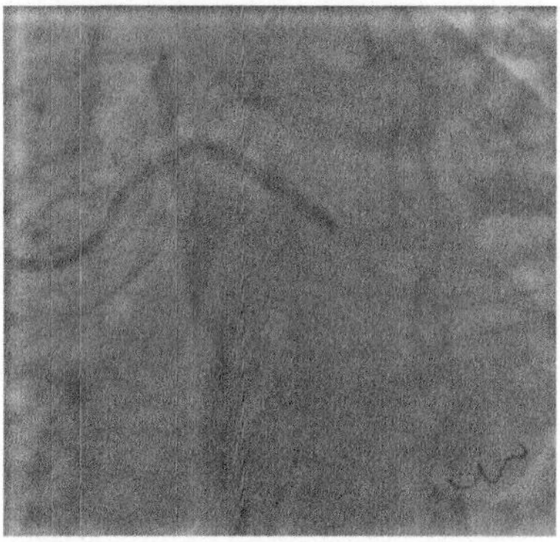

Figure 10.8g(viii) Proximal stent being deployed.

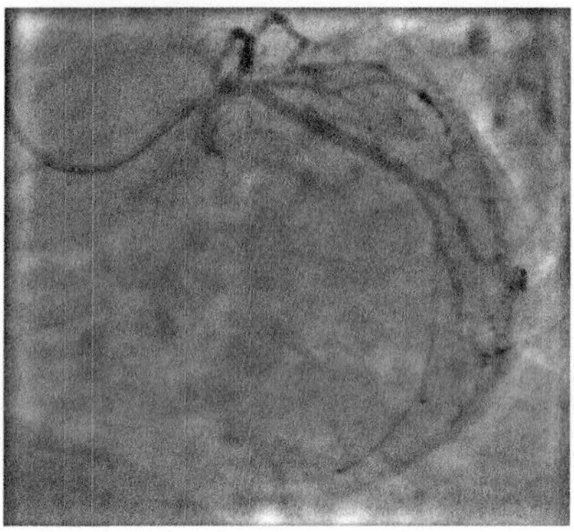

Figure 10.8g(ix) Final result. Successful PCI. The patient's ischemic mitral regurgitation recovered completely following PCI.

- In patients with a stenosis in ostial or proximal left main artery, requiring a percutaneous coronary intervention (PCI) to the LAD, a JL guide may be preferred over an extra-back up (XB or EBU) [Figures 10.8h(i–iii)]. Please see legends to figures 10.8h(i–iii) for details of the case.

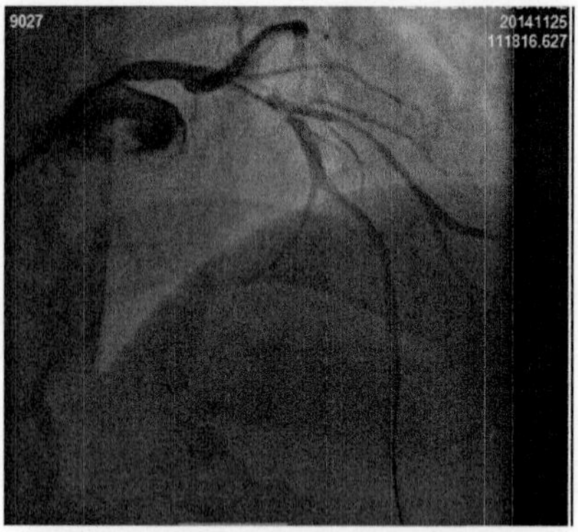

Figure 10.8h(i) A 6F Judkins Left coronary guide is used because of significant ostial left main stenosis for primary angioplasty in this 63-year-old patient with acute anterior myocardial infarction. A BMW wire is used to cross the occlusion in proximal LAD.

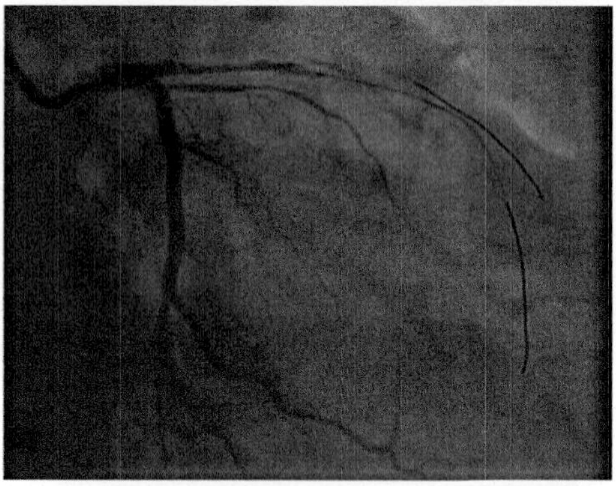

Figure 10.8h(ii) Second BMW wire is in diagonal. Stent in position in proximal LAD.

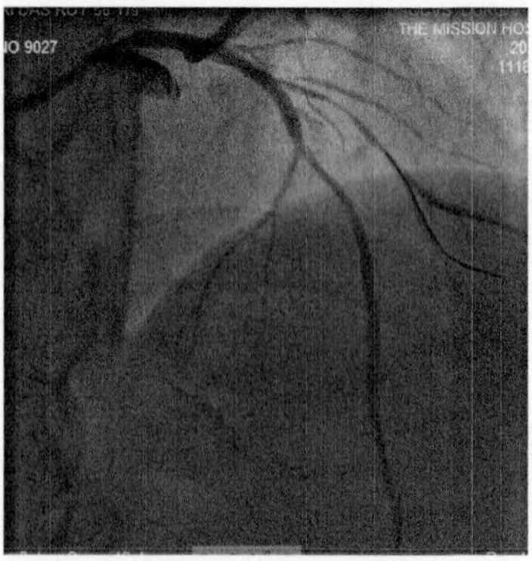

Figure 10.8h(iii) Stent deployed.

- With a long left main artery, an XB guide gives better support for left coronary interventions compared to a JL [Figure 10.8hx(i–vii)]. Please see legends to figures 10.8hx(i–vii) for details of the case.

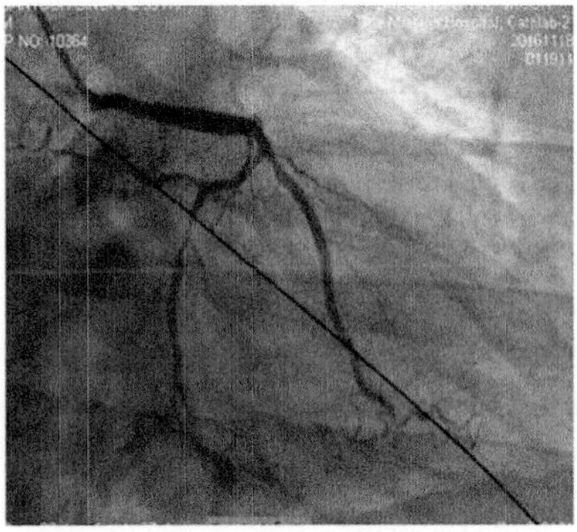

Figure 10.8hx(i) Flush occlusion of ostial left anterior descending artery (LAD) with long left main artery in a patient with acute ST elevation anterior myocardial infarction (AW STEMI).

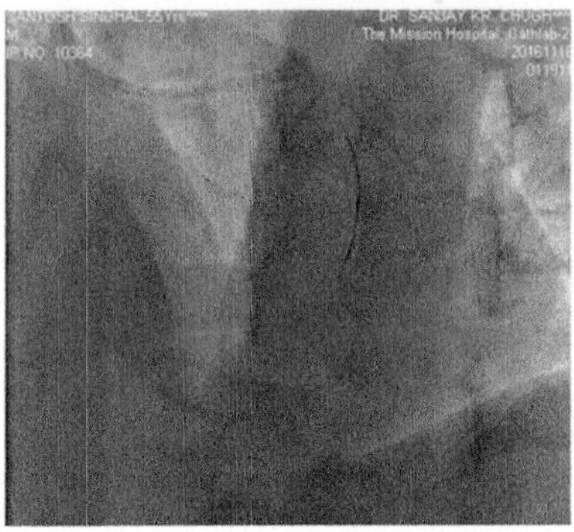

Figure 10.8hx(ii) An XB3.0 guide is used. A balance middle weight (BMW) wire crosses the lesion.

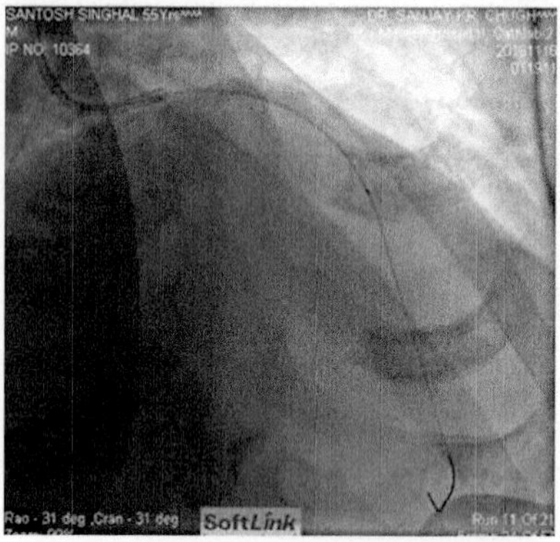

Figure 10.8hx(iii) Export (Medtronic™) thrombosuction in progress to get a visual on downstream anatomy of the artery.

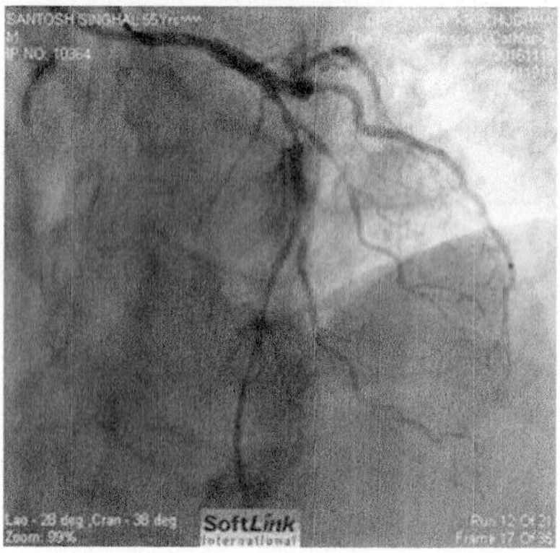

Figure 10.8hx(iv) Post thrombosuction, angiogram of left anterior descending artery (LAD).

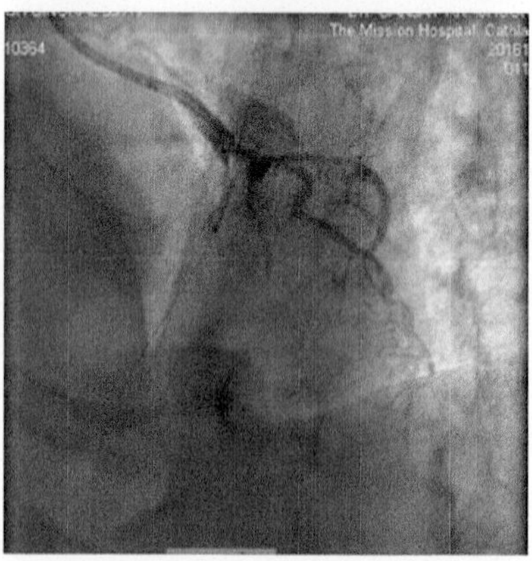

Figure 10.8hx(v) A 3 × 18 Xience V® stent is positioned at the ostial left anterior descending artery (LAD) in the left anterior oblique cranial projection which is sometimes the best view for a clear visual on the ostium, as in this case.

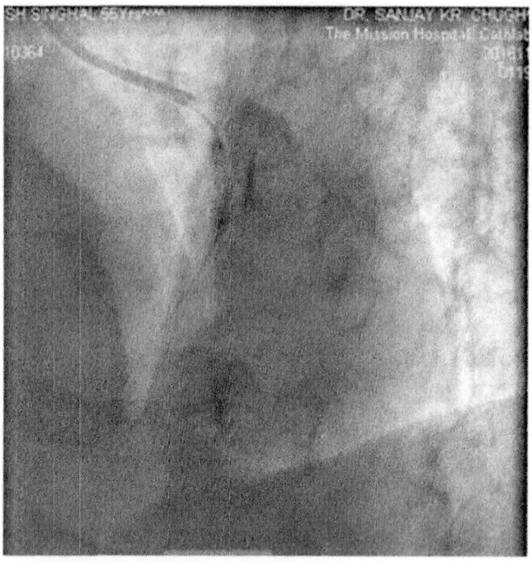

Figure 10.8hx(vi) Stent deployed.

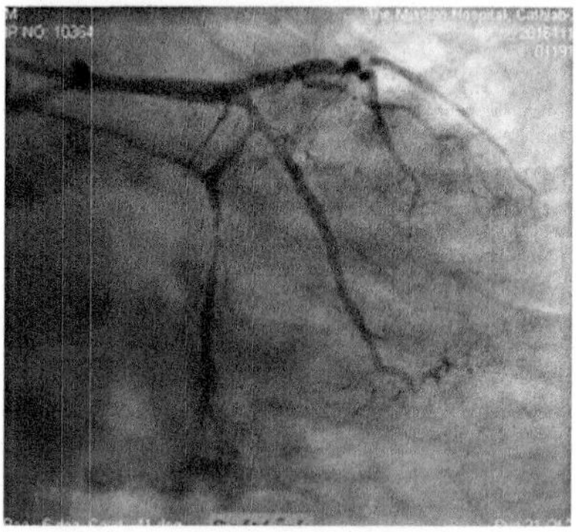

Figure 10.8hx(vii) Final result, successful PCI.

- Unfolded aortic arch can lead to anatomical rotation of the aortic root[42] making it difficult to hook the coronary as the ostium may be shifted from the usual expected position as also with a horizontal aorta. In a horizontal aorta, the coronary sinuses shift. Angioplasty of the right or left coronary artery in this situation can be challenging because the position of left posterior coronary sinus (LCS) shifts to lie above the anterior (right) coronary sinus (RCS) and the ostium of left main artery (LCAO) shifts to near 12 o'clock position in LCS. The right coronary ostium may also shift down to 6–7 o'clock position; sometimes with an acute upward bend in proximal right coronary artery, the Shepherd's crook right coronary (Please see Figure 7.6c(iii) in Chapter 7). Figure 10.8hy(i–xiii) shows the difficulty faced in PCI of LCX because of a 360° loop in right subclavian artery, and horizontal aorta, with a concomitant shift of LCS which lies above RCS, with LCAO at 12 O'clock position with take-off of left circumflex artery (LCX) at 90° to the left main coronary artery (LMCA). The procedure was completed from left radial artery because of less tortuous left subclavian artery. An XB or EBU shape is most suitable in this situation. Because of displacement of LCS, an XB3.0 and XB3.5 were unable to reach up to ostium of LMCA. An XB4.0 reached close to the LMCA ostium. Using buddy wire and angioplasty balloon, the XB4.0 GC tip was pulled-up, close to LMCA bifurcation, near to bifurcation, where the LCX takes-off at 90°. The case could be completed without difficulty. During removal of GC from LMCA, counter-clockwise rotation was used, again an angioplasty wire and balloon inserted in it, to prevent trauma to LMCA.

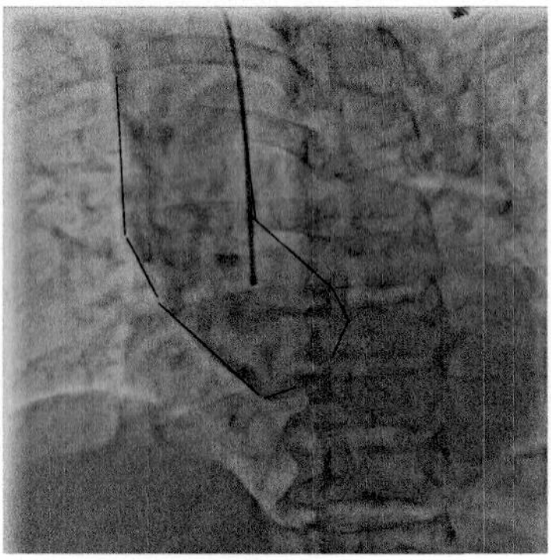

Figure 10.8hy(i)(a) Horizontal aorta.

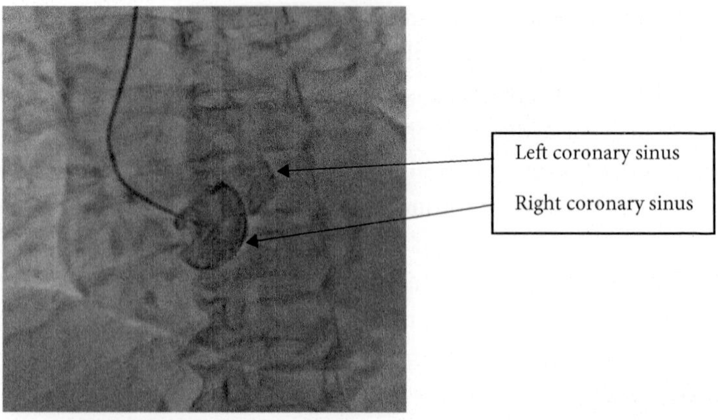

Figure 10.8hy(i)(b) The right coronary sinus below and left coronary sinus above in a horizontal aorta.

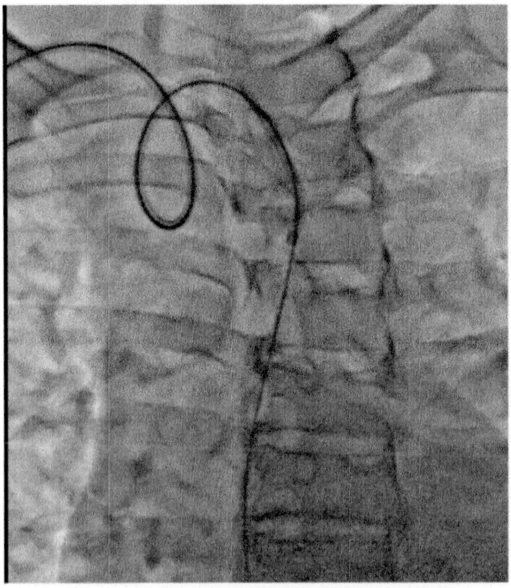

Figure 10.8hy(ii) 360° loop in right subclavian artery.

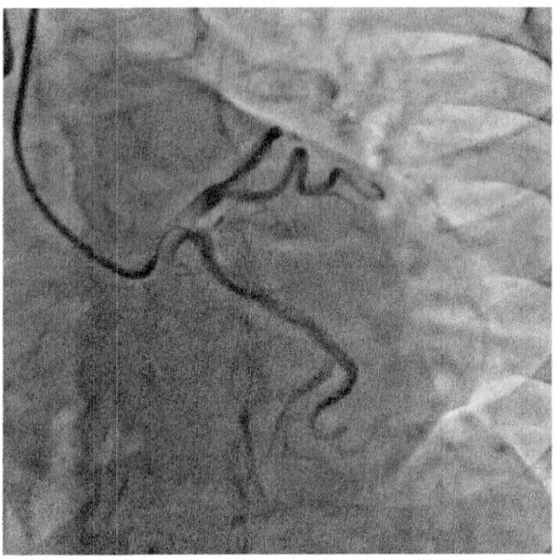

Figure 10.8hy(iii) A Judkins Left (JL)3 6F Guiding catheter barely hooks the left coronary artery. Culprit lesion is seen in proximal left circumflex artery.

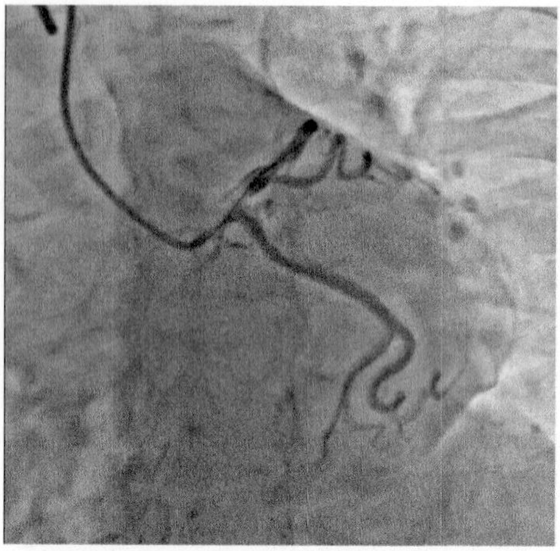

Figure 10.8hy(iv) Two run-through wires fail to turn 90° into left circumflex artery and proceed into left anterior descending artery.

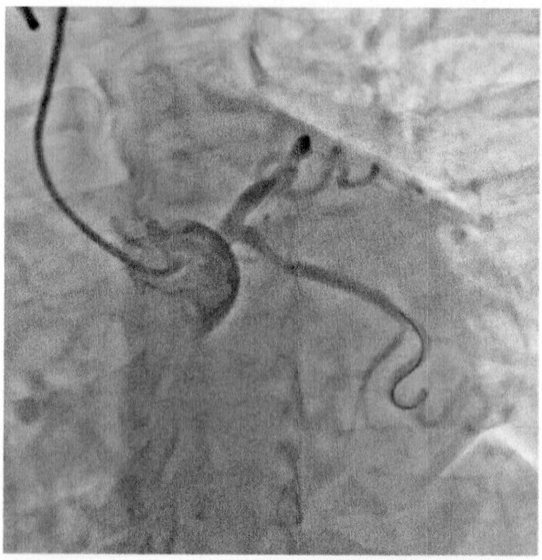

Figure 10.8hy(v) A run-through wire is successfully advanced into the left circumflex artery but the guide catheter (GC) is now disengaged from left coronary artery and stent could not be advanced. Attempts to advance the GC failed because of pull from the 360° loop in right subclavian artery [Figure 10.8hy(vi)(a-b)] which could only be straightened with a 0.035" or 0.038" Dacron angiographic guidewire [Figure 10.8hy(vi)(c)] to allow GC to be advanced. But that was not feasible with the angioplasty wire successfully in place in the left circumflex artery. So a decision was made to change the GC.

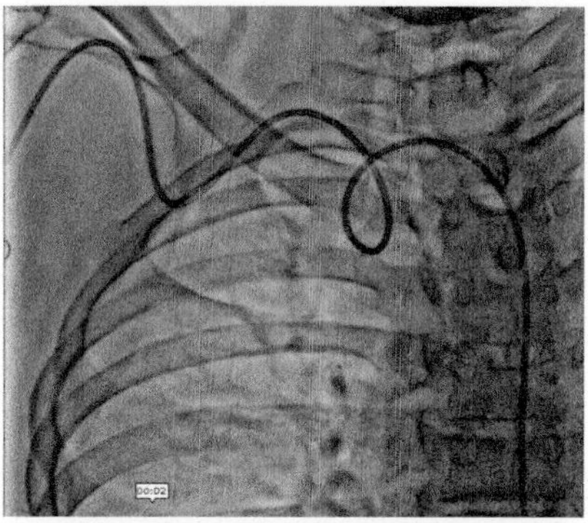

Figure 10.8hy(vi)(a) Tortuous right subclavian artery with 360° loop.

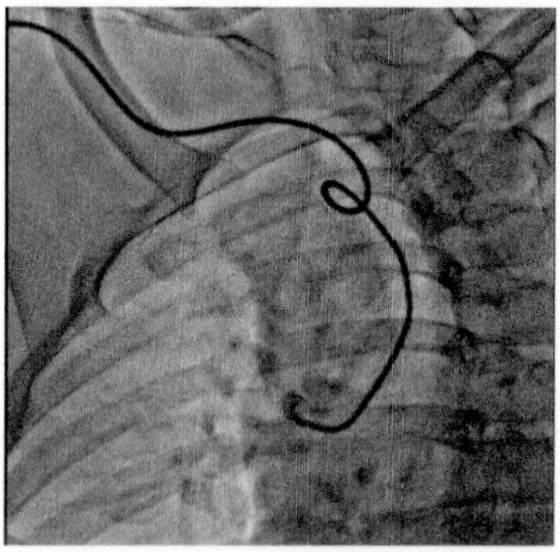

Figure 10.8hy(vi)(b) Catheter pulled up by the accordion effect of the 360° loop in right subclavian artery.

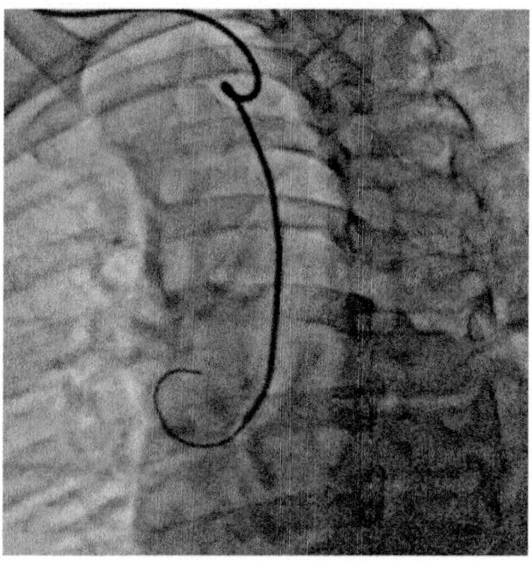

Figure 10.8hy(vi)(c) How the 360° loop in right subclavian artery is being straightened with a 0.038" Dacron angiographic guidewire to enable advancement of the catheter into coronary sinus to engage the coronaries.

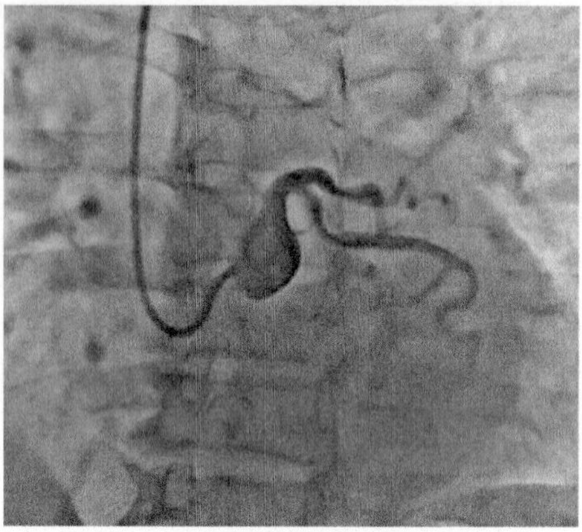

Figure 10.8hy(vii) An Amplatz Left (AL)1 guide catheter fails to engage the left coronary artery.

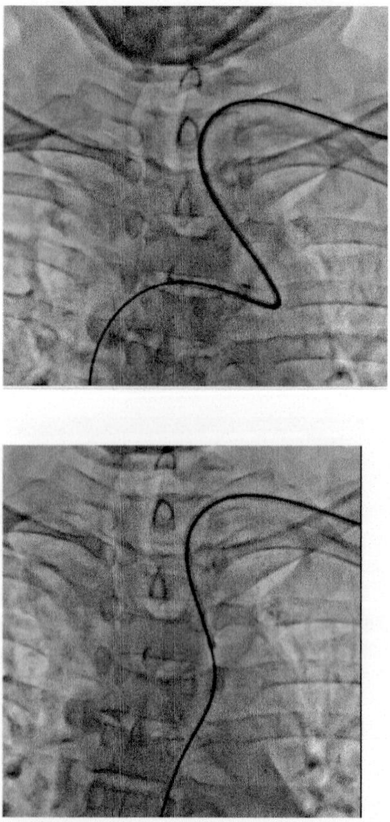

Figure 10.8hy(viii) Distal origin of left subclavian artery from arch of aorta and tortuosity of left subclavian which straightenst with the passage of angiographic guidewire.

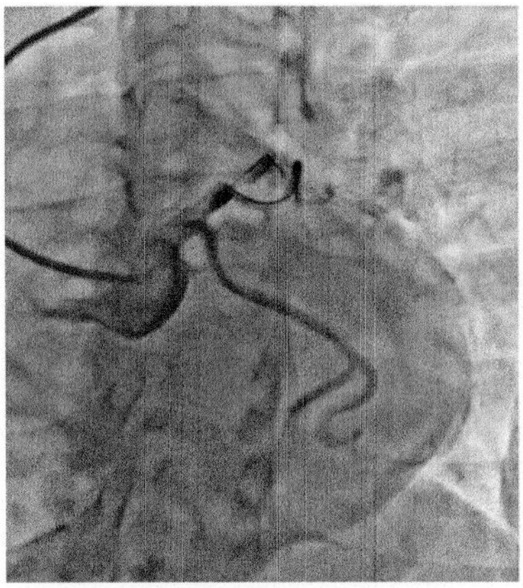

Figure 10.8hy(ix) XB4 guide catheter from left radial access unable to engage the left coronary artery. Angioplasty wires advanced in left anterior descending artery and first diagonal branch.

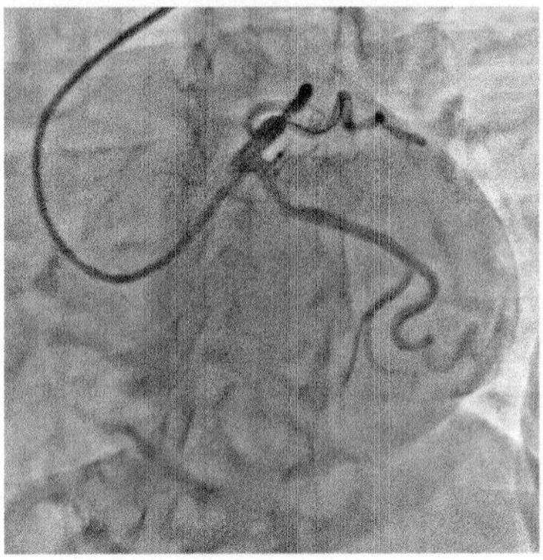

Figure 10.8hy(x) A balloon advanced over the wire is used to help engage the coronary with guide catheter.

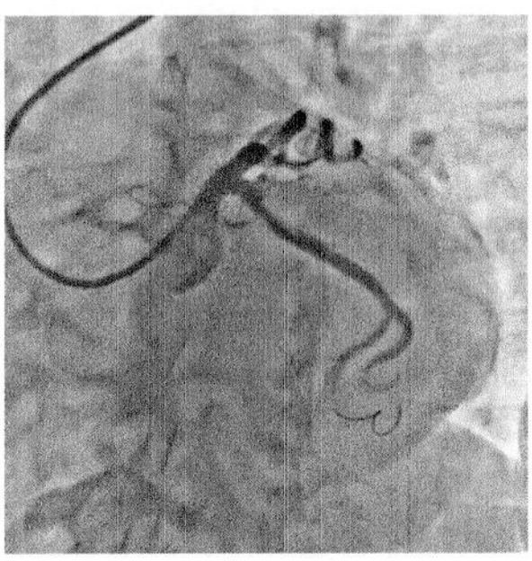

Figure 10.8hy(xi) The tip of XB4 guide catheter is now near to the ostium of left circumflex artery; a wire is now easily inserted into the left circumflex artery.

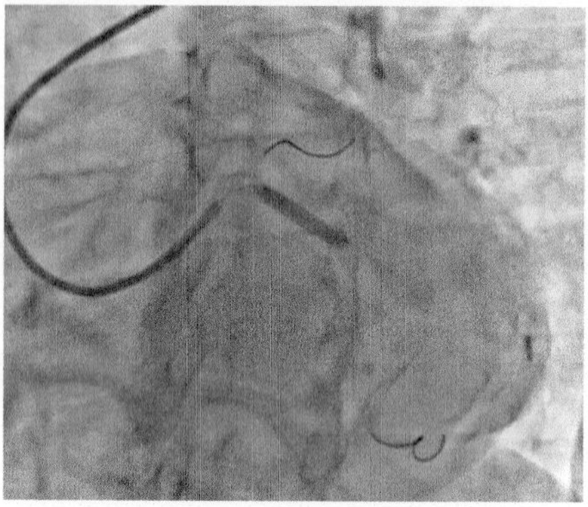

Figure 10.8hy(xii) Stent is deployed in left circumflex artery lesion.

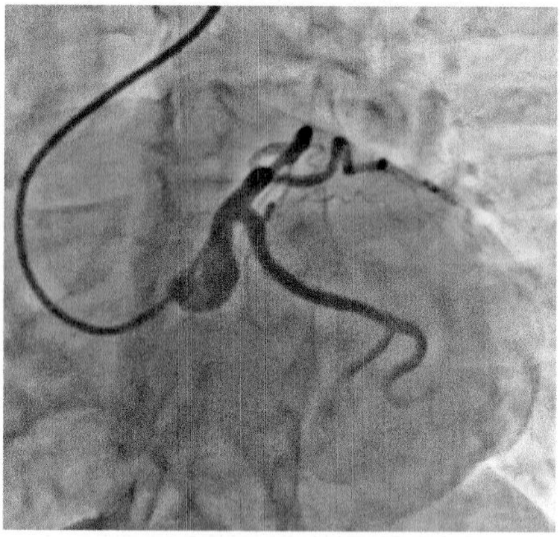

Figure 10.8hy(xiii) Final TIMI 3 flow in left circumflex artery.

Tips to facilitate engagement of the left coronary with GC.

The techniques of hooking coronaries are described in Chapter 8.

Some additional tips to hook the left coronary with XB/EBU or JL when usual techniques fail, are described here.

- Figures 10.8hz(i)(a-c) illustrate standard technique of counterclockwise rotation of XB guide to engage the LCA.
- If the standard technique of engagement fails, a reversed angiography 0.035" guidewire is used cautiously inside the GC till the middle of the curve of the XB GC to straighten its bend to hook the LCA as illustrated in Figure 10.8hz(ii)(a-c).

- Figures 10.8hz(iii)(a-c) show technique of engaging the LCA using XB3.0 GC, by rotating the GC clockwise at the level of the LCA in a patient with small aortic root.
- Rarely, an angioplasty wire can be used to help engage the GC by inserting it into LCA when the GC is aligned in the direction of, but still outside the LCA ostium.

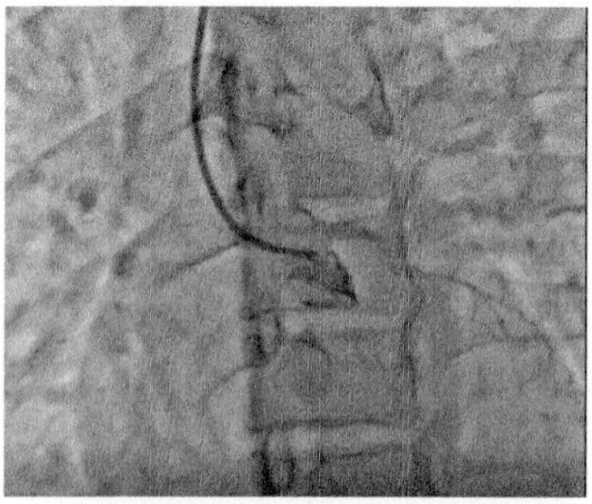

Figure 10.8hz(i)(a) Position of XB GC in the aortic root.

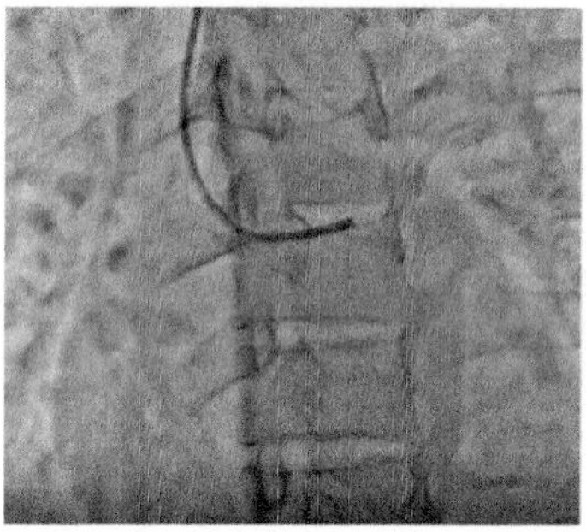

Figure 10.8hz(i)(b) Standard technique of counter-clockwise rotation of XB guide to engage the LCA.

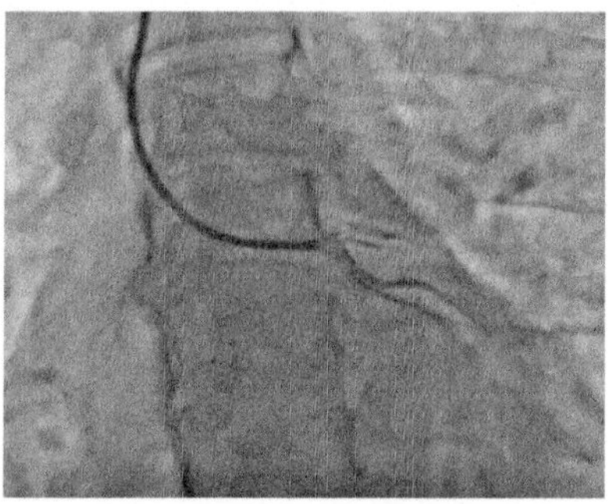

Figure 10.8hz(i)(c) LCA engaged successfully and angioplasty wire introduced into LCA (please see text for abbreviations).

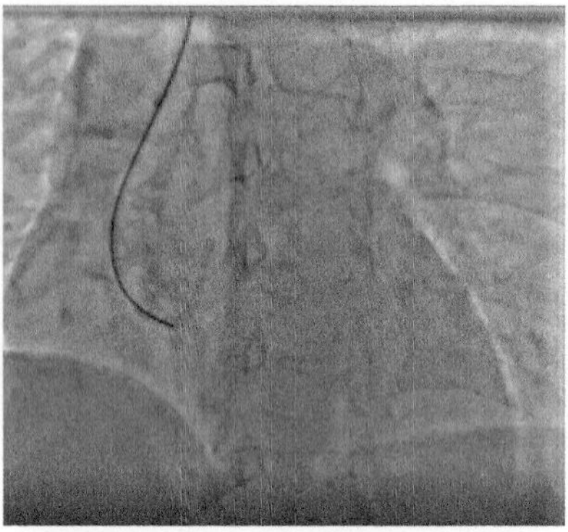

Figure 10.8hz(ii)(a) XB GC in the ascending aorta. The standard technique of engagement fails; the XB GC is rotated clockwise and pulled back to ascending aorta using an angiographic guidewire, which is removed.

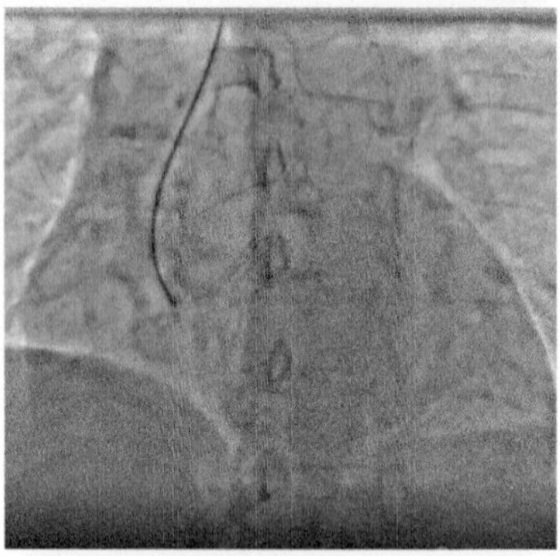

Figure 10.8hz(ii)(b) A reversed angiography 0.035" guidewire is introduced cautiously inside the GC till the middle of the curve of the XB GC to straighten the curve, while pushing the GC to bring the tip of XB GC to the level of ostium of the LCA.

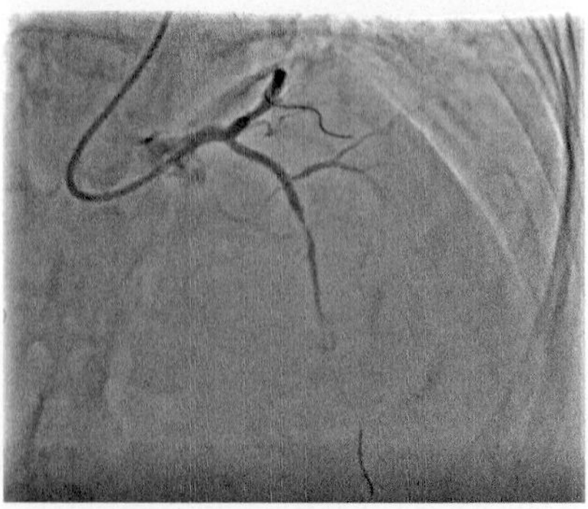

Figure 10.8hz(ii)(c) XB guide successfully engages the LCA.

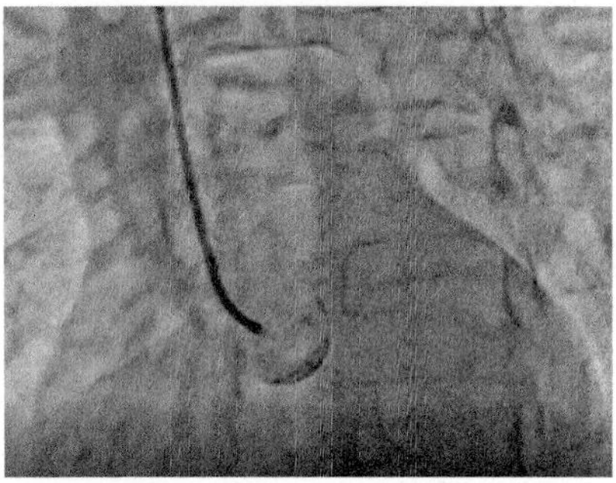

Figure 10.8hz(iii)(a) An XB GC is withdrawn into ascending aorta, with the GC tip at the level of LCA.

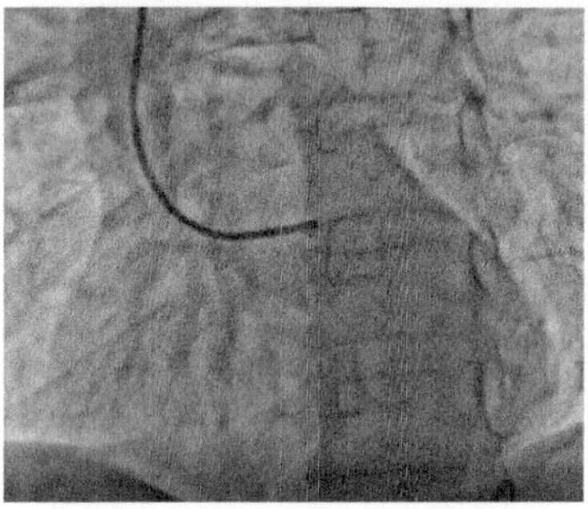

Figure 10.8hz(iii)(b) LCA is engaged by the XB 3.0 GC by rotating the GC clockwise at the level of the LCA, in a patient with small aortic root.

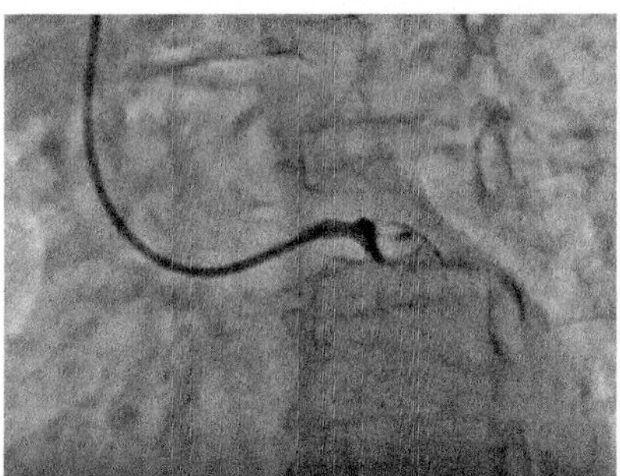

Figure 10.8hz(iii)(c) LCA is successfully engaged by XB guide catheter.

Enhancing Guide Support

Guide support can be enhanced using the following:

- With a second (buddy) angioplasty wire:
  i) To enhance guide support during angioplasty to LAD a second angioplasty wire can be inserted into the LCX [Figure 10.8i(i–iv)], or in the marginal branch for right coronary angioplasty.

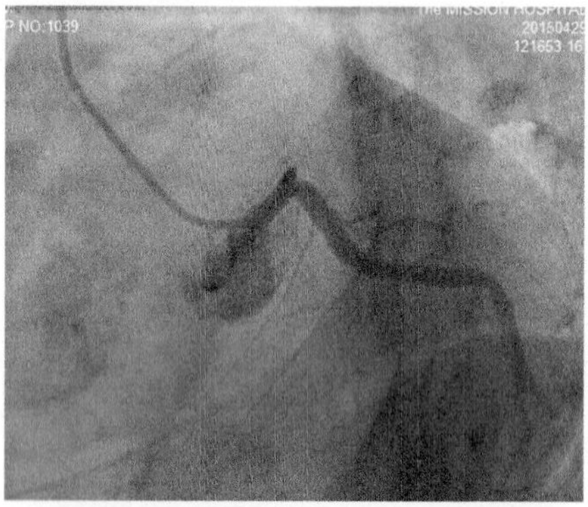

Figure 10.8i(i) Occluded ostial LAD. Patient presented with acute anterior myocardial infarction.

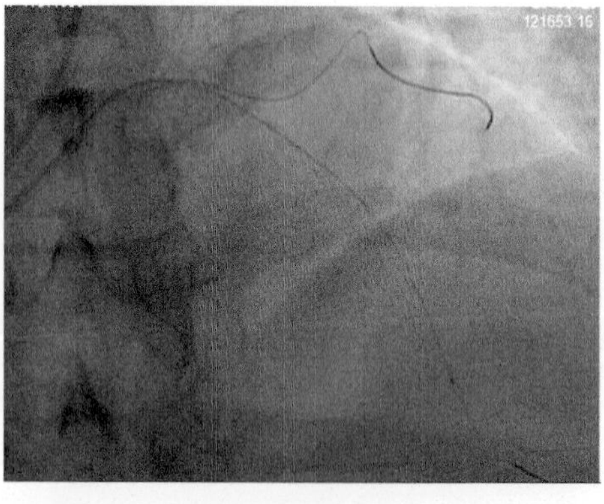

Figure 10.8i(ii) A balance middle weight (BMW) wire with support of a 1.5-mm balloon crosses the ostial left anterior descending artery occlusion. A second wire, a balance middle weight (BMW) wire is in the left circumflex to enhance guide support.

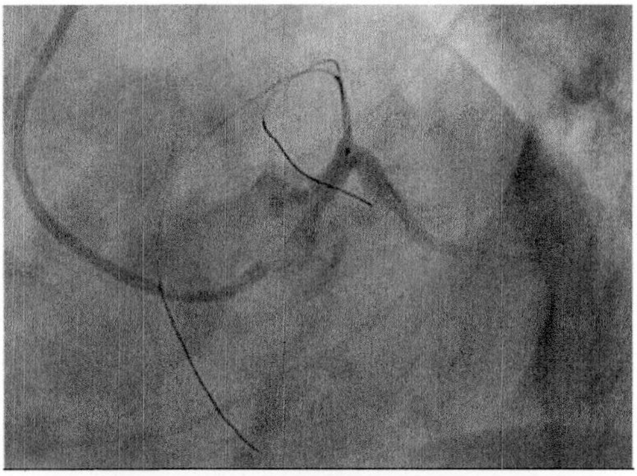

Figure 10.8i(iii) Stent in position at ostial LAD.

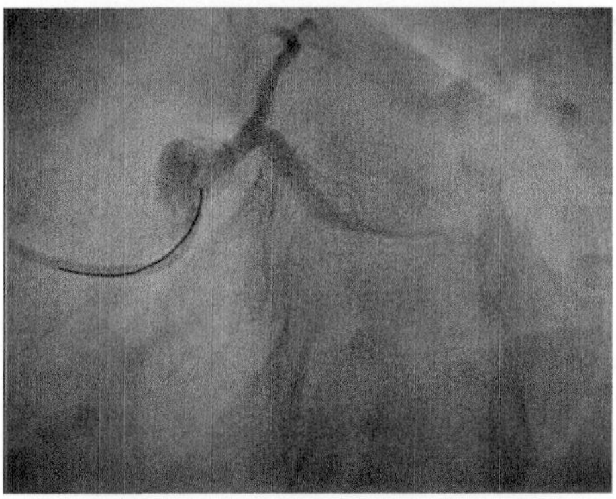

Figure 10.8i(iv) Final-TIMI-3 flow in LAD.

ii) Another example is shown in Figures 10.8j(i–iv) where a balloon had burst during post dilatation of the stent in the LAD [Figure 10.8j(i)]. The ruptured balloon was removed; a second balance middle weight (BMW) angioplasty (buddy) wire was inserted in the left anterior descending artery (LAD). Following this, a balloon was kept inflated at the site of perforation of the LAD on the first wire [Figure 10.8j(ii)]. Because the leak had not stopped after balloon inflation, a covered stent was then kept ready on the buddy (second) wire, just outside the Tuohy-Borst adapter and rapidly rail- roaded into the LAD [Figure 10.8j(iii)], as soon as the deflated balloon exited the Tuohy-Borst adapter on the first wire.

A rapid exchange was thus done without any significant pericardial leak developing. The coronary perforation was successfully and quickly sealed [Figure 10.8j(iv)]. The patient went home in 72 hours (Presented at Transcatheter Cardiovascular Therapeutics (TCT) 2007, Washington DC; at National intervention Council (NIC) Mid-Term Meet, Hyderabad, India, 2015 and Transradial Masterclass 2017, Cheshire, UK).

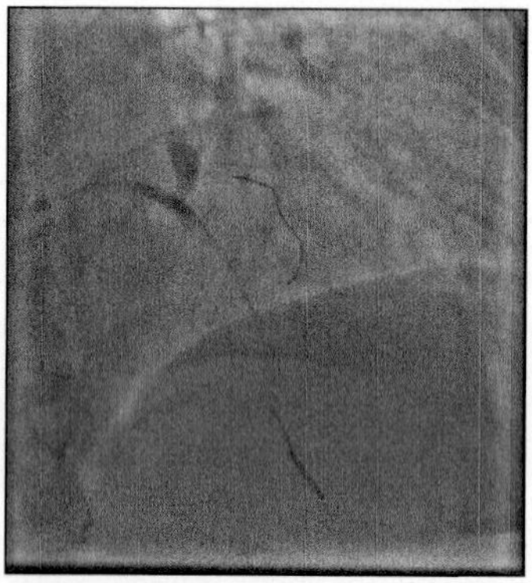

Figure 10.8j(i) Balloon had burst during post-dilatation of the stent in the LAD.

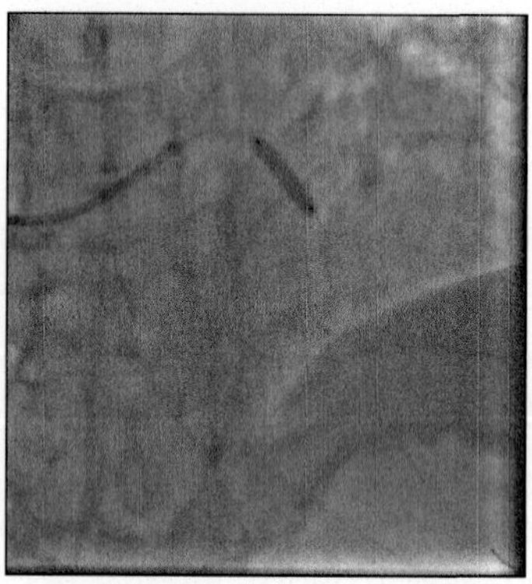

Figure 10.8j(ii) The ruptured balloon was removed; a second balance middle weight angioplasty (buddy)wire was inserted in the left anterior descending artery (LAD). Following this, a balloon was kept inflated at the site of perforation of the LAD on the first wire.

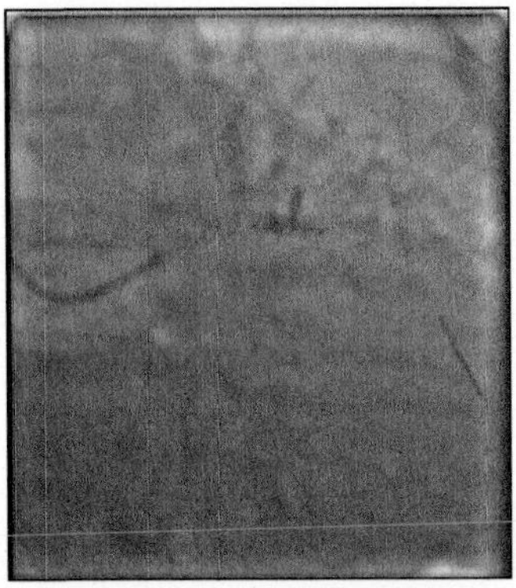

Figure 10.8j(iii) Because the leak had not stopped after balloon inflation, a covered stent was then kept ready on the buddy (second) wire, just outside the Tuohy-Borst adapter and rapidly railroaded into the LAD. As soon as the deflated balloon exited the Tuohy-Borst adapter on the first wire. A rapid exchange was thus done without any significant pericardial leak developing.

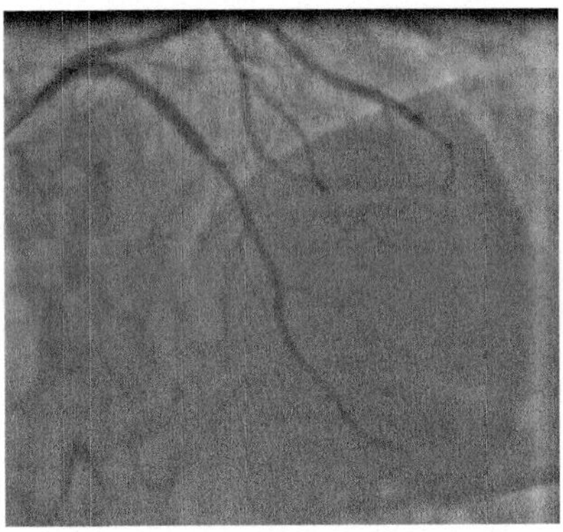

Figure 10.8j(iv) The coronary perforation was successfully and quickly sealed. The patient went home in 72 hours.

- A buddy wire can get trapped by the stent if it is not removed before stent deployment. In such a situation, as is done to retrieve a trapped jailed side-branch wire, the trapped wire can be removed by using a 1.5-mm deflated balloon over the buddy wire [Figure 10.8j(v)] by 'push-pull' which involves pushing on the balloon and pulling on the trapped wire [Figure 10.8j(vi)].

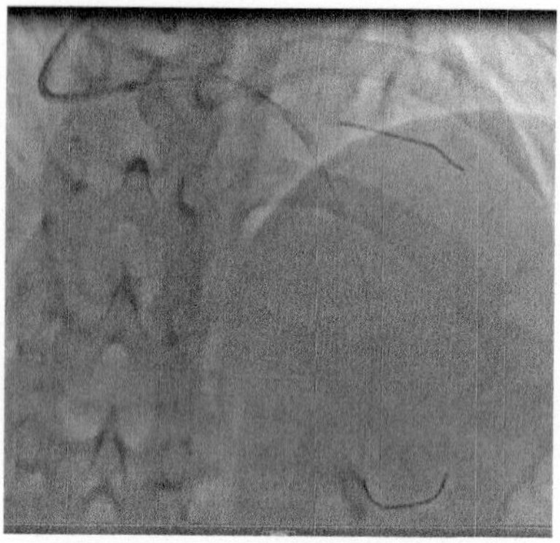

Figure 10.8j(v) A trapped side branch wire being removed by using a 1.5-mm deflated balloon over the side branch wire.

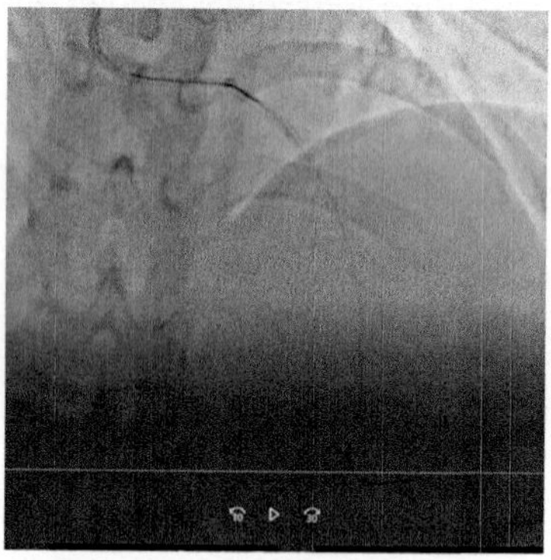

Figure 10.8j(vi) 'Push-Pull' technique involving pushing on the balloon and pulling on the trapped wire to be removed is seen at the tip of the balloon. The wire balloon assembly is then removed.

- A GuideLiner or Guidezilla™ catheter is useful to deliver a stent in tortuous or calcific vessels. In order to minimize trauma to the coronary artery, it should be introduced into the coronary artery over a balloon.

Aortic Anatomical Variations and Abnormalities

- **Dilated aortic root:** A bigger curve of Judkins left (JL5) or extra-backup (XB)/EBU (XB4/EBU4) or Amplatz left (AL2) is required to hook the left coronary artery [Figure 10.8g(i–ix)].

- **Unfolded aortic arch:** In elderly and long-standing hypertensives. The ostia of coronaries shift antero-posteriorly from the usual expected anatomical location (Figure 10.8k). Appropriate manipulation of catheter helps engage the coronary.

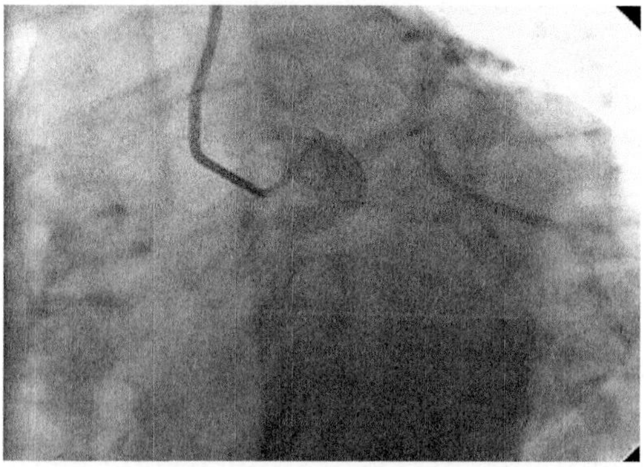

Figure 10.8k The ostia of coronaries shift antero-posteriorly from usual expected anatomical location.

- **Right-sided aortic arch**: With right-sided aortic arch in LAO (left anterior oblique) view, the image of the aortic arch looks like what it would in an AP (antero-posterior) view (Figure 10.8l). The 0.035" guidewire tracks into the descending aorta by default. To enter the ascending aorta, the guidewire has to be taken to the arch knuckle and pushed to deflect it into the ascending aorta. The Teflon guidewire usually fails; a 0.035" glidewire or a floppy, non-coated angioplasty wire can be used successfully (Figure 10.8m) as was done in this case.

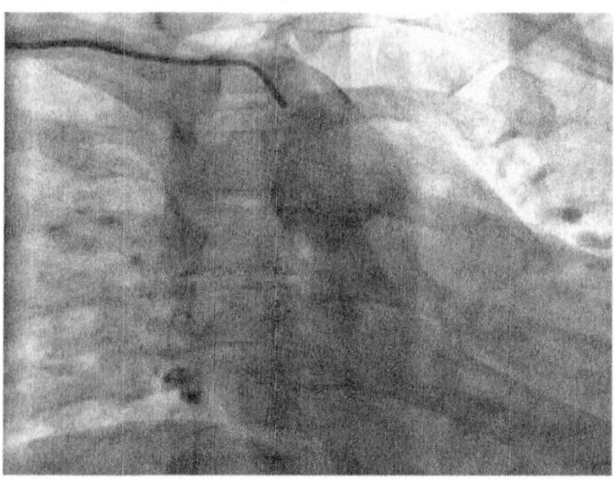

Figure 10.8l With right-sided aortic arch in left anterior oblique (LAO) view, the image of the aortic arch looks like what it would in an antero-posterior (AP) view.

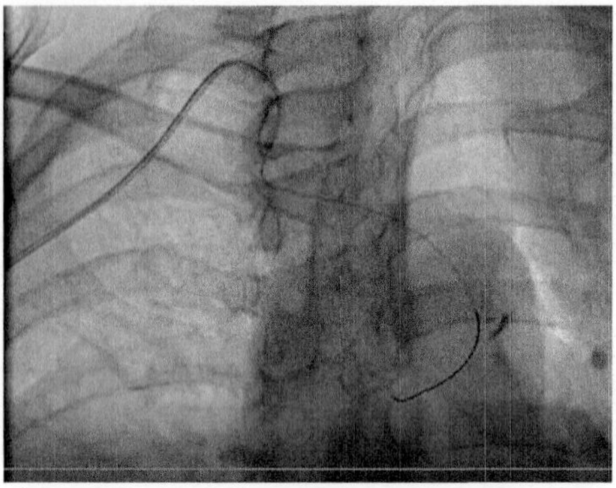

Figure 10.8m Angioplasty wire is deflected off the aortic knuckle to enter the ascending aorta.

Transradial Access in Women and Elderly

Figures 10.8m(i–xv) show how distal transradial access was gained in a short statured 145 cm chronic smoker, 80 yr old female with diagnosis of acute coronary syndrome whose right radial artery measured 1.4 mm, and had atheromatous plaque in her proximal right radial artery beyond the sheath. Severe radial artery spasm made passage of a 0.035" Terumo glidewire difficult. A check angiogram with 5 ml diluted contrast injected through a 20G Jelco® cannula used for puncture showed a short segment of stenosis and a long segment of severe spasm. The spasm abated with 100 mcg intra-arterial Nitroglycerine; 2 mg, Nicorandil; and 5 mg Diltiazem repeated twice intrarterially into the radial artery. Patient received mild sedation and analgesia with Intravenous 0.5 mg midazolam and 12.5 mcg of intravenous Fentanyl given slowly. A 0.014" BMW angioplasty wire was then negotiated into the radial artery. A 4F Diagnostic JL3.5 was then introduced over it and taken to the ascending aorta. In the ascending aorta, the angioplasty wire was exchanged for a Teflon 0.035" J-tipped angiography guidewire. A 6F JR 3.5 guide catheter then tracked on it to the ascending aorta. Angioplasty with 1 drug eluting stent to culprit critical proximal right coronary artery lesion was done successfully. This illustrative case highlights the challenges faced in transradial procedures in women related to smaller radials and how they may be successfully overcome.

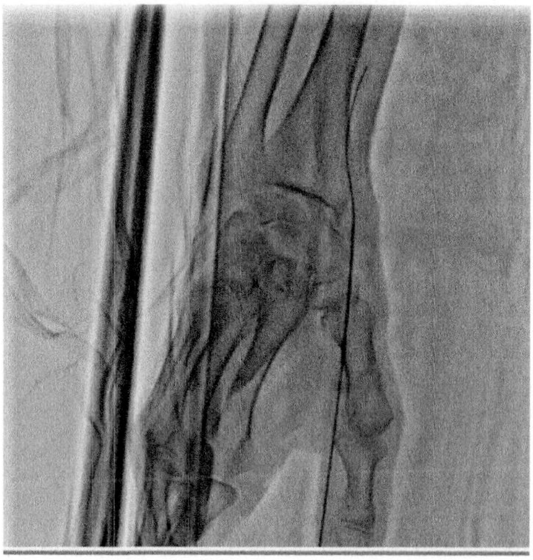

Figure 10.8m(i) Distal transradial artery punctured in a short-statured, 145-cm, chronic smoker, 80-year-old female with diagnosis of acute coronary syndrome whose right radial artery measured 1.4 mm. 0.018 glidewire of Terumo™ introducer sheath introduced through puncturing cannula could not be advanced.

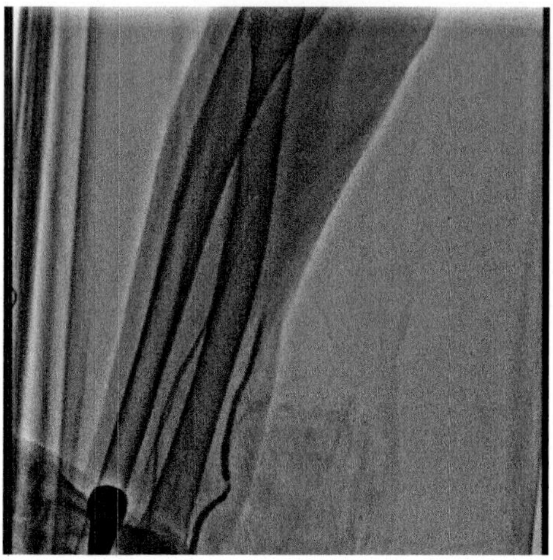

Figure 10.8m(ii) Check injection with contrast in radial artery shows atheromatous plaque with stenosis in her proximal right radial artery beyond the sheath.

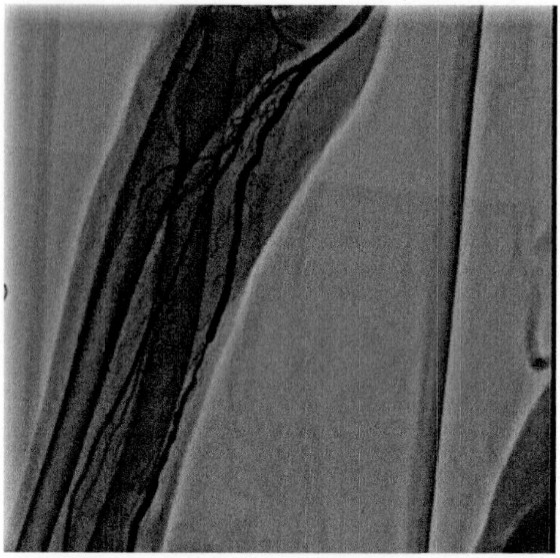

Figure 10.8m(iii) Long segment of spasm noted beyond sheath. Intra-arterial nitroglycerine, nicorandil and diltiazem given (see text for doses).

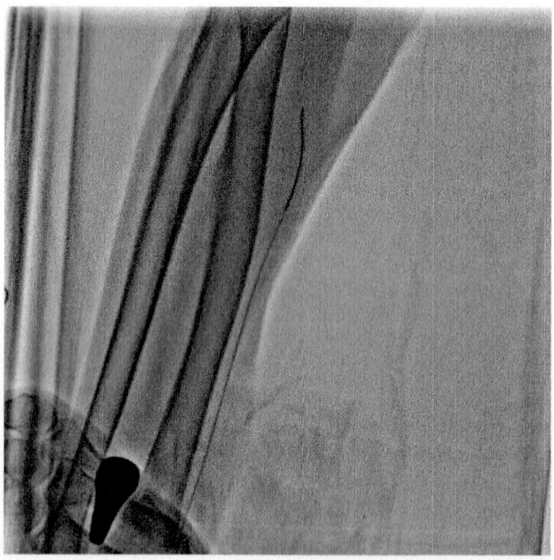

Figure 10.8m(iv) A 0.014" BMW angioplasty wire advanced through the stenosis and spasm segments of radial artery. A 6F Terumo™ sheath is advanced over the angioplasty wire.

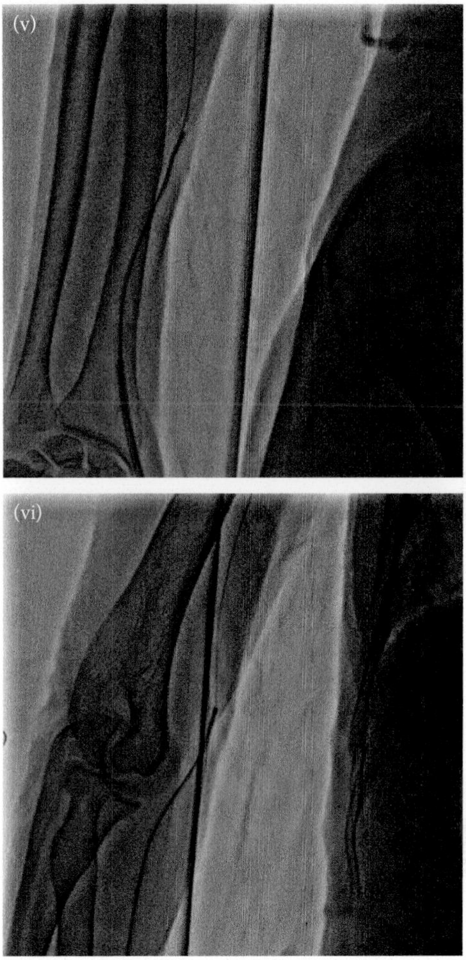

Figure 10.8m(v, vi) A 4F diagnostic JL 3.5 catheter (Cordis™).

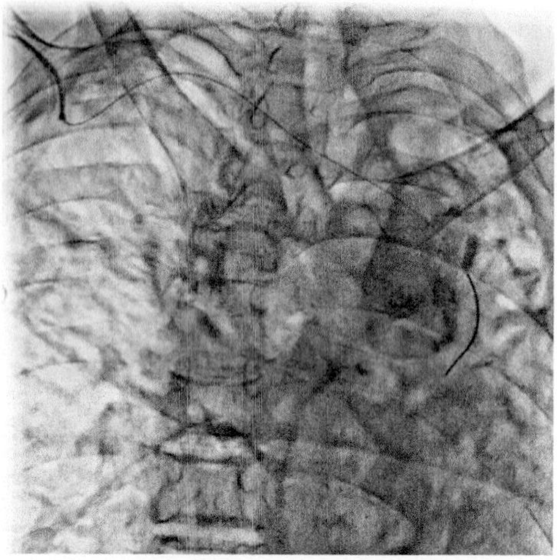

Figure 10.8m(vii) Angioplasty wire in ascending aorta.

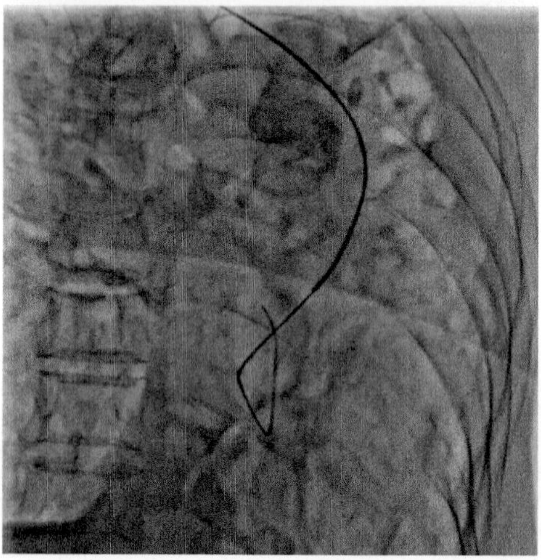

Figure 10.8m(viii) Diagnostic 4F, JL3.5 guiding catheter reaches ascending aorta over the angioplasty wire. Note the severe bend because of distal origin of the right brachiocephalic artery from an unfolded aorta.

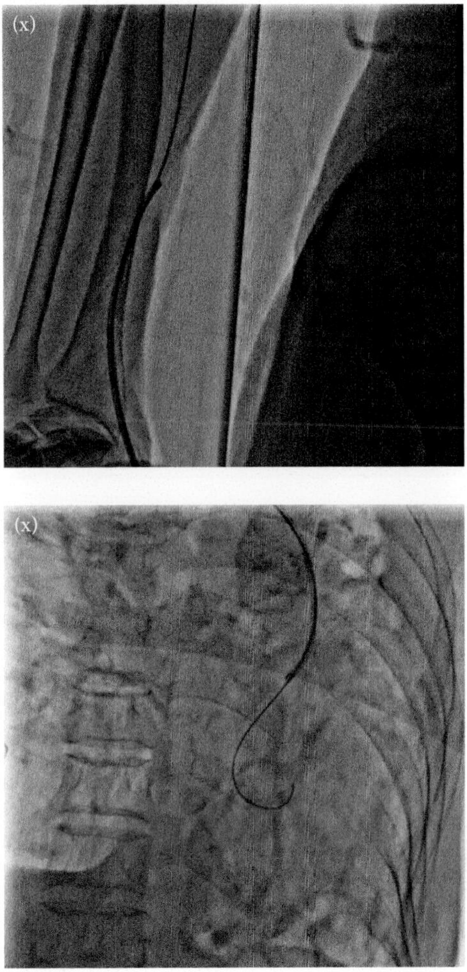

Figure 10.8m(ix, x) The angioplasty wire is now removed and a 0.035" J-tip Teflon woven angiographic guidewire is introduced. A 6F JR 3.5 guiding catheter then tracks on it to ascending aorta.

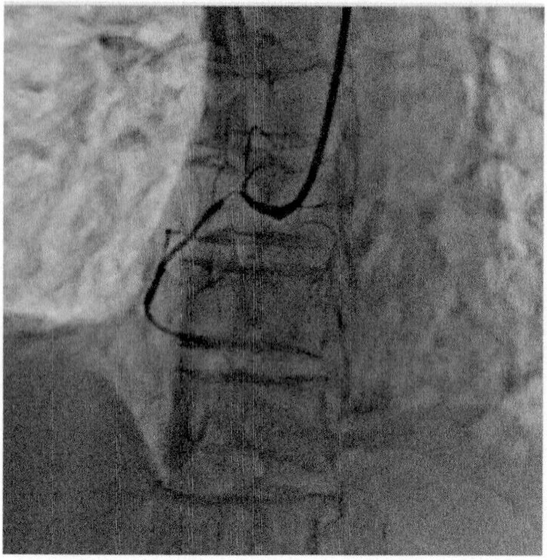

Figure 10.8m(xi) Critical stenosis in proximal right coronary artery (RCA). Please note presence of adventitial calcification in the artery adjacent to culprit lesion in RCA.

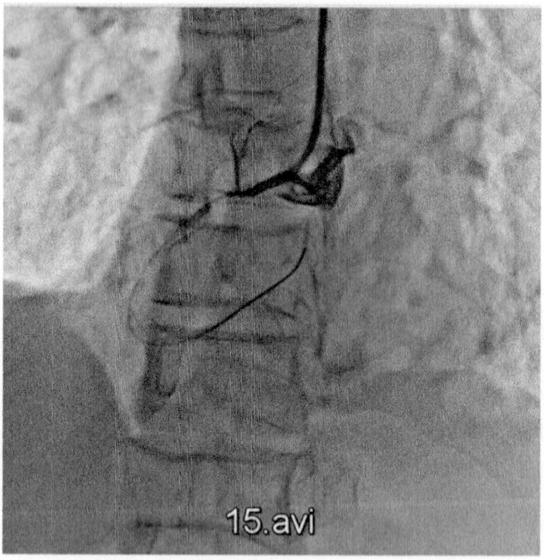

Figure 10.8m(xii) A run-through wire is used to cross the lesion.

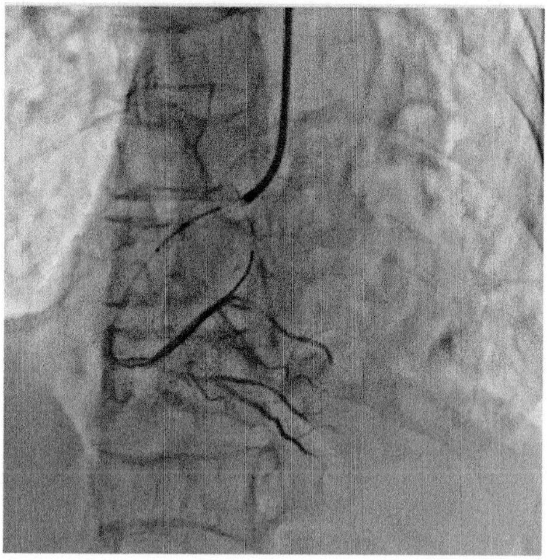

Figure 10.8m(xiii) 2.75 mm × 12 mm DES in position at the lesion.

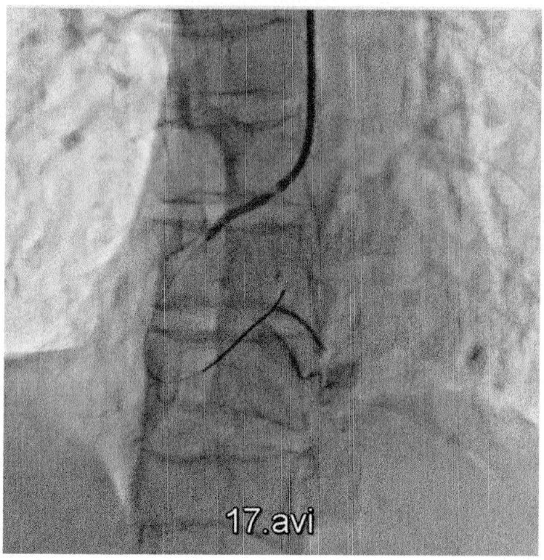

Figure 10.8m(xiv) Stent deployed at 12 atmospheres.

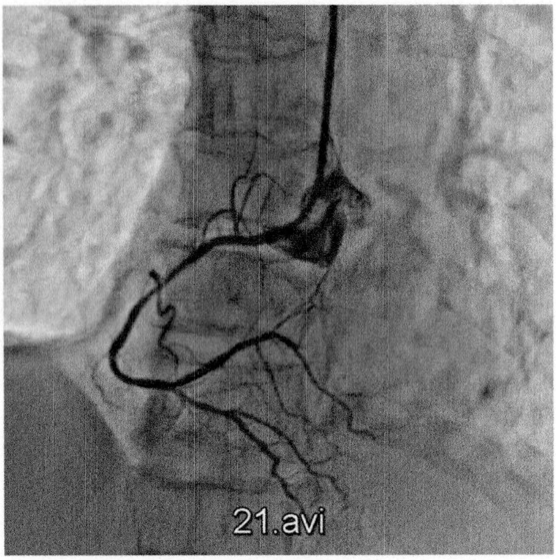

Figure 10.8m(xv) Final, TIMI 3 flow.

Small radials in women have higher risk of puncture failure,[14] radial spasm (9.5% in women vs 3.3% in men; $p < 0.001$)[42] and procedure failure leading to crossover to alternate access,[43–45] besides higher non-access-site bleeding.[31] SDRA is a factor for higher risk of RAS and crossovers[44] and is associated with higher risk of radial occlusion.[28]

In one observational study of the four forearm arteries in each arm; women were found more commonly to have at least one artery bigger than the remaining 3, compared to that in men. The following were the percentage of patients (F vs M) who were found to have at least one artery bigger than the other 3 in the various diameter categories: 1.5 mm [(17.1% (F) vs 7.8% (M)], 1.6 mm [(9.6% (F) vs 3.8% (M)] and 1.7 mm groups [(10.6% (F) vs 4.5% (M) groups ($p < 0.001$)] and 1.8-2.0 mm group [(42.8% (F) vs 29.7% (M), $p < 0.001$)].[45] This suggests that pre-procedure ultrasound may be beneficial for selecting the straightest and biggest forearm access artery to minimize procedure failure, crossover and patient discomfort.

Strategies to deal with SDRA are discussed above; in addition, a pre-procedure ultrasound of forearm arteries may be helpful in overcoming the challenges by pre-selection of a bigger forearm artery for access.

Studies related to transradial interventions in women and elderly are discussed in a separate chapter.

Tips for Transradial Primary Angioplasty in Acute Myocardial Infarction

Transradial (TR) primary angioplasty in ST elevation acute myocardial infarction (STE-AMI) or TR-PAMI is associated with reduction in all-cause mortality compared to transfemoral (TF) primary angioplasty in STE-acute myocardial infarction (PAMI).[46–49] In the RIVAL study,[46] with transradial angioplasty for ST elevation acute myocardial infarction (STE-AMI), there was a 40% relative risk reduction (RR) for death, myocardial infarction (MI), stroke, or non-CABG-related major ACUITY bleeding compared to PAMI via TF access. There was also a significant 61% RR reduction in the 30-day mortality (1.3% vs 3.2%, p = 0.006, Hazard ratio = 0.39).

In the RIFLE STEACS[47] randomized study on PAMI in which 1,001 STEMI patients were randomized to either radial or femoral access (1:1), there was a significant reduction in 30-day cardiac mortality (5.2 vs 9.2%, p = 0.02) and major adverse cardiac events (MACE).

The STEMI-RADIAL (ST Elevation Myocardial Infarction Treated by Radial or Femoral Approach–Randomized Multicenter Study Comparing Radial Versus Femoral Approach in Primary PCI) trial, randomized patients with STEAMI undergoing PAMI to TR or TF access (n = 348 and 359, respectively).[48] TR-PAMI was associated with 80% less bleeding and access-site complications compared with TF-PAMI (1.4% vs. 7.2%, p = 0.0001) at 30 days. Though there was no significant difference in MACE (3.5% vs. 4.2%, p = 0.7) or mortality (2.3% vs. 3.1%, p = 0.64) between the 2 groups; the composite rate of adverse events was also significantly lower in the TR-PAMI group (4.6% vs. 11.0%, p = 0.0028).

The MATRIX[49] (Minimizing Adverse Haemorrhagic Events by TRansradial Access Site and Systemic Implementation of angioX) study which enrolled Non-ST elevation Acute Coronary Syndrome (NSTEACS) (52%) as well as STEAMI (48%) also showed similar benefits of transradial interventions in NSTEACS, with 28% reduction in all-cause cardiovascular mortality and 33% reduction in net adverse cardiac events (NACE) [composite of death, MI or stroke and major (BARC3 or 5) bleeding].

In a meta-analysis of 12 randomized controlled trials (RCTs) in 5,124 patients of STE-AMI with transradial angioplasty,[50] in addition to a significant reduction in major bleeding [OR: 0.52 (95% CI 0.38–0.71), p < 0.0001 both] mortality and MACE were found to be significantly lower with TR PAMI compared to PAMI using TF access [OR 0.58 (95% CI: 0.43–0.79), p = 0.0005] and [OR 0.67 (95% CI: 0.52–0.86), p = 00.002].

The European Society of Cardiology (ESC) 2012 updated STEMI guidelines state that for Primary PCI for STEMI, transradial access is recommended, if performed by experienced operators (Class II a) which was recently upgraded to Class I for transradial intervention in acute coronary syndrome (ACS).[1]

A recently published study, the SAFARI–STEMI[52] study randomized a total of 2,292 patients (1,136 to radial and 1,156 to arm respectively; low risk patients with 93% in Killip class 1; mean age 61–62 years). Bivalirudin use was 88.1% in the TR and 92.4% in the TF arm; vascular closure device was used in 68.2% vs 5.5% in TF vs TF groups. The crossover in radial arm was 8% vs 2.3% in Femoral arm. In <80-year-old patients the crossover rate is expected to be less than 2%.[52] The trial was terminated prematurely after enrolling 2,292 patients with 99.6% having completed the 30-day follow-up The study showed no difference in mortality between TR-PAMI and TF-PAMI groups at 30 days. Similarly, the secondary outcomes of stroke, reinfarction and a composite of death, stroke, thrombosis and reinfarction, no difference was detected. No advantage to radial access was detected with regards to bleeding (using the TIMI and BARC) either (Please see Corollary to Chapter 17, Transradial Access Site Practice and Outcomes in Patients with Acute Coronary Syndromes, page 385).

The practical tips for PAMI[54] and illustrative cases are described here. *For a detailed review of literature, please refer to chapter 17 on 'Transradial access site practice and outcomes in patients with acute coronary syndromes'.*

- Heparin: The authors' practice is to withhold giving full-dose heparin until the coronary is hooked.[54] If it takes longer than a few minutes, we have the option to crossover to left radial artery or to femoral artery, without the risk of groin haematoma, which can be high when femoral artery puncture is attempted after full heparinization. This strategy also minimizes risk of extravasation in crossing a cubital loop, if encountered. This strategy is not associated with an increased risk of thrombus formation; but, on the other hand, puncturing the femoral artery after failure to gain radial access was found to be responsible for greater mortality in patients in whom crossover was done after administration of full anticoagulation.[41]

- Time to access, door-to-balloon (D2B) time and operator experience: Prompt revascularization[55] is recommended in acute myocardial infarction because time is muscle. In their proposed algorithm (Figure 10.9(a)) for transradial angioplasty in acute myocardial infarction, Rao et al. arbitrarily describe the time to access as 3 minutes, time to coronary angiogram as 10 minutes and time to achieving flow in coronary as 20 minutes[2] as acceptable. The author's (SKC) average of last 5 years from 1,000 trans-radial PAMI, average time to access, angiography and achieving flow in coronary was 54 seconds, 4.86 minutes and 12 minutes respectively. It has been suggested, from calculations that a >20 minutes delay in D2B time (achieving flow) would neutralize the mortality benefit of transradial access for PAMI.[55, 56] This exemplifies the role of experience which is an integral part of the class IA recommendation of the European Society of Cardiology for using transradial access for PAMI.[1] For details please refer to the chapter on: *'Transradial access site practice and outcomes in patients with acute coronary syndromes'.*
- Negotiating tortuosities: In acute myocardial infarction cases, because time is muscle; in order to save time, when negotiating radial, brachial or subclavian tortuosities, the authors prefer to use 0.014" angioplasty wire and combine it with a big breath taken by the patient to cross the tortuosities in subclavian artery. A deflated balloon is then advanced on this angioplasty wire, before advancing a GC on it After engaging the coronary artery with the GC, the same angioplasty wire which was used to negotiate tortuosities in the subclavian artery is used to cross the coronary lesion and the same balloon can be used for low pressure dilatation and dottering of the occluded vessel; unless the operator wants to do thrombectomy first.
- Venous access: It is the authors' practice in acute cases to cannulate forearm veins for venous access rather than at the level of the

wrists. With forearm access, wrists are free for crossover; thus minimizing delays,[54] should a crossover from the default right radial access to left radial access become necessary. This ensures a smooth transition in case cross-over to the contralateral arm artery is needed.

- Thrombosuction: Although data with thrombosuction in acute myocardial infarction does not support its routine use because it has no significant benefit on mortality[57]; the authors still use it in situations where there is tortuosity in the vessel and it is difficult to know the downstream anatomy of the coronary without getting a direct visual by removing thrombus; also in some situations

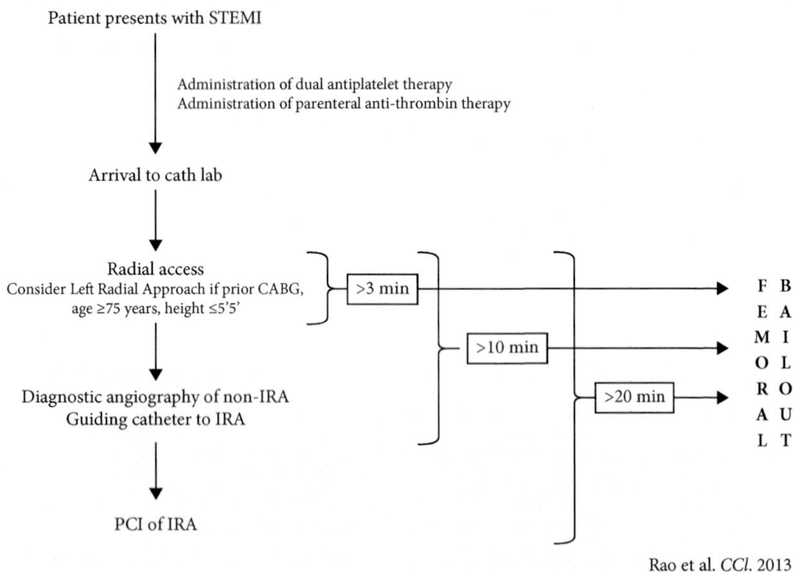

Figure 10.9a Proposed algorithm for transradial angioplasty in acute myocardial infarction, Rao et al.[2] arbitrarily describe the time to access as 3 minutes, time to coronary angiogram as 10 minutes and time to PCI as 20 minutes as being acceptable.

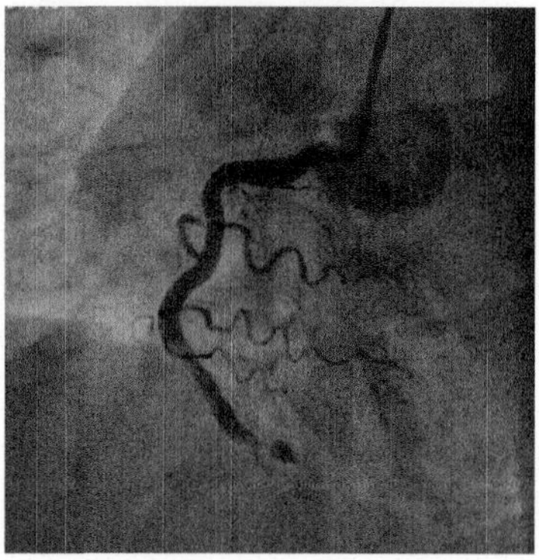

Figure 10.9b JR 3.5 guiding catheter engages right coronary artery which shows distal occlusion with thrombus.

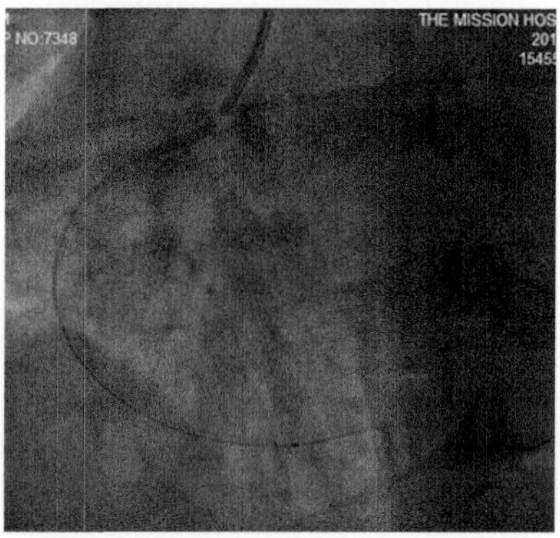

Figure 10.9c RCA–thrombectomy done with Export™ catheter.

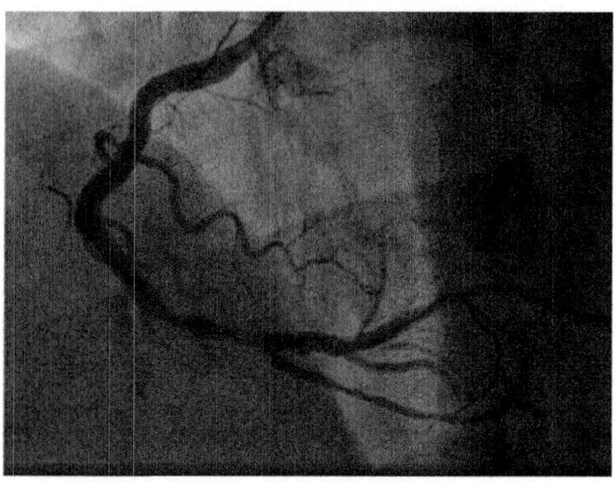

Figure 10.9d After export thrombosuction.

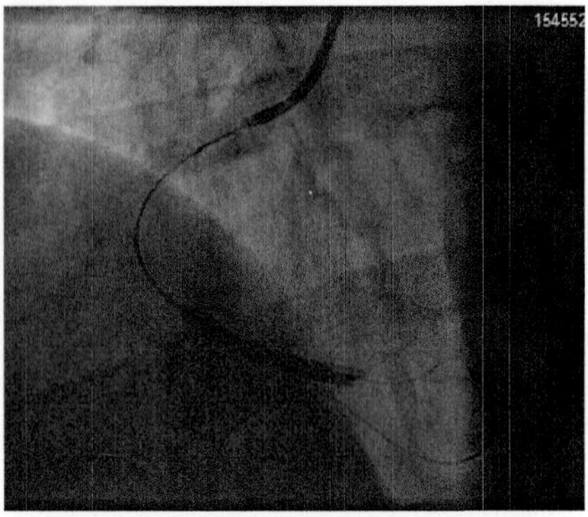

Figure 10.9e A second (buddy) BMW wire is inserted after thrombosuction and 2.75 × 28 mm Xience V® stent is positioned.

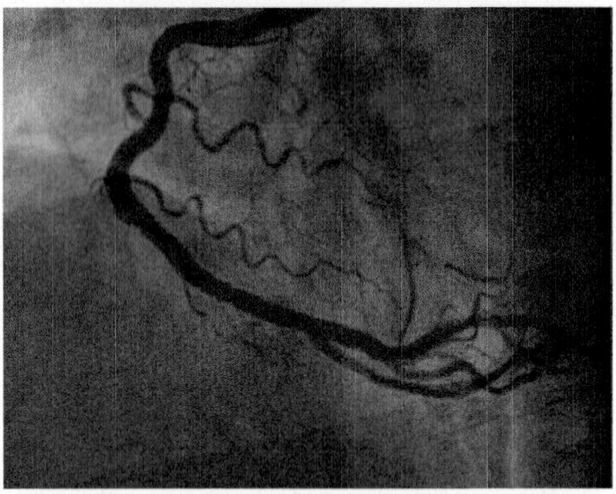

Figure 10.9f Final result: TIMI-3 flow in right coronary artery, after successful stent deployment.

it is difficult to assess the extent of stenosis to decide on an appropriate stent size without thrombectomy (Figure 10.9b–f).

- Export™ thrombus aspiration catheter is preferred by the authors for thrombosuction in such situations because of its lower cost and ease of use. It is 6F compatible but cannot be used in 6F guiding catheter with 2 wires. With 6F GC, the side-branch wire for PCI in bifurcation be inserted after thrombosuction of the main vessel is completed and Export™ thrombus aspiration catheter is removed (Figs 10.9b–f). However occlusions can be crossed with balloon support, even with another wire in a side branch or main vessel. [Figs 9i(A–D)] illustrates a case of PCI to occluded LAD; in which second wire is in LCX to maintain the engagement of LCA by the GC.

- Orienting the guide catheter (GC) to target vessel: If the guide catheter (GC) is oriented to the left circumflex in LAD interventions, the authors use the *crawling technique,* which was first described by them.[54] The first wire is inserted into whichever branch the wire tracks into (Figure 10.10a). This holds the GC in place. A 2nd BMW wire is then inserted into the LAD; the 1st wire is removed and introduced into the 1st diagonal (Figure 10.10b). This then orients the GC towards the LAD. The LAD wire is then advanced further and then the first wire is removed from 1st diagonal and inserted (Figure 10.10c) into the second diagonal which is relevant to the LAD lesion (Figure 10.10d).

  Thereafter the LAD lesion was pre-dilated, stented (BioMime™ 3 × 38 mm stent at 12 atmospheres Figure 10.10e) and finally post-dilated (3 × 12 mm NC balloon to 15 atmospheres) with good result (Figure 10.10f).

  Transvenous temporary pacing: Temporary pacing can be done transfemorally [Figure 10.11(a–e)] or through antecubital vein in the

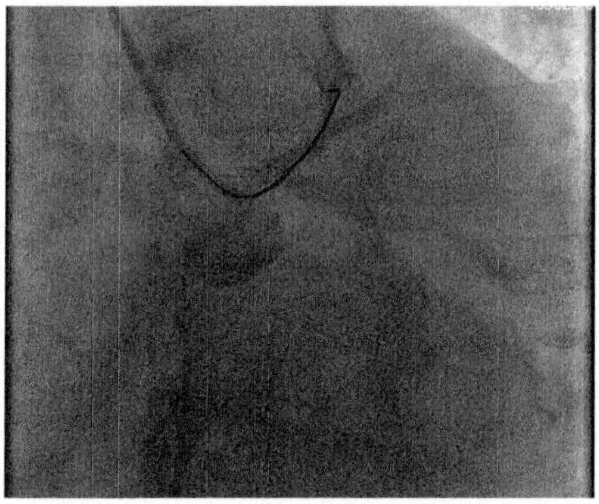

Figure 10.10a Illustrating our 'Crawling technique' being used for angioplasty to left anterior descending artery. The Judkins left (JL) 3.0 guide points to left circumflex. A BMW is inserted into whichever artery the wire tracks into.

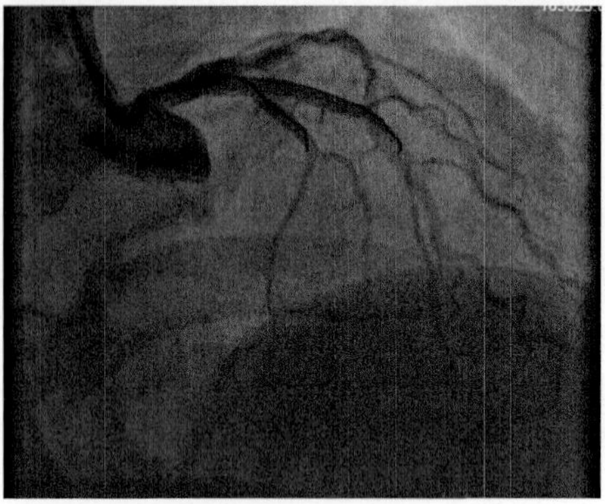

Figure 10.10b The second BMW wire is inserted into the LAD and the first wire is advanced into the first diagonal.

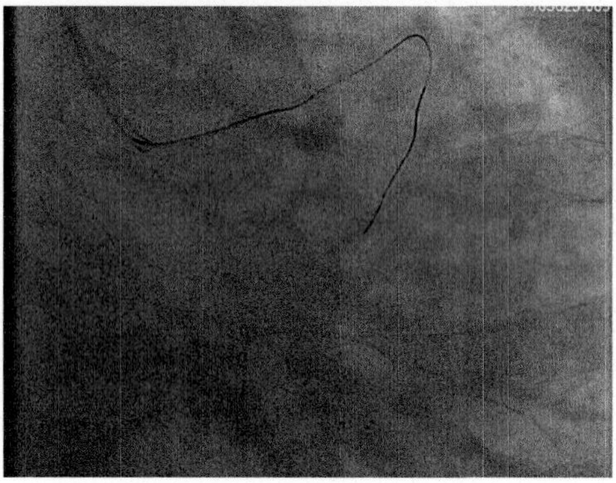

Figure 10.10c Again the LAD wire is advanced further and then the first wire is taken out from first diagonal and inserted into the second diagonal which is relevant to the culprit LAD lesion. The LAD lesion was then pre-dilated.

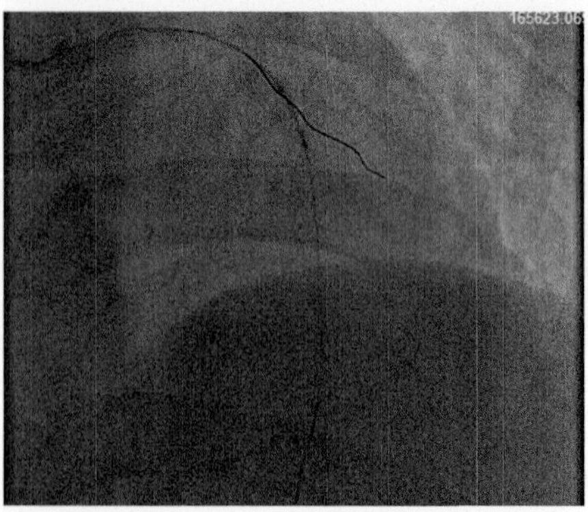

Figure 10.10d A BioMime™ 3 × 38 mm stent is in position at the lesion.

arm, just like a right heart catheter advanced through a sheath in the antecubital vein [Figure 10.11(f–h)].

- Thrombosuction: Although data with thrombosuction in acute myocardial infarction does not support its routine use because it has no significant benefit on mortality[57]; we still use it in situations where there is tortuosity in the vessel and it is difficult to know the downstream anatomy of the coronary without getting a direct visual by removing thrombus; also in some situations it is difficult to assess

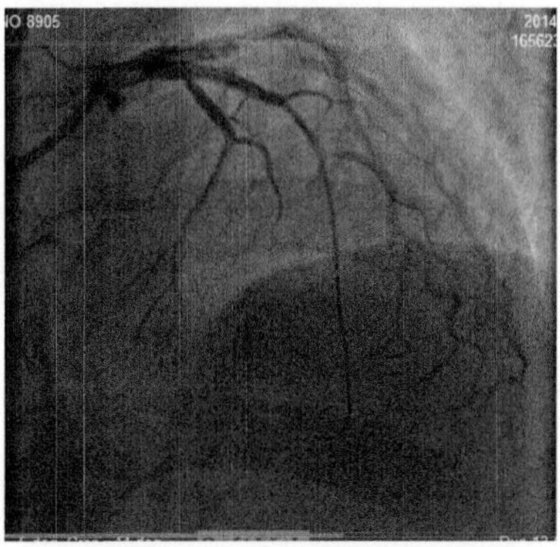

Figure 10.10e Angiogram after stent deployment and post-dilatation.

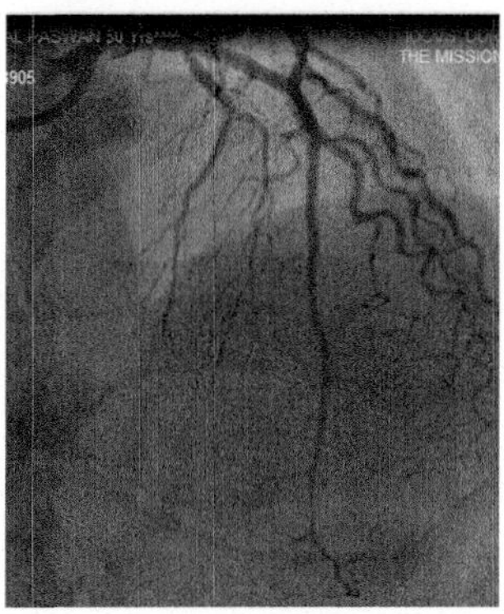

Figure 10.10f Final angiogram after removing wire shows TIMI 3 flow.

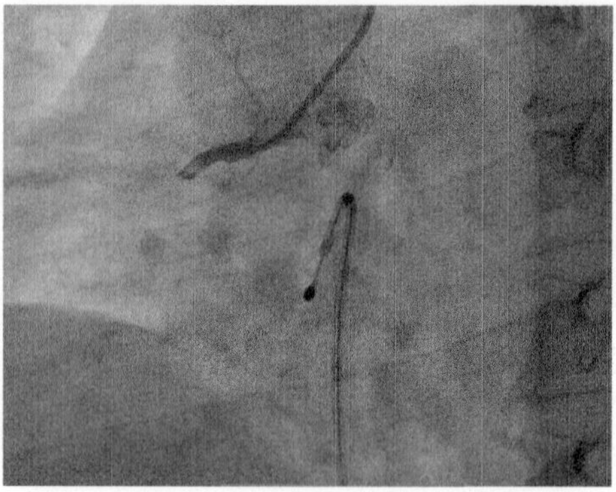

Figure 10.11a Patient with acute inferior STE acute myocardial infarction. A 6F Judkins right (JR) 3.5 guide catheter is used to engage the right coronary artery (RCA). Temporary pacemaker inserted as patient is in complete heart block.

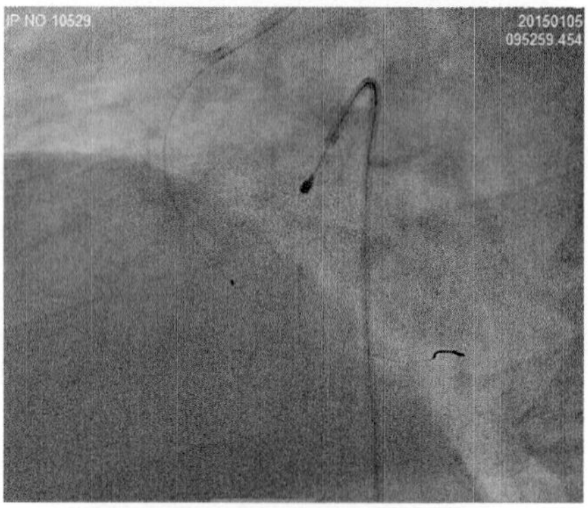

Figure 10.11b A BMW wire crosses the occlusion in RCA. Export thrombosuction in progress.

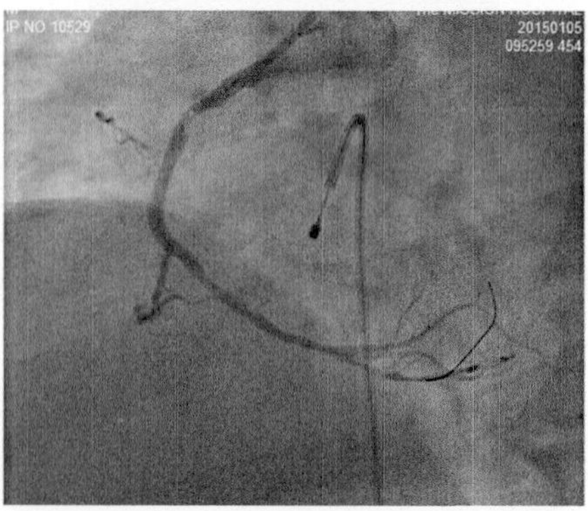

Figure 10.11c Post-thrombosuction angiogram shows focal RCA lesion.

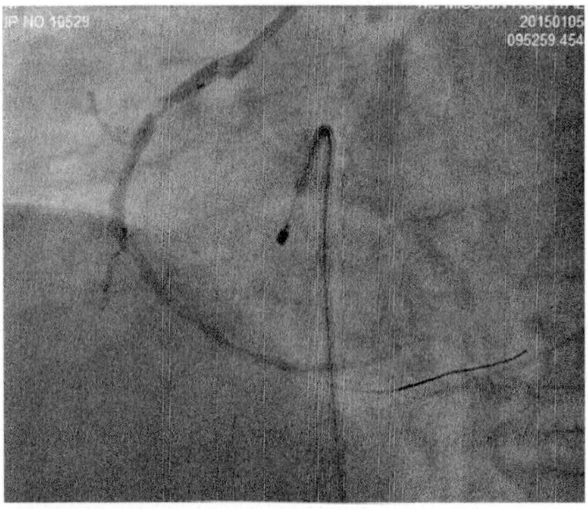

Figure 10.11d Stent in position.

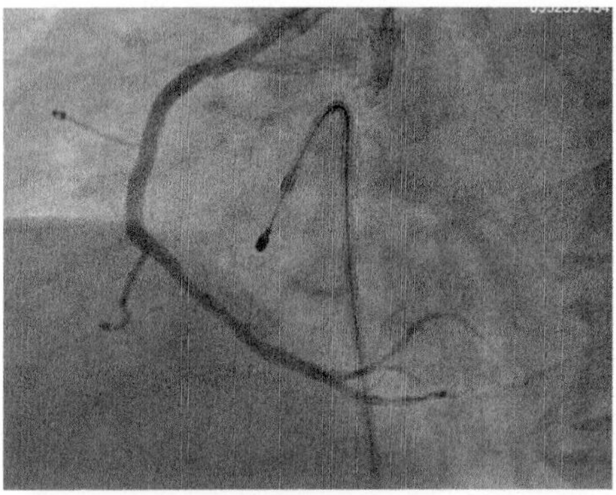

Figure 10.11e Final. TIMI-3 flow in RCA.

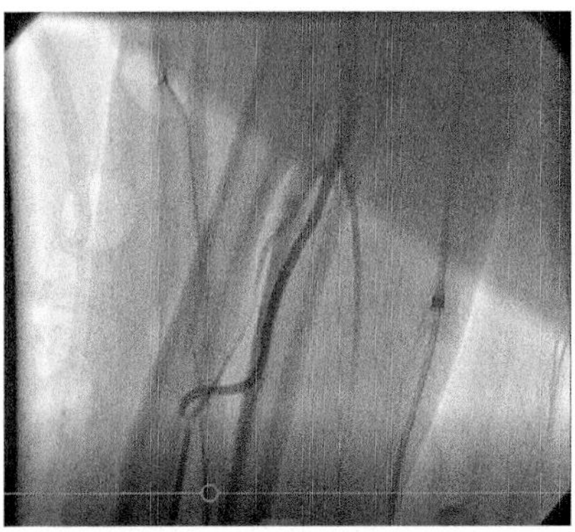

Figure 10.11f A sheath is inserted in antecubital vein of right forearm.

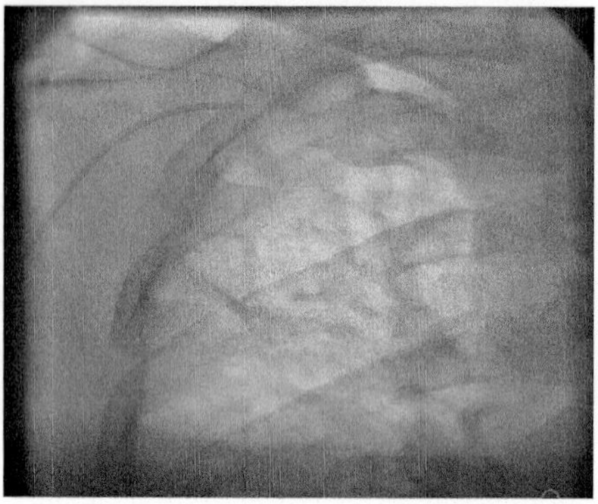

Figure 10.11g A Swan-Ganz catheter tracks up the arm to the right heart.

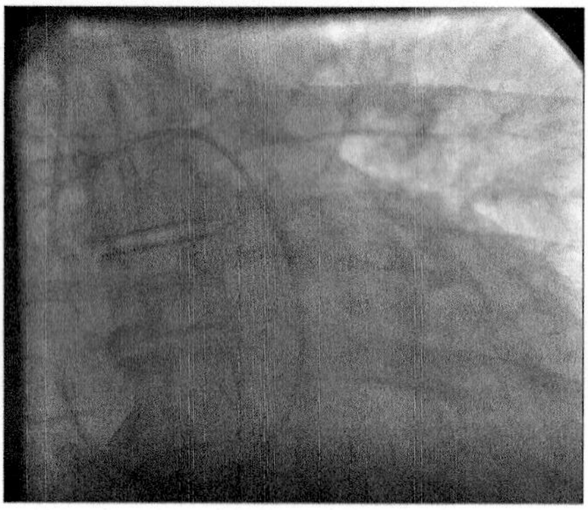

Figure 10.11h The catheter is in right pulmonary artery.

the extent of stenosis to decide on an appropriate stent size without thrombectomy (Figure 10.12a–d, 10.12e(i), 10.12e(ii), and 10.12f–g). Thrombosuction by Export aspiration catheter™ may be required to see the downstream anatomy of the coronary to choose appropriate stent size.

- Dealing with Shepherd's crook RCA: Transradial angioplasty of a Shepherd's crook RCA can be challenging in acute myocardial infarction. Tracking an Export thrombosuction catheter in a Shepherd's crook RCA is difficult. Two wires are sometimes used to enhance support. A run-through wire is preferred over a BMW wire in this situation. A balloon is sometimes used to cross the occluded vessel,

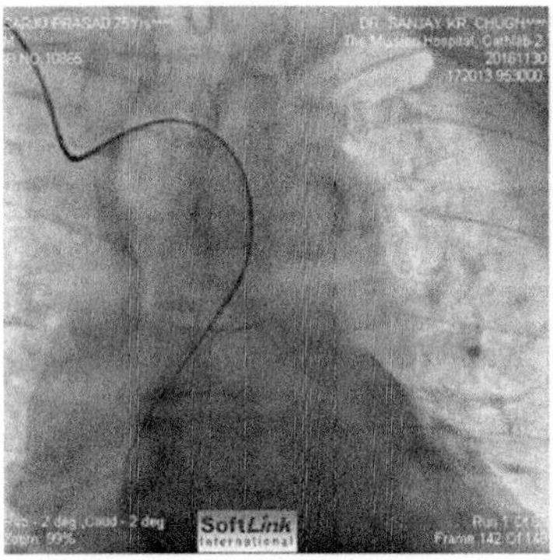

Figure 10.12a Guide catheter and wire negotiating the tortuous right subclavian artery.

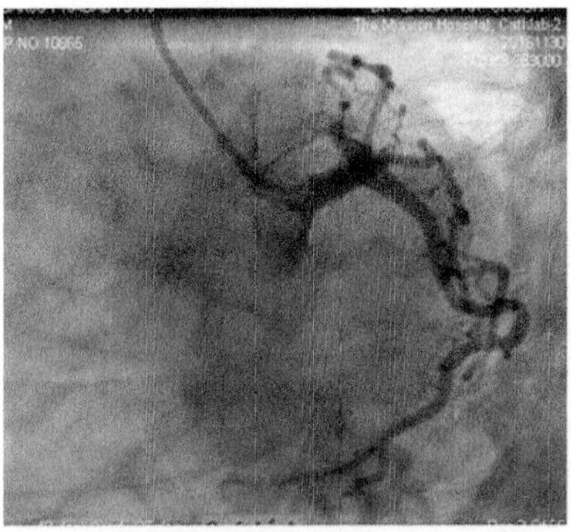

Figure 10.12b Occluded ostial left anterior descending artery [in left anterior oblique (LAO) caudal view] in a patient of acute anterior STE myocardial infarction.

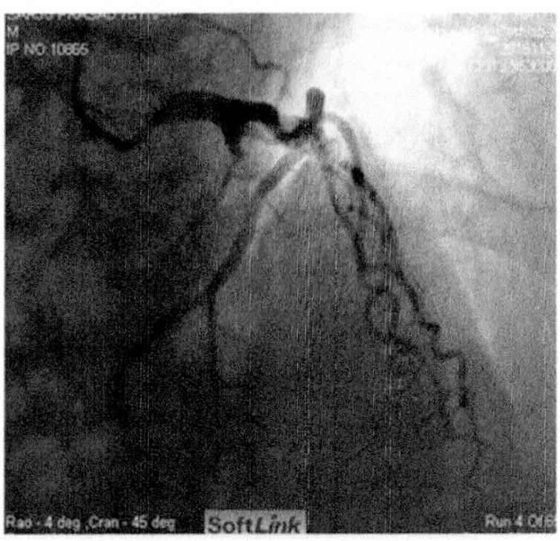

Figure 10.12c Occluded ostial left anterior descending artery seen in LAO cranial.

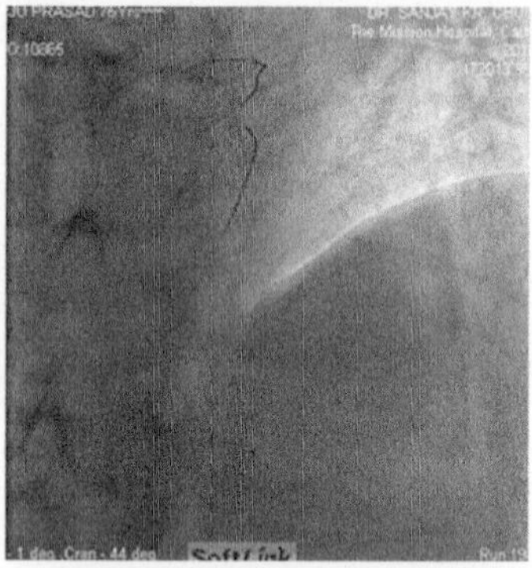

Figure 10.12d A balance middle weight (BMW) wire is in left circumflex artery (LCX) to enhance guide support. A BMW™, Runthrough™, Whisper™ and FielderXT™ wire failed to negotiate the bends in occluded ostial LAD. A Pilot-50™ successfully negotiated the tortuosity in ostial LAD and crossed the occlusion.

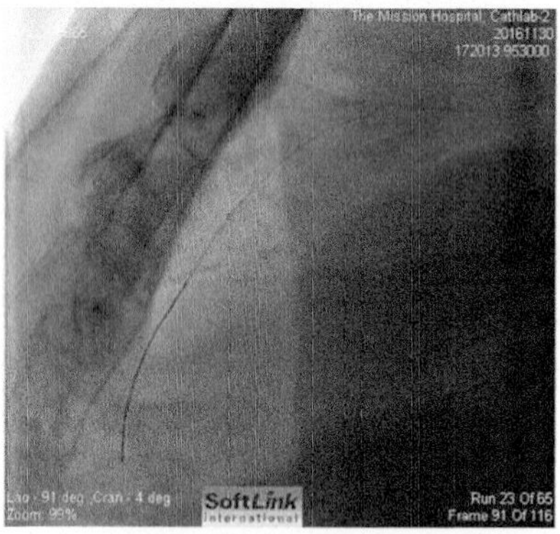

Figure 10.12e(i) Pilot-50 angioplasty wire is manipulated to distal LAD.

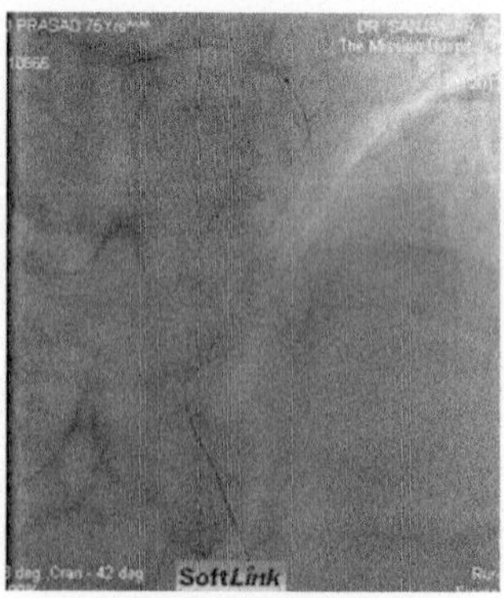

Figure 10.12e(ii) Export thrombosuction done to get a visual on downstream anatomy in LAD to decide on stent length.

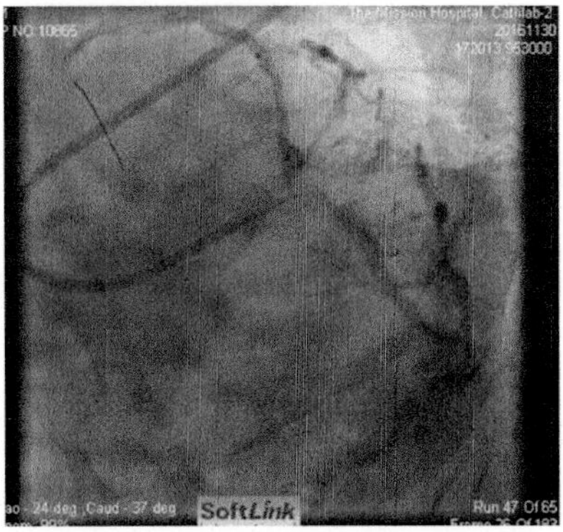

Figure 10.12f Post thrombosuction lesion and downstream vessel seen clearly. Stent in position.

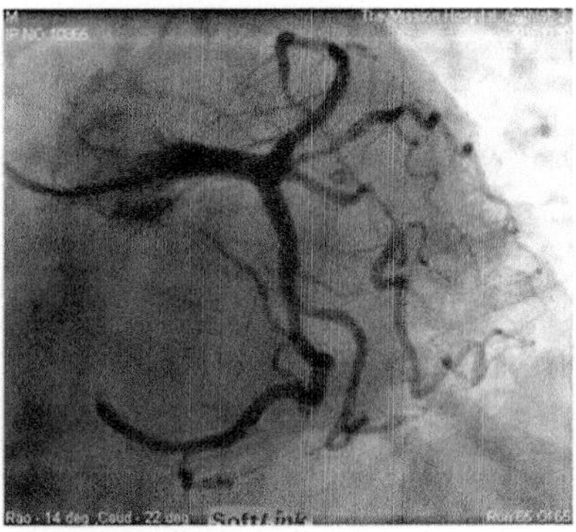

Figure 10.12g Final-TIMI-3 flow in LAD.

which also enhances support to the guide catheter [Figures 10.13(a–j)] and can be used to dotter the occluded artery to establish flow.

- PPUAA takes an average of 6.4 minutes to complete and is useful in reducing the risk of RA spasm, crossover to alternate access and procedure failure[17]; but may have logistical difficulties for primary angioplasty due to non-availability of ultrasound equipment and of sonologist in some centers.
- Cardiogenic shock: In patients with cardiogenic shock, the authors have used intra-aortic balloon pump (IABP) inserted

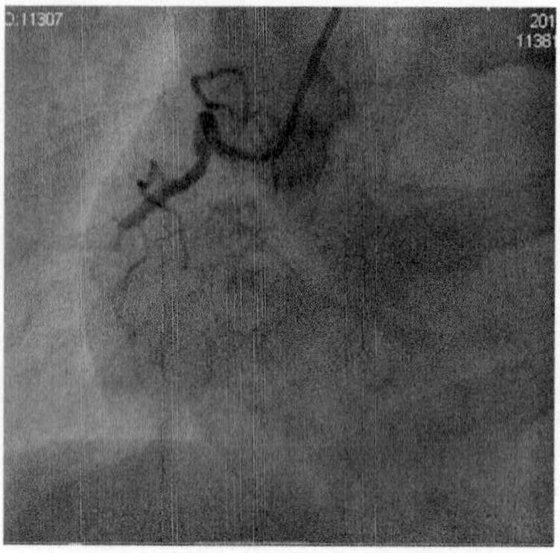

Figure 10.13a Shepherd's crook right coronary artery (RCA) occluded in mid segment. An AR2 guiding catheter is used. A 45-year-old male patient with acute ST-elevation inferior myocardial infarction with complete heart block. Temporary transvenous pacemaker inserted.

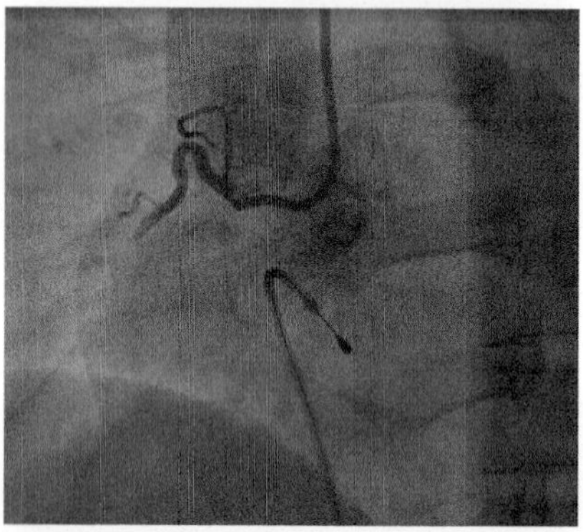

Figure 10.13b Two BMW wires; one in marginal branch to enhance support; the other is the main wire which is advanced to the occluded mid segment of RCA. Note the guiding catheter is changed to 6F Judkins right catheter because of operator preference, as the AR2 was not giving desired support.

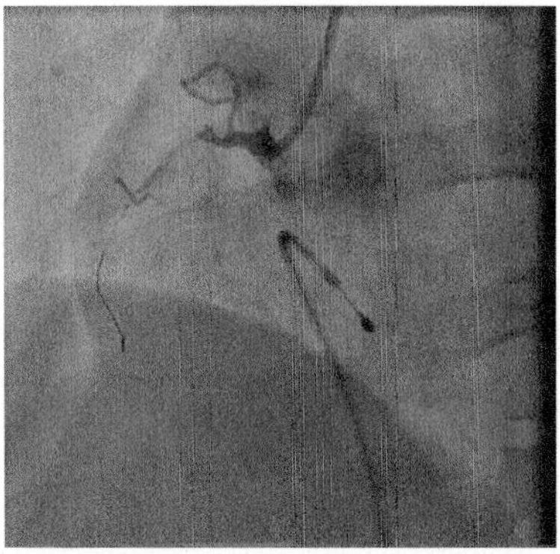

Figure 10.13c A balloon is used to enhance the push on the angioplasty wire (BMW) and also provides enhanced guide support in the Shepherd's crook RCA. The wire is in a marginal branch.

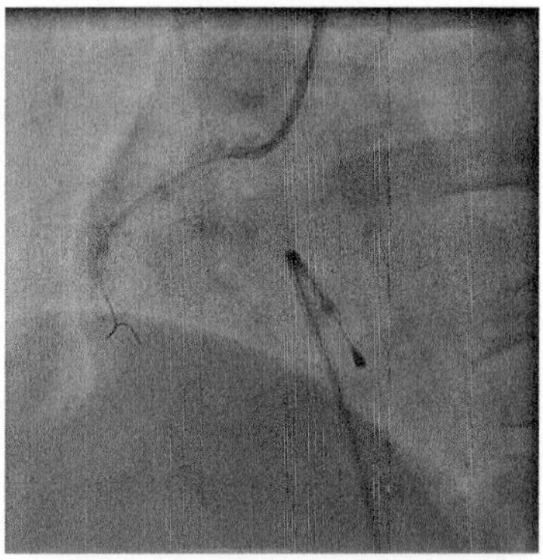

Figure 10.13d The same 2 × 12 mm balloon is used for pre-dilatation at site of occlusion.

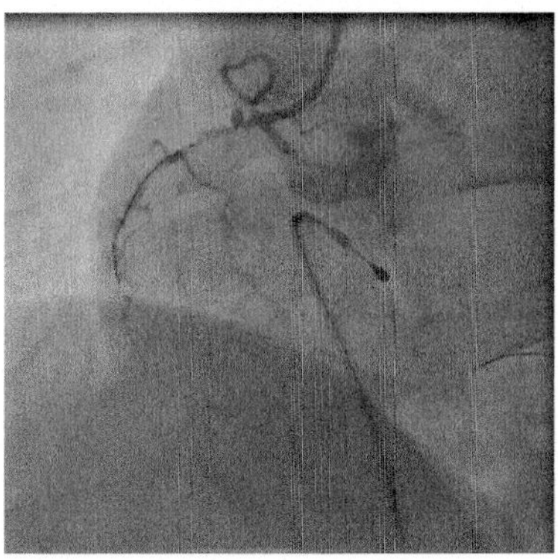

Figure 10.13e The BMW wire is advanced to distal RCA with support of a pre-dilatation balloon which also enhances guide support and allows the angioplasty BMW wire to track into distal RCA. Balloon is withdrawn to proximal RCA. There is no flow in the artery. Note concertina in proximal RCA.

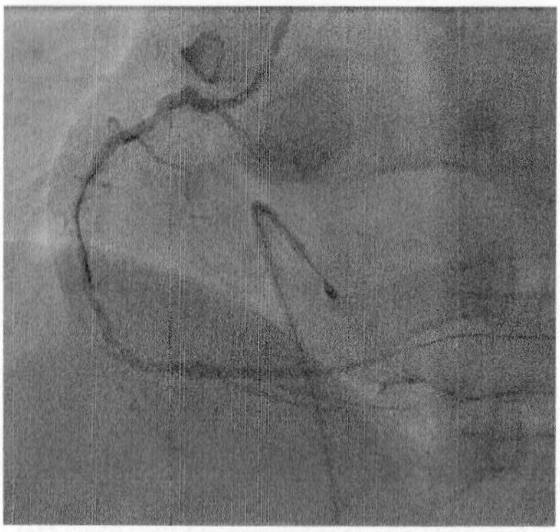

Figure 10.13f After pre-dilatation and intracoronary nitroglycerine, diffusely diseased right coronary artery is seen.

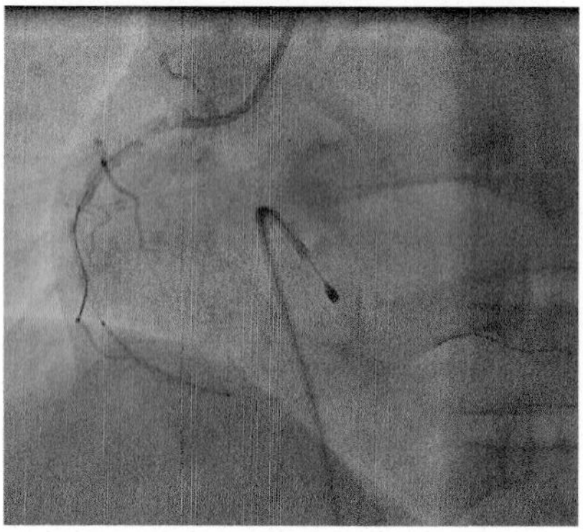

Figure 10.13g A second (buddy) wire is passed into RCA into the distal marginal branch. First stent in position in distal RCA.

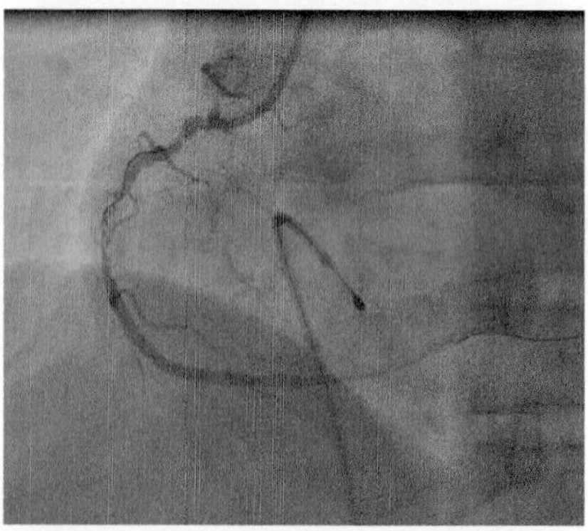

Figure 10.13h Second stent being deployed in mid-RCA.

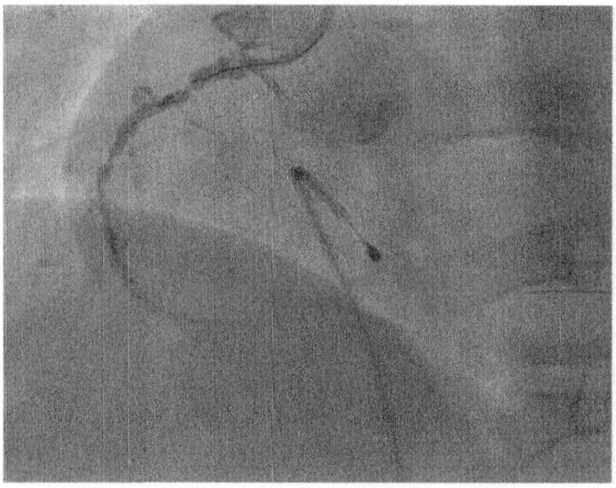

Figure 10.13i Third stent being deployed in proximal RCA.

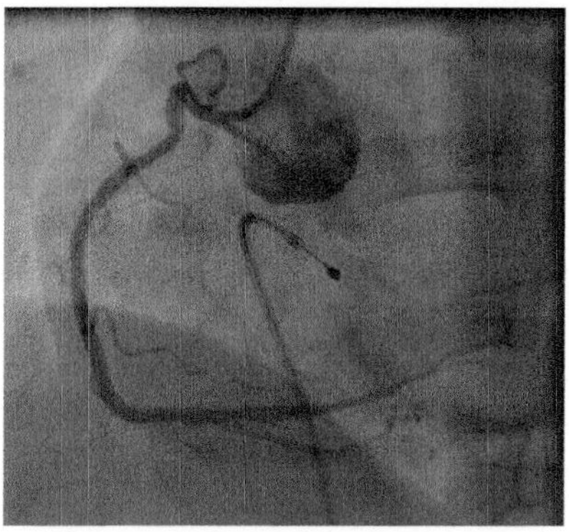

Figure 10.13j Final, TIMI3 flow in RCA.

transfemorally for transradial interventions (TRIs) because of prohibitive cost and non-availability of Impella® left ventricular assist device for left ventricular support, until recently. TRI is justified in patients requiring IABP [Figures 10.14(a–j)]; to avoid traumatizing both groins in order to minimize patient discomfort as well as risk of bleeding, since the sheath used for angioplasty is removed when patient is still on Gp2b/3a blockers and bleeding risk would therefore be high with transfemoral access (TFA) for angioplasty. The IABP balloon, on the other hand, comes out after the patient's haemodynamics improve, long after the GP2b/3a blocker infusion is over. Hence risk of groin haematoma is less. The same logic would be true for use of Impella via Femoral access.

- In a retrospective study of PAMI cases requiring IABP support, TRA was associated with a lower incidence of access-related bleedings (6.3% vs 18.7%, $p < 0.01$) and lower unadjusted NACE compared with PAMI via TFA (36.6% vs 57.4%, $p < 0.01$).[57]

Tips for TRI in Complex Lesions

TRI in complex lesions, transradial rotablation, chronic total occlusions, TRI in bifurcation lesions and left main disease are covered in details in separate chapters.

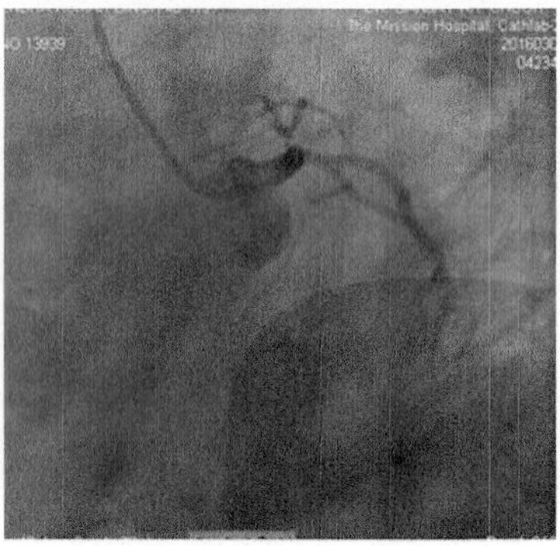

Figure 10.14a A 43-year-old patient of anterior wall myocardial infarction in cardiogenic shock. Balloon pump inserted. Transradial angiogram shows critical ostial left anterior descending artery (LAD) stenosis as culprit.

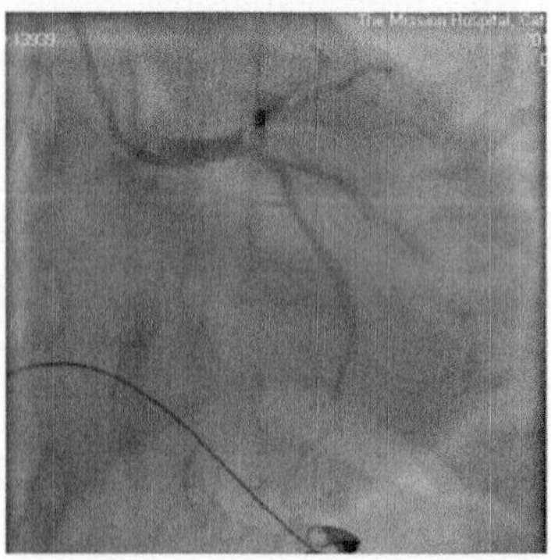

Figure 10.14b Ostial LAD stenosis seen in anteroposterior (AP) caudal view.

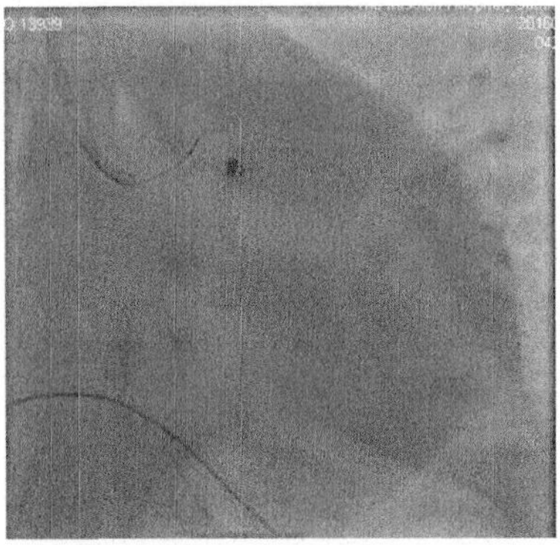

Figure 10.14c A balance middle weight (BMW) wire is used to cross the lesion. Note a 6F Judkins left (JL) 3.0 guiding catheter is used. An XB (extra backup) guide may be too aggressive and injure the ostial left anterior descending artery (LAD).

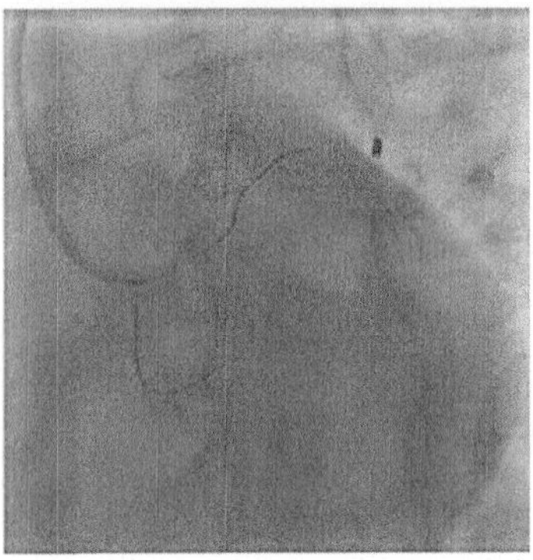

Figure 10.14d A second BMW wire is inserted in the first diagonal artery, after the wire in the main vessel is inserted all the way down into the distal LAD.

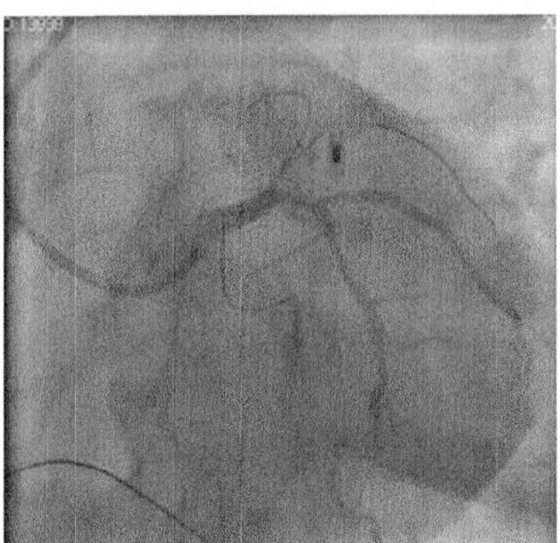

Figure 10.14e A 2-mm balloon is used to pre-dilate the ostial LAD lesion.

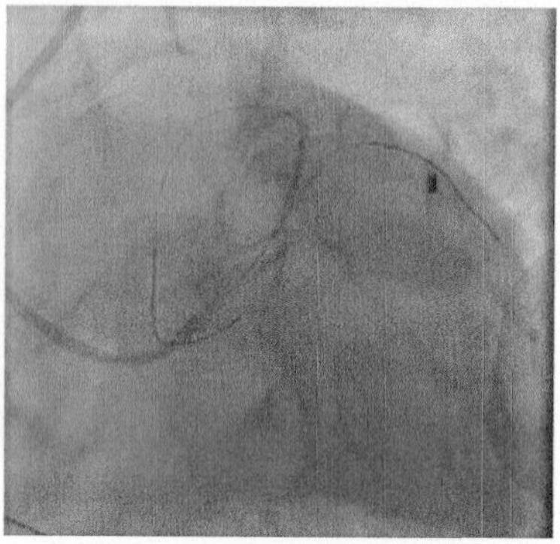

Figure 10.14f A Xience V® stent (3 × 18 mm) is in position.

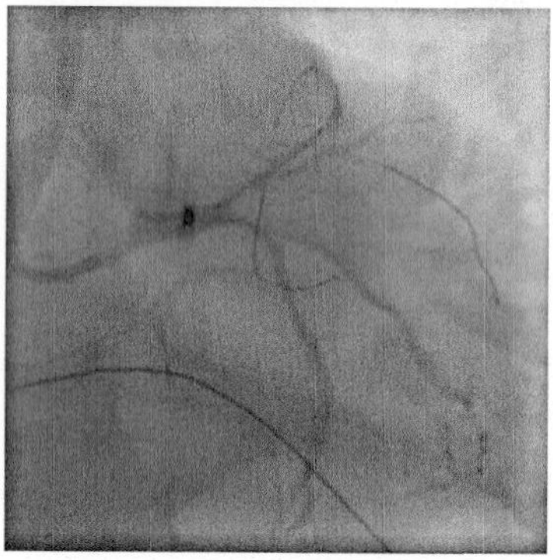

Figure 10.14g Stent positioned in ostial LAD.

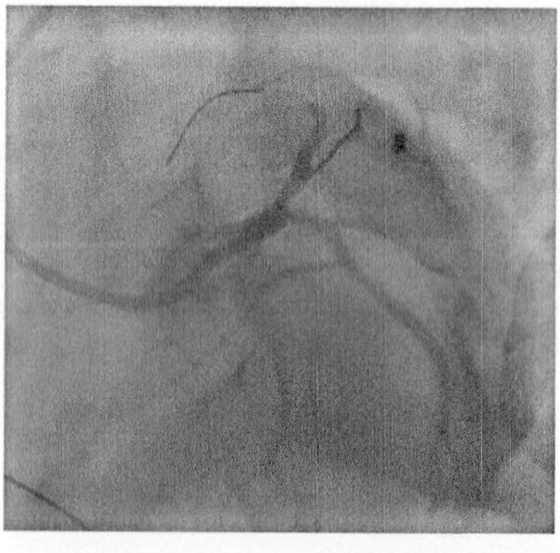

Figure 10.14h Post-stent deployment, LAD viewed in left anterior oblique (LAO) caudal view.

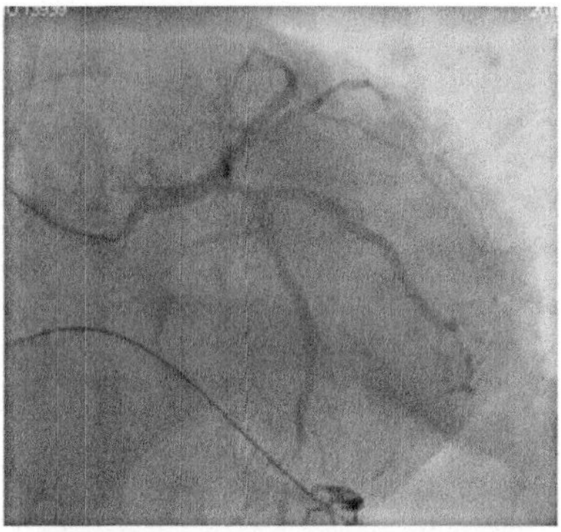

Figure 10.14i Final TIMI 3 flow in LAO caudal view.

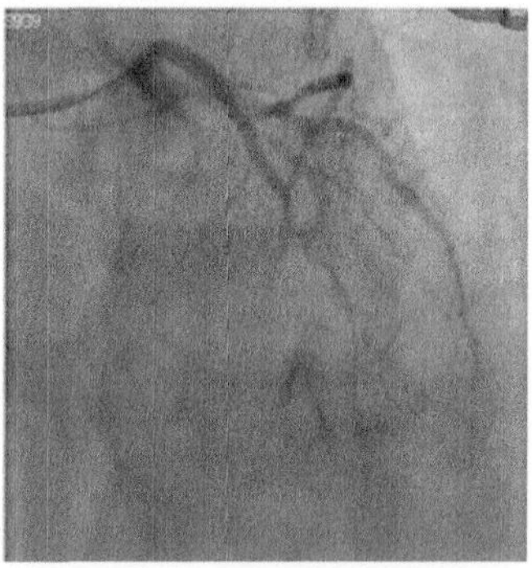

Figure 10.14j Final TIMI3 flow in anterior oblique with cranial projection.

- Bifurcation lesions [Figure 10.15(a–g)] and rotablation with ≥1.75 burr [Figure 10.16(a–i)] may require 7F guide catheter which can be used safely (*please see sheath sizing protocol above*) in patients with radial arteries ≥2.1 mm. Most bifurcation lesions can be managed with 6F guide catheter, even for double kissing crush [Figure 10.17(a–o)].

- TRI in post bypass grafts: Usually an Amplatz guide catheter is successful in engaging the SVGs from the left radial artery which is the authors Hence the authors' preferred access site in these cases.

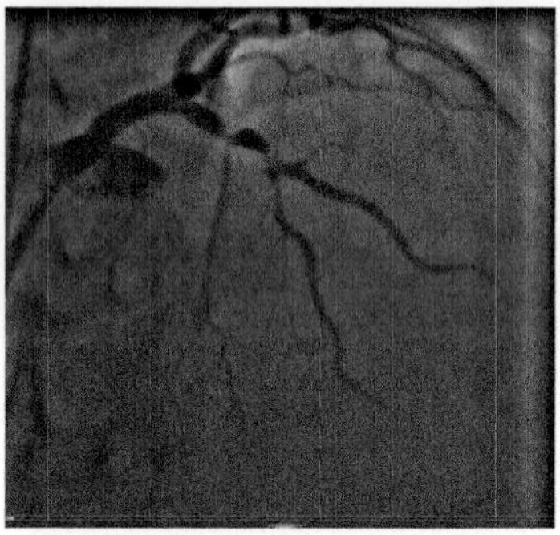

Figure 10.15a LAD, D1 lesion, Medina 1, 1, 1 bifurcation lesion.

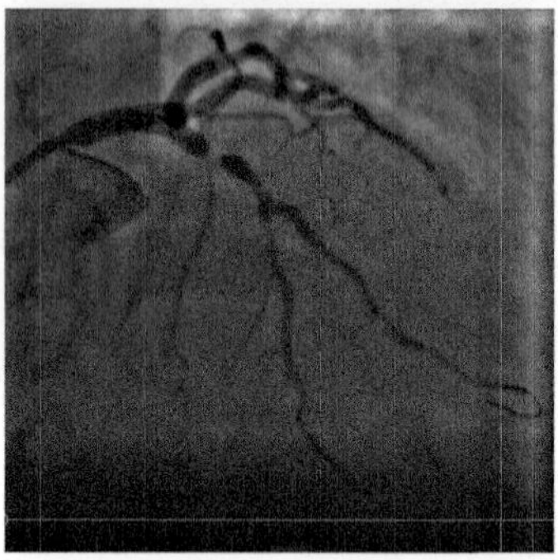

Figure 10.15b Wire in both LAD and large first diagonal.

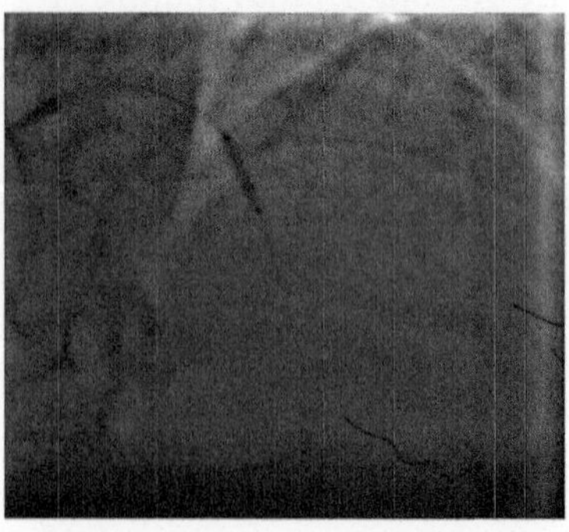

Figure 10.15c A 2.5-mm cutting balloon is inflated to 8 atmospheres in LAD at bifurcation.

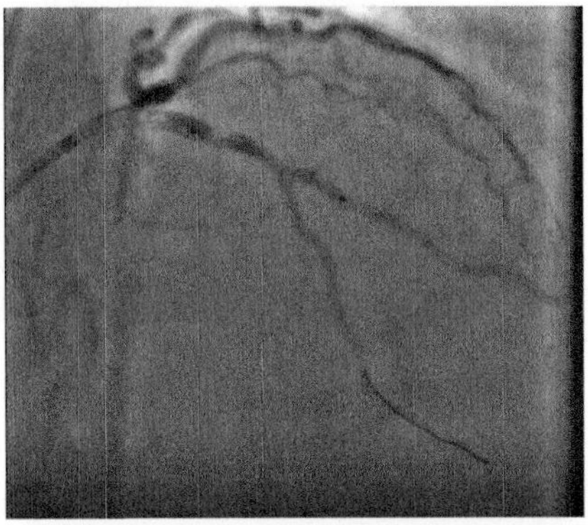

Figure 10.15d Stent being positioned from LAD mid to first diagonal (D1) across the bifurcation.

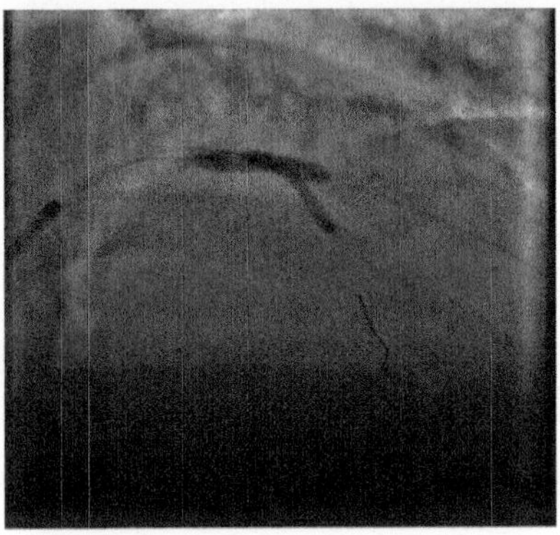

Figure 10.15e Kissing balloon dilatation at bifurcation after LAD and D1 wires were exchanged.

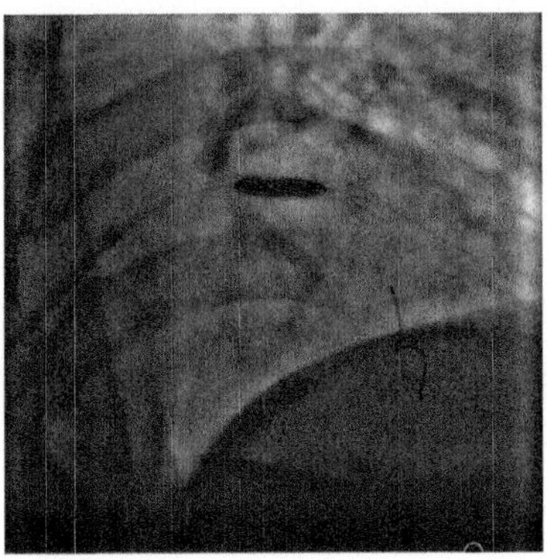

Figure 10.15f Post dilatation of LAD stent after LAD and D1 wires were exchanged before final kissing balloon dilatation.

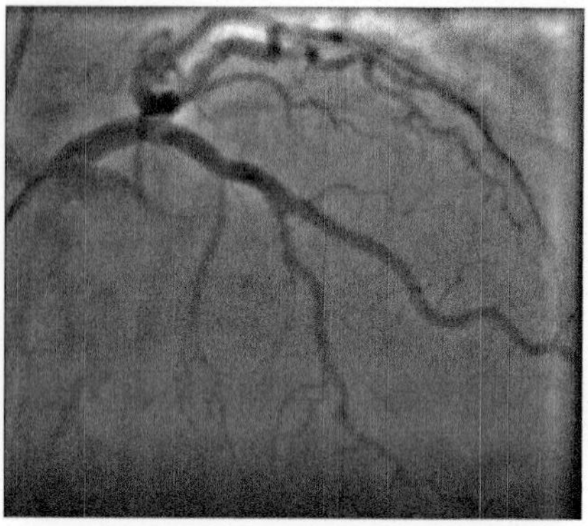

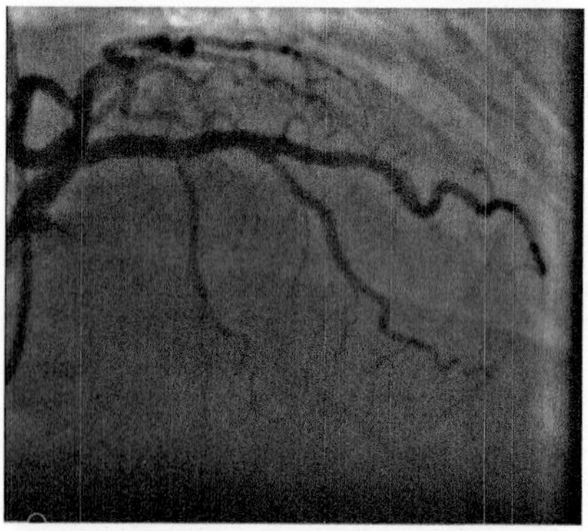

Figure 10.15g Final result, TIMI 3 flow.

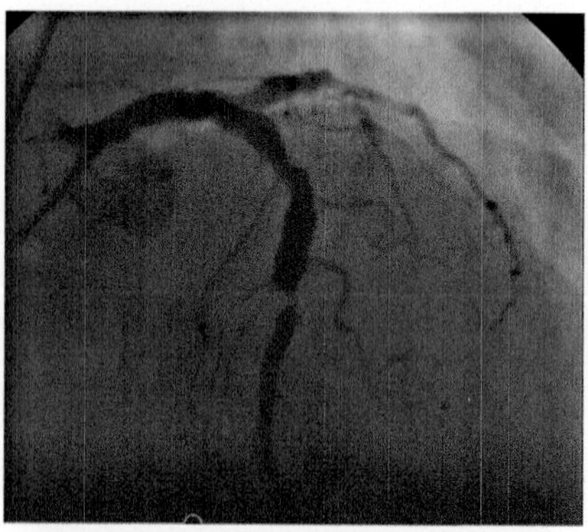

Figure 10.16a Ectatic LAD with critical calcific distal stenosis. An XB 3.5, 7F guide catheter is used.

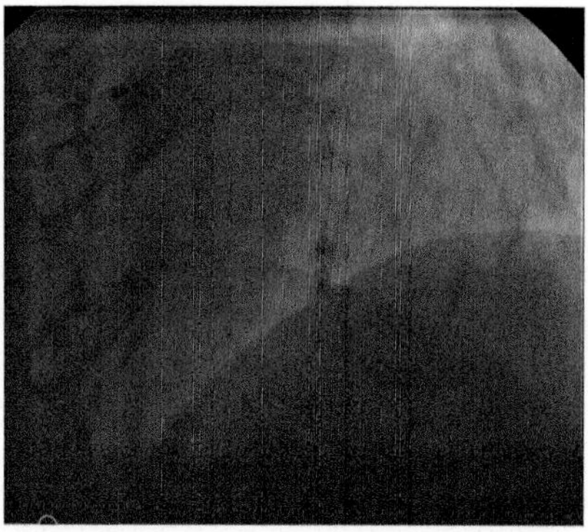

Figure 10.16b 2- and 2.5-mm non-compliant balloons failed to dilate the lesion.

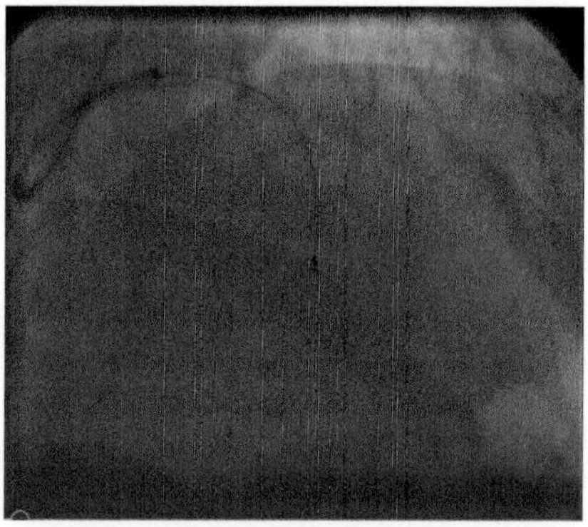

Figure 10.16c A 1.5-mm rotational atherectomy burr was used to debulk the lesion after the angioplasty wire was exchanged for a Rota C wire.

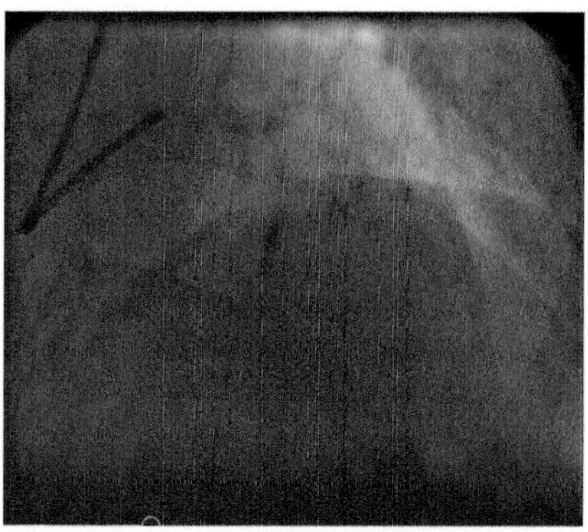

Figure 10.16d A 3-mm non-compliant (NC) balloon failed to dilate the lesion.

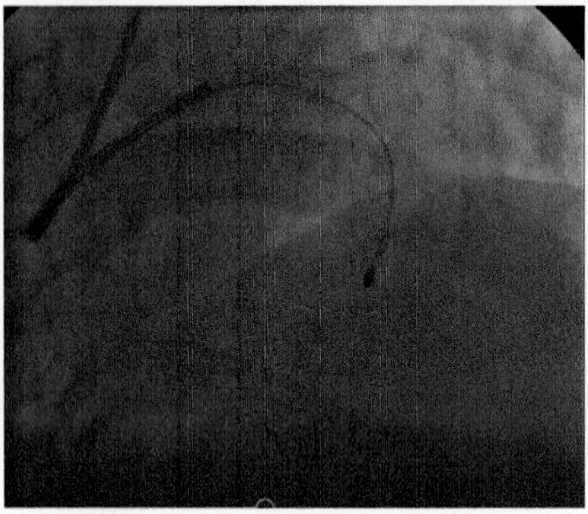

Figure 10.16e Several passes were made by a 1.75-mm burr to debulk the densely calcified lesion.

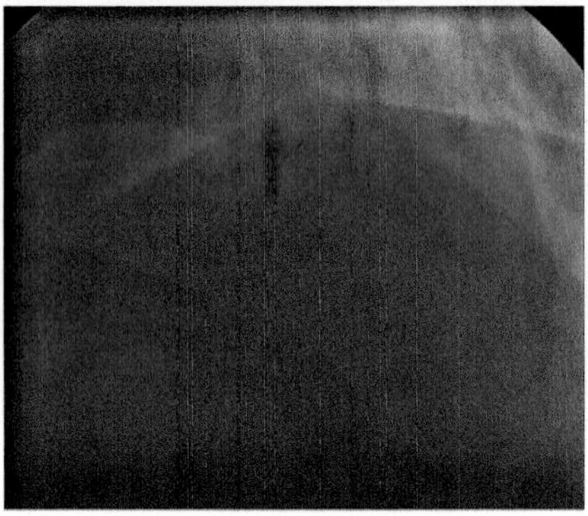

Figure 10.16f A 3-mm non-compliant (NC) balloon is now able to dilate the lesion.

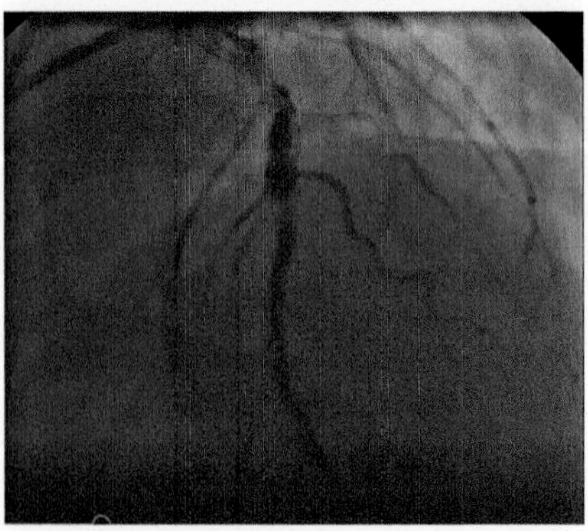

Figure 10.16g Stent in position.

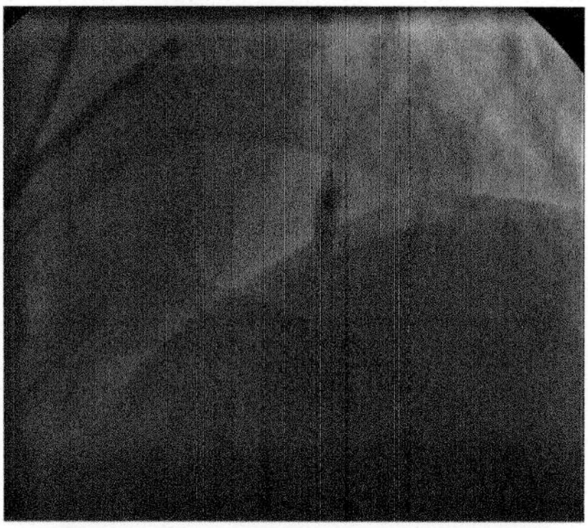

Figure 10.16h Stent post-dilatation done.

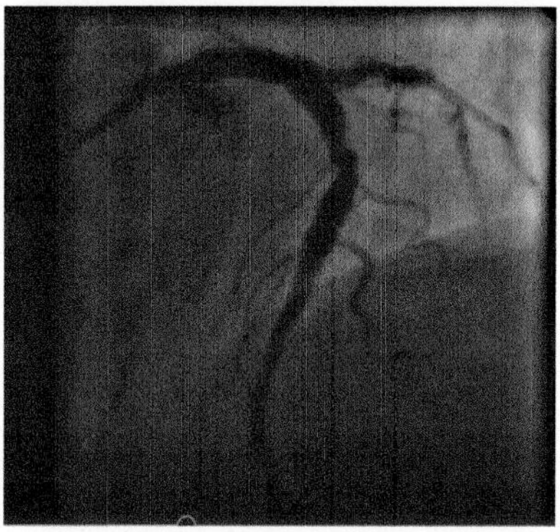

Figure 10.16i Final result, TIMI 3 flow.

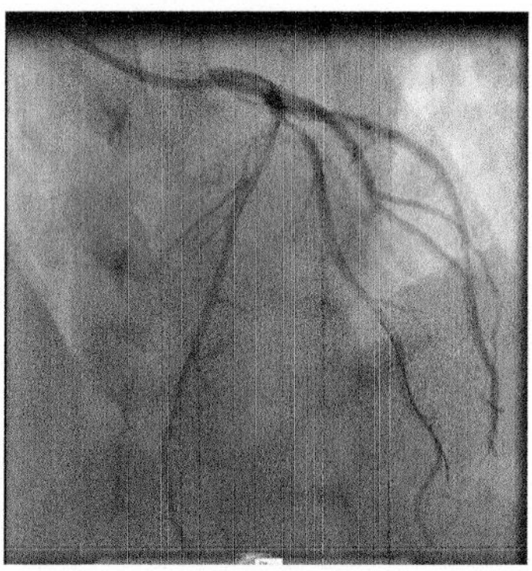

Figure 10.17a A Medina 0, 1, 1 bifurcation lesion with a large first diagonal (D1). Both left anterior descending artery (LAD) and first diagonal have a significant lesion. Both are wired. The LAD lesion has a pre-dilatation balloon in place.

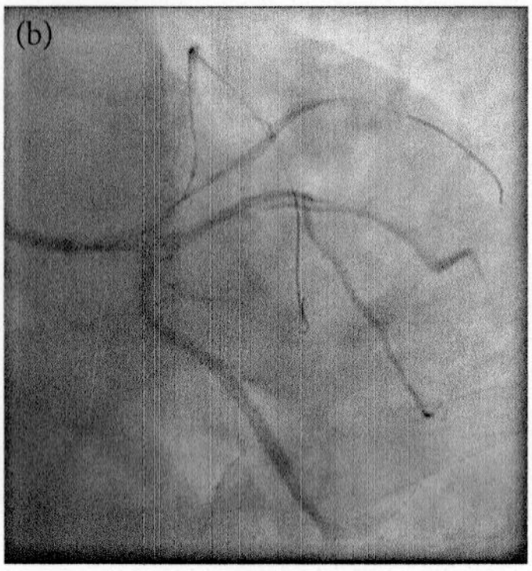

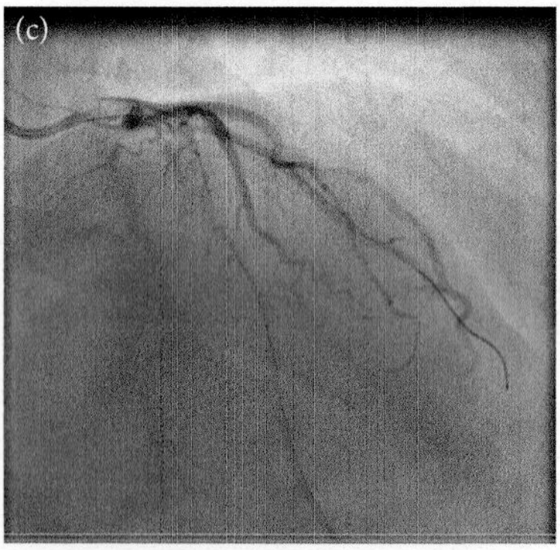

Figure 10.17b,c Stent in D1 and balloon in LAD.

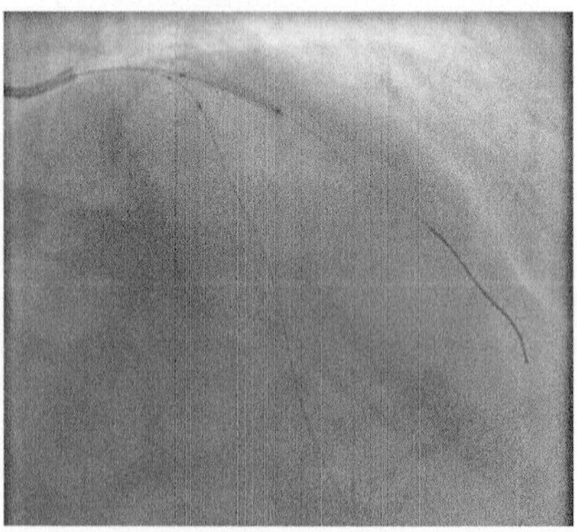

Figure 10.17d Stent deployed in D1.

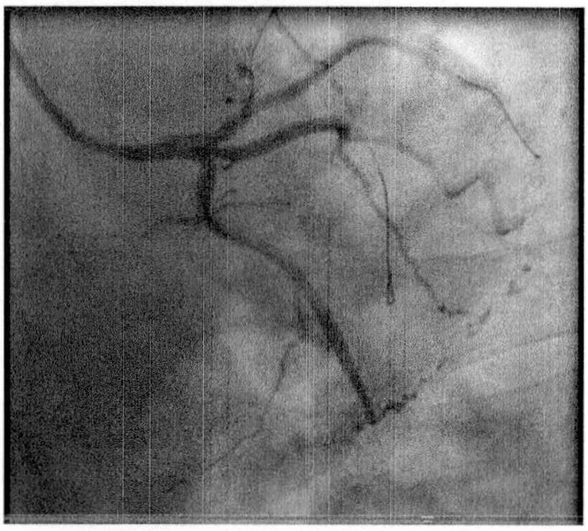

Figure 10.17e Post-stent deployment in D1.

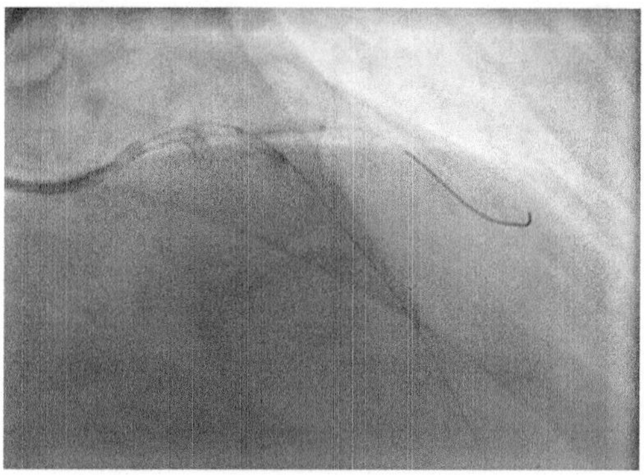

Figure 10.17f First kissing balloon (KB) in progress at LAD, D1 bifurcation.

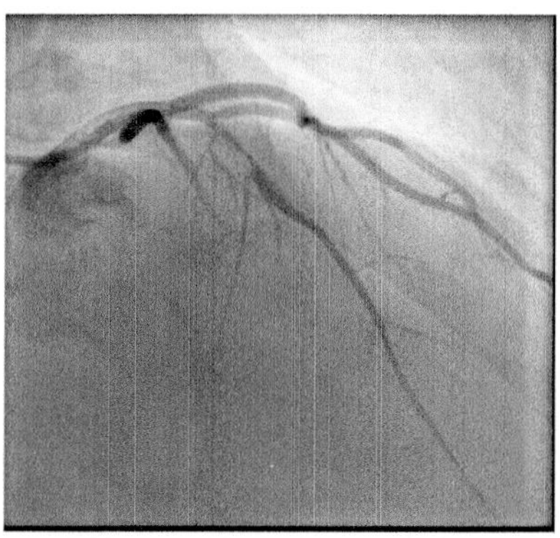

Figure 10.17g Post first kissing balloon (KB) angiogram.

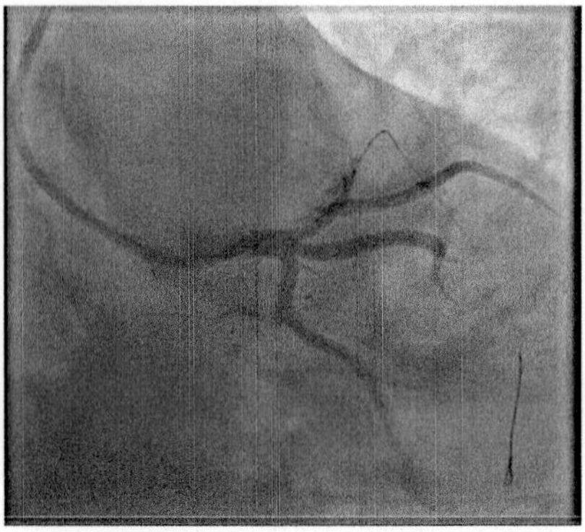

Figure 10.17h LAD stent in positon, D1 wire removed.

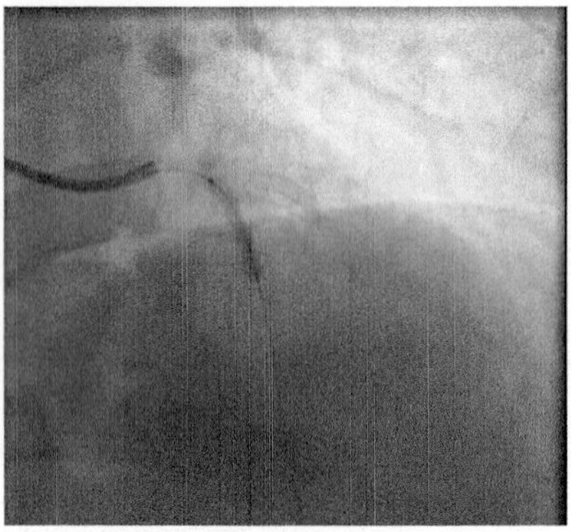

Figure 10.17i LAD stent deployed.

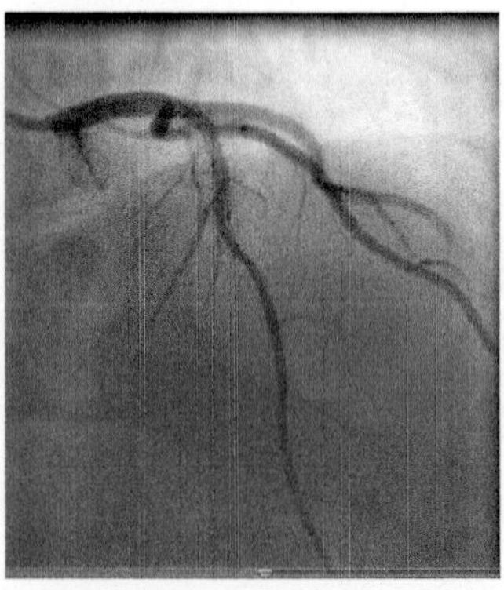

Figure 10.17j Post LAD stent deployment angiogram.

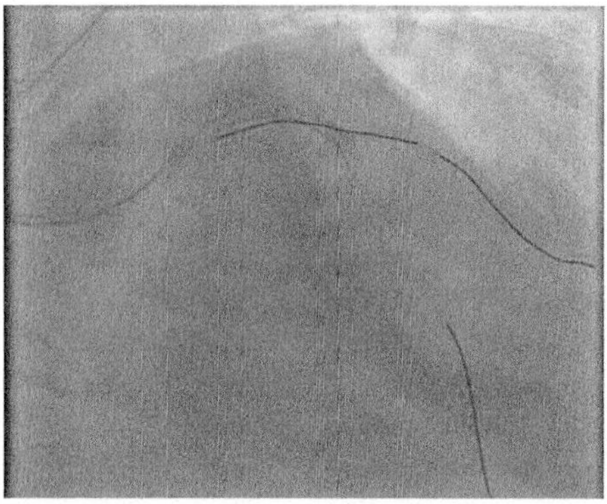

Figure 10.17k Side branch re-crossed with BMW; jailed side branch wire being pulled out.

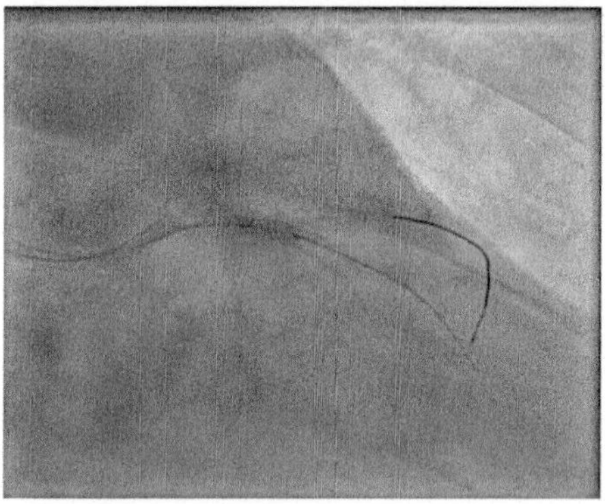

Figure 10.17l Post dilating LAD stent.

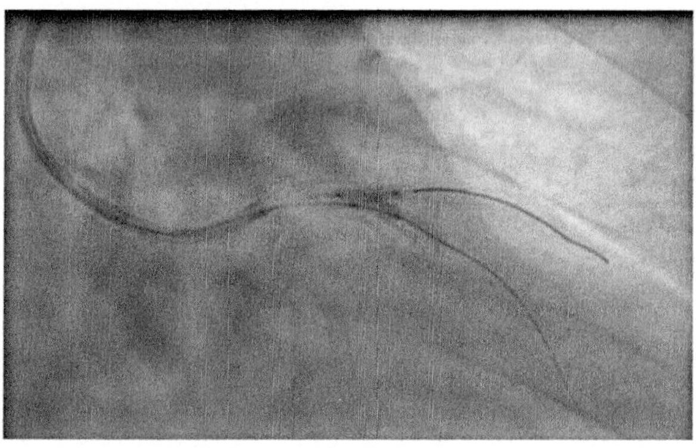

Figure 10.17m Final KB.

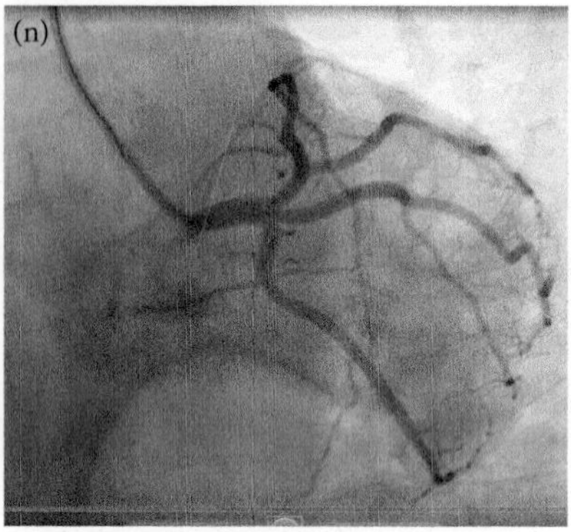

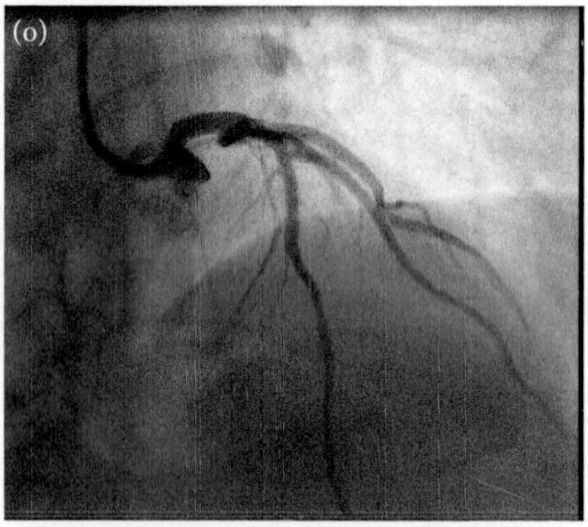

Figures 10.17n and 10.17o Final result, TIMI 3 flow.

In the short-statured patients and those with smaller aortic roots, an AR2 guide [Figure 10.2c(i–ix)] is usually successful; while in the larger aortic roots and taller subjects, an AL1 may be required [Figure 10.2d(i–viii)]. A multipurpose guide (MPA2) is sometimes required for engaging the SVG to right coronary artery (RCA) or obtuse marginal artery. A left internal mammary artery (LIMA) guide catheter successfully hooks the LIMA from left radial artery [Figure 10.2e(i–iii)]. A LIMA catheter is advanced via left radial artery to the site of LIMA origin from subclavian artery; after checking the position in antero-posterior (AP) view, LIMA is hooked easily in the left anterior oblique view (LAO), by gentle clockwise rotation. In LAO view, the LIMA ostium is seen anterior to catheter tip.

- Chronic total occlusions (CTOs): CTOs can be disobliterated successfully using 5F guide[28,30] and microcatheter [Figure 10.18 (a–j)], but usually require 6F or 7F GC. Transradial interventions in CTO and post bypass grafts is discussed in detail in Chapter 15.

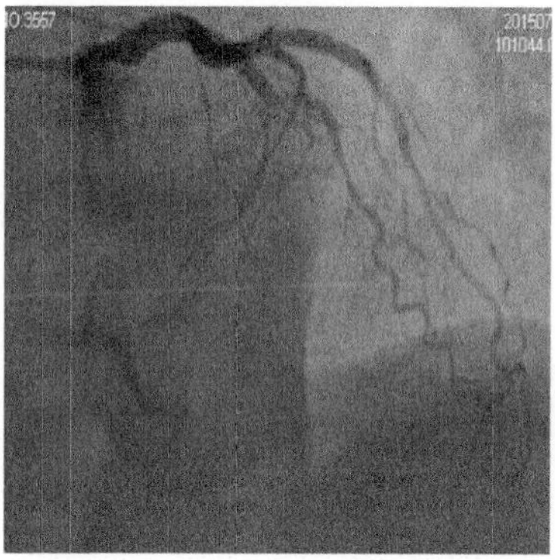

Figure 10.18a A chronic occlusion of proximal left anterior descending artery (LAD). A 5F, JL3.5 guiding catheter is used.

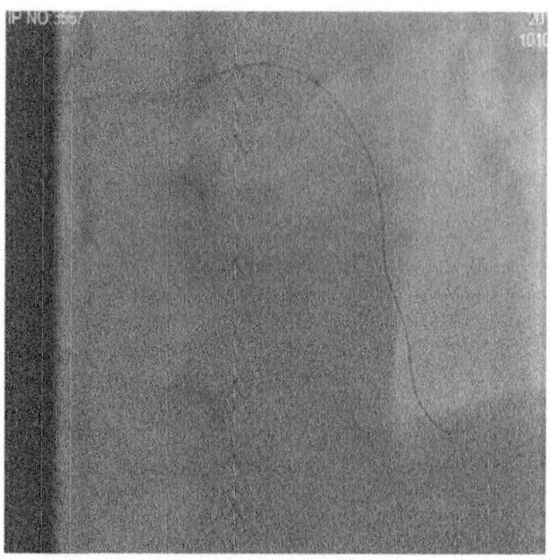

Figure 10.18b With the support of microcatheter, a miracle wire crosses the lesion.

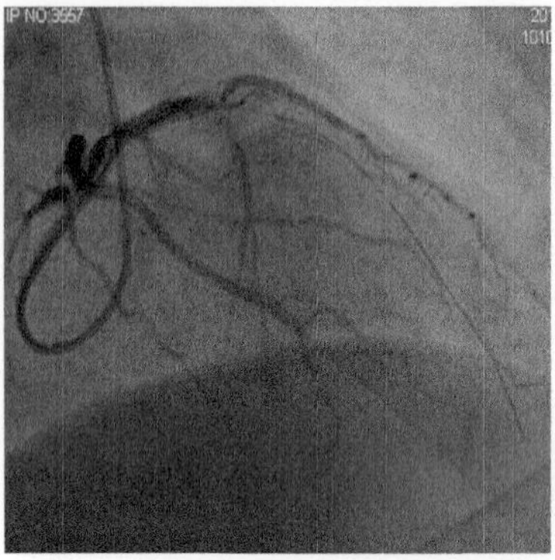

Figure 10.18c A 1.5-mm balloon is used to predilate the left anterior descending artery (LAD) at the site of occlusion.

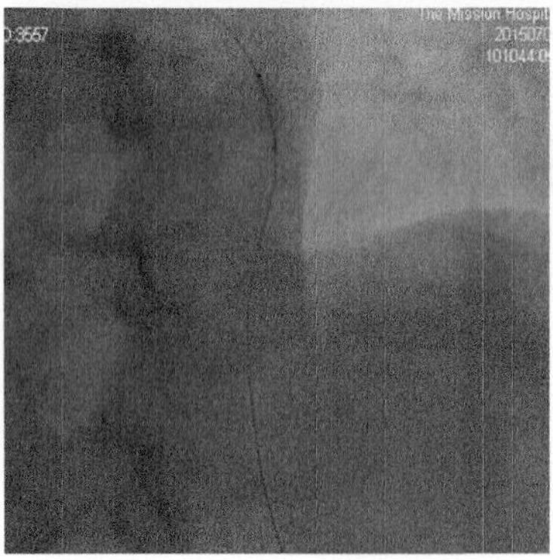

Figure 10.18d Check angiogram after pre-dilatation.

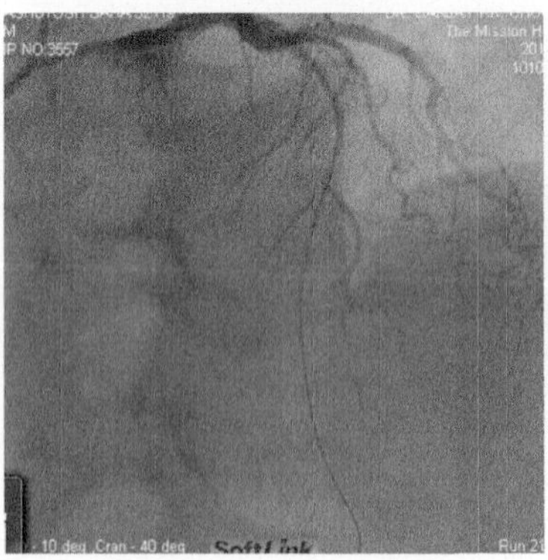

Figure 10.18e Further pre-dilatation along the length of LAD.

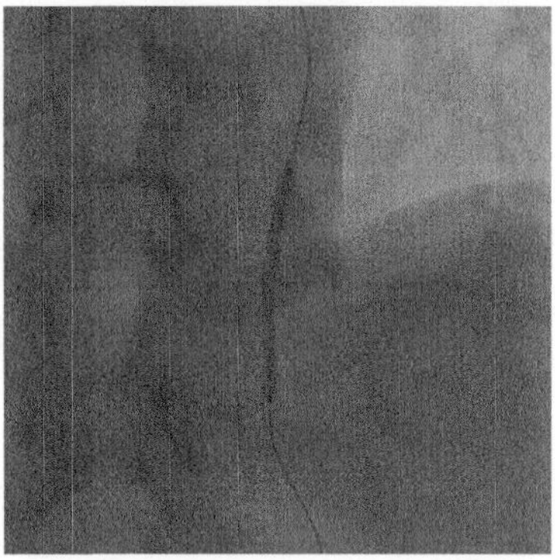

Figure 10.18f Distal stent deployed.

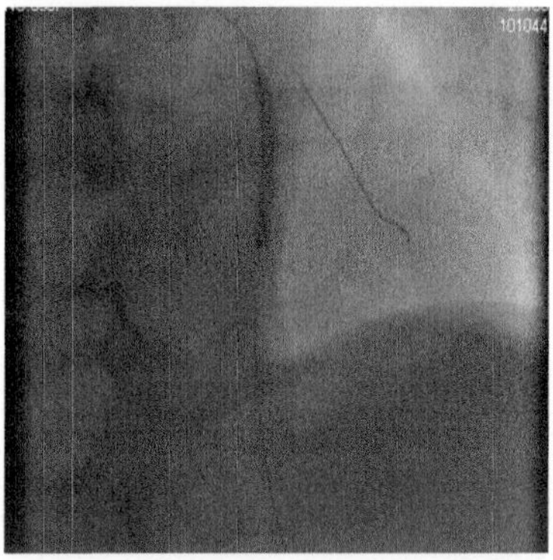

Figure 10.18g Stent deployed in mid LAD.

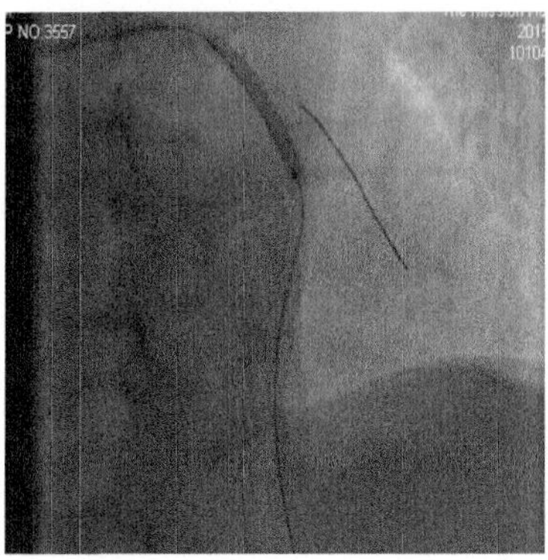

Figure 10.18h Proximal stent deployed.

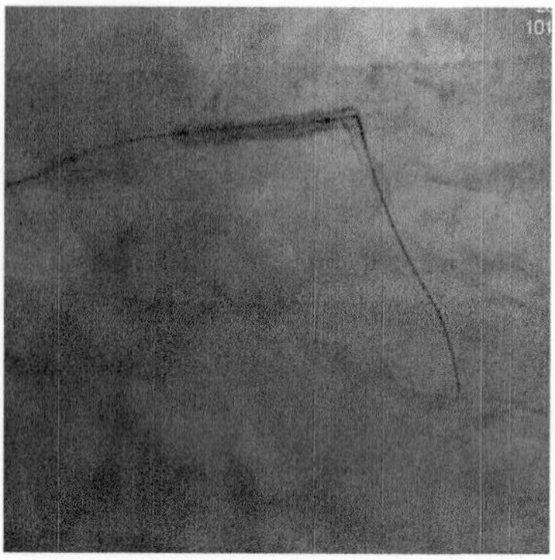

Figure 10.18i Post dilatation of stents using non-compliant (NC) balloon.

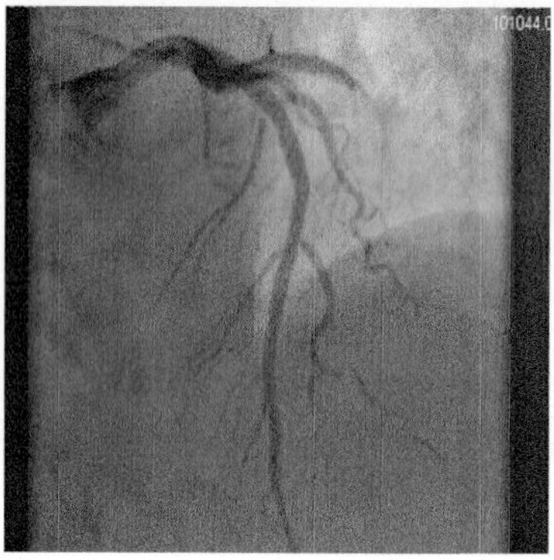

Figure 10.18j Final TIMI 3 flow in LAD.

Tips for Haemostasis

Haemostasis is discussed in details in the chapter on '*Haemostasis, Anticoagulation and the Anticoagulated*'. Haemostasis in snuffbox access are discussed in the chapter on '*Distal Transradial Interventions*'.

In this chapter, we present our tips and tricks for economical and effective haemostasis with a radial artery occlusion (RAO) rate comparable to that with non-occlusive haemostasis (RAO 3.4% using **b**andage-roll and **e**lastic bandage **t**echnique (BEST) for haemostasis (see below) vs 4.3%[58,59] using patent haemostasis). In the PROPHET[58] and PROPHET II[59] studies, 5F sheaths and catheters were used for diagnostic cardiac catheterization in stable patients and the assessment of RAO was not done using colour Doppler ultrasound. In the authors' registry (*see below*), which included 6F angioplasty in patients with average RAD of 1.78 mm'" patients undergoing primary transradial angioplasty and those with haemodynamic instability were included and colour Doppler ultrasound was used to assess RAO.

Manual compression and pneumatic device were compared for haemostasis after 5F radial procedures in the MEMORY trial and were found to have similar RAO.[60] The incidence of RAO was 12% with manual compression versus 8% with pneumatic devices using 5F sheaths with mean RAD of 2.8 mm. Manual compression is impractical and requires trained human resource which is difficult to procure and expensive; the pneumatic devices too cost $20 in the US and Rs 2000/ in India (~$30).

The authors' technique of haemostasis, using Gauze ball/bandage roll combined with Elastoplast or elastic bandage to compress the puncture site is economical (costs $1 for 3 patients) and has shown[61] radial occlusion rates similar to the pneumatic haemostasis devices (TR band®) with non-occlusive haemostasis, with very low rate of haematoma formation (1.4%).

Technique

A standard cotton bandage roll of 3 cm diameter × 5 cm length is placed over the site of puncture where the sheath exits the skin [Figure 10.19 (a–c)]. The sheath is then pulled out and a strip of elastic bandage measuring 15 cm long, 3 cm wide is stretched to full stretch (15cm → 27 cm) and wrapped around the wrist, covering half of the cotton bandage-roll [Figure 10.19(d–g)]; the second wrap covers the remaining bandage-roll; the third comes on top of both. This bandage is loosened after an hour and removed ≥12 hours later. After the bandage is loosened, patient is closely observed for any bleeding in the forearm manifest as early induration or visible swelling.

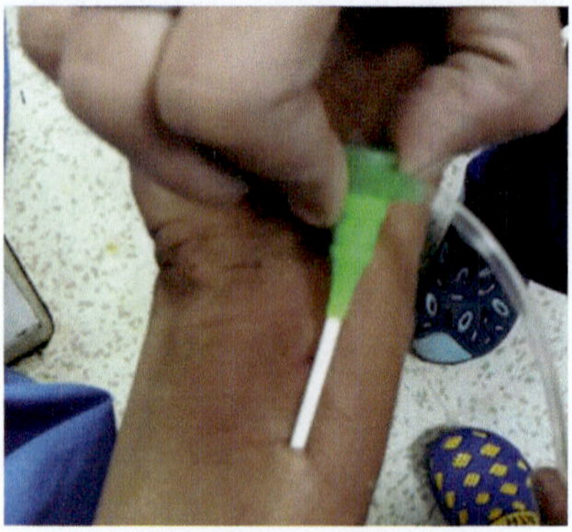

Figure 10.19a The sheath is pulled back by a centimetre.

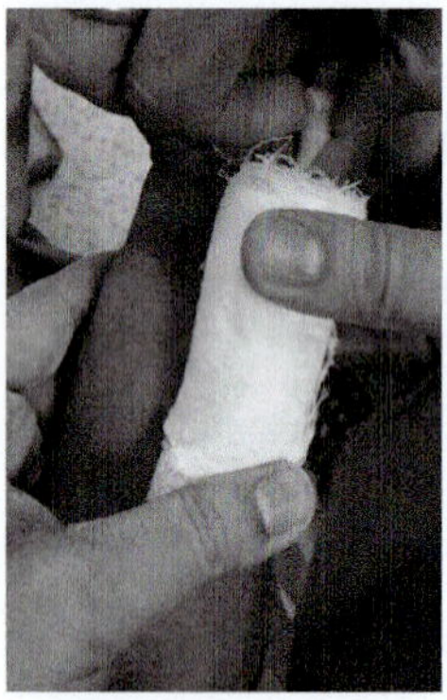

Figure 10.19b A standard cotton bandage roll 3 cm diameter × 5 cm length is placed over the site of puncture where the sheath exits the skin.

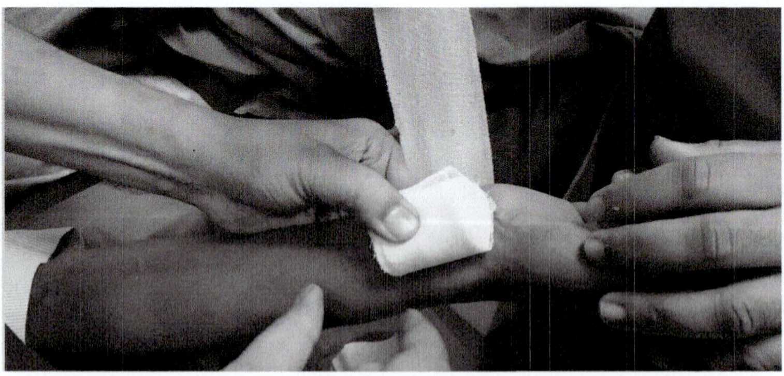

Figure 10.19c The sheath is then pulled out and an elastic bandage strip that is 15 cm long and 3 cm wide is stretched and wrapped around the wrist, covering half of the cotton bandage-roll.

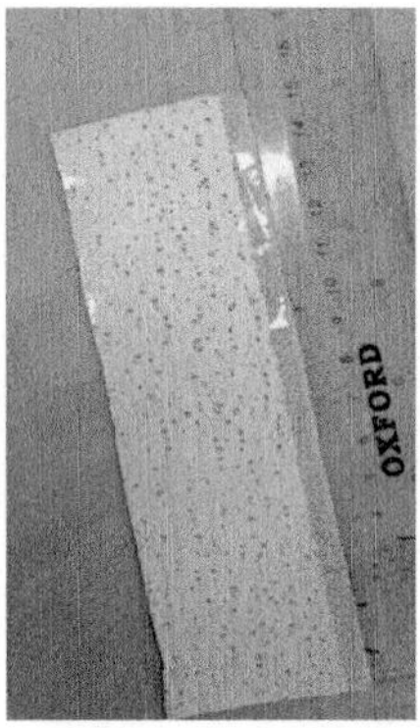

Figure 10.19d A strip of elastic bandage 15 cm long, 3 cm wide. Such strips are cut from the roll of elastic bandage. Three of such strips are usually required in each case.

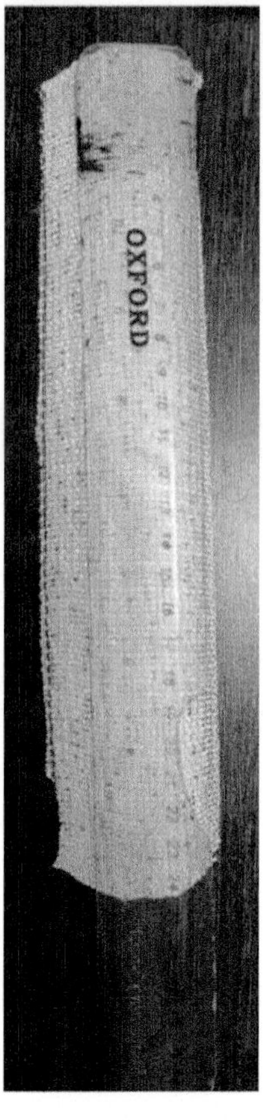

Figure 10.19e Strip of elastic bandage stretched to full length grows by 180% and becomes 27 cm.

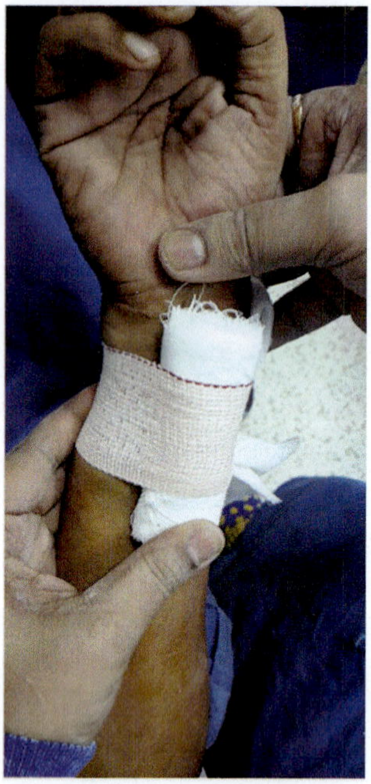

Figure 10.19f The second elastic bandage strip is wrapped around the wrist similarly and covers the remaining bandage-roll.

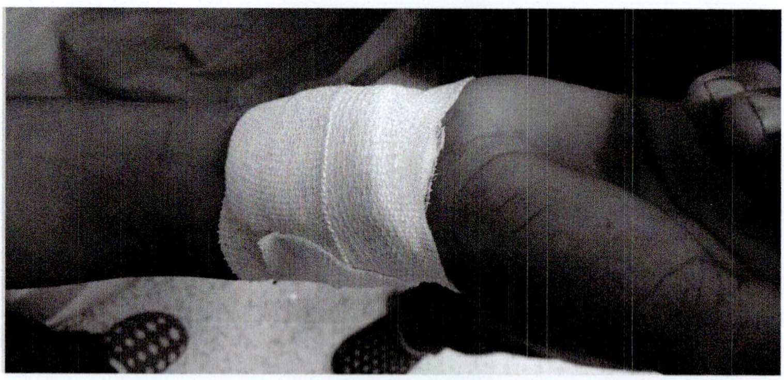

Figure 10.19g The third elastic bandage strip comes on top of both.
Acknowledgement:
Courtesy Dr Sanjay Kumar Chugh

Using this method, RAO rate in a real-world cohort (Comparison of distal versus standard transradial access as default: Insights from a colour Doppler study (The Distal Radial versus Transradial Access Study: D.A.T.A STARStudy[61]—of 972 (mean age 58.36 years; 75.1% M; 83.5% hypertensives, 57% diabetics, 65.9% tobacco abuse; mean RAD 1.78 mm) who underwent **coronary angiogram** (CAG) using 5F (n = 717), and 6F **percutaneous transluminal coronary angioplasty** (PTCA) (n = 255; 57 primary angioplasty) was 3.4%, without use of non-occlusive haemostasis. 40% RAO patients had had a second procedure (52% PTCA). Total 144 (14.8%) patients had more than 2 procedures through the same site. Repeat procedures are known to increase risk of RAO *(for details on RAO, please see separate chapter on radial artery occlusion).*

Practice of non-occlusive haemostasis requires trained nursing staff who can closely monitor the forearm to ensure early detection of bleeding from access site following deflation of pneumatic cuff to make the compression non-occlusive. This is difficult in our set up and so we use a bandage roll with elastic bandage compression as described, with equivalent results.

Conclusion

To conclude, a paradigm shift has occurred in interventional cardiology to not only radial, but forearm access. Survival benefit reported with transradial access compared to transfemoral access in patients with acute coronary syndromes and acute ST-elevation acute myocardial infarction and its feasibility in cardiogenic shock have made radial access extremely popular. However, there are difficulties and challenges with regard to puncturing smaller diameter radial arteries, or performing transradial angioplasty using 6F in patients with small diameter radial arteries as in women" which need to be overcome. Again, radial artery spasm, cubital loops, and tortuous radial, brachial and subclavian arteries pose a challenge. Guide support issues also occur in patients with complex coronary lesions, anomalous coronary origin or retro-esophageal right subclavian artery (RORSA) and with aortic anomalies (rotation, dilatation, horizontal lie, or right sided-arch). All these can be easily overcome using the tips and tricks discussed and primary angioplasty can also be performed by operators who are facile and have adequate experience with transradial interventions. Pre-procedure ultrasound is useful to select the biggest and straightest radial or ulnar artery for access, to minimize spasm, fluoroscopy time, and patient discomfort, while enhancing success. It also helps identify the SDRAs, in which, tricks to overcome the challenge of small arteries can be applied for successful transradial angiography and interventions with low complications and minimal patient discomfort. With the newer slender and sheathless techniques including the Railway Sheathless system™ by Cordis, with miniaturization of hardware, it is becoming increasingly possible to perform transradial interventions in the vast majority including smaller individuals. Distal transradial access is a new and upcoming area which needs further evaluation and is covered in a separate chapter on 'Distal Transradial Interventions'.

Acknowledgements

We acknowledge the help of Cath lab staff at Jaipur National University Hospital: Geetesh Joshi, Saurabh Dabral, Dwarika Prasad Sharma, Priyanka Kumari, and Poonam Jangid, and Staff of Cath lab of The Mission Hospital, Durgapur: Cath lab technicians Rajeeb Nandi and Uttam Bera; and Sudip Kesh, Coordinator, for help with illustrations.

References

1. Hamon M, Pristipino C, Di Mario C, et al. Consensus document on the radial approach in percutaneous cardiovascular interventions: position paper by the European Association of Percutaneous Cardiovascular Interventions and Working Groups on Acute Cardiac Care and Thrombosis of the European Society of Cardiology. *EuroIntervention*. 2013;8:1242–51.
2. Rao SV, Tremmel JA, Gilchrist A, et al. Best practices for transradial angiography and intervention: a consensus statement from the society for cardiovascular angiography and intervention's transradial working group. *Catheter Cardiovasc Interv*. 2014;83(2):228–36.
3. Shah B, Bangalore S, Feit F, Fernandez G, Coppola J, Attubato MJ, Slater J. Radiation exposure during coronary angiography via transradial or transfemoral approaches when performed by experienced operators. *Am Heart J*. 2013;165(3):286–92.
4. Jang JS, Jin HY, Seo JS, Yang TH, Kim DK, Kim DI, Cho KI, Kim BH, Park YH, Je HG, Kim DS. The transradial versus the transfemoral approach for primary

percutaneous coronary interventions in patients with acute myocardial infarction: a systemic review and meta-analysis. *Eurointervention.* 2012;8(4):501–10.

5. Arzamendi D, Ly HQ, Tanguay JF, Chan MY Chevallereau P, Gallo R, Ibrahim R, L'Allier P, Levesque S, Gosselin G, Deguise P, Joyal M, Gergorie J, Bonan R, Crepeau J, Doucet S. Effect on bleeding, time to revascularization, and one year clinical outcomes of the radial approach during primary percutaneous coronary intervention in patients with ST-segment elevation myocardial infarction. *Am J Cardiol.* 2010; 106:148–54.
6. Dehghani P, Mohammad A, Bajaj R, Hong T, Suen CM, Sharieff W, Chisholm RJ, Kutryk MJ, Fam NP, Cheema AN. Mechanism and predictors of failed transradial approach for percutaneous coronary interventions. *JACC Cardiovasc Interv.* 2009;2(11):1057–64.
7. Jolly SS, Yusuf S, Cairns J, et al. Radial versus femoral access for coronary angiography and intervention in patients with acute coronary syndromes (RIVAL): a randomized, parallel group, multicenter trial. *Lancet.* 2011; 77:1409–20.
8. Burzotta F, Trani C, Mazzari MA, et al. Vascular complications and access crossovers in 10,676 transradial percutaneous coronary procedures. *Am Heart J.* 2012; 163:230–8.
9. Secco GG, Marinucci L, Uguccioni L, Parisi R, Uguccioni S, Fattori R. Transradial versus transfemoral approach for primary percutaneous coronary interventions in elderly patients. *J Invasive Cardiol.* 2013;25(5):254–56.
10. Dehghani P, Mohammad A, Bajaj R, Hong T, Suen CM, Sharieff W, Chisholm RJ, Kutryk MJ, Fam NP, Cheema AN. Mechanism and predictors of failed transradial approach for percutaneous coronary interventions. *JACC Cardiovasc Interv.* 2009;2(11):1057–64.
11. Brzezinski M, Luisetti T, London MJ. Radial artery cannulation: a comprehensive review of recent anatomic and physiologic investigations. *Anesth Analg.* 2009;109(6):1763–81.
12. Fujii T, Masuda N, Tamiya S, Shima M, Toda E, Ito D, Nakazawa G, Matsukage T, Ogata N, Morino Y, Tanabe T, Ikari Y. Angiographic evaluation of right upper-limb arterial anomalies: implications for transradial coronary interventions. *J Invasive Cardiol.* 2010;22(11):536–40.
13. Valsecchi O, Vassileva A, Musumeci G, Rossini R, Tespili M, Guagliumi G, Mihalcsik L, Gavazzi A, Ferrazzi P. Failure of transradial approach during coronary interventions: anatomic considerations. *Catheter Cardiovasc Interv.* 2006;67(6):870–8.
14. Guedes A, Dangoise V, Gabriel L, et al. Low rate of conversion to transfemoral approach when attempting both radial arteries for coronary angiography and percutaneous coronary intervention: a study of 1,826 consecutive procedures. *J Invasive Cardiol* 2010;22(9):391–7.
15. Ball WT, Sharieff W, Jolly SS, et al. Characterization of operator learning curve for transradial coronary interventions. *Circ Cardiovasc Interv* 2011;4(4):336–41.
16. Dehghani P, Mohammad A, Bajaj R, et al. Mechanism and predictors of failed transradial approach for percutaneous coronary interventions. *JACC Cardiovasc Inter.* 2009;2(11):1057–64.
17. Kumar Chugh S, Chugh S, Chugh Y, Rao SV. Feasibility and utility of pre-procedural ultrasound imaging of the arm to facilitate transradial coronary diagnostic and

interventional procedures (PRIMAFACIE-TRI). *Catheter Cardiovasc Interv.* 2013;82:64–73.

18. Chugh SK, *Tips and tricks for transradial coronary angioplasty*, CSI Cardiology Update, Jaypee Publishers, 2014.
19. Filho JR, Assad JA, Zago AC, et al. Comparative study of the use of diltiazem as an antispasmodic drug in coronary angiography via the trans radial approach. *Arq Bras Cardiol.* 2003;81(1):54–58.
20. Chugh SK, Chugh Y, Chugh S. How to tackle complications in radial procedures: tip and tricks. *Indian Heart J.* 2015;67(3):275–81.
21. Kim SH, Kim EJ, Cheon WS, et al. Comparative study of nicorandil and a spasmolytic cocktail in preventing radial artery spasm during transradial coronary angiography. *Int J Cardiol.* 2007;120(3):325–30.
22. Impact of anticoagulation levels on outcomes in patients undergoing elective percutaneous coronary intervention: insights from the STEEPLE trial. *Eur Heart J.* 2008;29:462–71.
23. Saito S, Ikie H, Hosokawa G, Tanaka S. Influence of the ratio between radial artery inner diameter and sheath outer diameter on radial artery flow after transradial coronary intervention. *Catheter Cardiovasc Interv.* 1999;46(2):173–8.
24. Elmahdy MF, Hassan M, Elquindy A. Role of vascular ultrasound scanning in repeated trans-radial coronary artery intervention (prospective randomized study). *Catheter Cardiovasc Interv.* 2017.
25. Kwan TW, Cherukuri S, Huang Y, et al. Feasibility and safety of 7F sheathless guiding catheter during transradial coronary intervention. *Catheter Cardiovasc Interv.* 2012;80(2):274–80.
26. Douglas F and Mamas MA. Transradial sheathless approach for PCI. *Curr Cardiol Rep.* 2015;17:47.
27. Mamas M, D'Souza S, Hendry C, Ali R, Iles-Smith H, Palmer K, El-Omar M, Fath-Ordoubadi F, Neyses L, Fraser DG. Use of the sheathless guide catheter during routine transradial percutaneous coronary intervention: a feasibility study. *Catheter Cardiovasc Interv.* 2010;75(4):596–602.
28. Chugh SK, Chugh Y, Chugh S. *Slender transradial interventions, in update in interventional cardiology*, 2017, pp. 26–36, Edited by AB Mehta, Jaypee Publishers.
29. Chugh K, Chugh S, Chugh Y. Addressing the challenges of access of small radial and ulnar arteries in transradial and transulnar interventions: Insights from a color Doppler study. *JACC.* 2014;63(12):A442.
30. Chugh SK, Chugh Y, Chugh S. Safety and feasibility of 5Fr Glidesheath slender for complex transradial interventions in small diameter radial arteries. *Indian Heart J.* 2017;69:3,405–6.
31. Lo TS, Nolan J, Fountzopoulos E, et al. Radial artery anomaly and its influence on transradial coronary procedural outcome. *Heart.* 2009;95(5):410.
32. Schiano P, Barbou F, Chenilleau MC, Louembe J, Monsegu J. Adjusted weight anticoagulation for radial approach in elective coronarography: the AWARE coronarography study. *EuroIntervention.* 2010;6:247–50.
33. Gilchrist IC. Is the Allen's test accurate for patients considered for transradial coronary angiography? *J Am Coll Cardiol.* 2006;48:1283–88.

34. Chugh Y, Chugh S, Chugh S. A paradigm shift toward forearm arterial access requires establishing preprocedure adequacy of hand collateralization or patency of collateralizing forearm arteries. *J Invasive Cardiol.* 2016;28(4).
35. Shah RM, Patel D, Abbate A, et al. Comparison of transradial coronary procedures via right radial versus left radial artery approach: a meta- analysis. *Cath Cardiovasc Interv.* 2016;88:1027–33.
36. Rashid M, Lawson C, Potts J, et al. Incidence, determinants, and outcomes of left and right radial access use in patients undergoing percutaneous coronary intervention in the United Kingdom: a national perspective using the British Cardiovascular Intervention Society (BCIS) dataset. *JACC Cardiovasc Interv.* 2018;11(11):1021–33.
37. Sanjay Chugh and Yashasvi Chugh. To BAT or not to BAT. *J Invasive Cardiology.* 2014;26(8):E120–21.
38. Bertrand OF, Rao SV, Pancholy S, et al. Transradial approach for coronary angiography and interventions: results of the first international transradial practice survey. *JACC CardiovascInterv.* 2010;3(10):1022–31.
39. Chugh SK, Panwar RB, Kasliwal RR, Trehan N. Taming the tiger: a single center experience using a new catheter for transradial coronary angiography. *Cath Cardiovasc Intervent.* 2006;67:788–38.
40. Chugh SK. Transradial right or left? *Indian Heart J.* 2008;60(1 Suppl A):A27–35.
41. Jokhi P, Talwar S. Transradial percutaneous coronary intervention in acute myocardial infarction: in search of a consensus. *J Indian Med Assoc.* 2009;107(9):598, 600–1.
42. Tips and tricks to overcome challenging anatomies during radial approach. In: Chandra and Sethi (Eds) *NIC Handbook of Interventional Cardiology.* Jaypee Publishers, 2015, pp. 24–41.
43. Pandie S, Mehta SR, Cantor WJ, et al. Radial versus femoral access for coronary angiography/intervention in women with acute coronary syndromes: insights from the RIVAL trial (Radial Vs femorAL access for coronary intervention). 2015;8(4):505–12.
44. Rao SV, Hess CN, Barham B, et al. A registry-based randomized trial comparing radial and femoral approaches in women undergoing percutaneous coronary intervention: the SAFE-PCI for Women (Study of Access Site for Enhancement of PCI for Women) trial. *JACC Cardiovasc Interv.* 2014;7(8):857–67.
45. Chugh S, Chugh Y. Transradial PCI in women: zeroing in on crossovers. *JACC Cardiovasc Interv.* 2015;8(4):638.
46. Chugh SK, Chugh Y, Chugh S. Overcoming the challenge of transradial interventions in women: insights from a color Doppler study. *J Am Coll Cardiol* 2014;64(11): B240.
47. Jolly SS, Yusuf S, Cairns J, Niemelä K, Xavier D, Widimsky P, Budaj A, Niemelä M, Valentin V, Lewis BS, Avezum A, Steg PG, Rao SV, Gao P, Afzal R, Joyner CD, Chrolavicius S, Mehta SR; RIVAL trial group. Radial versus femoral access for coronary angiography and intervention in patients with acute coronary syndromes (RIVAL): a randomised, parallel group, multicentre trial. *Lancet.* 2011;377(9775):1409–20. doi: 10.1016/S0140-6736(11)60404-2. Epub 2011 Apr 4.
48. Romagnoli E, Biondi-Zoccai G, Sciahbasi A, et al. Radial versus femoral randomized investigation in st-segment elevation acute coronary

syndrome: the RIFLE-STEACS (Radial Versus Femoral Randomized Investigation in ST-Elevation Acute Coronary Syndrome) study. *J Am Coll Cardiol.* 2012;60(24):2481–89.

49. Bernat I, Horak D, Stasek J, Mates M, Pesek J, Ostadal P, Hrabos V, Dusek J, Koza J, Sembera Z, Brtko M, Aschermann O, Smid M, Polansky P, Al Mawiri A, Vojacek J, Bis J, Costerousse O, Bertrand OF, Rokyta R. ST-segment elevation myocardial infarction treated by radial or femoral approach in a multicenter randomized clinical trial. The STEMI-RADIAL trial. *J Am Coll Cardiol.* 2014;63:964–72. doi:10.1016/j.jacc.2013.08.1651
50. Radial versus femoral access and bivalirudin versus unfractionated heparin in invasively managed patients with acute coronary syndrome (MATRIX): final 1-year results of a multicentre, randomised controlled trial. Lancet. September 08, 2018;392(Issue 10150):P835–P848.
51. Komócsi A, Aradi D, Kehl D, et al. Meta-analysis of randomized trials on access site selection for percutaneous coronary intervention in ST-segment elevation myocardial infarction. *Arch Med Sci.* 2014;10(2):203–12.
52. Le May Michel, Wells George, So Derek. Safety and efficacy of femoral access vs radial access in ST-segment elevation myocardial infarction, the SAFARI-STEMI randomized clinical trial. JAMA Cardiol. 2020;2 doi: 10.1001/jamacardio.2019.4852. Published online January.
53. Chugh, Y., Chugh, S., & Chugh, S. K. Post-the SAFARI STEMI study: Is there still a debate on radial vs. femoral access in STEMI?. Indian heart journal, 72(5), 466–468. https://doi.org/10.1016/j.ihj.2020.08.006
54. Chugh SK, Chugh Y, Chugh S. *Tips & tricks for primary angioplasty through the radial approach in ST segment elevation acute myocardial infarction in STEMI update*, Chopra and Mehta (Eds). Jaypee Publishers, 2016.
55. Windecker S, Kolh P, Alfonso F, et al. 2014 ESC/EACTS Guidelines on myocardial revascularization. The Task Force on Myocardial Revascularization of the European Society of Cardiology (ESC) and the European Association for Cardio-Thoracic Surgery (EACTS) Developed with the special contribution of the European Association of Percutaneous Cardiovascular Interventions (EAPCI). *Eur Heart J.* 2014;35(37):2541–19.
56. Wimmer NJ, Cohen DJ, Wasfy JH, Rathore SS, Mauri L, Yeh RW. Delay in reperfusion with transradial percutaneous coronary intervention for ST-elevation myocardial infarction: might some delays be acceptable? *Am Heart J.* 2014;168(1):103–9.
57. Mongeon FP, Belisle P, Joseph L, et al Adjunctive thrombectomy for acute myocardial infarction; a Bayesian meta-analysis. *Circ Cardiovasc Interv.* 2010;3:6–16.
58. Romagnoli E, De Vita M, Burzotta F, et al. Radial versus femoral approach comparison in percutaneous coronary intervention with intraaortic balloon pump support: The RADIAL PUMP UP Registry. *Am Heart J.* 2013;166(6):1019–26.
59. Pancholy S, Coppola J, Patel T, Roke-Thomas M. Prevention of radial artery occlusion-patent hemostasis evaluation trial (PROPHET study): a randomized comparison of traditional versus patency documented hemostasis after transradial catheterization. *Catheter Cardiovasc Interv.* 2008;72(3):335–40.

60. Pancholy SB, Bernat I, Bertrand OF, Patel TM. Prevention of radial artery occlusion after transradial catheterization: the PROPHET-II randomized trial. *JACC Cardiovasc Interv*. 2016;9(19):1992–99.
61. Petroglou D, Didagelos M, Chalikias G, et al. Manual versus mechanical compression of the radial artery after transradial coronary angiography: the MEMORY multicenter, randomized trial. *J Am Coll Cardiol Intv*. 2018;11:1050–58.
62. Chugh Y, Kanaparthy NS, Piplani S, Chugh S, Shroff A, Vidovich M, Nolan J, Mamas M, Chugh SK. Comparison of distal radial access versus standard transradial access in patients with smaller diameter radial Arteries (The distal radial versus transradial access in small transradial ArteriesStudy: D.A.T.A - S.T.A.R study). Indian Heart J. 2021 Jan-Feb;73(1):26–34. doi: 10.1016/j.ihj.2020.11.002. Epub 2020 Nov 11. PMID: 33714406

11

Radial Access for Transradial Procedures: Right versus Left

C. Raghu, Sunita Chugh, and Sanjay Kumar Chugh

Background

Trans-radial access has gained popularity because of its advantages over femoral access.[1] Although there may be operator preference or patient-related and technical reasons for choosing right or left radial; the merits and demerits of one over the other have been debated until recently. Studies comparing left versus right radial access are discussed in this chapter. Practical tips and illustrations relating to left versus right radial access are presented in the chapter on 'Tips and tricks for transradial interventions (TRIs)'.

Operator Preference

Conventionally, most operators prefer to use right radial artery (RRA) because of convenience of operating from the right side of the patient with RRA access. With the shift of paradigm to forearm access, right ulnar (RU) and right distal radial access (DRRA) are equivalent alternatives,[2–4] even then, the operator might prefer to cross-over to left radial if he is unable to secure access or complete the procedure from the right side. Some operators on the other hand prefer to access the left radial because it is easier to engage the coronaries using femoral catheters from left side.

Technical Reasons for Using Left Radial Access

Even though the RRA is the default for most trans-radial operators there are situations where an operator may prefer to use left radial artery for technical reasons,[5] as with:

- Failed RRA access
- Post-coronary artery bypass grafts (CABG) requiring angiography or intervention
- In patients with occluded or small diameter right radial artery (SDRA)
- Known anatomical anomalies on the right such as cubital loop or radial bifurcation anomaly
- A tortuous calcific Shepherd crook right coronary artery requiring intervention since the guide support is better from the left radial access (LRA).
- Severe tortuosity in the subclavian which makes catheter manipulation difficult as subclavian tortuosities are more on the right compared to left side[6] (Figure 11.1)

Role of Pre-procedure Ultrasound of Arm Arteries

In 2007 the Indian Heart Journal supplement[5] published the largest series of left TRIs, from our registry in which we described the technique of left radial puncture and shared our experience regarding choice of side based on technical and patient-related issues; the most important technical issue being a preference to access the biggest and straightest forearm artery based on pre-procedure ultrasound of arm arteries (PPUAA).[7]

In PPUAA, diameter of bilateral radial and ulnar artery is measured, and a colour Doppler imaging is done at cubital fossa to see if the radial and ulnar artery arises normally from brachial. This helps in identifying cases with 'parallel' radial and ulnar arteries; a fifth of whom have type 3 bifurcation[8] which can lead to procedure failure. For details of PPUAA, please see chapter on 'Role of Colour Doppler Ultrasound in Trans-radial Interventions'.

In the first consensus publication on TRIs[9] in 2009; on the subject of 'Transradial interventions: right or left' there was consensus regarding

	Subclavian tortuosity		Radial Vascular Complications		Stroke/TIA	
Studies	RRA N (%)	LRA N (%)	RRA N (%)	LRA N (%)	RRA N (%)	LRA N (%)
Kawashima et al. (2004) [8]	2 (0.9%)	0	0	0	NR	NR
Fernández-Portales et al. (2006) [9]	10 (5.8%)	1 (0.5%)	NR	NR	NR	NR
Santas et al. (2009) [10]	NR	NR	1 (0.3%)	3 (0.9%)	NR	NR
Kanei et al. (2011) [11]	NR	NR	0	4 (4.3%)	NR	NR
Sciahbasi et al. (2011) [12]	125 (16.2%)	65 (8.4%)	0	0	1 (0.1%)	0
Freixa et al. (2012) [13]	16 (32%)	3 (6%)	0	4 (8%)	NR	NR
Norgaz et al. (2012) [14]	44 (8.8%)	15 (3%)	12 (2.4%)	6 (1.2%)	0	0
Pacchioni et al. (2012) [15]	NR	NR	NR	NR	0	0
Dominici et al. (2013) [16]	NR	NR	NR	NR	2 (1%)	2 (1%)
Hu et al. (2013) [17]	NR	NR	4 (0.6%)	0	1 (0.1%)	0
Kado et al. (2014) [18]	NR	NR	NR	NR	NR	NR
Fu et al. (2015) [19]	NR	NR	0	0	0	0
	187/1541	83/1552	17/2767	17/2779	4/2140	2/2140
Total	12%	5%	0.6%	0.6%	0.2%	0.1%
P value (Fisher's Exact test)	<0.0001		1.0		0.68	

Figure 11.1 Subclavian tortuosity and procedural complications with Right & Left Radial. Subclavian tortuosity is reported to be more with RRA $P < 0.001$.[6]

the patient and technical issues regarding choice of side, which are presented below.

Patient-Related Issues

- Patient preference for LRA, in some right-handed patients because they can then use their right hand immediately after procedure.
- Right forearm haematoma from previous procedure
- Arm deformity on right side from previous orthopedic surgery
- Scar on right forearm from previous burn.
- After surgery for right sided breast malignancy and or radiotherapy

Fluoroscopy Time, Radiation Exposure, and Procedure Time: Right Versus Left Radial Access

Transradial Approach (Left Versus Right) and Procedural Times During Percutaneous Coronary Procedures (TALENT) Study

The TALENT study randomized 1540 patients equally to RRA or LRA for both angiography and angioplasty[10] and showed that:

- LRA is associated with shorter fluoroscopy time and reduced dose adsorbed by patients compared with the RRA. Radiation dose was more with right as compared to left in another study[11]
- The advantage of LRA is more pronounced when dealing with elderly patients and may be abolished with increased experience

OPERA Study

The OPERA study also showed radiation exposure (44mREMS versus 33 mREMS, P = 0.04) and fluoroscopy time (370 sec versus 349 sec, P = 0.09) both to be more with right radial access (Figure 11.2).[11] There was

Study name	Std diff In means	Lower limit	Upper limit	Z-Value	p-Value	Right radial	Left radial	Relative weight
	Statistics for each study					**Fluoroscopy time (min)**		
Kawashima et al	0.448	0.258	0.638	4.615	0.000	5.00 ±3.3	3.70 ±2.5	14.10
Sciahbasi et al	0.081	−0.022	0.183	1.542	0.123	3.78 ±2.9	3.54 ±3.0	23.37
Freixa et al	0.075	−0.317	0.467	0.375	0.707	8.90 ±9.1	8.30 ±6.7	5.01
Norgaz et al	0.137	0.013	0.261	2.168	0.030	3.08 ±2.6	2.76 ±2.0	20.76
Dominici et al	0.088	−0.105	0.281	0.893	0.372	6.16 ±4.1	5.81 ±3.8	13.87
Hu et al	0.131	0.024	0.237	2.409	0.016	3.80 ±3.3	3.40 ±2.8	22.80
Diagnostic procedures	**0.156**	**0.061**	**0.252**	**3.205**	**0.001**	4.06 ±3.2	3.65 ±2.8	
Farnandez-portales et al	0.434	0.217	0.650	3.924	0.000	5.50 ±3.9	3.95 ±3.3	17.02
Santas et al	0.000	0.204	0.204	0.000	1.000	5.00 ±3.3	5.00 ±5.0	17.47
Kanei et al	−0.194	−0.480	0.092	−1.330	0.184	9.20 ±6.7	10.5 ±6.7	14.47
Sciahbasi et al (PCI)	0.070	0.079	0.220	0.918	0.359	15.6 ±12.5	14.7 ±13.2	19.42
Pacchioni et al	0.607	−0.027	1.241	1.876	0.061	3.90 ±1.3	3.21 ±1.0	6.10
Kado et al	0.050	−0.342	0.442	0.252	0.801	10.9 ±8.0	10.5 ±7.9	11.06
Fu et al	0.406	0.120	0.691	2.781	0.005	8.80 ±3.5	7.40 ±3.4	14.47
Diagnostic & Interventional Procedures	**0.161**	**−0.023**	**0.344**	**1.714**	**0.087**	10.04 ±7.3	9.27 ±7.7	
Overall	**0.157**	**0.072**	**0.242**	**3.634**	**0.000**	5.76 ±4.4	5.25 ±4.2	

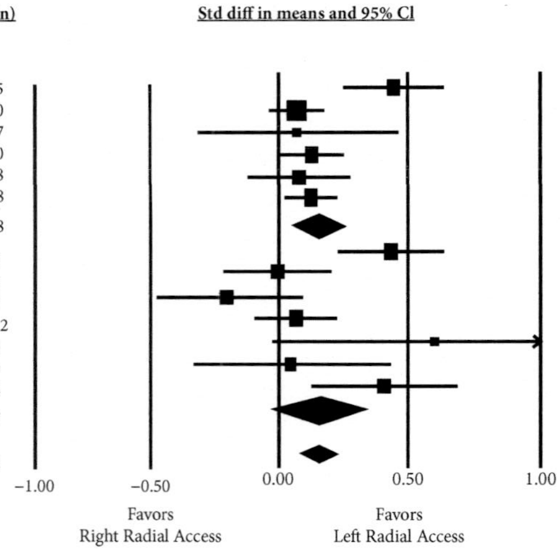

Figure 11.2 Meta-analysis for fluoroscopy time in right versus left radial access, shows less fluoroscopy time with left radial.[6]

a significant increase in external radiation exposure using the RRA versus LRA (head: median: 6.12 [interquartile range (IQR): 2.6–16.6] mRems versus median: 12.0 [IQR: 6.4–22.0] mRems, $p = 0.02$; thyroid: median: 10.10 [IQR: 4.3–25] mRems versus median: 18.70 [IQR: 11.0–38] mRems, $p = 0.001$).[12]

Procedure Time, Number of Catheters Used, and Cross-Over to Alternate Access

Procedure time for LRA versus RRA access (43.8 ± 20.6 minutes versus 37.7 ± 21.6 minutes; $p = 0.049$) has also been reported to be more with LRA because of more numbers of catheters required for LRA (2.2 ± 1 versus 1.4 ± 0.7, $p < 0.0010$) versus RRA access[13] (Figure 11.3). A meta-analysis of 12 studies including 6450 patients half of which had procedure through left radial artery[6] showed more cross over with right compared to left (Figure 11.4).

Risk of Brain Injury (Cerebral Microemboli) During Diagnostic Angiography

Risk of brain injury (cerebral microemboli) during diagnostic angiography[14] has been reported to be more with RRA (Figure 11.5) and with > 2 catheter usage (Figure 11.6).[14]

Operator Discomfort

Operator discomfort has been reported to be more with LRA (Figure 11.7) as bending over to operate from left wrist from the right side of the patient hurts the back of the operator. Discomfort was reported with the LRA during access (LRA: 22% versus RRA: 4%; $p = 0.017$), but not during procedure (LRA: 10.0% versus RRA: 4.0%, $p = 0.43$). This difference was almost entirely noted in obese patients (LRA: 30.0% versus RRA: 3.7%, $p = 0.005$).[15] In obese patients LRA can be especially strenuous.

Study name	Std diff In means	Lower limit	Upper limit	Z-Value	p-Value	Procedure Time (min) Right radial	Procedure Time (min) Left radial	Relative weight
Kawashima et al	0.410	0.220	0.600	4.235	0.000	13.7 ±6.4	11.4 ±4.8	18.85
Sciahbasi et al	0.000	−0.102	0.102	0.000	1.000	16.0 ±9.0	16.0 ±10.0	24.56
Freixa et al	−0.259	−0.653	0.134	−1.291	0.197	16.2 ±12.4	19.3 ±11.5	9.06
Norgaz et al	0.019	−0.105	0.143	0.304	0.761	8.6 ±5.2	8.5 ±4.1	23.21
Hu et al	0.146	0.040	0.253	2.696	0.007	14.1± 6.3	13.2 ±6.9	24.32
Diagnostic procedures	0.094	−0.050	0.238	1.277	0.201	13.5 ±7.1	13.0 ±6.9	
Farnandez-portales et al	0.462	0.245	0.679	4.173	0.000	11.0 ±7.0	8.0 ±6.0	
Santas et al	0.000	−0.204	0.204	0.000	1.000	28.0 ±12.0	28.0 ±12.0	22.57
Kanei et al	−0.289	−0.576	−0.002	−1.973	0.048	37.7 ±21.6	43.8 ±20.6	23.07
Sciahbasi et al (PCI)	0.073	−0.076	0.223	0.958	0.338	46.1 ±26.9	44.0 ±26.6	19.75
Pacchioni et al	0.062	−0.558	0.682	0.197	0.844	10.7 ±3.0	10.5 ±3.4	25.09
Diagnostic & Interventional Procedures	0.072	−0.164	0.307	0.595	0.552	33.1 ±19.2	31.7 ±18.4	9.52
Overall	0.088	−0.035	0.211	1.400	0.162	18.8 ±10.3	18.1 ±10.0	

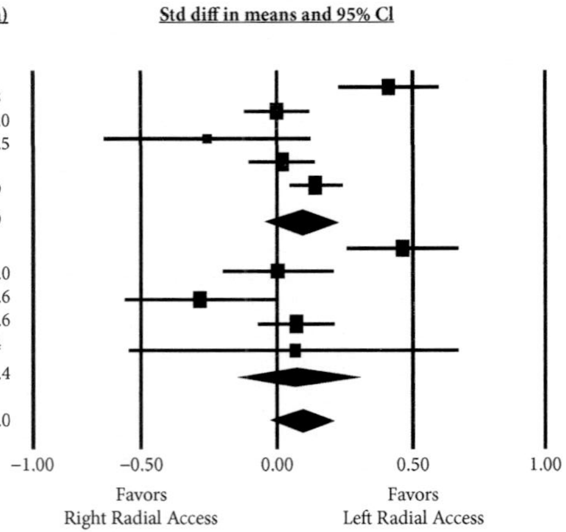

Figure 11.3 Meta-analysis for procedure time in right versus left radial access, showing less procedure time with left radial.[6]

Study name	Odds ratio	Lower limit	Upper limit	Z-Value	p-Value	Right radial	Left radial	Relative weight
	Statistics for each study							
Kawashima et al	5.659	0.658	48.833	1.576	0.115	5/210	1/233	4.13
Sciahbasi et al	0.664	0.235	1.875	−0.773	0.439	6/770	9/770	16.42
Freixa et al	0.375	0.069	2.031	−1.138	0.255	2/50	5/50	6.61
Norgaz etal	1.116	0.583	2.136	0.331	0.741	20/500	18/500	36.26
Hu et al	0.897	0.471	1.711	−0.329	0.742	18/700	20/700	36.58
Diagnostic procedures	0.941	0.604	1.467	−0.267	0.789	51/2230	53/2253	
Farnandez-portales et al	3.025	0.944	9.690	1.863	0.062	11/171	4/180	21.82
Santas et al	0.870	0.574	1.317	−0.660	0.509	50/280	61/305	48.30
Kanei et al	2.786	0.285	27.265	0.880	0.379	3/101	1/92	8.02
Kado et al	1.000	0.135	7.392	0.000	1.000	2/50	2/50	10.00
Fu et al	3.128	0.616	15.886	1.375	0.169	6/100	2/100	13.86
Diagnostic & Interventional Procedures	1.517	0.754	3.052	1.170	0.242	72/702	70/727	
Overall	1.080	0.742	1.570	0.401	0.688	123/2932	123/2980	

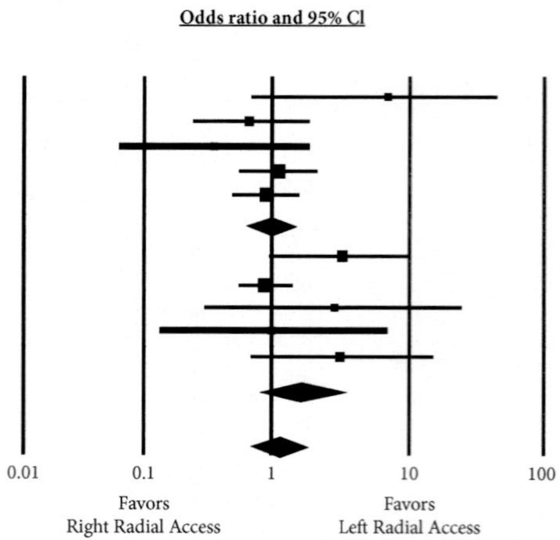

Figure 11.4 Meta-analysis for cross over rate or procedure failure, showing more procedure failure and cross-over with RRA access.[6]

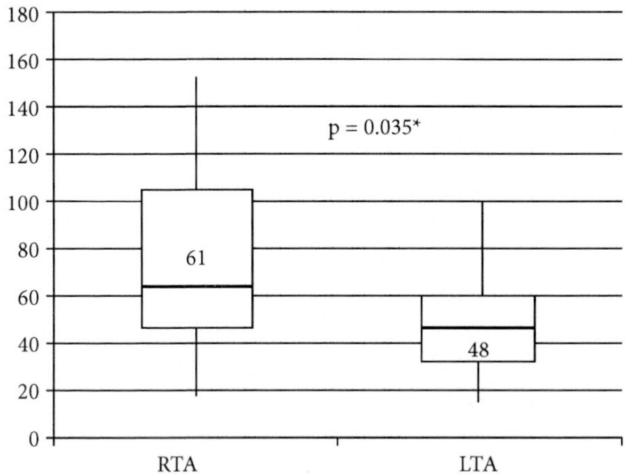

Figure 11.5 Occurrence of cerebral microemboli according to vascular access site, showing less cerebral microemboli with left radial.[14]

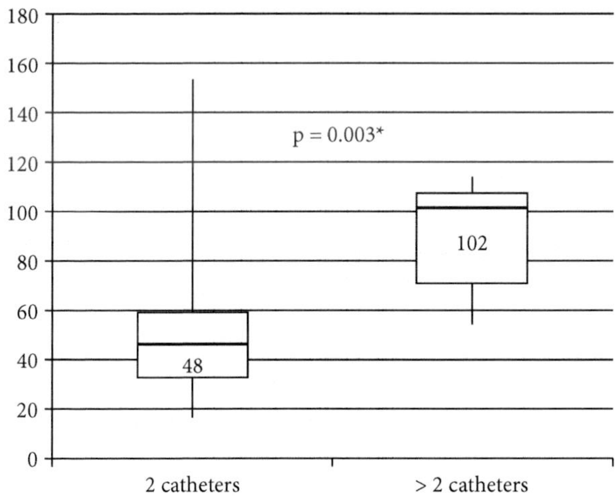

Figure 11.6 Occurrence of microemboli according to the number of catheters employed, showing more cerebral microemboli with use of >2 catheters.[14]

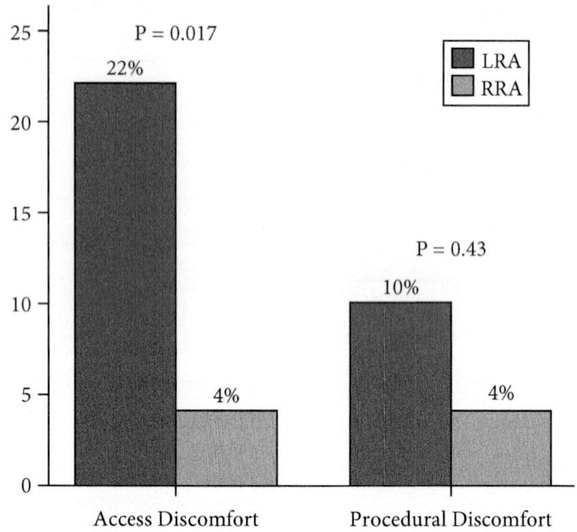

Figure 11.7 Moderate to severe operator discomfort (>4 on a 0 to 10 scale) during access and procedure expressed in percentage.[15]

Vascular Complications

Vascular complications with right and left radial (incidence of stroke and TIA) was not found to be different with left and right radial access in a recent meta-analysis (Figure 11.1).[6] However, in the elderly, especially >75 years, stroke may be more with RRA compared to LRA. In a propensity match analysis, LRA was associated with a significant decrease in in-hospital stroke (OR: 0.52, 95% CI: 0.37–0.82; $p = 0.005$).[16]

Limitation and Disadvantage of LRA for TRI

The limitation and disadvantage of using LRA are non-availability of LRA for further CABG or AV fistula for future dialysis in patients with chronic renal disease. Severe obesity other than straining the back of the operator makes LRA difficult and is likely to be less successful.

Conclusions from Recent Publications on Right Versus Left Radial Access

The following are conclusions from recent publications on RRA versus LRA:

- Subclavian tortuosity is reported to be more with RRA ($p < 0.001$)[6]
- Fluoroscopy time, radiation exposure more with RRA access[11]
- Procedure time and cross-over to alternate access more with RRA access[6]
- More number of catheters were required for angiography via LRA versus RRA access; a single catheter was more common in the right radial group (73% versus 18%, $p < 0.001$)[13]
- Risk of brain injury (cerebral microemboli) during diagnostic angiography is more with RRA access[14]
- Operator discomfort more with LRA
- Vascular complications: Stroke and TIA are no different[6]

Conclusion

To conclude, performing an angiogram or angioplasty via LRA is less technically challenging and hence easier; but may be inconvenient to the operator because it could cause back pain because it requires the operator to bend over the patient. Subclavian tortuosity being less on the left side also makes the performance of the procedure less challenging especially in the elderly. For the same reasons, radiation exposure and fluoroscopy time are less with LRA access; though number of catheters required and procedure time may be more. Although cerebral microembolism is more using RRA, incidence of stroke and TIA are not different in RRA versus LRA.

In the elderly, especially those above 75 years, it is worthwhile considering LRA especially as subclavian tortuosity and the risk of stroke may be less with LRA.

For details of practical aspects and tips and tricks related to left versus right transradial procedures please see chapter on 'Tips and Tricks for Trans-radial Interventions'.

References

1. Jolly SS, Amlani S, Hamon M, et al. Radial versus femoral access for coronary angiography or intervention and the impact on major bleeding and ischaemic events: a systematic review and meta-analysis of randomized trials. *American Heart Journal.* 2009;157:132–40.
2. Gokhroo R, Kishor K, Bhanwar R, Bisht D, Gupta S, Avinash A. Ulnar artery interventions non inferior to radial approach: Ajmer Ulnar Artery (AJULAR) intervention working group study results. *The Journal of Invasive Cardiology.* 2016;28:1–8.
3. Orazio Valsecchi MD, Angelina Vassileva MD, Alberto Francesco Cereda MD, Paolo Canova MD, Keisuke Satogami MD, Luigi Fiocca MD, Giulio Guagliumi MD. Early clinical experience with right and left distal transradial access in the anatomical snuffbox in 52 consecutive patients. *The Journal of Invasive Cardiology.* 2018 (Epub Ahead of Print).
4. Kiemeneij F. Left distal transradial access in the anatomical snuffbox for coronary angiography (ldTRA) and interventions (ldTRI). *EuroIntervention.* 2017;13(7):851–57. doi:10.4244/EIJ-D-17-00079.
5. Chugh SK. Transradial right or left? *Indian Heart J.* 2008;60 (1 Suppl A):A27–35.
6. Shah RM, Patel D, Abbate A, et al. Comparison of transradial coronary procedures via right radial versus left radial artery approach: a meta-analysis. *Catheterization and Cardiovascular Interventions.* 2016:88:1027–33.
7. Kumar Chugh S, Chugh S, Chugh Y, Rao SV. Feasibility and utility of pre-procedural ultrasound imaging of the arm to facilitate transradial coronary diagnostic and interventional procedures (PRIMAFACIE-TRI). *Catheterization and Cardiovascular Interventions.* 2013;82:64–73.
8. Hamon M, Pristipino C, Di Mario C, et al. Consensus document on the radial approach in percutaneous cardiovascular interventions: position paper by the European Association of Percutaneous Cardiovascular Interventions and Working Groups on Acute Cardiac Care and Thrombosis of the European Society of Cardiology. *EuroIntervntion.* 2013;8:1242–51.
9. SK Chugh. Consensus on which transradial access for diagnostic and interventional coronary and non-coronary procedures: left or right? *Journal of the Indian Medical Association (JIMA).* 2009;107(09):589–91.
10. Sciahbasi A, Romagnoli E, Burzotta F, et al. Trans radial approach (left vs right) and procedural times during percutaneous coronary procedures: TALENT study. *American Heart Journal.* 2011;161:172–79.
11. Belle E, EricVicaut J, on behalf of The OPERA Investigators. Ischemia-modified albumin levels predict long-term outcome in patients with acute myocardial infarction. The French Nationwide OPERA study. *American Heart Journal.* 2010;159(4):570–76.
12. Herman Kado, Ambar M. Patel, Siva Suryadevara, et al. Operator radiation exposure and physical discomfort during a right versus left radial approach for coronary interventions a randomized evaluation. *JACC: Cardiovascular Interventions.* 2014;7(7).
13. Kanei Y1, Nakra NC, Liou M, Vales LL, et al,. Randomized comparison of transradial coronary angiography via right or left radial artery

approaches. *The American Journal of Cardiology*. 2011;107(2):195–7. doi:10.1016/j.amjcard.2010.08.065.

14. Andrea Pacchioni, Francesco Versaci, Antonio Mugnolo, et al. Risk of brain injury during diagnostic coronary angiography: comparison between right and left radial approach. *International Journal of Cardiology* 2013;167:3021–26.
15. Herman Kado, Ambar M. Patel, Siva Suryadevara, et al. Operator Radiation Exposure and Physical Discomfort During a Right Versus Left Radial Approach for Coronary Interventions A Randomized Evaluation. JA CC: Cardiovascular Interventions Vol. 7, No. 7, 20 14
16. Rashid M, Lawson C, Potts J, et al. Incidence, determinants and outcomes of left and right radial access use in patients undergoing percutaneous coronary intervention in the United Kingdom, a national perspective using the British Cardiovascular Intervention Society (BCIS) dataset. *JACC: Cardiovascular Interventions*. 2018; Epub ahead of print.

12

Transradial Approach for Complex Coronary Interventions

Yves Louvard, Thomas Hovasse, Philippe Garot, and Hakim Benamer

The transradial route for percutaneous coronary intervention (PCI) is now used in more than 95% of cases in many centres worldwide as a result of the gradual adoption of the most complex techniques for the radial approach. This involves technological adjustments, comprehension of the technical issues associated with the transradial route, and simplification of the strategies implemented to treat complex coronary artery disease.

We present here a series of real-life clinical situations in order to illustrate the feasibility of transradial PCI in patients with complex coronary lesions.

Provisional Side-branch Stenting (LAD/D1 Bifurcation)

Patient 1 was a 70-year-old man with controlled arterial hypertension who presented with exertional chest pain that he had experienced for several days in addition to spontaneous pain at night. He was admitted to the Coronary Care Unit (CCU) with a normal EKG and normal troponin levels. Right transradial angiography performed with a 5-Fr diagnostic catheter revealed a single significant lesion in the LAD/Diagonal bifurcation (Figure 12.1(i–viii)). The angiogram showed a single diagonal artery with extensive vascular bed and a proximal bifurcation involving the first septal artery. Preserving the patency of this artery was judged to be crucial. The bifurcation was an LAD 1, LAD 2, Dg1 type, and 0, 1, 0 according to the Medina Classification (Figure 12.2).[1] There were no other significant coronary lesions.

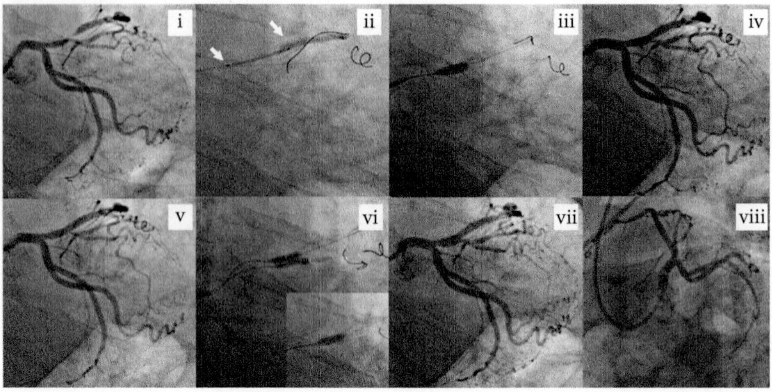

Figure 12.1 (i–viii) Transradial approach of LAD Diagonal bifurcation stenting.

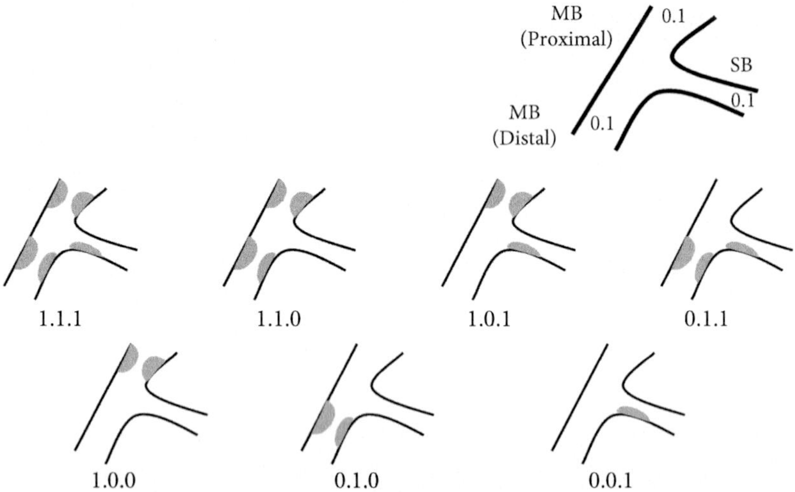

Figure 12.2 Medina bifurcation classification: a significant lesion is coded 1.

PCI was performed using the Provisional SB strategy (strategy B in the MADS classification) (Figure 12.3)[2] via the right radial approach with a Radifocus Terumo radial introducer and a 6F EBU 3.5 guiding-catheter (Launcher Medtronic). Two BMW 0.014" were inserted into the two distal branches. The lesion was pre-dilated using a 12 × 2 mm balloon allowing complete coverage of the lesion and of an 8-mm segment

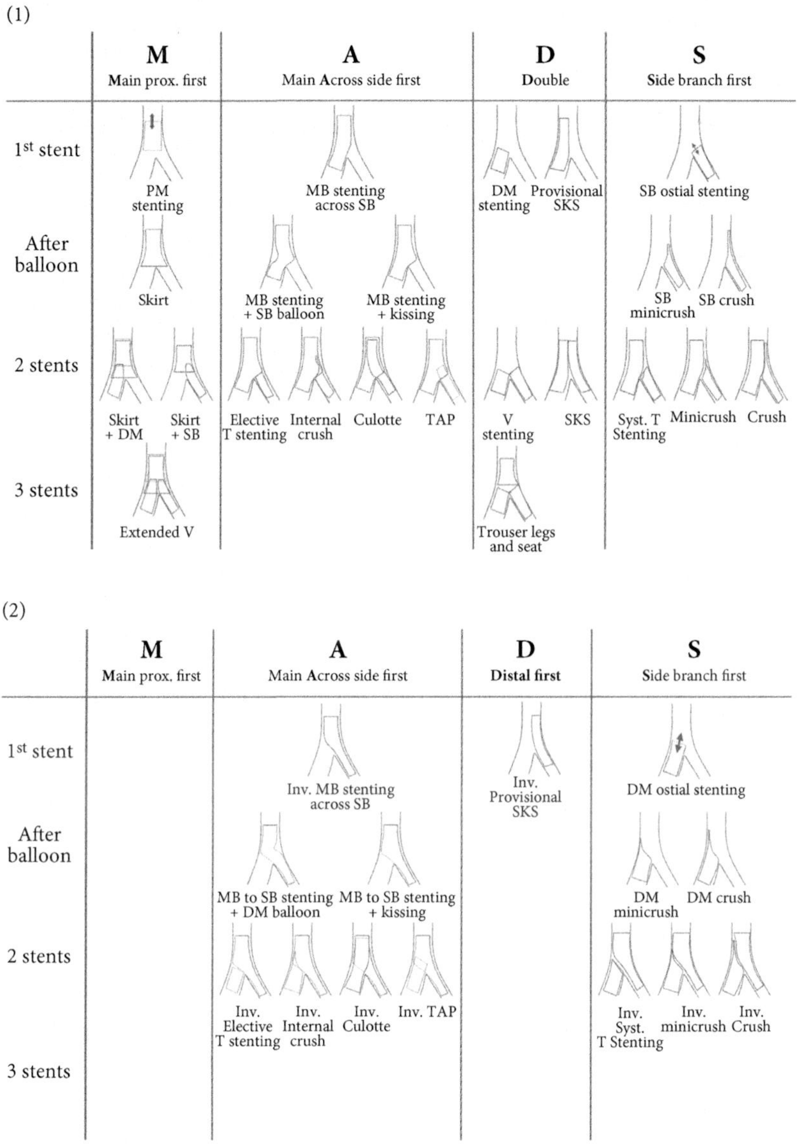

Figure 12.3 MADS classification of treatment based on final stent positions and strategy defined by the position of the first stent. Wire and balloon manipulations are not represented: (1) straight techniques, (2) inverted techniques where the SB is treated as the main branch, (3) description of provisional SB stenting strategy (see text).

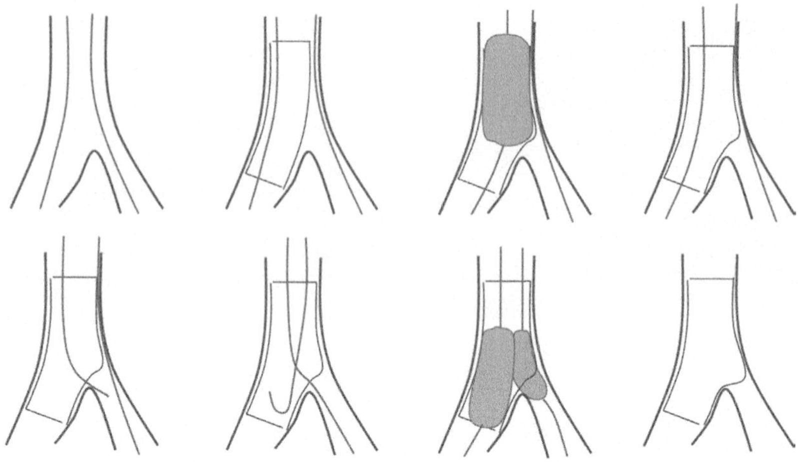

Figure 12.3 Continued

proximal to the *diagonal.* A 3 × 13 mm Cypher, which matched the diameter of the distal segment, was implanted 8 mm proximal to the diagonal, resulting in complete lesion coverage (12 atm) (Figure 12.1(ii)).

In order to restore the initial diameter of the proximal segment, a 3.5 × 9 mm balloon was inflated proximally with the distal marker positioned opposite the carena (16 atm) using the proximal optimization technique (POT) (Figure 12.1(iii)).[3,4] The LAD wire was inserted into the Diagonal using the pull-back technique whereby a pre-shaped wire penetrates the side-branch through the most distal stent strut.[5] The Diagonal wire shaped into a short loop was subsequently released and advanced into the distal LAD (Figure 12.1(v)). As the result in the ostium of the diagonal was considered inadequate, kissing balloon inflation was performed with two short balloons, a 2.5 mm Maverick in the diagonal and a 3 × 9 mm in the LAD, inflated at 7 and 10 atm, respectively (Figure 12.1(vi)).[6] POT was performed again with the short 3.5 × 9 mm balloon in order to eliminate the oval distortion in the proximal segment of the stent caused by Kissing (Figure 12.1(vi)).The stenting result achieved in all three segments of the bifurcation was excellent (Figures 12.1(vii) and 12.1(viii)).

This case illustrates the evidence-based principles of bifurcation treatment: (1) The number of stents as well as stent overlapping should be kept to a minimum. (2) Stents should be deployed carefully in order to avoid

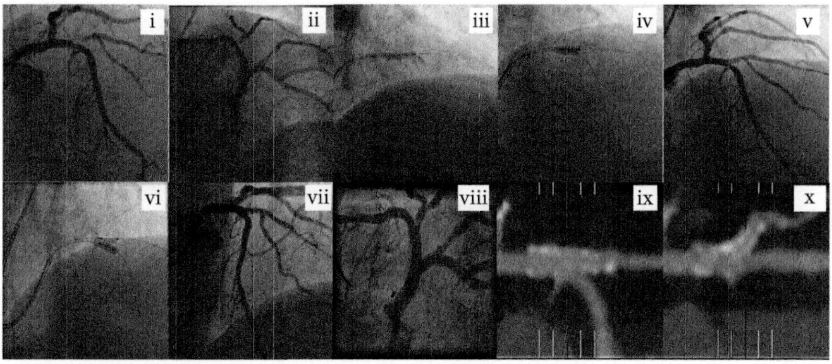

Figure 12.4(i–x) Inverted provisional stenting strategy.

malposition. (3) The anatomy of the bifurcations should be preserved, hence protecting their function. [Finet's law: Prox. diameter = (distal diam. + SB diam.) × 0.678.][7]

Inverted Provisional Side-branch Stenting (LAD/D1 Bifurcation)

Patient 2 was a 65-year-old woman treated for hypertension who presented with spontaneous chest pain of a few minutes' duration. She was admitted to the CCU where the EKG showed persistent T-wave inversion in the anterior leads.

Right transradial coronary angiography was carried out with a 5F diagnostic catheter and revealed the presence of a lesion in the LAD/Diag. bifurcation, type LAD1, LAD2, Diag 1; 1, 0, 1 (Medina classification). The diagonal was a single, large-diameter branch. In addition, a moderate lesion was visualized in the first left marginal branch.

PCI was subsequently performed via the right transradial route using a 6 F introducer (Terumo) [Figure 12.4(i–x)]. The patient agreed to be enrolled in the EBC 2 trial (PI: D. Hildick-Smith) comparing single versus double stenting in true bifurcation lesions with long lesions in large side branches (>2.5 mm). She was randomized to receive a single stent, and the operators selected the inverted provisional stenting strategy (Figure 12.3(2)). Using an EBU 3.5 Launcher Medtronic guiding catheter, 2 BMW 0.014" *wires were* inserted into the two branches beginning with the most difficult one, namely the diagonal, in order to avoid wire twisting during rotation (Figure 12.4(iii)). A Nobori 3.5 × 18 mm was implanted directly from the diagonal to proximal LAD at 8 atm. The diameter was chosen to match those of the diagonal (approximately 3.2 mm) and the proximal LAD (close to 4 mm). A 3.5 × 8 mm balloon was inflated at 24 atm (POT) in order to avoid the risk of malapposition in the proximal segment [Figure 12.4(iv)]. The result obtained in the LAD was considered unsatisfactory [Figure 12.4(v)]. Given the absence of any dissection in the diagonal, the diagonal wire was inserted into the LAD next to the carena using the pull-back technique. The LAD wire was subsequently released and advanced into the diagonal. Kissing balloon inflation was carried out using a 3.5 × 8 non-compliant balloon (Hiryu, Terumo) in the LAD and a 3 × 8 mm in the diagonal [Figure 12.4(vi)].[8]

Excellent results were achieved in all three segments of the coronary bifurcation [Figures 12.4(vii) and 12.4(viii)]. Three years later, *Coroscan* examination confirmed the persistence of these results [Figures 12.4(ix) and 12.4(x))].

This case is a good illustration of how to limit the number of stents in a coronary bifurcation. This technique is frequently implemented in the distal left main and requires careful selection of a stent which is able to accommodate two potentially very distinct diameters.[9] In cases of poor results, the provisional strategy can be completed by implantation of a second stent using the T or TAP technique[11] or the Classic Culotte strategy[12] or even Internal Crush, with final kissing balloon inflation performed in all cases.

The latest versions of the dual-stenting techniques starting with the side branch (inverted Culotte or mini DK Crush) are compatible with 6F guiding catheters and can be carried out via the transradial route (Figure 12.8).

LMCA/LAD/D2/LCX Trifurcation

Patient 3 was a 50-year-old male with no documented risk factors. He presented with increasingly frequent exertional chest pain. The EKG and biological findings were normal. Coronary angiography performed via

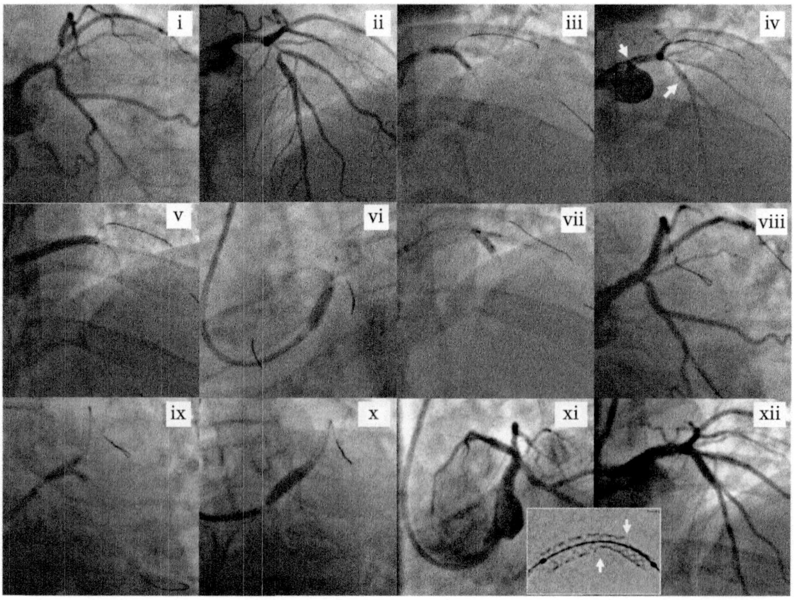

Figure 12.5(i–xii) Left main, LAD, circumflex artery bifurcation stenting.

the right transradial route with a 5F diagnostic catheter revealed a single significant lesion involving the distal left main, the LAD, the proximal Circumflex, and the first and second diagonal branches. Given the small size (diameter) of the first diagonal branch, the trifurcation was LM, LAD1, Cx1, Diag2; 0, 1, 1, 1 (Medina Classification) [Figure 12.5(i–xii)].

The treatment selected was coronary angioplasty with provisional SB stenting[13] rather than bypass surgery given the patient's age and his unwillingness for bypass surgery. The procedure was performed via the right radial route using a 6 F 3.5 EBU guiding-catheter (Launcher, Medtronic). Three 0.014" guide wires (Runthrough NS Terumo) were inserted into the second diagonal, the LAD, and the circumflex. The lesion was predilated from the left main to the LAD with a 2.5 × 20 mm balloon (Figure 12.5(iii)). A 3 × 28 mm Nobori stent was subsequently implanted from the left main ostium to the LAD at 10 atm (Figure 12.5(iv)). The stent delivery balloon was inflated to 20 atm proximal to the diagonal (pseudo POT) (Figure 12.5(v)). A 4 × 15 mm balloon was then used to carry out POT in the left main (Figure 12.5(vi)). The diagonal and

LAD wires were subsequently exchanged and kissing balloon inflation was performed with short 2.5 mm and 3 mm balloons (Figure 12.5(vii)). As the angiographic result was considered inadequate in the circumflex (Figure 12.5(viii)), the LAD and circumflex wires were exchanged and kissing inflation was performed in the LAD and Circumflex with 2 NC short 3.5 mm balloons (Figure 12.5(ix)). Repeat POT was carried out in the LM with a 4.5 × 10 Hiryu balloon (Figure 12.5(x)). The results were excellent in all treated segments. Stent enhancement shows the three diameters of the stent from post diagonal LAD to proximal LM with metal projection inside the Diagonal ostium (Figures 12.5(xi) and 12.5(xii)).

LMCA Stenting via Small Radial Artery, Post-Cardiac Arrest, Cardiogenic Shock

Patient 4 was a 48-year-old male admitted to the Interventional Cardiology Department directly from the MICU after he was cardioverted and resuscitated from cardiac arrest in a swimming pool. The patient had no documented risk factors. He was intubated, ventilated, and sedated; he presented with cardiogenic shock and was administered a continuous infusion of small-dose adrenalin which restored his systolic pressure to approximately 90 mmHg. The EKG showed significant diffuse ST segment depression. Following insertion of a transfemoral intra-aortic balloon for counter pulsation, a right radial puncture was made without difficulty.[14] Coronary angiography was subsequently performed using a 5F sheath (Figure 12.6(i–vi)).

Contrast injection in the left coronary artery (LCA) revealed a severe diffuse lesion in the left main and a lesion in the second diagonal branch (Figure 12.6(i)). Due to significant catheter friction, a 4F guiding catheter was used for right coronary artery (RCA) angiography which showed a tight lesion in the 2nd segment (Figure 12.6(ii)). Contrast injection performed with a 4F guiding catheter showed a small radial artery arising from the upper segment of a brachial artery (Figure 12.6(iii)). A second contrast injection below the elbow showed no anastomosis between the small brachio-radial vessel and the brachio-ulnar one.

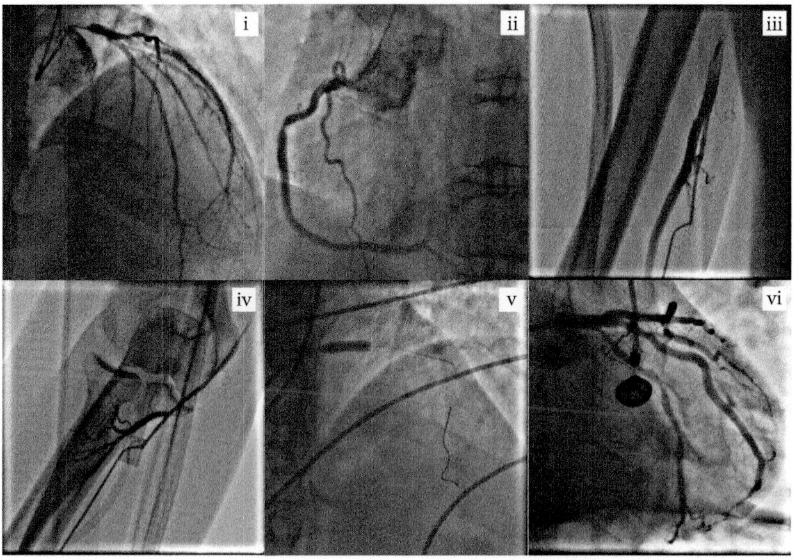

Figure 12.6(i–vi) Transradial treatment of a Left Main lesion after a resuscitated cardiac arrest.

In the absence of any data regarding the patient's neurological status, the decision was made to dilate the left main via the right transradial route using a sheathless SPB 3.5 Asahi guiding-catheter. The 4F guiding-catheter was used to insert a long 0.035" guide wire in the ascending aorta. After removing (withdrawing) the 5F sheath, a 6Fsheathless guiding-catheter was positioned in the left main coronary artery (Figure 12.6(v)). Subsequently, a 0.014" wire was inserted into the LAD and a 4 × 12 mm XIENCE stent was implanted following Quantitative Coronary Analysis (QCA). The stent was deployed immediately proximal to the circumflex with an excellent angiographic result (Figure 12.6(vi)). After a few days of therapeutic hypothermia, the patient awoke without any neurological sequelae.

The technical difficulties and procedural failure associated with the transradial approach are often attributable to abnormalities of the radial artery. Such anomalies have been well documented in autopsy series[15] as well as in reports of transradial PCI.[16,17] The origin of the radial artery is often located high up in the brachial or even axillary region. In 25% of cases,

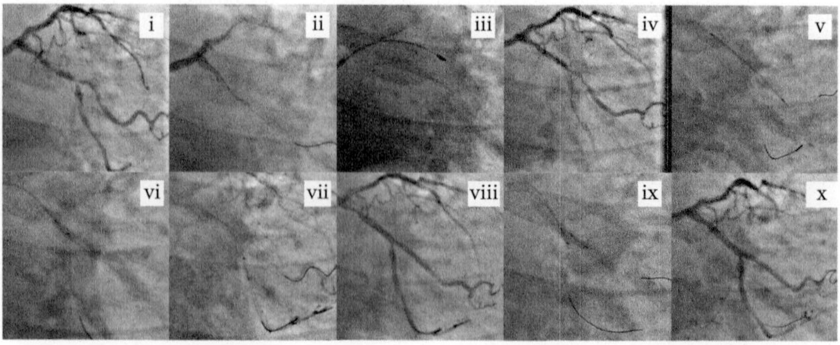

Figure 12.7(i–x) Transradial rotational atherectomy in a calcified circumflex artery bifurcation.

these frequently very thin arteries form an anastomosis with the brachio-ulnar vessel which can be simple or in the shape of a complex loop unsuitable for transradial puncture. Congenital abnormalities such as proximal loops or high radial origin are generally not bilateral.[18]

This case illustrates the use of sheathless guiding-catheters; 6F and 7 F sheathless GW have the diameter of a 4 Fr and 7 Fr sheath, respectively. In addition to their reduced diameters, the Asahi GW has an excellent hydrophilic coating.[19]

Rotablation of Calcific LCx with Bifurcation Stenting

Patient 5 was an 82-year-old male with hypertension and dyslipidemia presenting with exertional chest pain. Stress MRI revealed the presence of myocardial ischaemia in the antero-apical and lateral territories. Coronary angiography was carried out via the right transradial route with a 5F diagnostic catheter and showed much calcified coronary arteries and a long lesion in the mid-LAD involving the second diagonal branch which was subsequently treated using a long stent. The diagonal branch was protected with a wire. The right coronary artery was free of any tight lesion.

During the final part of the procedure, the operators treated a complex lesion in the Circumflex bifurcation (Circ 1, Marg 1, Marg 2; Medina classification 1, 1, 1) (Figure 12.7(i–x)). Another lesion was visualized in proximal circumflex artery. The main distal segment of the bifurcation had a long stenosis, whereas the ostial lesion in the SB was short and followed by another tight, short distal lesion, and the bifurcation was heavily calcified.

The initial strategy involved implantation of a long stent from the proximal circumflex to the first marginal through the second marginal following balloon predilatation. An EBU 4 guiding catheter was positioned in the left main and an 0.014" BMW wire was easily inserted into the first marginal (Figure 12.7(ii)). However, placement of an identical wire in the second marginal branch proved impossible and implementation of a CTO technique combining a Finecross microcatheter (Terumo) with an XT Fielder wire proved also unsuccessful.

Subsequently, the operators decided to perform rotational atherectomy rather than balloon predilatation towards the first marginal (Figure 12.7(iii)). A 1.5 mm burr was used to prepare the lesion proximal to the first marginal. The XT wire supported by the Finecross catheter was in turn easily inserted into the second marginal (Figure 12.7(iv)).

The microcatheter was used to exchange the XT guidewire for a 0.014" BMW (Figure 12.7(v)). A 3 × 38 mm Xience Stent was implanted from the proximal circumflex to the first marginal (Figure 12.7(v)). POT was carried out with a short 3.5 mm balloon (Figure 12.7(vi)). Following guide-wire exchange and predilatation of the second marginal branch, a short stent (2.5 × 8 mm XIENCE) was deployed in the distal lesion (Figure 12.7(viii)) at a sufficient distance from the ostium. The result was considered inadequate in the ostium of the second marginal branch (Figure 12.7(vii)). Final kissing balloon inflation was performed with two NC 3 × 8 mm balloons. Satisfactory final results were achieved in all three segments of the coronary bifurcation (Figure 12.7(x)).

This case shows that, as with the transfemoral approach, the transradial approach can be used by experienced operators in complex multi-vessel disease. Rotablator was used as an alternative technique in this particular bifurcation case where one of the distal branches could not be accessed by a wire. This is also an illustration of how CTO techniques can

Cath. Size	Devices	Techniques	Radial compatibility*
5F	Ballons ≤ 5 mm Microcatheter Stents ≤ 4.5 mm IVUS Rota 1.25 mm	No kissing balloon	100%
6F	All coronary balloons All coronary stents Cutting/scoring balloon Rota ≤ 1.75 mm Most protection devices Tornus	Kissing balloons (compliant or NC) 2 microcatheters Microcatheter and monorail B. Anchoring balloon	86.9%
7F	Angioguard Rota 2 mm	Kissing stent Microcatheter and IVUS	76.9%
8F	Rota > 2 mm		64.7%

Figure 12.8 Compatibilty of interventional devices for complex TRI with French size of guiding catheters

be implemented via the transradial route. A 6F GW can accommodate a 1.75 mm Rotablator burr.

Figure 12.8 shows the compatibility between guiding-catheters, devices and the technical strategies applied during complex procedures as well as their feasibility in a population of French patients treated by transradial PCI.

Conclusion

Obviously, the few examples provided here do not illustrate all the potentially complex coronary angioplasty cases.

The transradial route can also be used in patients with multi-vessel disease under FFR guidance, as well as in chronic coronary occlusions via both radial arteries in most cases, and in alcohol septal ablation for hypertrophic obstructive cardiomyopathy.

Although the management of complex coronary situations via the transradial route requires a learning period even for experienced transfemoral operators, the setup of proctoring programmes and the availability of dedicated devices have considerably reduced this learning phase.

The authors thank Mrs Catherine Dupic for expert translation and preparation of the manuscript.

References

1. Medina A, Suarez de Lezo J, Pan M. A new classification of coronary bifurcation lesions. *Rev Esp Cardiol.* 2006; 59:183.
2. Louvard Y, Thomas M, Dzavik V, Hildick-Smith D, Galassi AR, Pan M, Burzotta F, Zelizko M, Dudek D, Ludman P, Sheiban I, Lassen JF, Darremont O, Kastrati A, Ludwig J, Iakovou I, Brunel P, Lansky A, Meerkin D, Legrand V, Medina A, Lefèvre T. Classification of coronary artery bifurcation lesions and treatments: time for a consensus! *Catheter Cardiovasc Interv.* 2008;71(2):175–83.
3. Mylotte D, Routledge H, Harb T, Garot P, Hovasse T, Benamer H, Unterseeh T, Chevalier B, Morice MC, Louvard Y, Lefèvre T. Provisional side branch-stenting for coronary bifurcation lesions: evidence of improving procedural and clinical outcomes with contemporary techniques. *Catheter Cardiovasc Interv.* 2013;82(4):E437–45.
4. Finet G, Derimay F, Motreff P, Guerin P, Pilet P, Ohayon J, Darremont O, Rioufol G. Comparative analysis of sequential proximal optimizing technique versus kissing balloon inflation technique in provisional bifurcation stenting: fractal coronary bifurcation bench test. *JACC Cardiovasc Interv.* 2015;8(10):1308–17.
5. Alegria-Barrero E, Foin N, Chan PH, Lindsay AC, Di Mario C. Choosing the right cell: guidance with three-dimensional optical coherence tomography of bifurcational stenting. *Eur Heart J Cardiovasc Imaging.* 2012;13(5):443.
6. Murasato Y, Finet G, Foin N. Final kissing balloon inflation: the whole story. *EuroIntervention.* 2015;11(Suppl V):V81–5.
7. Finet G, Gilard M, Perrenot B, Rioufol G, Motreff P, Gavit L, Prost R. Fractal geometry of arterial coronary bifurcations: a quantitative coronary angiography and intravascular ultrasound analysis. *EuroIntervention.* 2008;3(4):490–8.
8. Mylotte D, Hovasse T, Ziani A, Lefèvre T, Dumonteil N, Louvard Y, Carrie D. Non-compliant balloons for final kissing inflation in coronary bifurcation lesions treated with provisional side branch stenting: a pilot study. *EuroIntervention.* 2012;7(10):1162–9.
9. Foin N, Sen S, Allegria E, Petraco R, Nijjer S, Francis DP, Di Mario C, Davies JE. Maximal expansion capacity with current DES platforms: a critical factor for stent selection in the treatment of left main bifurcations? *EuroIntervention.* 2013;8(11):1315–25.
10. Koo BK, Kang HJ, Youn TJ, et al. Physiologic assessment of jailed side branch lesions using fractional flow reserve. *J Am Coll Cardiol.* 2005;46(4):633–7.
11. Burzotta F, Gwon HC, Hahn JY, Romagnoli E, Choi JH, Trani C, Colombo A. Modified T-stenting with intentional protrusion of the side-branch stent within

the main vessel stent to ensure ostial coverage and facilitate final kissing balloon: the T-stenting and small protrusion technique (TAP-stenting). Report of bench testing and first clinical Italian-Korean two-centre experience. *Catheter Cardiovasc Interv.* 2007;70(1):75–82.

12. Chevalier B, Glatt B, Royer T, Guyon P. Placement of coronary stents in bifurcation lesions by the 'culotte' technique. *Am J Cardiol.* 1998;82(8):943–9.
13. D'Ascenzo F, Iannaccone M, Giordana F, Chieffo A, Connor SO, Napp LC, Chandran S, de la Torre Hernández JM, Chen SL, Varbella F, Omedè P, Taha S, Meliga E, Kawamoto H, Montefusco A, Chong M, Garot P, Sin L, Gasparetto V, Abdirashid M, Cerrato E, Biondi-Zoccai G, Gaita F, Escaned J, Hiddick Smith D, Lefèvre T, Colombo A, Sheiban I, Moretti C. Provisional vs. two-stent technique for unprotected left main coronary artery disease after ten years follow up: a propensity matched analysis. *Int J Cardiol.* 2016;211:37–42.
14. Bernat I, Abdelaal E, Plourde G, Bataille Y, Cech J, Pesek J, Koza J, Jirous S, Machaalany J, Déry JP, Costerousse O, Rokyta R, Bertrand OF. Early and late outcomes after primary percutaneous coronary intervention by radial or femoral approach in patients presenting in acute ST-elevation myocardial infarction and cardiogenic shock. *Am Heart J.* 2013;165(3):338–43.
15. Rodríguez-Niedenführ M, Vázquez T, Nearn L, Ferreira B, Parkin I, Sañudo JR. Variations of the arterial pattern in the upper limb revisited: a morphological and statistical study, with a review of the literature. *J Anat.* 2001;199(Pt 5):547–66.
16. Lo TS, Nolan J, Fountzopoulos E, Behan M, Butler R, Hetherington SL, Vijayalakshmi K, Rajagopal R, Fraser D, Zaman A, Hildick-Smith D. Radial artery anomaly and its influence on transradial coronary procedural outcome. *Heart.* 2009;95(5):410–5.
17. Burzotta F, Brancati MF, Trani C, Tommasino A, Porto I, Niccoli G, Leone AM, Coluccia V, Di Noi P, Crea F. Impact of radial-to-aorta vascular anatomical variants on risk of failure in trans-radial coronary procedures. *Catheter Cardiovasc Interv.* 2012;80(2):298–303.
18. Burzotta F, Brancati MF, Porto I, Saffioti S, Aurigemma C, Niccoli G, Leone AM, Coluccia V, Crea F, Trani C. Comparison of right and left upper limb arterial variants in patients undergoing bilateral transradial procedures. *Circ Cardiovasc Interv.* 2015;8(12).
19. Cheaito R, Benamer H, Hovasse T, Tritar A, Hage F, Garot P, Lefèvre T, Unterseeh T, Chevalier B, Morice MC, Louvard Y. Feasibility and safety of transradial coronary interventions using a 6.5-F sheathless guiding catheter in patients with small radial arteries. *Catheter Cardiovasc Interv.* 2015;86(1):51–8.
20. Watt J, Oldroyd KG. Radial versus femoral approach for high-speed rotational atherectomy. *Catheter Cardiovasc Interv.* 2009;74(4):550–4.

13

Transradial Approach for Left Main and Bifurcation Stenting

Tapan Ghose

F. Kiemeneij and colleagues are credited with the pioneering work on transradial coronary interventions.[1] The initial paper was presented as a poster in American College of Cardiology (ACC) meeting in 1993. Before this, Radner described radial artery cutdown approach in 1948.[2] Subsequently Campeau described the percutaneous entry to radial artery for diagnostic coronary angiography in 1948.[3] Over the years, the experience with transradial coronary intervention has become very popular because of patient comfort, early ambulation, less bleeding, and shorter hospital stay. More recently, various scientific societies have endorsed radial as a default route for primary angioplasty because of mortality benefit.[4]

Bifurcation lesion angioplasty is performed in 15–20% of cases in large series.[5] In angioplasty era, up to 50% cases the side branch compromise used to occur.[6] Subsequently, bifurcation angioplasty and stenting was successfully performed. Transradial route, DK crush technique with final kissing balloon inflation has brought down the rate of repeat revascularization to a very low level (5%).[7] However, transradial stenting of both left main (LM) and non-left main lesions have specific challenges, like catheter size limitation, poor back up support, simultaneously requiring placement of 2 balloon or 2 stents. The cross over to femoral route remains an issue.[8]

Evidence for Transradial Non-left Main Coronary Artery (Non-LMCA) Bifurcation Intervention

The impact of trans-femoral (TF) versus transradial (TR) route on bifurcation angioplasty was addressed in the subanalysis of Coronary

Bifurcation Stenting (COBIS) registry data base.[9] This is a retrospective study involving 16 major interventional centres in Korea. The inclusion criteria were bifurcation lesion treated with at least one drug-eluting stent (DES), main vessel diameter ≥2.5 mm and side branch diameter ≥2.0 mm. Cardiogenic shock, ST segment myocardial infarction (STEMI) intervention and LCMA intervention were excluded. 1,668 patients' data were analysed. TR approach was used in 503 (30%) patients.

At baseline patients in the TR group were less likely to have dyslipidemia, peripheral artery disease, chronic renal disease and acute coronary syndrome (ACS) at presentation. Presence of true bifurcation and GP IIbIIIa inhibitors usage was higher in TR group. Usage of IVUS and 2 stents were higher in TF group. 10.9% (53) patients received 2 stents. T stenting (85.5%), crush (7.2%), culotte (1.8%) and V stenting (5.3%) were the various techniques used.

In the TF group 26 (20.3%) patients received 2 stents. The techniques of stenting were T stenting (29.8%), crush (40.3%), culotte (3%) and V (16.9%) stenting.

A total of 424 pairs were created after propensity matching. Good distinction (C. statistic 0.869 for propensity score model) was created. There was no significant difference at baseline clinical, angiographic and procedural parameters except a few. TR group patients were less likely to have chronic renal disease or peripheral artery disease. There was no significant differences between TF and TR groups for procedural success in the main vessel (99.6% vs 98.6%, $P = 0.08$) and side branches (62.6% vs 66.7%, $P = 0.11$). Over a mean follow up duration of 22 months cardiac death or myocardial infarction (MI) (1.8% vs 2.2%, $P = 0.45$), TLR (4.0% vs 5.2%, $P = 0.22$) and major adverse cardiovascular events (MACE) (5.2% vs. >7.0%, $P = 0.11$) did not differ significantly between TR and TF groups respectively. Sub group analysis showed no difference in outcome between TR and TF group on the occurrence of MACE. The authors concluded that TR percutaneous Coronary Intervention (PCI) in feasible alternative in bifurcation stenting procedure.

The impact of TR or TF route on true bifurcation angioplasty was reported in another study.[10] The authors reported the immediate and 55 ± 22 months follow up data in 805 consecutive patients{TF (n = 297), TR (n = 508)}. Using logistic regression 249 propensity match pairs were created. The demographic, angiographic and procedural variables were similar except less prior PCI, multi-vessel disease and left main coronary artery (LMCA) bifurcation in TR group (all $p < 0.05$). Angiographic success and fluoroscopy time was similar. Bleeding Academic Research Consortium (BARC)defined bleeding was lower in TR group (3.9% vs 9.1%, $p \leq 0.01$). Long-term safety was similar. Cardiac death, MACE, MI, target vessel revascularization (TVR), stent thrombosis was not different between the TR and TF groups. Dedicated radial centres have reported good immediate and 30 days outcome of bifurcation intervention in ACS and STEMI lesions.[20] Figures 13.11–13.20 show step-by-step approach of transradial bifurcation stenting using dedicated bifurcation stent.

Transradial LCMA Intervention

Several studies reported the feasibility and safety of LMCA intervention through TR route. In a single-centre experience involving 80 patients of LMCA intervention TR route was used in 34% of patients.[11]The PCI indications, lesion locations were similar in between TR and TF groups. However, TR group had higher LV ejection fraction.

In TF group patients' larger diameter sheath 7F and 8F were used and more patient required Intra Aotic Balloon Pump (IABP). Other parameters such as procedural time, fluoroscopy time, and contrast utilization were similar. Procedural success, in hospital outcome and 6 months MACE were similar in between TR and TF groups. One patient in femoral group had vascular complication (5.7%).

One retrospective study (n = 131) from Taiwan reported the utility of LMCA PCI in 2008.[12] 116 (88.5%) patients were treated through TR approach and 15 (11.5%) patients were treated through TF approach. Angiographic and procedural success were achieved in all {114 (98.3%) vs 14 (93.3%) $P = 0.876$}. TF group patients required more debulking procedures, larger guiding catheter and had larger minimal lumen diameter (MLD) following PCI. TR group had less in-hospital MACE (7.8% vs 33.3%, $P = 0.003$). Vascular complication was lower in TR group (1.7% vs 26.6%, $p < 0.001$). 6 months MACE was lower in TR group (8% vs 23%, P = 0.299). The author concluded that TR PCI in LM is associated with lower vascular complication compared to TF route.

The largest experience of TR vs TF LMCA PCI was reported by Yang et al. in 2010.[13] 821 consecutive patients were treated via TR (n = 353) or TF (n = 468) route. Clinical and angiographic features were similar between groups except TR group patients had less unstable angina and had less bifurcation disease requiring 2 stents. Procedural time and success rate (97% TF vs 96% TR, $p = 0.57$) were similar. Hospital stay and bleeding (0.6% vs 2.8%, $p = 0.02$) were less in TR group. Using propensity score model (n = 254 matched pair), over mean 17 months follow up duration, the rates of CV death (1.2% vs 2.0%, $p = 0.48$), non-fatal MI (4.7% vs 2.4%, $p = 0.16$), stent thrombosis (0.8% vs 2.8%, $p = 0.10$) and TVR (6.0% vs 6.7%, $p = 0.72$) were similar in TR and TF groups respectively. Only 43% of the total unprotected left main (UPLM) were treated via TR approach in spite in spite of high operator experience (80% transradial). The authors concluded that TR PCI of UPLM disease is associated with similar procedural success shorter hospital stay, reduced bleeding and comparable late clinical safety and efficacy parameters.

All of these single-centre observational studies results point to similar short- and intermediate-term outcome when performed by skilled radial operators (80% PCI through TR approach). Shorter hospital stay and less TIMI major and minor bleeding are additional advantages which allows aggressive antiplatelet and antithrombotic therapy.

LM Bifurcation Disease

Randomized controlled trial data in this setting has not been reported yet.

Left main bifurcation Oxford Rome (LABOR) study included 467 patients from 2 large volume tertiary care PCI centres.[14] 53% were treated via TR approach. Transradial LMCA PCI increased gradually over time (9% in 2005 to 91% in 2013) in consonant with the increased operator experience. In TF group patients true bifurcation lesions were more (60% vs 40%, $p = <0.001$), were more frequently treated with larger catheters, required less radiation. Double stents were more commonly used in TF group. The authors point out that more multi vessels PCI in TR group may explain higher radiation exposure. IVUS guidance and rotational atherectomy usage were similar. TF group had more haemodynamic support device usage. Over a period of 1 year follow up duration there was no difference in ischaemic complications.

One multicentre registry COBIS II reported results of 853 UPLMCA PCI from 18 Korean centres.[15] TR approach was used in 25% of cases. These patients were less likely to have ACS, chronic renal disease and true bifurcation lesion. IVUS usage, double stent technique, final kissing balloon inflation were significantly higher in TF group. The procedural success was similar. Bleeding was less in TR group. Over a mean follow up duration of 35 months the MACE rate was similar between the two approaches.

Thus, the largest published experience in LMCA PCI results is available in Asian and European patients. The evidence suggests that in experienced hands the TR approach to LMCA PCI is associated with similar in hospital and intermediate-term outcome. Less bleeding in this situation is an advantage. However, patients with haemodynamic instability, large plaque burden, foreseeable requirement of haemodynamic support device, debulking device, ACS at presentation still are better treated via TF approach Figures 13.1–13.10 show stepwise transradial LMCA bifurcation stenting using T stenting technique.

Prevailing Trends of Bifurcation and LMCA PCI

Overall, there is a growing trend of TR approach in bifurcation PCI all over the globe. European bifurcation club (EBC) annually reviews and updates the data base.[16] Consensus document is published from time to time.[17] Evidence suggests that 6F catheter can be used in most bifurcation lesions. 7F or even 8F sheath have been used through TR route. Sheathless 6.5, 7.5 and 8.5 F guiding catheters are available. The outer diameters are similar and inner diameter is larger in these catheters. This results in poor back up support. The 7.5F sheath less guiding catheter have smaller outer diameter (2.49 mm) than 6F introducer sheath (2.62 mm). In contrast, however, any guide catheter of operator's choice can be used with the 'Sheathless Railway System' from Cordis. Slender sheaths are also available where the outer diameter is reduced by 1F sized, keeping the inner diameter constant.[18]

At this point of time, the hardware does not limit the use of TR approach of bifurcation PCI stenting in left main and non-left main location if performed by skilled operators.[19,20] Cardiogenic shock, ACS

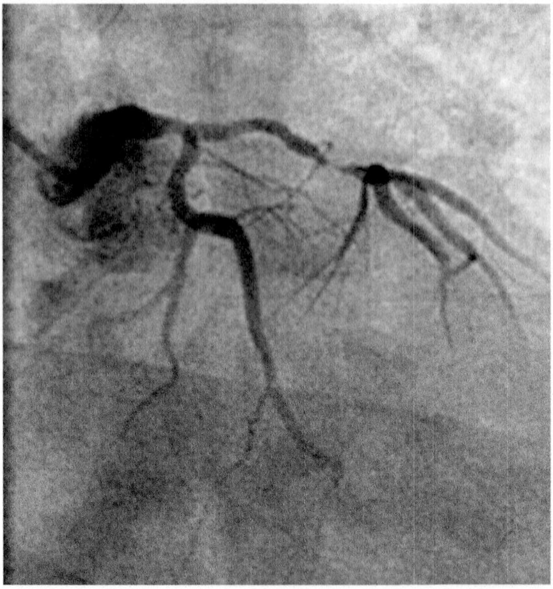

Figure 13.1 RAO caudal view of LCA(LMCA 50%, proximal LAD 80-95% (Medina 1.0.0) stenoses.

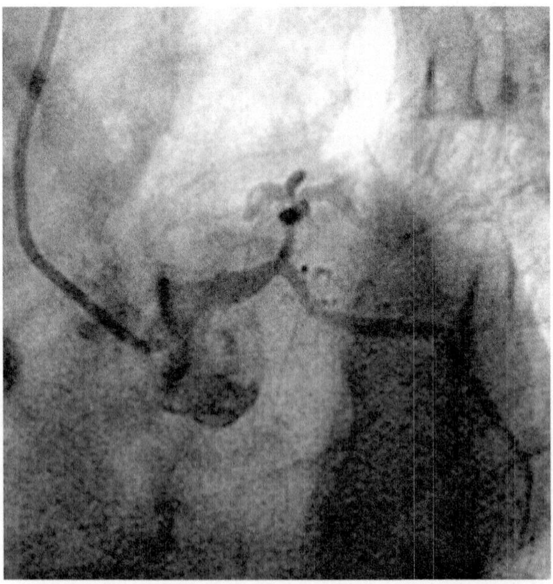

Figure 13.2 LAO caudal view of LCA showing 50% distal LMCA stenosis (Medina 1.0.0).

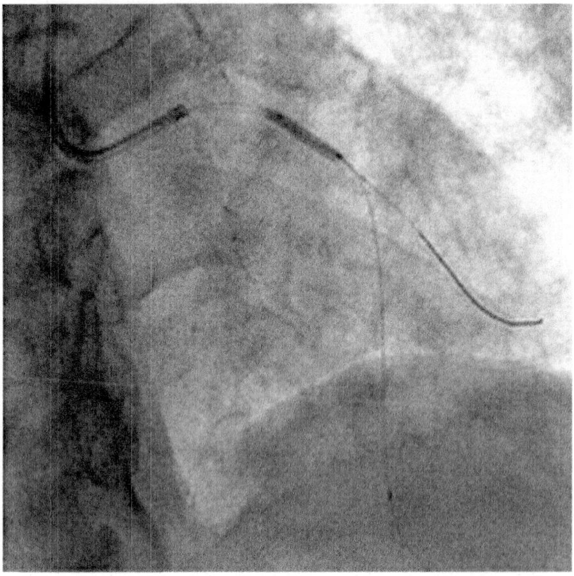

Figure 13.3 LAD and D1 crossed. Balloon dilatation.

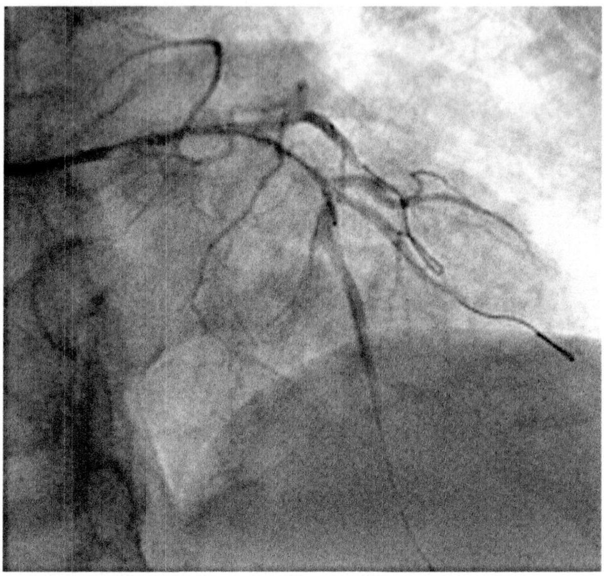

Figure 13.4 Synergy 3.5X38 mm stent from LMCA body up to mid lad across the D1 origin.

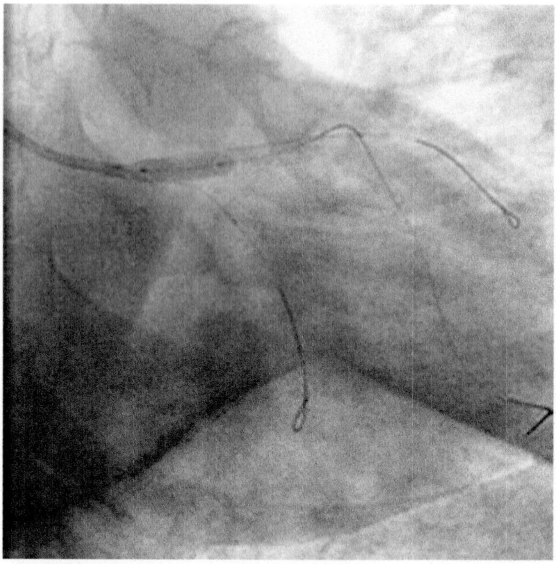

Figure 13.5 Proximal optimization technique.

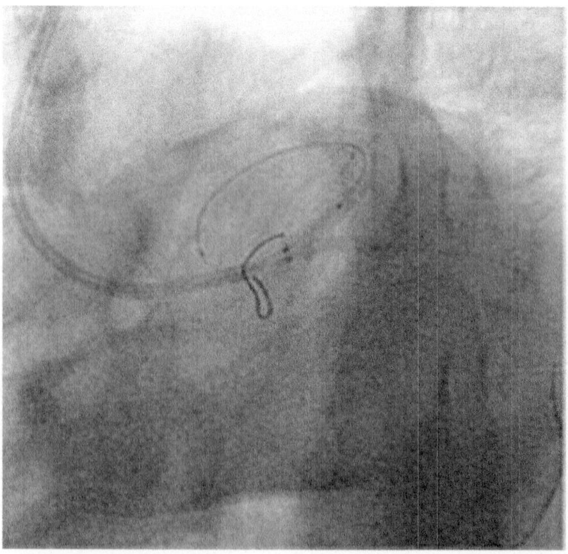

Figure 13.6 Kissing balloon dilation.

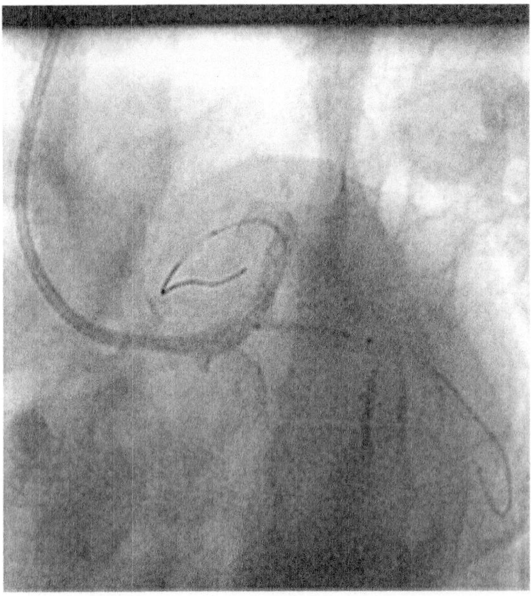

Figure 13.7 Provisional stentingof Lcx (2.5 × 16mm).

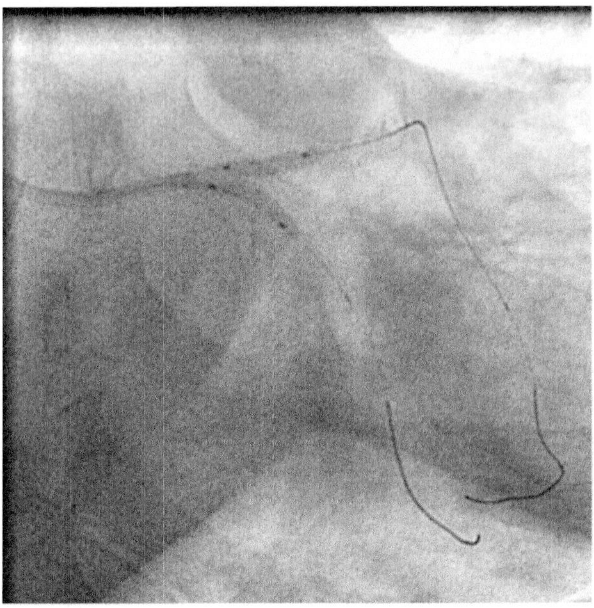

Figure 13.8 Final kissing balloon inflation (FKBI).

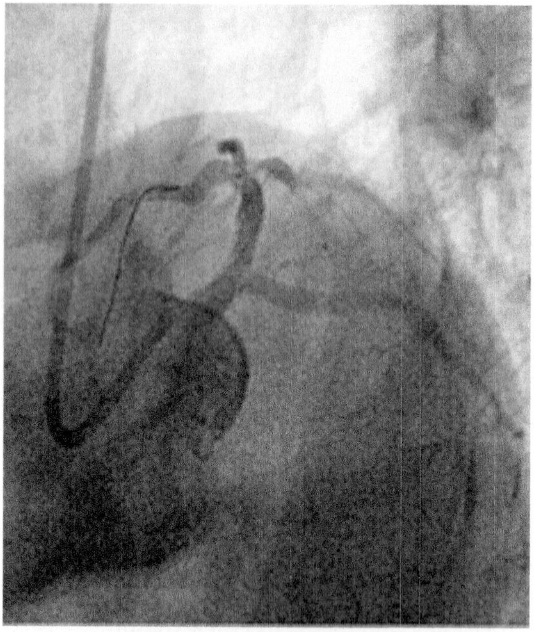

Figure 13.9 Final result in LAO Caudal view.

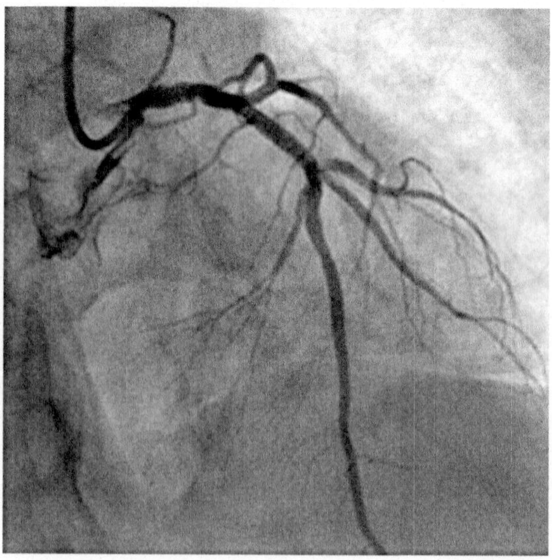

Figure 13.10 Final result in AP Cranial view.

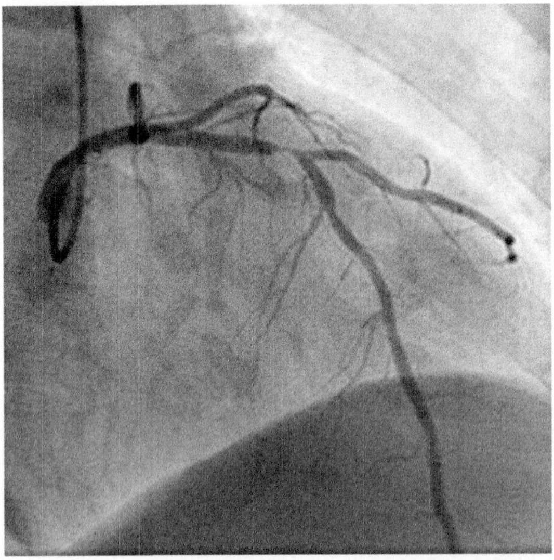

Figure 13.11 LAD,D1 95% stenosis Medina 1.1.1.

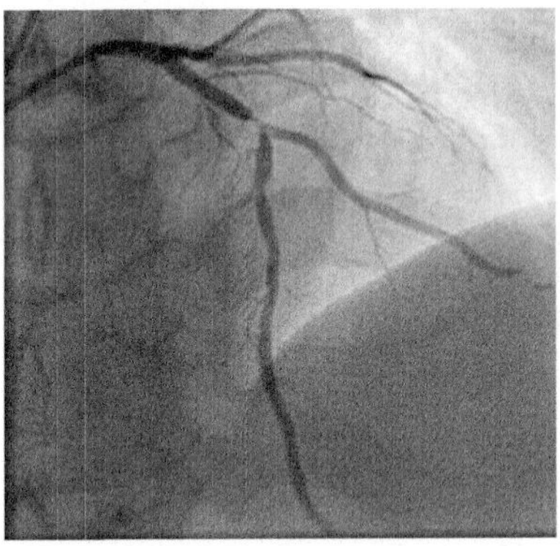

Figure 13.12 AP Cranial view showing lesion.

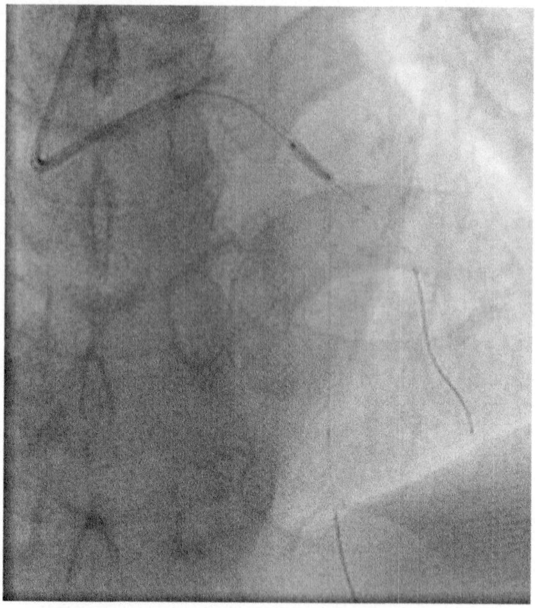

Figure 13.13 LAD,D1 crossed, Balloon dilation of D1.

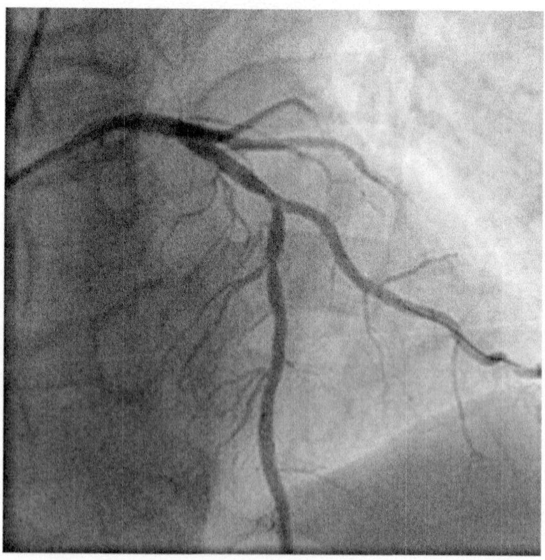

Figure 13.14 Post balloon dilation of D1.

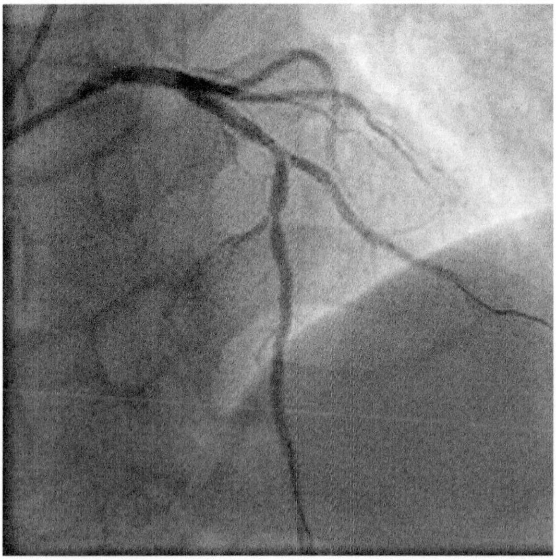

Figure 13.15 Biomime Branch 3.5-3 × 19 stent deployed in main to side.

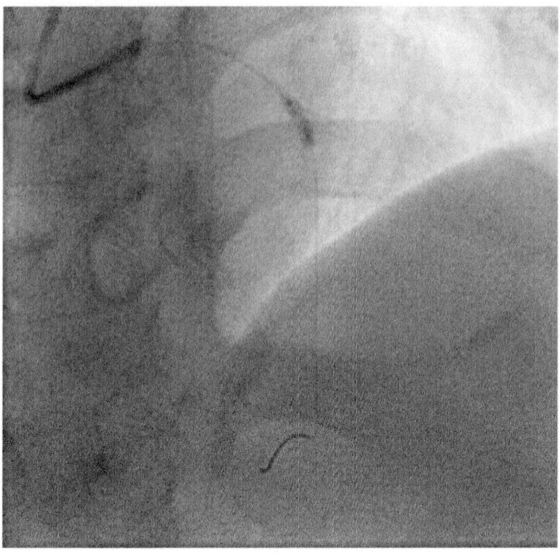

Figure 13.16 Side-branch wire out; inflated balloon in main vessel.

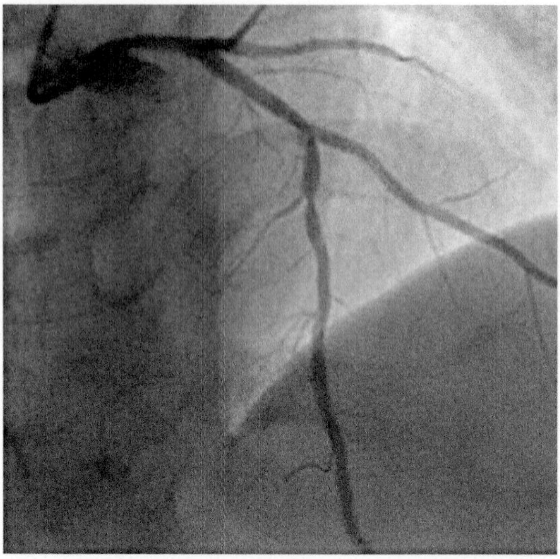

Figure 13.17 Post-balloon result.

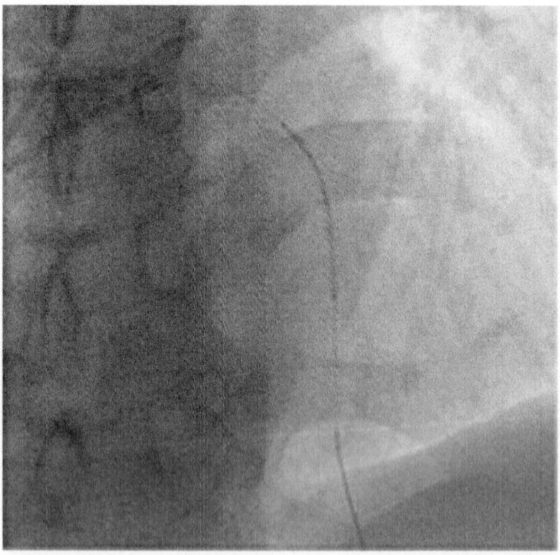

Figure 13.18 Evermime 3.5 × 37 mm stent in main vessel. Side-branch wire is out.

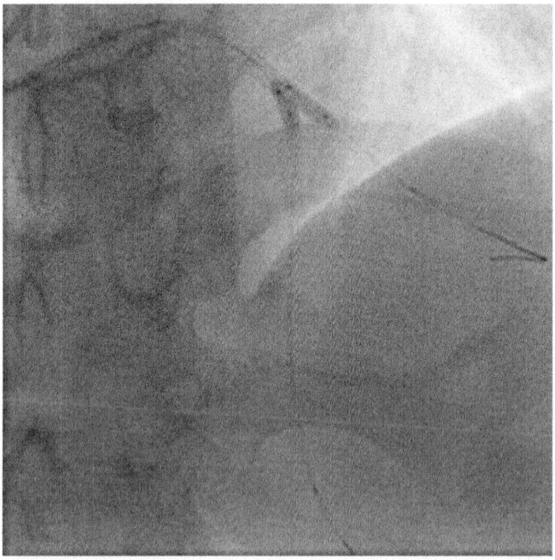

Figure 13.19 Final kissing balloon inflation (FKBI).

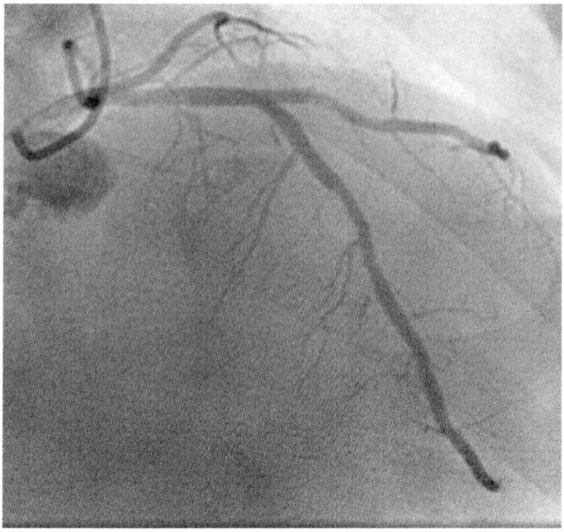

Figure 13.20 Final result (Cullote technique).

at presentation, haemodynamic instability, need for larger (>1.75) atherectomy burr would still be treated by TF approach.

References

1. Kiemeneij F, Laarman GJ. Percutaneous transradial artery approach for coronary stent implantation. *Cathet Cardiovasc Diagn.* 1993;30:173–78.
2. Radner S. Thoracal aortography by catheterization from the radial artery; preliminary report of a new technique. *Acta Radiol.* 1948;29:178–80.
3. Campeau L. Percutaneous radial artery approach for coronary angiography. *Cathet Cardiovasc Diagn.* 1989;16:3–7.
4. Hamon M, Pristipino C, Di Mario C, et al. Consensus document on the radial approach in percutaneous cardiovascular interventions: position paper by the European Association of Percutaneous Cardiovascular Interventions and Working Groups on Acute Cardiac Care and Thrombosis of the European Society of Cardiology. *EuroIntervention.* 2013;8:1242–51.
5. Stankovic G, Lassen JF, Hildick-Smith D, et al. The EuroIntervention coronary bifurcation treatment supplement. *EuroIntervention.* 2015;11(suppl V):V9–11.
6. Meier B, Gruentzig AR, King III SB, et al., Risk of side branch occlusion during coronary angioplasty. *Am J Cordiol.* 1984;53(1):10–14.
7. Chen SL, Thang JJ, Han Y, Jing Kan, et al. Double kissing crush versus provisional stenting for left main distal bifurcation lesions, D. K Crush – v randomized trial. *J Am Coll Cardiol.* 2017;70:2605–17.
8. Lefevre T, Girasis C, Lassen JF. Differences between the left main and other bifurcations. *EuroIntervention.* 2015;11(suppl V):V106–10.
9. Chung S, Her SH, Song PS, et al. Trans-radial versus trans-femoral intervention for the treatment of coronary bifurcations: results from Coronary Bifurcation Stenting Registry. *J Korean Med Sci.* 2013;28:388–95.
10. Gao Z, Xu B, Yang Y, et al. Transradial versus transfemoral method of two-stent implantation for true bifurcation lesions: comparison of immediate and long-term outcomes. *J Interv Cardiol.* 2014;27:99–107.
11. Ziakas A, Klinke P, Mildenberger R, et al. Comparison of the radial and femoral approaches in left main PCI: a retrospective study. *J Invasive Cardiol.* 2004;16:129–32.
12. Hsueh SK, Hsieh YK, Wu CJ, et al. Immediate results of percutaneous coronary intervention for unprotected left main coronary artery stenoses: transradial versus transfemoral approach. *Chang Gung Med J.* 2008;31:190–200.
13. Yang YJ, Kandzari DE, Gao Z, et al. Transradial versus transfemoral method of percutaneous coronary revascularization for unprotected left main coronary artery disease: comparison of procedural and late-term outcomes. *JACC Cardiovasc Interv.* 2010;3:1035–42.
14. De Maria GL, Burzotta F, Trani C, et al. Trends and outcomes of radial approach in left-main bifurcation percutaneous coronary intervention in the drug-eluting stent era: a two-center registry. *J Invasive Cardiol.* 2015;27:E125–36.

15. Chung S, Yang JH, Choi SH, et al. Transradial versus transfemoral intervention for the treatment of left main coronary bifurcations: results from the COBIS (Coronary Bifurcation Stenting) II registry. *J Invasive Cardiol.* 2015;27:35–40.
16. Lassen JF, Burzotta F, Banning AP, Lefevre T, Darremont O, Hildick Smith D, et al. Percutaneous coronary intervention for the left main stem and other bifurcation lesions: 12th consensus document for the European Bifurcation Club. *EuroIntervention.* 2018;13(13):1540–53.
17. Burzotta F, Lassen JF, Banning AF, Banning AF, Lefevre T, Hidick-Smith D, Chieffo A, et al. *EuroIntervention.* 2018;14(1):112–20.
18. Slender PCI via transradial approach. In: *Transradial Approach for Percutaneous Interventions.* Zhou, Y., Kiemeneij, F., Saito, S., Liu, W. (Eds.) Springer, (Switzerland), 2017, pp. 245–52. doi:10.1007/978-94-017-7350-8-22.
19. Ghose T. Transradial bifurcation angioplasty using bioresorbable vascular scaffold and kissing balloon technique. *J Am Coll Cordiol.* 2016;67(16 SUPPLS): pp S147. doi:10.1016/j.jacc.2016.03.262.
20. Ghose T, Kachru R, Sood R, Khan WU, Mishra N, Hussain S, Jamie Baba IA, Jabeen S, Joshi A, Immediate and thirty day results of bifurcation angioplasty performed in a dedicated radial centre. Submitted abstract TCT 2018 and Cardiological Society of India Annual meeting 2018.

14
Transradial Rotablation

Fuminobu Yoshimachi

Introduction

The evolution of drug-eluting stents (DES) has not only reduced the risk of acute stent failure; it also has reduced the long-term rate of re-intervention and has improved clinical outcomes with percutaneous coronary intervention (PCI). However, the unsolved problems still remain. The selection of the access site is considered to be one of them.

Transradial intervention (TRI) is superior to transfemoral intervention (TFI) in terms of less bleeding complications, reduced patient discomfort with shorter duration of bed-restriction following treatment, shorter duration of hospital stay, and reduced cost. For these reasons, TRI has become a popular procedure all over the world.[1] Of course there are some limitations of TRI; the most serious one is the limitation of the small size of radial artery compared to the size of guiding catheter (GC) or sheath.

Further, a calcified lesion still remains a formidable challenge for percutaneous coronary intervention (PCI). While, insufficient expansion of the stent in presence of dense coronary calcification may cause poor outcome; high-pressure post-dilatation may be associated with risk of coronary perforation. In order to solve this problem, rotablation or rotational atherectomy (Figure 14.1) (Boston Scientific Corporation, USA) has been used effectively since the bare-metal stent (BMS) era.[2]

With this background, the effective usage of rotablation or rotational atherectomy for TRI is described here.

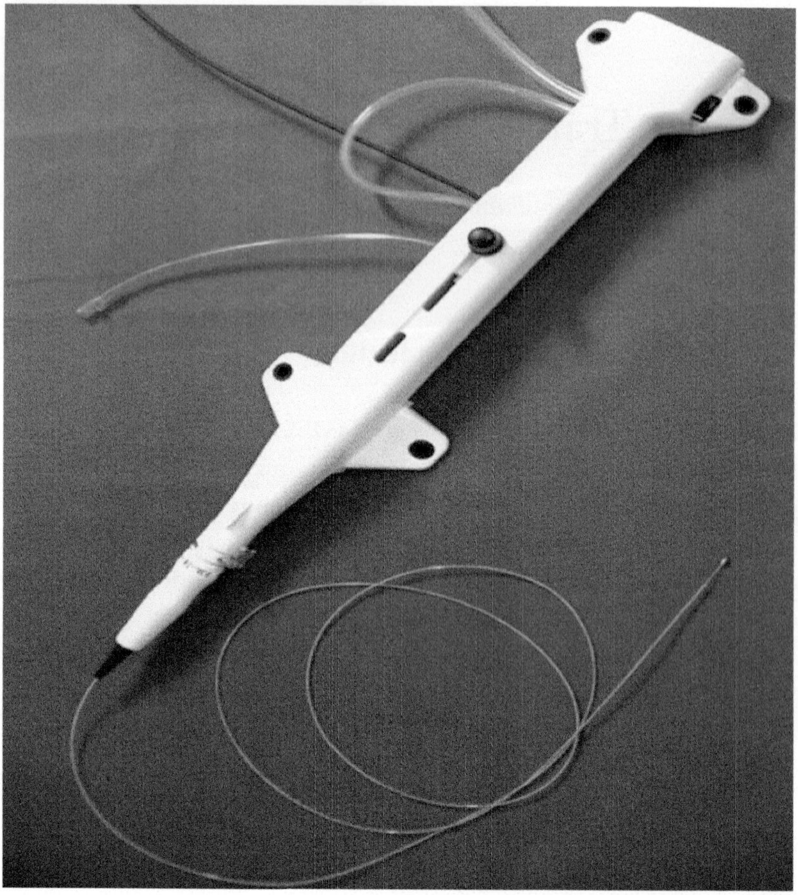

Figure 14.1 Rotablator.

Overcoming the Limitation of Small Radial Artery (RA) Diameter

The most serious limitation of TRI is the size of GC for small size of radial artery. GC or sheath equal to or smaller than 6F size has been used for most TRI cases.

Larger size of GC is considered ideal for Rotablation. For this reason, a larger size GC has been sometimes been used sheathlessly in the past.[3]

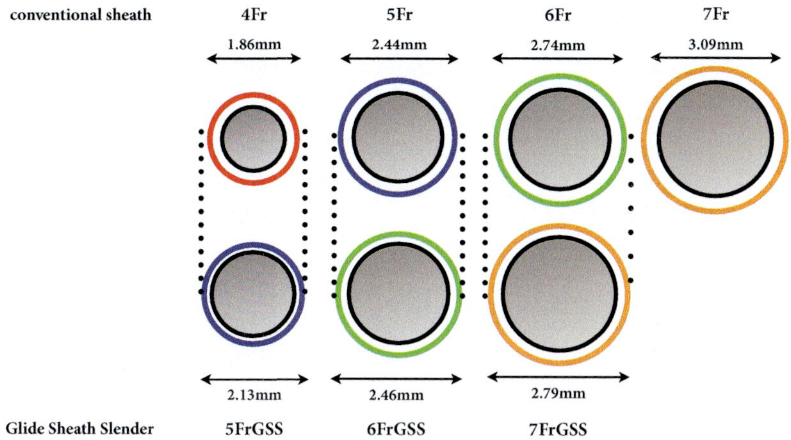

Figure 14.2 Glide sheath slender: Inner diameter is the same, but outer diameter is one French smaller. It expands the indication of Trans Radial Intervention.

Lately, Glidesheath Slender (GSS) (Terumo, Japan) is available for use.[4–5] The outer diameter of this 7 French sheath is almost the same size as 6 French size of conventional sheath because of the wall thickness of that is thinner (Figure 14.2). By using this device, TRI is performed with 6Fr or 7Fr GC without any limitation regarding the selection of devices and techniques even in small diameter radial arteries for PCI.

The Burr Size of Rotablator

Debulking can be performed in most cases using a small sized burr compatible with small size of GC; bigger burr size is usually not necessary in most of the cases except particular diseases such as Kawasaki disease.

By contrast, big burr may increase the risks of coronary perforation, slow flow or no reflow. The role of Rotablation is for lesion modification to enable optimal stent deployment and adequate post-dilatation; its objective is not to create a big lumen.

There are several reports that outcome of transradial rotablation is the same as TFI.[6,7]

Table 14.1 Burr size compatibility

Vessel size	Manufacturers recommendations	Real world
1.25mm	6Fr	5Fr
1.50mm	6Fr	5Fr
1.75mm	7Fr	6Fr
2.00mm	8Fr	7Fr
2.15mm	8Fr	8Fr
2.25mm	9Fr	8Fr
2.50mm	9Fr	9Fr

Table 14.2 Burr to artery ratio (%) in drug eluting stent (DES) era more than 50% area is enough as preparation for DES

Vessel size	Adequate size of Burr	Burr/vessel
2.00mm	1.25mm	63%
2.25mm	1.25mm	56%
2.50mm	1.25mm	50%
2.75mm	1.50mm	55%
3.00mm	1.50mm	50%
3.25mm	1.75mm	54%
3.50mm	1.75mm	50%
3.75mm	2.00mm	53%
4.00mm	2.00mm	50%

The manufacturer recommends 6Fr GC for 1.5 mm, 7Fr GC for 2.0 mm, and 8Fr GC for 2.25 mm of burr. But in actual clinical setting 5Fr GC is compatible with 1.5 mm, 6Fr GC is compatible with 1.75 mm, and 7Fr GC is compatible with 2.00 mm. Larger than 2.15 mm burr is not used in daily practice (Table 14.1).

Excessive over expansion is not necessary in DES era, and smaller burr to artery ratio is ideal for DES compared to BMS. Hence, 1.5 mm burr and 5F GC for 3 mm vessel, 1.75 mm burr and 6F GC for 3.5 mm vessel, and 2.0 mm burr and 7F GC for 4 mm are compatible (Table 14.2).

Slender Catheter Usage via Radial Artery for Rotablation

Although it is difficult to check the blood pressure through the tip of the GC and inject contrast medium during rotablation because of the small space between slender GC and Rotablator burr, there have been no clinical issues in our experience.

Furthermore, it is difficult to upsize the rotablator burr, with use of 5F GC for 1.5 mm burr (Figure 14.3(i)). We can check the effect of Rotablation by using optical coherence tomography (OCT) after rotablation (Figure 14.3(ii)).[8]

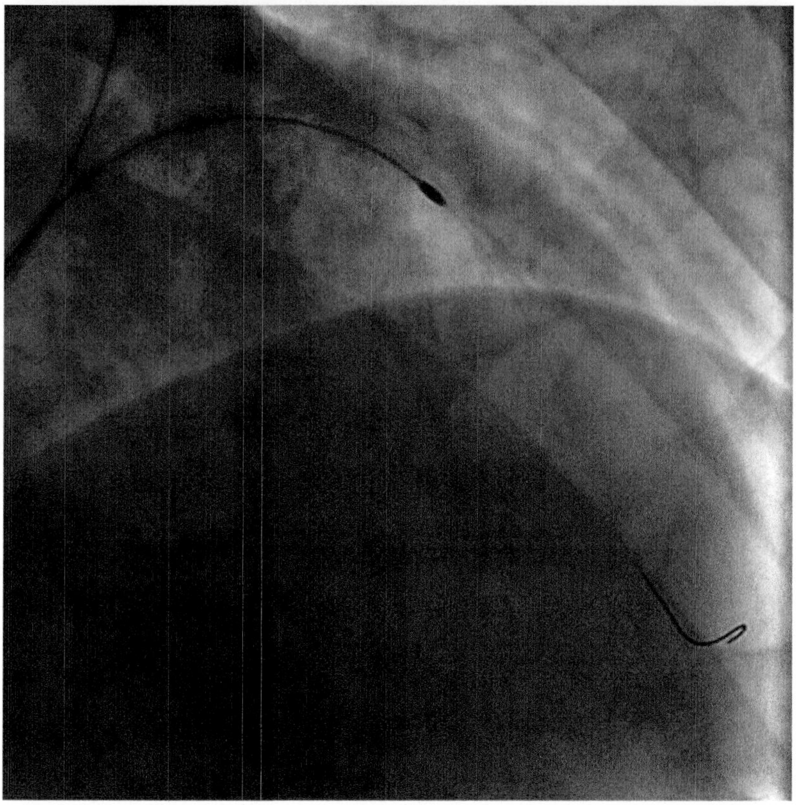

Figure 14.3(i) Rotablator for severe calcification in left anterior descending artery (LAD) with 5Fr Guiding Catheter and 1.50 mm Burr for Trans Radial Intervention.

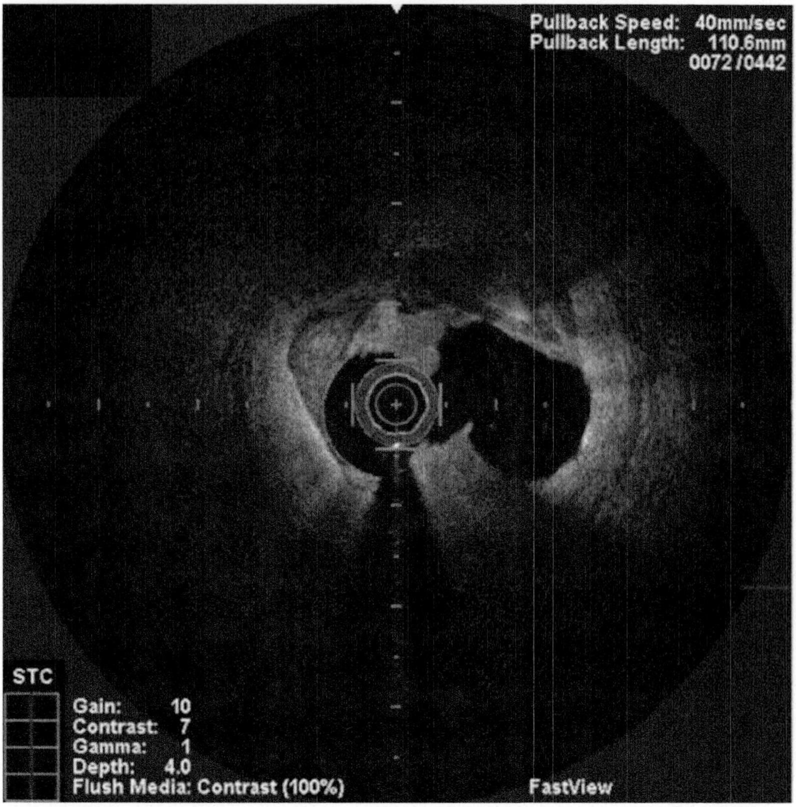

Figure 14.3(ii) 1.5 mm crack was observed after using 1.50 mm Burr by Optical Coherence Tomography (OCT).[8]

A Slender GC is associated with less back-up support for Rotablation.

Because some degree of back up support is needed for rotablation, it is important to create the so called 'power position', which is to make loop with GC by rotating, and pressing the GC to the other side of aorta and make it coaxial with the coronary, in order to have extra back-up support, which is necessary for rotablation.[9] This technique enables to have great pushability, however, the pull-back force is weak due to flexible slender GC. 'Stuck burr' must be prevented by avoiding pushing the burr forcefully.[10]

A recent large real-world single centre registry (n = 66; 72% radial and 28% femoral) showed that it is feasible to perform PCI with rotablation via RA access with very high success rates, lower access site complications

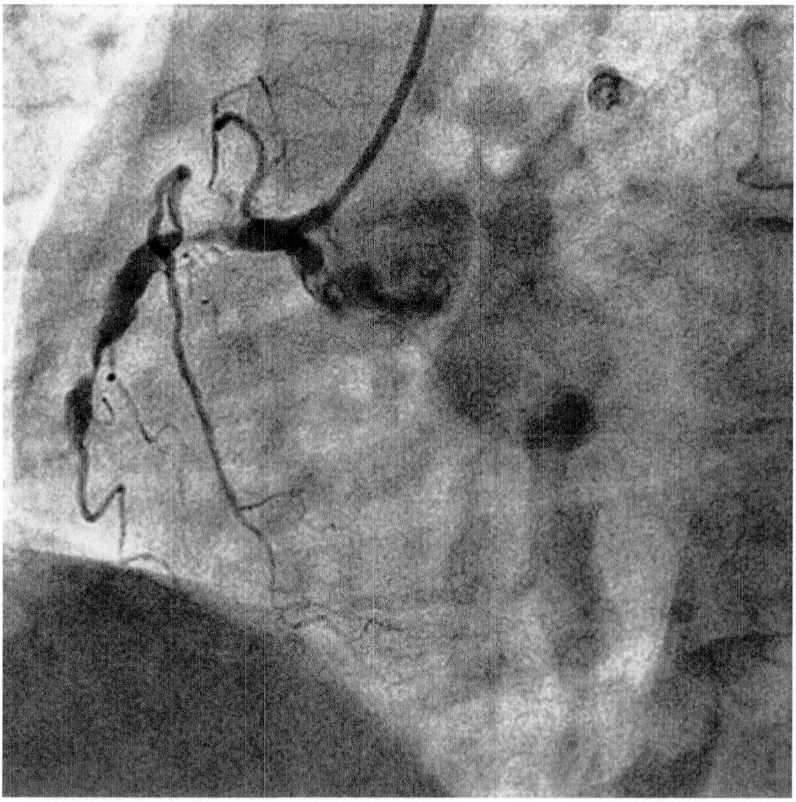

Figure 14.4(i) Chronic Total Occlusion (CTO) of Right Coronary Artery (RCA).

(6.1% versus 16.2, $p = 0.02$) and similar in-hospital and long-term outcomes (MACE events 2.2 versus 0.0%, $p = 0.20$ and 17.8 versus 12.2%, $p = 0.27$ respectively) compared to femoral procedure. In-hospital complications were twice more common with femoral than with radial access (18.9 versus 9.0%, $p = 0.03$); major bleeding (BARC score >2) was 4.1% versus 0 in femoral versus radial patients ($p = 0.002$).[11]

Conclusion

TRI is useful and effective for the patients and the indication is expanding with the development of GSS and other low-profile PCI devices. There

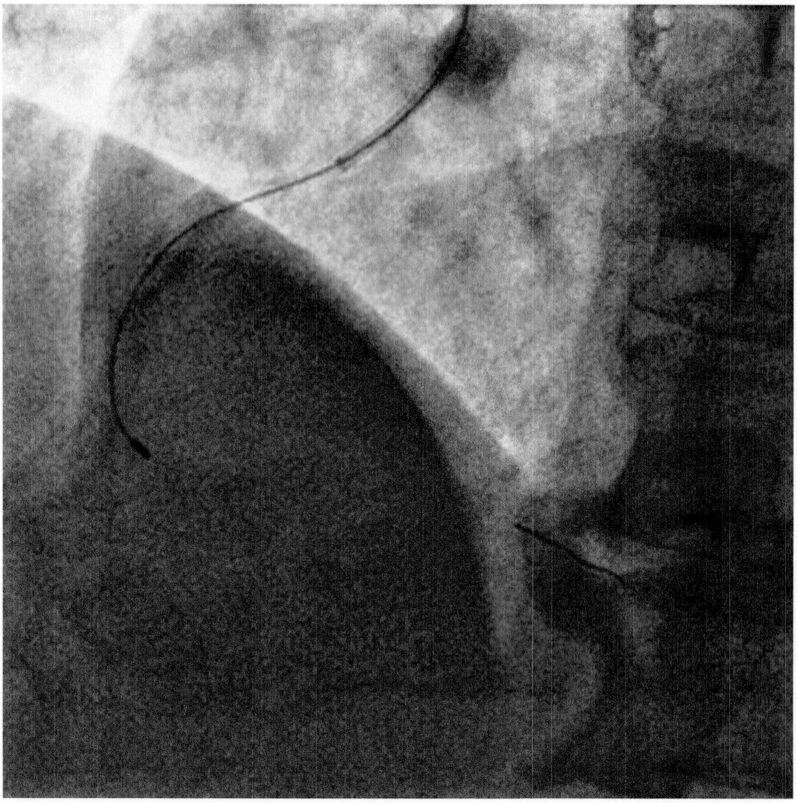

Figure 14.4(ii) Rotablator 1.5 mm Burr was used after crossing the Guidewire because of severe calcified lesion.

is no reason to hesitate to use Rotablator when treating calcified lesions including chronic total occlusion by TRI (Figures 14.4(i), 14.4(ii), and 14.4(iii)). We believe that using Rotablator in order to have better stent expansion will gain long-term patency.

After finding severe calcification by angiography and/or imaging devices such as OCT or intravascular ultrasound (IVUS), even if one physician or assistant in cath lab thinks that Rotablation is required, that should be considered to be an indication for Rotablation.

After finding severe calcification by angiography and/or imaging devices such as OCT or intravascular ultrasound (IVUS), even if one physician or assistant in cath lab thinks that Rotablation is required, that should be considered to be an indication for Rotablation.

Comparing with Manufacturer's recommendations and real world.

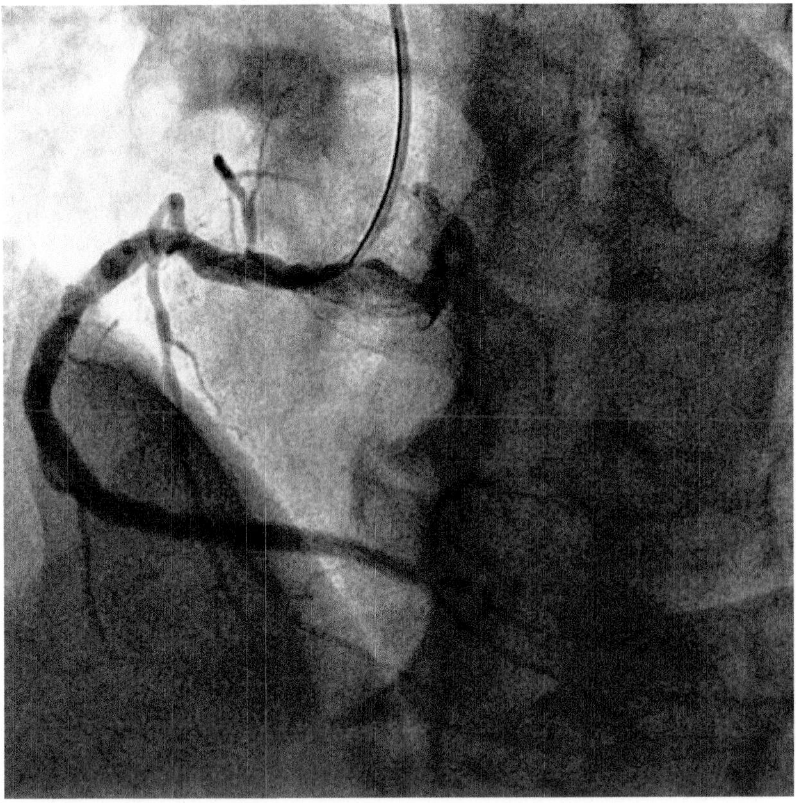

Figure 14.4(iii) Final angiography.

References

1. Bertrand OF, et al. Transradial approach for coronary angiography and interventions: results of the first international transradial practice survey. *JACC Cardiovasc Interv*. 2010;3(10):1022–31.
2. Henneke KH, et al. Impact of target lesion calcification on coronary stent expansion after rotational atherectomy. *Am Heart J*. 1999;137(1):93–9.
3. Lozano I, et al. Rotational atherectomy through radial access with a 7.5 fr sheathless guiding catheter. *Rev Esp Cardiol*. 2011;64(3):247–8.
4. Yoshimachi F, et al. Safety and feasibility of the new 5 Fr Glidesheath Slender. *Cardiovasc Interv Ther*. 2016;31(1):38–41.
5. Aminian A, et al. Initial experience with the Glidesheath Slender for transradial coronary angiography and intervention: a feasibility study with prospective radial ultrasound follow-up. *Catheter Cardiovasc Interv*. 2014;84(3):436–42.
6. Yin WH, et al. Transradial versus transfemoral rotablation for heavily calcified coronary lesions in contemporary drug-eluting stent era. *J Geriatr Cardiol*. 2015;12(5):489–96.

7. Kotowycz MA, et al. Rotational atherectomy through the radial artery is associated with similar procedural success when compared with the transfemoral route. *Coron Artery Dis*. 2015;26(3):254–8.
8. Attizzani GF, et al. Optical coherence tomography assessment of calcified plaque modification after rotational atherectomy. *Catheter Cardiovasc Interv*. 2013;81(3):558–61.
9. Kiemeneij F, et al. Focus on maximal miniaturisation of transradial coronary access materials and techniques by the Slender Club Japan and Europe: an overview and classification. *EuroIntervention*. 2015;10(10):1178–86.
10. Kaneda H, et al. Trapped rotablator: kokesi phenomenon. *Catheter Cardiovasc Interv*. 2000;49(1):82–4.
11. Garner D, Balakrishnan Nair S, Patel B, et al. 66 Comparison between transradial and femoral approach for rotational atherectomy in contemporary practice - a large single centre experience. *Heart*. 2014;100(Suppl 3):A37–38.

15

Trans-Radial Interventions in Chronic Total Occlusions and Post-CABG Patients

Charan Lanjewar, Dhiraj Kumar, and Prafulla Kerkar

Introduction

Ever since the first TR coronary angiogram in 1989 by Campeau et al.[1] and first transradial percutaneous intervention (PCI) was performed in 1993 by Kiemeneij,[2] there has been a phenomenal development of transradial interventions (TRI). There is robust data to prove that TR approach is superior to TF approach at least in ST elevation myocardial infarction (STEMI) patients. Many randomized trials prove that the access site complications are lesser with TR than TF approach.[3–5] The meta-analyses go even a step further and show mortality benefit.[6] All this data has made radial approach the default approach of PCI as per the European Society of Cardiology 2017 guidelines for STEMI.[7] However, there has been a variable adoption of radial approach among different countries. In US it is around 16–25% as per latest Cath PCI registry data, which is a far cry from, as early as 2008 when it was a paltry 3%. The British Registry quotes rates of more than 75% of PCI done by radial route and it is more than 80% in France and similar rates in Japan [8]. In India, as per the recent National Intervention Council (NIC), TRI are being performed as the default approach in 13% patients, however there is no subgroup analysis in this group particularly TRI in chronic total occlusion (CTO) and post-coronary artery bypass grafting (CABG) group (Please also see NIC/WARIS data in Chapter1, page-2).

PCI in CTO and post-CABG interventions are an evolving field of interventional cardiology. According to standard practice of the majority of CTO dedicated centres and operators, PCI in CTO is attempted using large bore guide catheters (GC) and TF approach (TFA). Yet TRI is a valuable alternative to TFA, which has been shown to reduce vascular complications and possibly better clinical outcomes.[8] However, the advantages of TRI might be offset by disadvantages regarding backup support in treatment of complex CTO.

With increasing adoption of radial PCI increasing number of operators are comfortable in using CTO and post-CABG PCI trans-radially. This document is an attempt to fill the gaps in knowledge and practice by focusing on the available data.

Trans-radial Interventions in CTO

Definition of CTO

Coronary CTOs are defined as coronary lesions with thrombolysis in myocardial infarction (TIMI) grade 0 flow of at least 3-month duration. Estimation of the occlusion duration is based on first onset of angina symptoms, prior history of myocardial infarction in the target vessel territory, or comparison with a prior angiogram. Technical success of CTO PCI is defined as successful CTO revascularization with achievement of <30% residual diameter stenosis within the treated segment and restoration of TIMI grade 3 ante grade flow.

There is enough evidence which suggests that low J-CTO score has higher rate of success of CTO PCI. J-CTO score is a score to evaluate the difficulty and rates of crossing the lesion.[9]

(1) Entry shape—blunt or tapered
(2) Calcification—present or absent
(3) Bending > 45 degrees—present or absent
(4) Occlusion length more than or less than 20 mm
(5) Previously failed lesions.

1 point is added for each adverse factor.

Category of difficulty: Easy = 0, Intermediate = 1, Difficult = 2, Very difficult ≥ 3.

As interventionists all over the world are adopting radial PCI, increasingly more interventionists are attempting radial approach. However, although the radial route offers advantages of lack of vascular complications and patient comfort there are significant technical limitations including access size, inadequate support for hardware for crossing and negotiating different hardware across lesion, spasm of radial artery with long procedure times and steep learning curve.

We reviewed multiple trials, registries and meta-analysis for trans-radial interventions in CTO. PCI results in CTO overall are similar for trans-radial PCI and trans-femoral PCI with success rates varying from 69% to 93%. Overall, rate of access-site complications is just 1% and crossover rates of 5.8%.[10]

Role of Pre-procedural Doppler

Prior to TRI CTO PCI it is recommended to perform a radial Doppler. Average radial diameter (RAD) in Indians[11,12] is 1.9 ± 1.12mm (for right radial) and 1.8 ± 0.29mm (for left radial) in males and 1.7 ± 0.2 mm in females[12] (Please refer to Table 6.1, Chapter 6, page 53.) It is prudent to use 7F guide catheter when radial artery ultrasound colour Doppler shows an artery size ≥ 2mm as the success increases with a 7F guide use as it provides better support.[11] With RAD ≥ 1.7 mm, 6F guide catheter can be used.

Pre-procedural assessment of forearm arteries using Doppler helps in assessing diameter and tortuosity of forearm vessels and helps in improving success rates in radial procedures. Such a strategy helps in improving rates of successful radial access and guide-catheter engagement rates of 97.5% in comparison to no imaging in which rates were 93%.[12] Also, a 7F when used in radial PCI is associated better outcomes in CTO.

Sheath Selection

Use of hydrophilic coated sheaths, which are shorter in length (7–10 cm) and slender provide lesser radial spasm.[13] Respecting the sheath to artery ratio is also important. RA inner diameter to the sheath outer diameter ratio should be close to or equal to 1: to prevent severe flow reduction post procedure.[14]

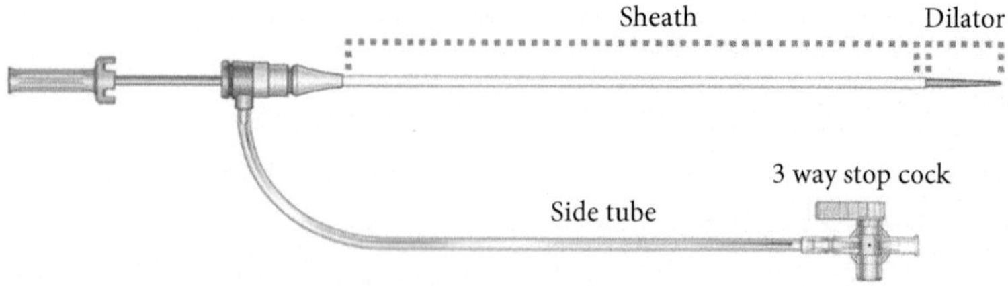

Figure 15.1 Ideal glide sheath by Terumo™ thin and short with hydrophilic exteriors.

The Glidesheath slender sheaths (Figure 15.1) can accomodate a 7F guide catheter in a 6-7F sheath, which has outer diameter of 6F and can also accomodate rotablation burrs upto 1.75mm. (Please refer to Table 14.1, page 338, Chapter 14) or intravascular ultrasound (IVUS) catheters. It has been observed by Tanaka et al. that failed cases of TRI CTO had a higher prevalence of the usage of guiding catheters (GC) less than 7F.[10] Any 5F-7F GC of operator's choice can be used with the 'Railway sheathless system™' from Cordis.

As sheathless guides up to 8F have same outer diameter as routine radial 6F sheath, they can be used wherever extra backup is needed. 8F provides 3 times more backup as compared to 6F catheter. Dautev and Ribero described the detailed procedure of use of sheathless GC and found favourable RA patency rates as compared to conventional approach. In the end at 5 months follow up, one symptomatic and 3 asymptomatic RA occlusions were found thus making it feasible to use large sized guide catheters in those with complex CTO lesions.[15]

Spasmolytic Cocktail and Anticoagulation

Spasmolytic 'cocktails' used judiciously after sheath insertion, with each catheter exchange and prior to sheath removal is of paramount importance in preventing spasms.

Spasmolytic agents commonly used include 1–5 mg of intra-arterial injection of Verapamil or Diltiazem.[16] The use of nitroglycerine (100 mcg) alone versus verapamil (1.25 mg) with nitroglycerine showed a similar reduction in incidence of radial artery spasm when compared to placebo.[17] Additionally, Nicorandil and Verapamil were found to be equally effective; unlike phentolamine which was inferior in its action.[18]

With regards the choice of anticoagulation there has been a raging debate about the ideal parenteral anticoagulant during PCI. After many trials it is now firmly established Heparin is the default anticoagulant in patients undergoing PCI with the sole exception on heparin-induced thrombocytopenia (HIT) when Bivalirudin may be preferred. Heparin dose in PCI is 100 U/kg.[19,20] ACT should be checked and maintained at >250 during the procedure.

Pre-procedural and Access Site Assessment and Proposed Recommendations

- Pre-procedural angiogram to be carefully analysed in two orthogonal views and J-CTO scoring to be done.
- Preprocedural radial artery Doppler to assess size and bifurcation anomaly anomaly may be performed.
- 7F radial access for arteries with RAD ≥ 2.0mm and 6F access for arteries with RAD ≥ 1.7mm (Please refer to page 151, and Figure 10.3 in Chapter 10).
- Hydrophilic sheaths to be used in radial access.
- When using 7F and 8F GC sheathless approach should be considered specially when ante grade dissection re-entry and rotational atherectomy with > 1.5mm burr is being considered. The Railway sheathless system™ by Cordis allows GC (≤7F) of choice to be used.
- Spasmolytic cocktails of verapamil or Diltiazem and or nitroglycerine should be used routinely after sheath placement.
- Heparin is the anticoagulant of choice in a dose of 100 U/kg in all trans radial PCI except heparin-induced thrombocytopenia (HIT).
- Sheath or catheter with Radial artery to sheath/catheter O.D with ratio >1:1 should preferably be avoided wherever possible.

Transradial CTO PCI Procedural Aspects

It is desirable for operators with at least annual experience of 50 radial PCI and 15 CTOs should undertake CTO PCI from trans-radial route. Also, it is important that TRI CTO should be performed in high volume trans-radial centre. In the setting of TRI CTO interventions operators must focus their attention on materials and compatibility [Please see Table 12.8 (Chapter 12) & 14.1(Chapter 14)].

Guide selection is very important for stability and often extra back up (EBU) 3.5, 3.75 cm for left coronary cannulation and for RCA cannulation, Amplatz Left, short tip Amplatz Right, Multipurpose is a good enough catheter to be used. Generally, the opposite radial access for CTO involving RCA gives more support.

Although overall radial PCI in CTO has similar rates of procedural success, but certain subsets are associated with increased failure. Radial CTO PCI is associated with more frequency of strategy changes (0.7 versus 0.5) in comparison to trans-femoral. Also, failure of delivery of various devices like balloon or stents was observed with TRI.[10] With the newer innovative devices and techniques including micro catheters, IVUS, anchoring technique, retrograde approach using collateral channels, sub-intimal tracking, and mother and child technique there has been an improvement in complex transradial CTO PCI. All these advances can be applied with TRI with 6F GC except IVUS with simultaneous micro catheter.[10]

Those with severe calcification, flush total occlusion of RCA ostium, long segment 20 mm occlusion, blunt stump, proximal cap ambiguity and J-CTO score ≥ 3 should be best attempted through femoral approach.

Antegrade Approach

Specific technical details are beyond the scope of this document. However, broad outlines are provided as follows and there is no difference as far as guidewire and crossing technique of CTO is concerned compared to TFA.[21]

1. First Wire to be Tried

We feel that the single transradial access may be taken and ante grade escalation strategy may be used. This includes the polymer coated Fielder XT, XTR, XTA wire (Asahi Intec, Japan), Wizard-7,8 (Lifeline,

Japan), Gaia 1 (Lifeline, Japan) Gentle manipulation of these wires may allow the passage of these guidewires through microchannels in the CTO.

The CTO PCI success is enhanced by the use of microcatheter which can provide support to the guidewire while attempting to manipulate across the CTO and for guidewire exchanges.

2. Single Wire Ante Grade CTO Technique

A hydrophilic floppy wire with tapered tip supported by a microcatheter, the guidewire tip with a short curve is gently advanced and rotated to find microchannels which offer no resistance. Tapered polymer coated guidewires that are generally preferred are the Fielder XT (Asahi Intec, Aichi, Japan) series wires (Fielder XT with tip load of 0.8 gm, Fielder XT-R with tip load of 0.6 gm and Fielder XT-A with tip load of 1.0 gm). The operator should attempt crossing the CTO with the Fielder XT wire for at least 10–15 min before changing the wire. Next in line comes Miracle 3,6,12 and Conquest Pro, Gaia series wires.

Figure 15.1(a-p) (*Courtesy Dr Sanjay Chugh*) illustrates use of microcatheter and Fileder XT wire used for successful PCI in a CTO in the RCA using slender techniques with 4F Glidesheath Slender (GSS) and 5F guide catheter. Because of traversing a narrow radial with type 3 bifurcation with 5F guide catheter (see legends to figures), this patient had a small remote forearm extravasation which was managed successfully by compression with a sphygmomanometer cuff inflated to above systolic pressure and deflated for a few seconds every 3 min (see Chapter 14 for details). Alternatively, the cubital loop can be traversed using an angioplasty wire in these situations (see Chapter 10). As is illustrated in the case, because of risk of extravasation, it is best to crossover to alternate access (such as to the contralateral radial, ulnar or rarely femoral) in the face of such radial anomaly. On 2 years follow-up post-PCI, the patient is asymptomatic and well. For further case illustrations on CTO, please see Chapter 10 (Figure 10.18 (a-j)), under 'Tips and Tricks for Transradial Interventions'.

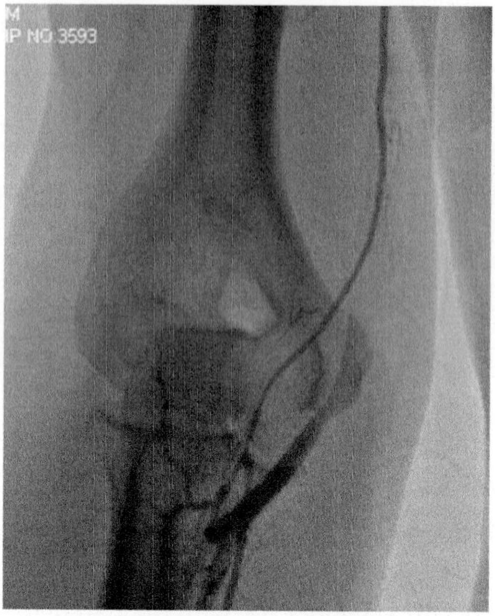

Figure 15.1a A high up origin of radial (type 3 bifurcation) with cubital loop. Access done via right radial with 4 F glide sheath slender (GSS). Test injection of contrast done through 5F Amplatz left (AL1) guide catheter (GC) (*Courtesy Dr Sanjay Chugh*).

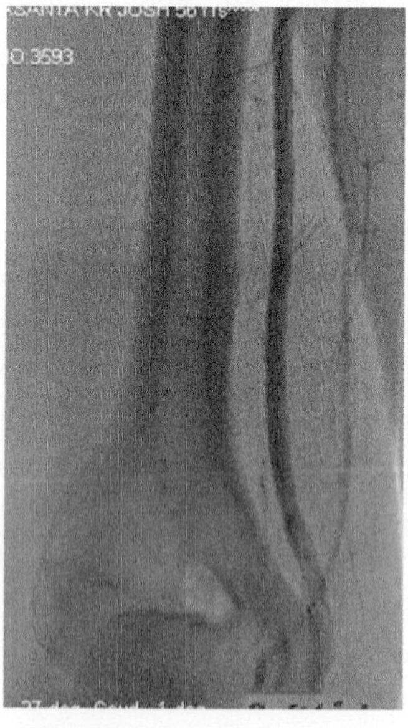

Figure 15.1b Selective injection into radial artery shows high origin of radial from brachial (Type3 bifurcation) (*Courtesy Dr Sanjay Chugh*).

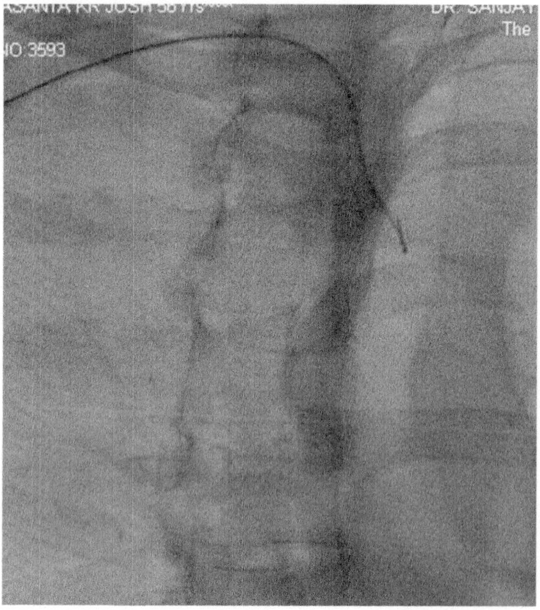

Figure 15.1c Guide catheter reaches arch of aorta via narrow right radial negotiated using balance middle weight (BMW™) angioplasty wire (*Courtesy Dr Sanjay Chugh*).

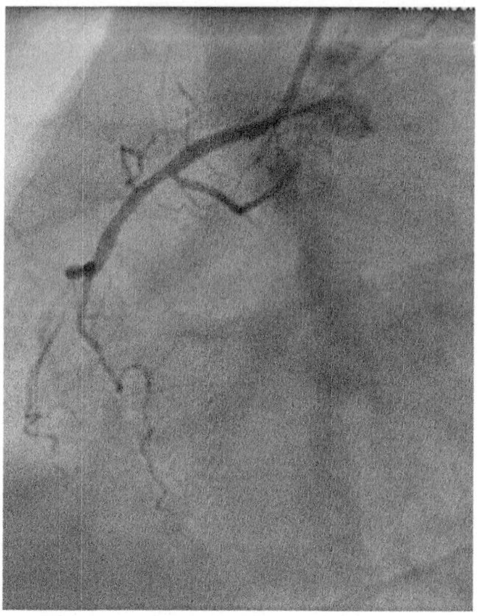

Figure 15.1d Guide catheter changed to 5F Judkins Right (JR) 3.5 GC because AL1 GC could not be advanced. Angiogram shows a chronic total occlusion (CTO) of mid right coronary artery (RCA) (*Courtesy Dr Sanjay Chugh*).

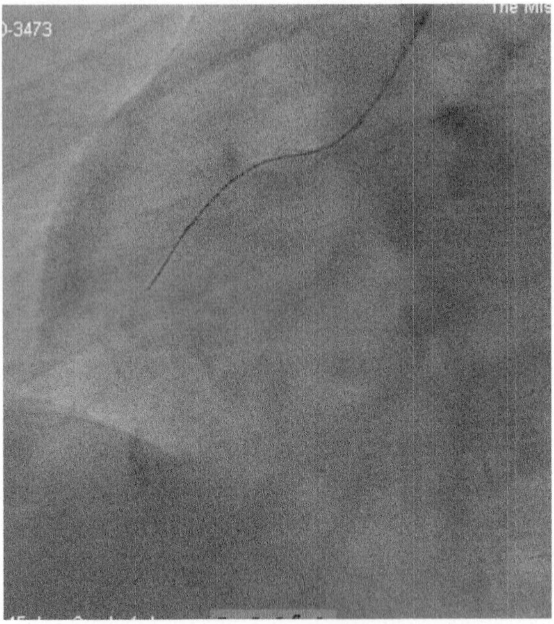

Figure 15.1e A Fielder XT™ wire with Fine cross™ micro catheter is used to cross the lesion. Micro catheter enhances guide support (*Courtesy Dr Sanjay Chugh*).

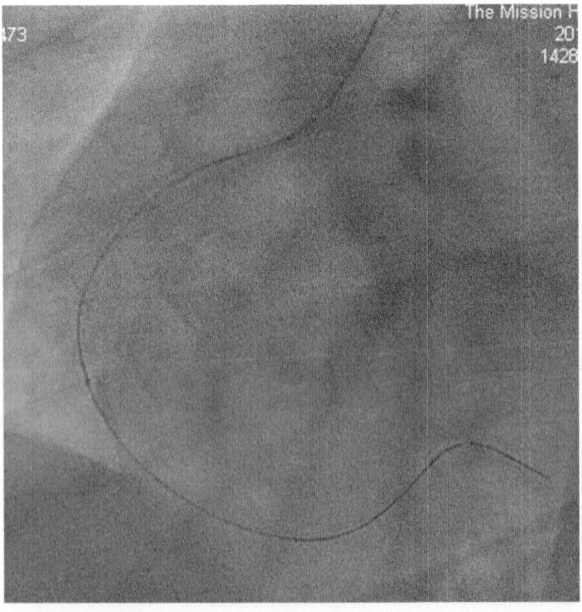

Figure 15.1f Wire crosses the CTO lesion (*Courtesy Dr Sanjay Chugh*).

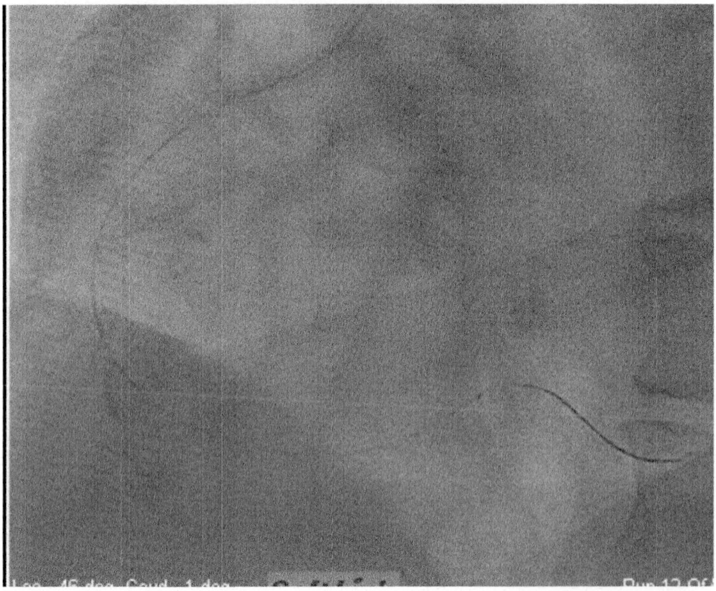

Figure 15.1g Finecross™ is adavanced and wire is exchanged for balance middle weight (BMW™) (*Courtesy Dr Sanjay Chugh*).

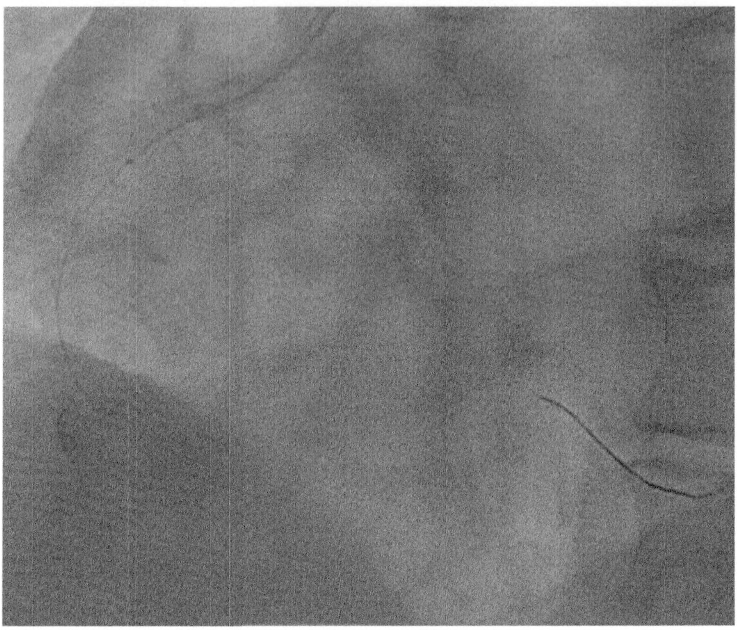

Figure 15.1h Microcathter is removed by connecting indeflator to microcatheter and inflation device is maintained at 8-10 atm (*Courtesy Dr Sanjay Chugh*).

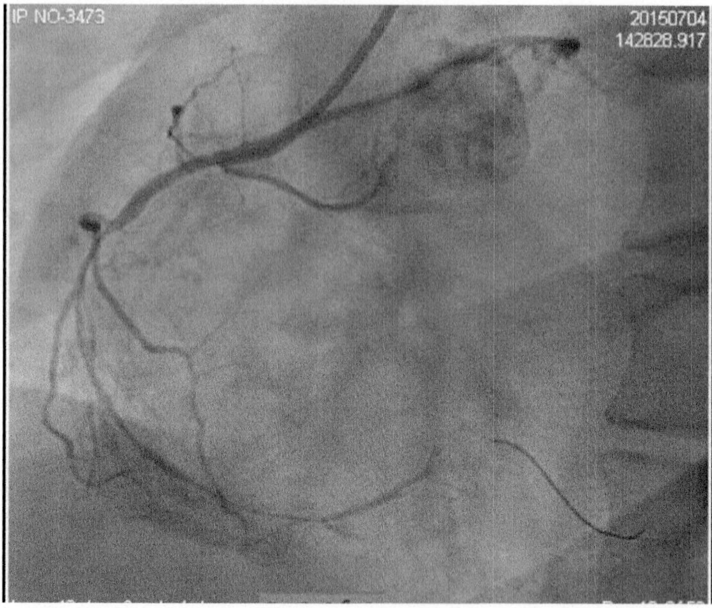

Figure 15.1i After pre-dilatation with 1.5 mm balloon (*Courtesy Dr Sanjay Chugh*).

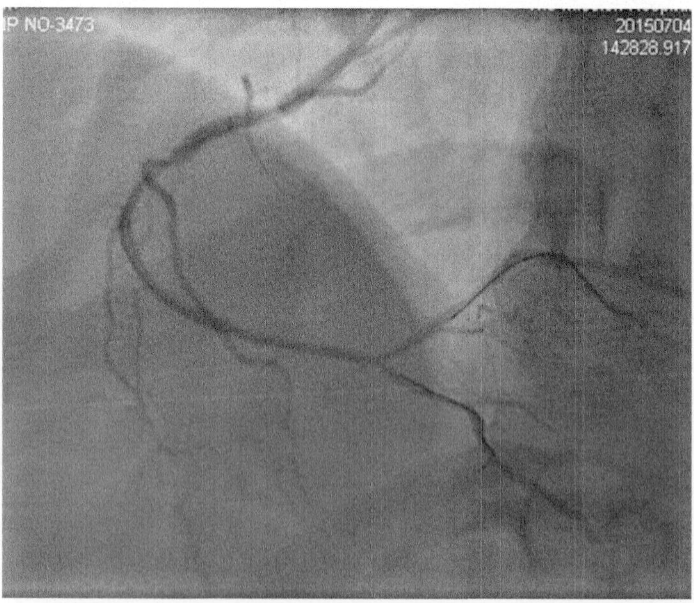

Figure 15.1j After second BMW wire into Posterior descending artery and predilatation of RCA with 2.0 and 2.5 mm balloons (*Courtesy Dr Sanjay Chugh*).

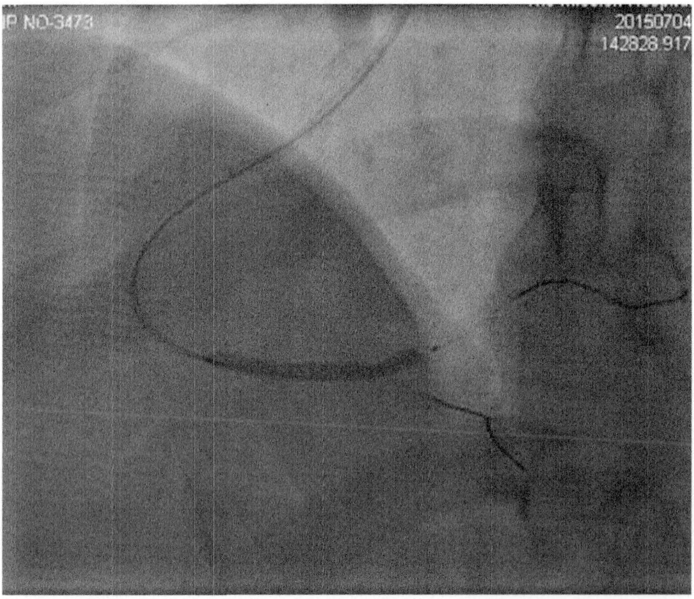

Figure 15.1k First stent is deployed distally (*Courtesy Dr Sanjay Chugh*).

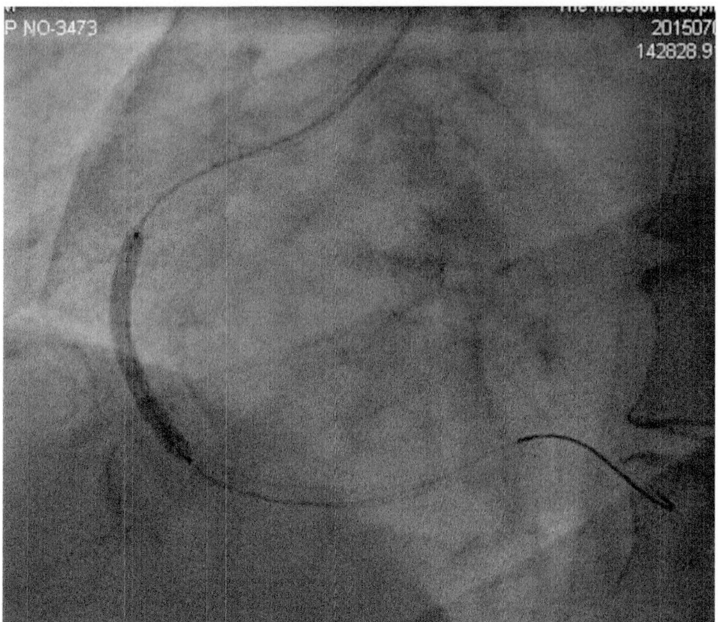

Figure 15.1l Second stent is deployed (*Courtesy Dr Sanjay Chugh*).

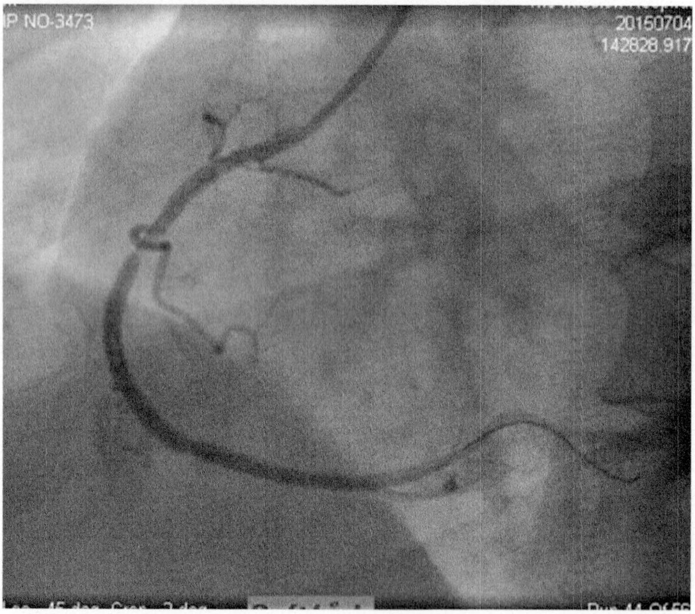

Figure 15.1m Post stenting angiogram shows a gap between the two stents (*Courtesy Dr Sanjay Chugh*).

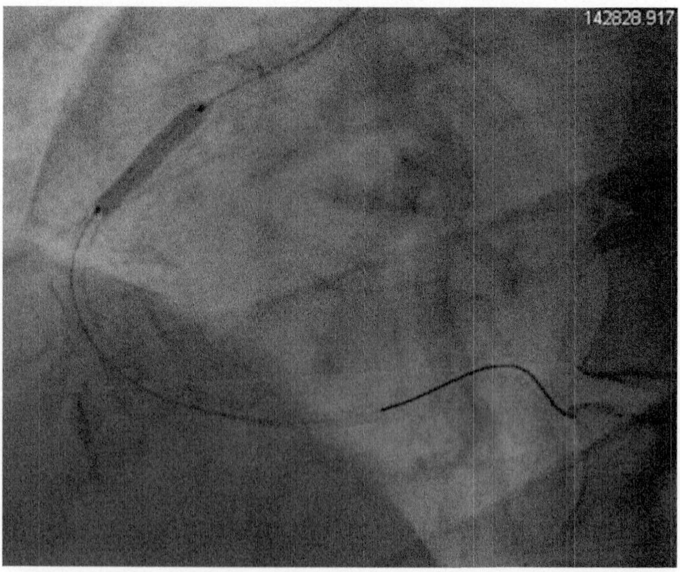

Figure 15.1n Third stent is deployed in proximal RCA (*Courtesy Dr Sanjay Chugh*).

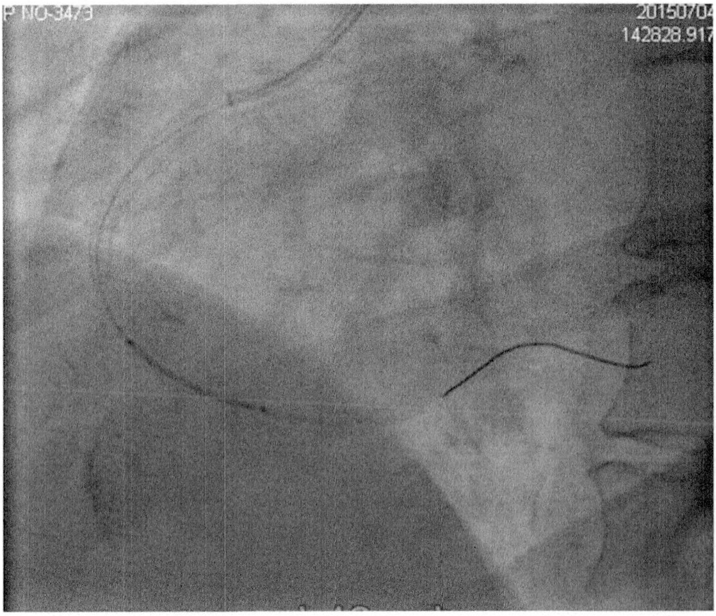

Figure 15.1o Fourth stent is deployed in gap between first and second stents (*Courtesy Dr Sanjay Chugh*).

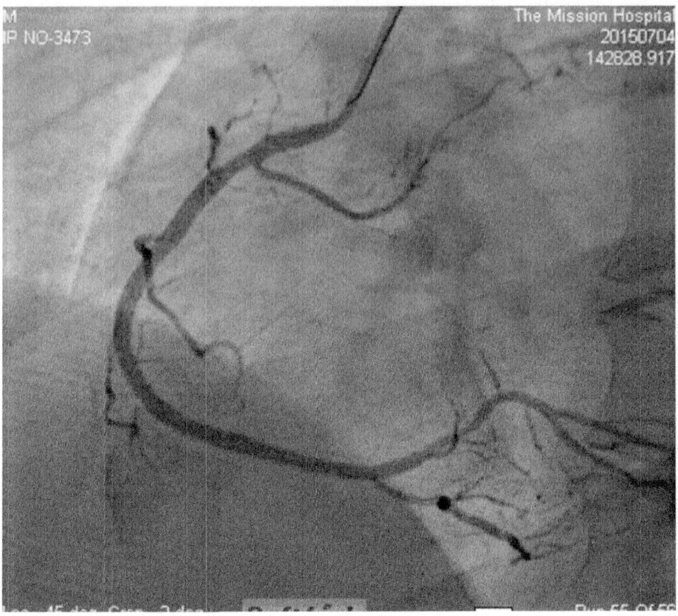

Figure 15.1p Final angiogram after post-dilatation shows TIMI-3 flow (*Courtesy Dr Sanjay Chugh*).

3. Dual Injection/Hybrid Approach

Once such techniques fail then additional femoral or radial access is taken and dual injection is performed.[22]

4. Complex Antegrade Techniques

Complex antegrade techniques, are used by experienced operators transradially. when the usual techniques are unsuccessful. IVUS guided CTO PCI can be used if the initial guidewire fails to cross the CTO and causes a sub-intimal dissection. Generally, these techniques need more guide support and must be attempted by expert operators. Additional methods like balloon trapping and sub-intimal tracking and re-entry (STAR) may be required.

Retrograde Approach

Transradial approach is used by experienced transradial CTO operators for retrograde crossing of CTO. Rinfret et al. have successfully shown retrograde recanalization of CTO through transradial route.[22] The retrograde approach[22] is attempted with a soft polymer-jacketed guidewire (Pilot 50, Fielder FC or more rarely Fielder XTR). While there is scanty data on attempting retrograde PCI transradially, Rinfret et al[23]. could use the radial access to cross in 83% patients and success overall in 88%. This excellent success rate however was counterbalanced by a 15% rate of wire perforations.

Safety

Access-site complications are significantly higher in TFA versus TRI (11.3% versus 3.5%); while early major adverse cardiac events (MACE) rates[24] as well as contrast volume, procedure time and radiation dose were all similar in transradial CTO PCI compared to transfemoral approach.[25] The FORT CTO study also reported radial access to be non-inferior to femoral access, with lower access-site complications.

Summary of Suggested Recommendations for Procedural Aspects of TRI for CTO PCI

- Operators with annual experience of at least 50 transradial PCI and 15 CTO PCI may undertake trans-radial CTO PCI.
- In patients with suitable anatomy for TRI and severe peripheral vascular disease (PVD) where TFA is not possible TRI CTO PCI should be default approach.
- Antegrade escalation is the default first approach to be used in transradial CTO PCI.
- Tapered tip polymer wire to engage micro-channels is the first wire to be tried.
- Trans radial CTO PCI should be attempted in selected patients with favourable characteristics like tapered tip CTOs, JCTO score less than 3, short segment (<20 mm), no proximal cap ambiguity, especially where 7F can be used.
- After ante grade escalation fails hybrid approach should be used.

Caution should be Exercised in the Following Subsets of Patients while Attempting TRI CTO

- Complex methods like balloon trapping, sub-intimal dissection, and re-entry through transradial approach, hybrid approach
- Transradial CTO PCI should not be attempted in those patients with CKD stage 3 and above who may need an AV fistula in the arm in future
- Retrograde CTO should not be attempted transradially.
- If extremely complex methods are to be attempted, they should be performed by expert operators (more than 1000 PCIs in total and more than 100 TRI CTO PCI) after due counselling to the patient explaining risks and benefits in a centre with cardiac surgery back-up.

Transradial Approach for Post-CABG Patients

With increasing popularity of radial PCI overall there has been a recent interest in radial PCI post-CABG patients. At least 10% of PCIs are performed in post-graft patients. Patients with previous CABG have multi-vessel coronary artery disease and may have associated diffuse atherosclerosis involving different vascular territories, such as the iliac and femoral arteries, therefore, RA could be an effective strategy to reduce access-site complications in this setting.[26] On the other hand, radial artery access could entail longer procedure times, for those with less experience, and is technically more demanding. There is limited data on post-CABG trans-radial PCI. Current review is an endeavour to review the available evidence and define best practices.

Access site selection *(please refer to Table 15.1 for abbreviations)*:

Left radial is a more optimal approach so that left internal mammary artery graft (LIMA) can be cannulated. For saphenous venous graft (SVG) PCI 7F guides are more advisable if use of embolic protection device is contemplated. If stable guide cannulation cannot be achieved then crossover to femoral route may have to be done. On an average cross over rate was found to be around 4.7%. The vascular site access complication rates were 2.3% for RA route and femoral route is 5.8%.[27]

Right RA is preferred for native PCI in post-CABG patients and right internal mammary artery graft (RIMA) intervention. Although better as far as access site complications are concerned, radial PCI is associated with greater contrast volume, procedure time and radiation exposure to operator.[28]

Guide catheter selection[26] *(please refer to Table 15.1* for abbreviations*)*:

- SVG: For SVG on right side of ascending aorta, right radial access with MPA or JR are better used to cannulate. On the contrary, for grafts arising from left side or anteriorly from the aorta left radial route provides easy access and Amplatz left and sometimes even Judkins left can help in cannulation with good backup[27] (Figure 15.2(a) shows an angiogram of SVG to right coronary artery (RCA), using an Amplatz right (AR2) catheter from left radial artery (LRA), showing a critical stenosis.
- LIMA grafts: IMA or modified IMA are preferred; though, JR 3.5 or JR 4 guide catheter can be used. Please see Chapter 10 'Tips and Tricks for Transradial Interventions: Under TRI in Post-bypass Grafts' (Figures 15.2e (1–3)) Experienced operators can not only hook all coronary bypass grafts, except RIMA, easily and quickly; graft angioplasty can also be done in most cases via left radial access (Figures 15.2a–c).

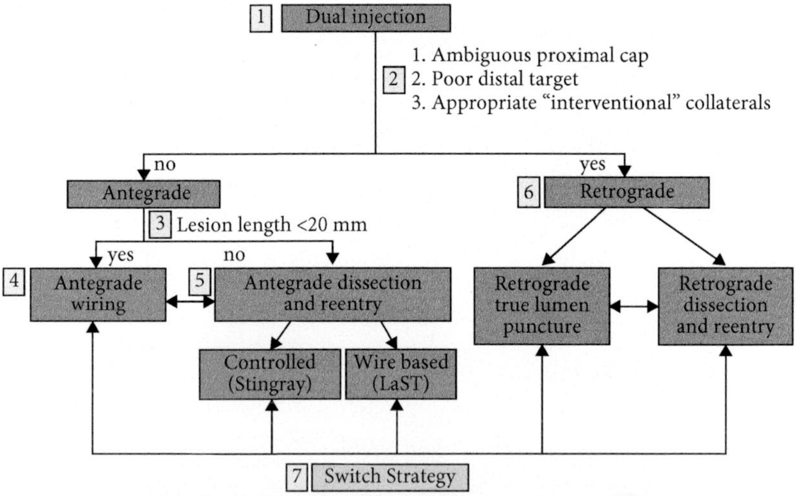

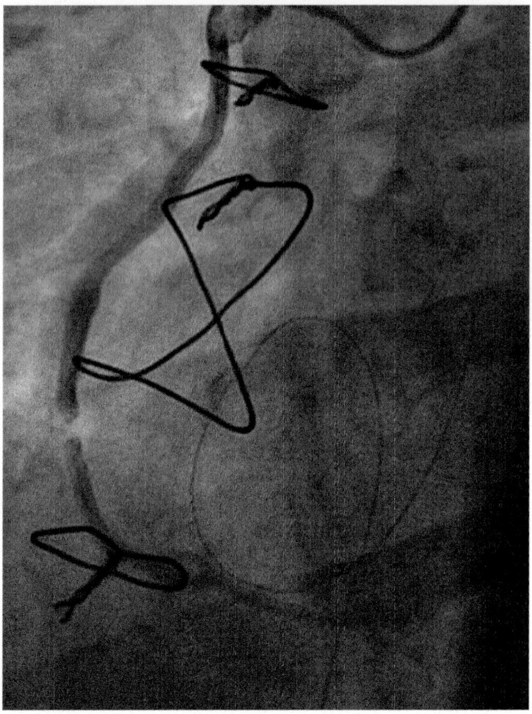

Figure 15.2a Angiogram of SVG to right coronary artery (RCA) using an Amplatz right (AR2) catheter from left radial artery (LRA) shows a critical stenosis. (Courtesy Dr Sanjay Chugh)

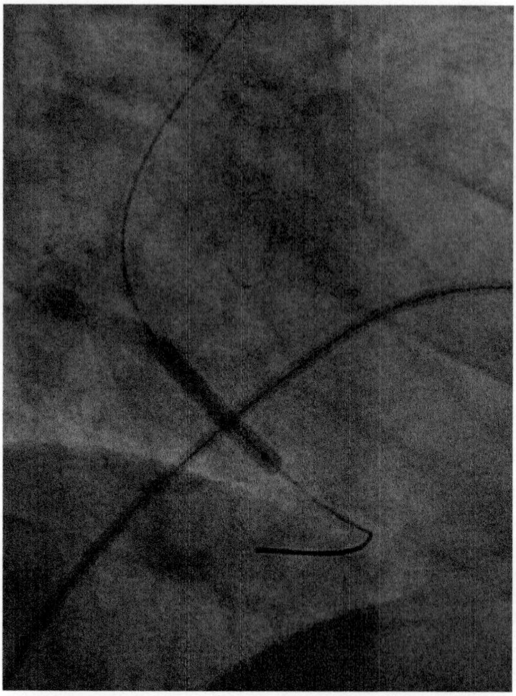

Figure 15.2b Direct stenting of the lesion using an AL1 Guide catheter via left radial access. A transvenous temporary pacemaker lead is inserted in the right ventricle for complete heart block (*Courtesy Dr Sanjay Chugh*).

- For RIMA grafts, as the takeoff is at 90-degree angle to Rt. subclavian artery: over the wire cannulation with IMA guide is more advisable.
- Native vessels: Usual guides used and decided by operator.
- SVG PCI: Is feasible transradially; sometimes there is need for 7F access for distal embolic protection device. Some failures are reported by inexperienced operators because of poor guide support.[29]

Spider filter™ embolic protection device can be used with 6F and using left radial access, SVG PCI can be performed safely with experience. For further case illustrations please see Figures 10.2c (i–ix) and 10.2d in Chapter 10, 'Tips and Tricks for Transradial Interventions: Under TRI in Post-bypass Grafts'.

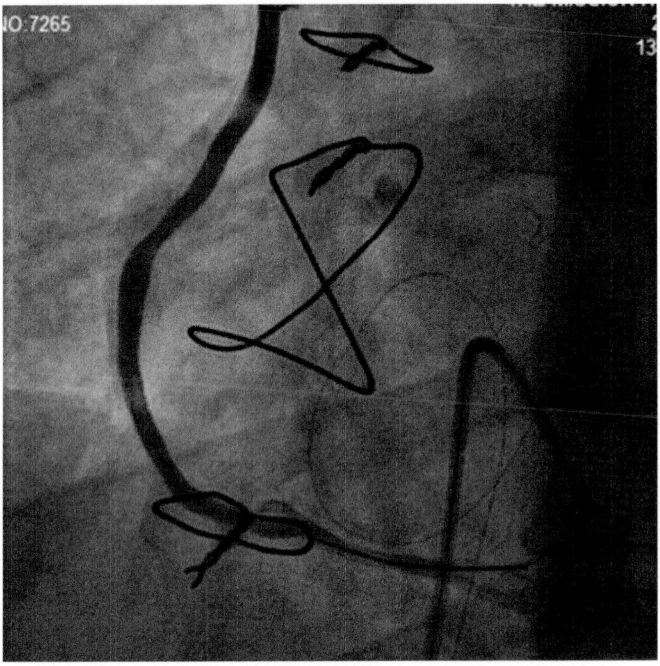

Figure 15.2c Final TIMI 3 flow (*Courtesy Dr Sanjay Chugh*).

Lesions Subsets to Avoid

TRA should not be used in post-graft CTOs and radial bypass grafts. In patients presenting with ACS when previous grafts are not known and those having radial bypass grafts. While bilateral IMA grafts may be attempted bi-radially or transfemorally; Operator experience and comfort should guide the choice of access route in patients with ACS, when details of previous grafts are not known.

Suggested Recommendations for Post-CABG TRI

- In patients with severe PVD or severe aortic disease where TFA is not possible TRA post CABG should be default approach.
- Left radial to be used for LIMA and SVG interventions.

Table 15.1 ACCESS site selection based on grafts to be intervened upon[26]

Pattern of coronary grafting	Suggested primary approach	Comments	Alternative approach
LIMA	Left Radial	Documented faciliation compared to femoral approach	
LIMA + RIMA	Right and left Radial or Femoral	Avoid to attempt contralateral radial cannulation in the presence of severe atherosclerosis of the Arotic arch and subclavian arteries	Right Radial and combined Left Radial if necessary (discuss with the patient its preference for post-catheterization course: double forearm compression versus single femoral)
LIMA + RIMA + RA	Femoral		
LIMA + SVG(s)	Left Radial	Consider aortography to obtan SVG visualization and to facilitate proper catheter selection	
SVG(s)	Right Radial or Left Radial	Left radial probably easier, advisable during the learning curve	
Any graft combination + GEA	Femoral		

LIMA = left internal mammary artery; RIMA = right internal mammary artery; SVG = saphenous vein graft; GEA = right gastroepiploic artery.

- TRI can be performed in native artery interventions in post-CABG patients.
- Transradial to be used with caution in post-CABG patients presenting with ACS, and Transradial interventions for CTOs in post-CABG patients.

Conclusion

In conclusion, as a stock analyst, trans-radial CABG PCI could be given a 'buy' recommendation as a 'long-term investment'. To increase the proportion of radial PCI in CABG, we will require additional operator proficiency, new equipment, and unequivocal confirmation about equipoise when it comes to radiation dose, contrast use, and procedure time. Continued growth of CTO PCI along with improvement in femoral access may well leave this a niche PCI procedure in a 50/50 radial/femoral zone; however, use of TRI in post-CABG grafts and CTO is increasing with experience.

References

1. L Campeau, "Percutaneous radial artery approach for coronary angiography," *Cathet Cardiovascular Diagn*, vol. *16*, no. 1, pp. 3–7, 1989.
2. Ferdinand Kiemenji and Gert Jan Laarman, "Percutaneous transradial artery approach for coronary stent implantation," *Cath and Cardiovas Diagn*, vol. *30*, no. 1, pp. 173–78, 1993.
3. I Bernat, D Horak, and J Stasek, "ST-segment myocardial infarction treated by radial or femoral approach in a multicenter randomized clinical trial," *J Am Coll Cardiol*, vol. *63*, no. 1, pp. 964–72, 2014.
4. SS Jolly, Y Salim, and J Cairns, "Radial versus femoral access for coronary angiography and intervention in patients with acute coronary syndromes (RIVAL): a randomized clinical trial," *Lancet*, vol. *377*, no. 1, pp. 1409–20, 2011.
5. E Ramagnoli, G Biondi-Zoccai, and A Sciahbasi, et al. "Radial versus femoral randomized investigation in ST-segment elevation acute coronary syndrome: the RIFLE-STEACS study," *J Am Coll Cardiol*, vol. *60*, no. 1, pp. 2481–9, 2012.
6. W Karrowni, A Vyas, and B Giaconimo, "Radial versus femoralaccess for primary percutaneous interventions in ST-segment elevation myocardial infarction patients: a meta-analysis of randomized controlled trials," *J Am Coll Cardiol Intv*, vol. *6*, no. 1, pp. 814–23, 2013.
7. B Ibanez, S James, and S Agewall, "2017 ESC Guidelines for the management of acute myocardial infarction in patients presenting with ST-segment elevation: the Task Force for the management of acute myocardial infarction in patients presenting with ST-segment elevation of the European Society," *European Heart Journal*, vol. 39, no. 2, pp. 119–77, 2017.
8. SV Rao, J Tremmet, IC Gilchrist, et al. "Best practices for transradial angiography and interventions: a consensus statement from the society for cardiovascular angiography and intervention's transradial working group," *Catherter Cardiovasc Interv*, vol. *83*, pp. 228–36, 2014.

9. Y Morino, M. Abe, T Morimoto, et al. "Predicting successful guidewire crossing through chronic total occlusion," *J Am Coll Cardiol Intv*, vol. *4*, no. 2, pp. 214–20, 2011.
10. Tanaka Y, Moriyama N, and Ochiai T, "Transradial coronary interventions for complex chronic total occlusions," *J Am Coll Cardiol Intv*, vol. *10*, no. 3, pp. 235–43, 2017.
11. S Beniwal, K Bhargava, and S. Kaushik, "Size of distal radial and distal ulnar arteries in adults," *Indian Heart J*, vol. *66*, no. 1, pp. 506–09, 2014.
12. Chugh SK, Chugh S, Chugh Y, and Rao SV, "Feasibility and utility of pre-procedure ultrasound imaging of the arm to facilitate transradial coronary diagnostic and interventional procedures (PRIMAFACIE-TRI)," *Catheter Cardiovasc Interv*, vol. *82*, no. 1, pp. 64–73, 2013.
13. Saito S, Tanaka S, Hiroe Y, and Miyashita Y, "Usefulness of hydrophilic coating on arterial sheath introducer in transradial coronary intervention," *Catheter Cardiovasc Interv*, vol. *56*, no. 1, pp. 328–32, 2002.
14. Saito S, Hajimei I, and Hosokawa G, "Influence of the ratio between radial artery inner diameter and sheath outer diameter on radial artery flow after transradial coronary intervention," *Catheter Cardiovasc Interv*, vol. *46*, no. 1, pp. 173–78, 1999.
15. R Dautov and Barbosa Ribero H, "Effectiveness and safety of the transradial 8 French sheathless approach for revascularization of chronic total occlusions," *Am J of Cardiology*, vol. *118*, no. 6, pp. 785–89, 2016.
16. J Rosencher, A Chaib, and F Barbou. How to limit radial artery spasm during percutaneous coronary interventions: the spasmolytic agents to avoid spasm during transradial percutaneous coronary interventions (SPASM3) study. *Catheter Cardiovasc Interv*, vol. *84*, no. 5, pp. 766–71, 2014.
17. J Coppola, T Patel, and T Kwan, "Nitroglycerin, nitroprusside, or both, in preventing radial artery spasm during transradial artery catheterization," *J Invasive Cardiol*, vol. *18*, no. 4, pp. 155–58, 2006.
18. SH Kim, EJ Kim, and W Cheon, "Comparative study of nikorandil and a sposmolytic cocktail during tansradial coronary angiography," *Int J Cardiol*, vol. *120*, no. 1, pp. 325–30, 2007.
19. M Valimigli, E Frigoli, and S Leonardi, "Bivalirudin or unfractionated heparin in acute coronary syndromes," *N Engl J Med*, vol. *373*, no. 1, pp. 997–1009, 2015.
20. D Erlinje, E Omerovic, O Frobert, et al. "Bivalirudin versus heparin monotherapy in myocardial infarction," *N Engl J Med*, vol. *377*, no. 1, pp. 1132–42, 2017.
21. MC Lim, "Antegrade techniques for chronic total occlusion," *Curr Cardiol Reviews*, vol. *11*, no. 1, pp. 285–90, 2015.
22. ES Brilakis, JA Grantam, S Rinfret, et al., "A percutaneous treatment algorithm for crossing coronary chronic total occlusions," *J Am Coll Cardiol Intv*, vol. *5*, no. 4, pp. 367–79, 2012.
23. S Rinfret, D Joyal, and GM Nguyen, "Retrograde recanalization of chronic total occlusions from the transradial approach; early Canadian experience," *Catheter Cardiovasc Interv*, vol. *78*, no. 1, pp. 366–74, 2011.
24. S Rathore, A Hakeem, and M Pauriah, A comparison of the transradial and the transfemoral approach in chronic total occlusion percutaneous coronary intervention. *Catheter Cardiovasc Interv*, vol. *73*, pp. 883–87, 2009.

25. F Burzotta, M Vita, and T Lefvre, "Radial approach for percutaneous coronary interventions in chronic total occlusions: technical issues and data review," *Catheter Cardiovasc Interv*, vol. *01*, no. 01, pp. 1–11, 2013.
26. T Kinnaird, R Andersen, and S Gallaghar, "Transradial access site and outcomes in 58,870 patients undergoing percutaneous coronary intervention with a previous history of coronary bypass surgery," *J Am Coll Cardiol*, vol. *11*, no. 5, pp. 482–91, 2018.
27. S Rigattiri, A Schiabasi, and EL Brilakis, "Meta-analysis of radial versus femoral artery approach for coronary procedures in patients with previous coronary artery bypass grafting," *Am J Cardiol*, vol. *117*, no. 8, pp. 1248–55, 2016.
28. F Burzotto, C Trani, M Hammon, et al., "Transradial approach for coronary angiography and interventions in patients with coronary bypass grafts: tips and tricks," *Catheter Cardiovasc Interv*, vol. *72*, no. 1, pp. 263–72, 2008.
29. Bundhoo SS, Earp E, and Ivanauskiene T, "Saphenous vein graft percutaneous coronary intervention via radial artery access: safe and effective with reduced hospital length of stay," *Am Heart J*, vol. *164*, no. 4, pp. 468–72, 2012.

16

Transradial Intravascular Ultrasound (IVUS) and Optical Coherence Tomography (OCT)

B. Dixit, M. A. Azeez Asad, and P. C. Rath

Introduction

Even after decades of its introduction, coronary angiography is the most frequently utilized imaging approach for both diagnosing coronary artery disease (CAD) and for guiding coronary interventions.[1] Currently, intravascular ultrasound (IVUS) is emerging as the preferred intracoronary imaging modality to guide interventional procedures. One of the primary limitations of IVUS is low spatial resolution.[2] Optical coherence tomography (OCT) is an optical counterpart of IVUS that utilizes infrared light to look inside the coronary arteries with 10-fold superior resolution compared to IVUS. This technology appears to have higher sensitivity and specificity for classifying the various forms of atherosclerotic plaques.[3,4]

Transradial access has increasingly become the preferred approach for percutaneous coronary intervention (PCI) due to a shorter recovery time, diminished bleeding risk, and lack of severe access-site complications. With continued innovation and production of improved guiding catheters, through 6F or 7F sheath (Please refer to Table 7.3, page 87, Chapter 7, for requisite Guide catheter sizes), the TR approach is a reasonable alternative to transfemoral access for PCI and other adjunctive diagnostic strategies, such as IVUS and OCT of complex coronary anatomy.

IVUS Imaging Technology

IVUS uses high-frequency ultrasound to envisage the coronary arteries to a depth of 10 mm with a resolution of 100–150 μm.[5] Two kinds of IVUS systems available for clinical use include 'a mechanical single-element rotating transducer' and 'the solid-state electronic phased array transducer'.[5]

IVUS Image Interpretation

The comparative echolucency of the media vis-à-vis the intima and adventitia produces a trilaminar three-layered 'Bright–Dark–Bright appearance' (Figure 16.1).

Applications of IVUS—Current Practices

The evidence for IVUS in coronary imaging comes from prospective as well as retrospective studies showing potential clinical benefit to patients.[5] IVUS gives additional information over conventional angiography concerning lumen and arterial dimensions, plaque type and distribution, and vascular remodelling.[6] By the most recent American

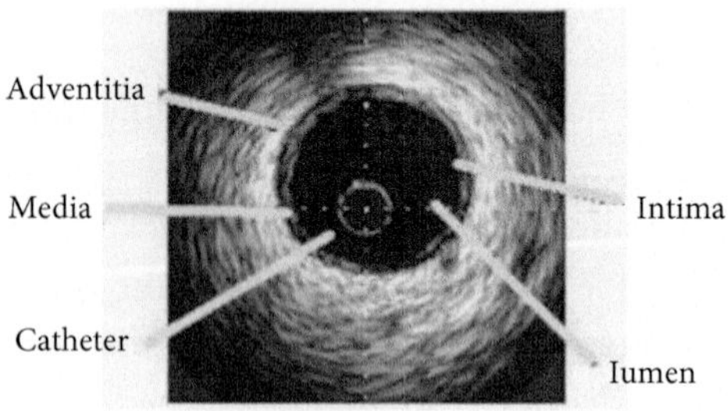

Figure 16.1 IVUS image depicting the trilaminar appearance of wall of normal coronary artery.[42]

Table 16.1 ACC/AHA Guidelines for Use of IVUS[7]

Recommendations	Class of Recommendation	Level of Evidence
IVUS for assessment of 'angiographically indeterminate' left main coronary artery disease	II a	B
IVUS for the assessment of other (non-left main) 'angiographically intermediate' stenoses	II b	B
IVUS to determine the mechanism of in-stent restenosis	II a	C
IVUS for the mechanism of stent thrombosis	II b	C
IVUS post cardiac transplantation (vasculopathy)	II a	B
IVUS for coronary stent implantation guidance	II b	B
IVUS for routine lesion assessment and revascularization is not planned	III—No Benefit	C

College of Cardiology/American Heart Association (ACC/AHA) guidelines, IVUS can be utilized to assess intermediate lesions, mechanism and reason behind in-stent re-stenosis and stent thrombosis, allograft vasculopathy, and for guidance of intracoronary stent implantation (Table 16.1).[7]

IVUS in Angiographic Non-left Main Intermediate Lesions

Lesion severity can be assessed more accurately by IVUS than angiography, but this role has been largely supplanted by fractional flow reserve (FFR).[8] Majority of the intermediate lesions involving non left main coronary arteries with a mean luminal area (MLA) $\geq 4.0\ mm^2$ are functionally not significant and may be left alone.[9–11] For MLA < $4.0\ mm^2$, functional assessment with FFR is advised. If functional assessment is not feasible, such lesions tend to be haemodynamically significant in vessels with larger reference diameter and IVUS obtained percentage area stenosis more than 60%, more than 80% plaque burden, and more than 20 mm lesion length.[12]

IVUS in Angiographic Left Main Intermediate Lesions

For assessment of intermediate left main coronary artery lesions, FFR again is the favoured procedure. Nonetheless, if IVUS obtained left main coronary artery MLA is more than or equal to 6.0 mm^2, intervention may be safely deferred in these patients. MLA $\geq$ 6.0 mm^2 is not functionally related with ischaemia. These patients tend to have better outcomes. If the MLA < 6.0 mm^2, one should strongly consider FFR or noninvasive stress testing before intervention.[13–16]

IVUS for PCI

The most important role of IVUS is in planning, preparing, and optimizing PCI strategy. Pre-intervention IVUS is used for precise measurements of the reference luminal dimensions as well as lesion length for exact stent diameter and length. If IVUS shows more than 180–270° calcium deposition, the patient may require debulking strategies like cutting balloons or rotational atherectomy.[17] Post PCI evaluation is used to detect complications of intervention like dissection and malapposed or underexpanded stents. Side branch assessment can also be done with IVUS. If side branch MLA is ≥2.4 mm^2, side branch PCI is usually not necessary. On the other hand, if the MLA of the side branch is smaller than that, FFR of the side branch, along with clinical judgement, maybe useful.[18]

In patients with stent re-stenosis, IVUS helps in understanding the mechanism behind it, whether it is related to intimal hyperplasia or due to mechanical complications like stent underexpansion, malapposition, or stent fracture.

In PCI of chronic total occlusions, with antegrade approach, IVUS can be utilized to guide re-entry of the wire from the false lumen towards the true lumen.[19]

OCT—Imaging Technology

OCT is an intra-coronary imaging technology analogous to IVUS; it however uses infrared light, with wavelengths around 1,300 nm, in place of ultrasound. Images are produced by quantifying the magnitude and echo time delay of a reflected backscattered light signal.[20] The emitted light source is split by an interferometer into reference and sample beams.[20,21] OCT needs a blood-free space; blood scatters light and disrupts the images. The study artery is made free of blood for a few seconds, by intracoronary injection of saline or preferably contrast.[22]

OCT Imaging Interpretation

Among the available intravascular imaging modalities, OCT gives us distinctively detailed images of superficial coronary plaque components (Figure 16.2). Based on histological analysis of autopsy specimens, there are three general plaque types: fibrous plaque, fibro-calcific plaque, and lipid rich plaque. Lipid-laden plaque is identified by low-intensity, irregular signal having indistinct and uneven borders. Fibrous plaque is identified by high-intensity signals that are homogeneous (Figure 16.2A). Calcified plaque (Figure 16.2B) appears as low-intensity heterogenous signals with sharp borders and 'textured' appearances.

TCFA, or thin-cap fibroatheroma, is defined as a homogenous region in the vessel wall with a low refractive index, separated from the lumen by a thin capsule (less than 65 μm) having a high refractive index.

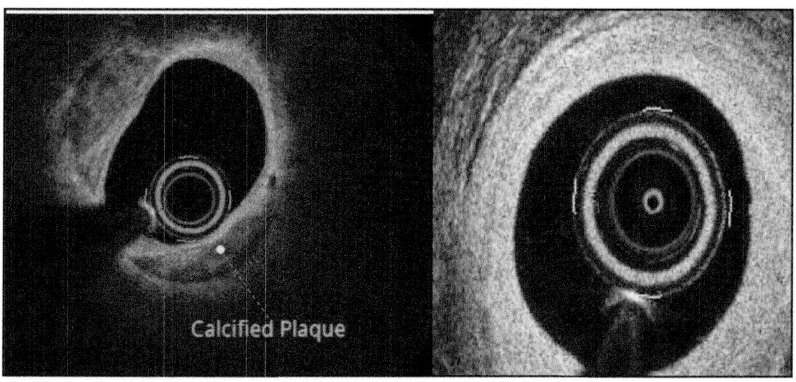

Figure 16.2 Plaque types on OCT: (A) calcified plaque; (B) fibrous plaque.

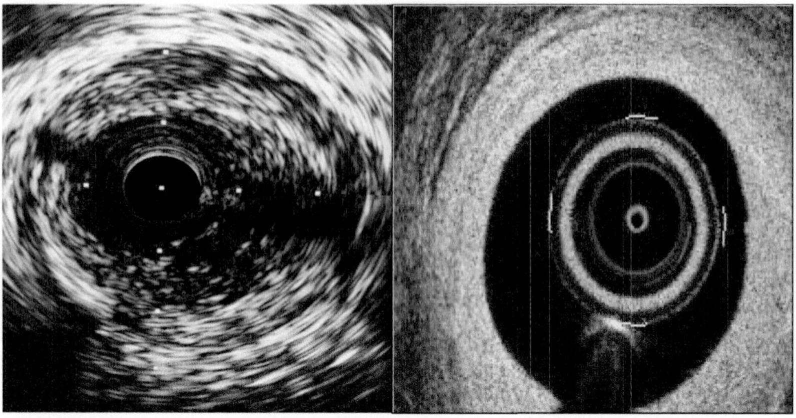

Figure 16.2A Fibrous plaque—IVUS and OCT.

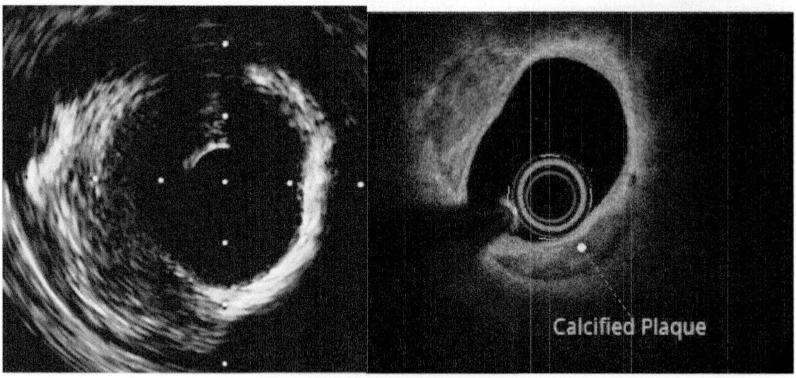

Figure 16.2B Calcified plaque—IVUS and OCT.

Identification of Thrombus by OCT

OCT is helpful to not just identify thrombus but also differentiate between red and white thrombus. This has been established histopathologically by various studies.[23] OCT has higher sensitivity than IVUS to detect thrombus.[24,25] Thrombus on OCT is identified by a protrusion into the vessel lumen, with attenuated signal. White thrombus is platelet-rich and has low backscatter. Red thrombus is platelet-poor and has high-backscattering projections into the vessel lumen, with signal-free shadowing (Figure 16.3).[26]

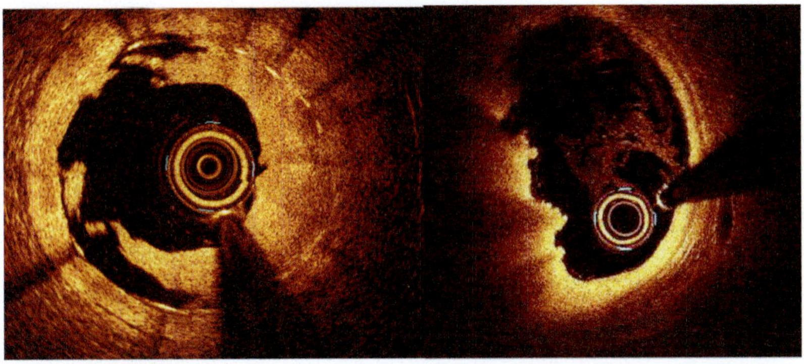

Figure 16.3 White thrombus and red thrombus on OCT.

Table 16.2 Comparison of IVUS and OCT—IMAGE Acquisition Technique[43]

	OCT	IVUS
Resolution (Axial)	12–15 μm	100–200 μm
Beam Width	20–40 mm	200–300 mm
Frames per second	100 frames per second	30 frames per second
Pullback Speed	20 mm per second	0.5–1 mm per second
Maximum Scan Diameter in mm	10	15
Tissue Penetration in mm	1.0–2.0	10
Lateral Sampling in mm	19	225
Blood Clearing	Required	Not necessary

Detection of Vulnerable Plaque—From IVUS to OCT

IVUS findings suggest that coronary vessels increase in size in relation to plaque area. Functionally significant luminal stenosis does not appear until at least 40% of the internal elastic lamina area is occupied by the lesion.[27] A direct relationship was observed between markers of atherosclerosis seen on IVUS, and cardiovascular events.[28,29] The PROSPECT study was a large multi-centric study that showed a significant association between non-culprit artery plaque characteristics defined by IVUS and future coronary events.[30,31] With OCT, we have

Table 16.3 Advantages and Disadvantages of OCT and IVUS[44]

Relative advantage/ disadvantage	OCT	IVUS
Resolution	Excellent Resolution	Poor resolution
Penetration	Low tissue penetration	High tissue penetration
Visualization (Please see Figures 16.4 to 16.6)	Good visualization of metal and polymer stents, strut coverage, and apposition	Can't differentiate thin neointima, or small dissections or malappositions
	Good imaging of lipid, calcium, fibre, thrombus	Good imaging of fibre, calcium; Poor for thrombus, lipids
Biovascular scaffold (Please see Figure 16.7)	Better for BVS struts	
Plaque burden measurement	Not very good	Excellent for plaque burden
Contrast load	Adds contrast load 10–15 ml per run	No contrast necessary

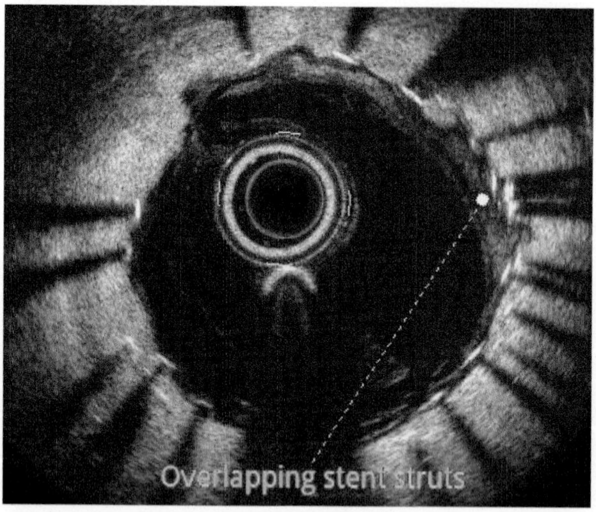

Figure 16.4 Post stent implantation—Overlapping stents—OCT.

better delineation of thin fibrous caps. These along with full circumferential extension of the necrotic cores are markers of vulnerable plaques (Figure 16.8).[32]

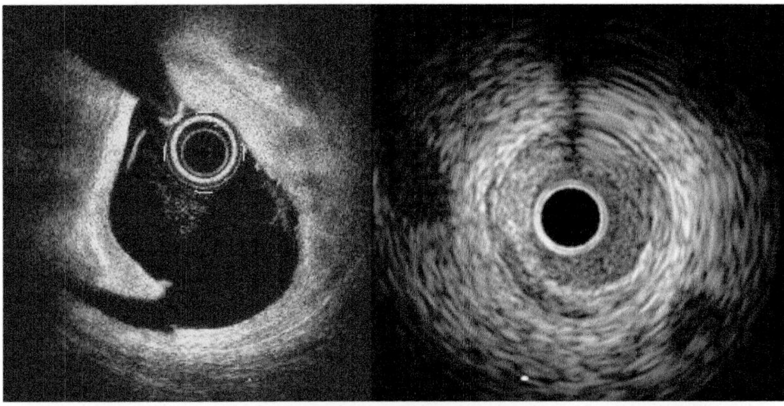

Figure 16.5 Edge dissection during stent implantation—OCT vs. IVUS.

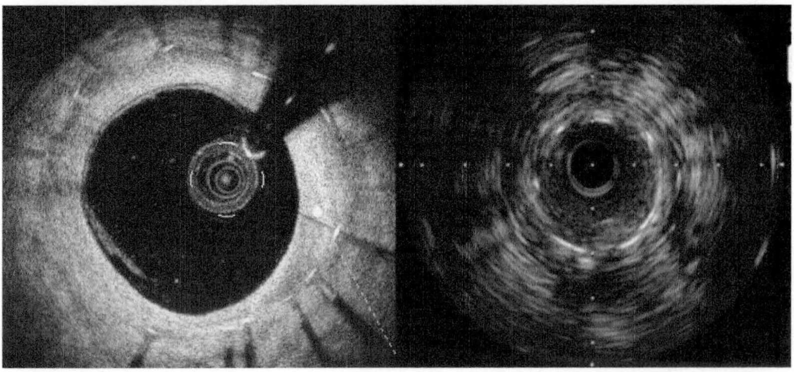

Figure 16.6 In-stent restenosis—OCT vs. IVUS.

OCT in PCI

OCT can be utilized to measure the exact reference vessel dimensions, plus minimal luminal diameter of the lesion and lesion length. OCT is probably more precise when compared to IVUS for assessing intermediate lesions, although it is unlikely to replace FFR.[33] Pre-PCI assessment of lesion, for instance, lipid and calcium content, presence of dissection or thrombus can predict myocardial infarction after the PCI.[34] Post-intervention, OCT can be used to identify stent malapposition, tissue prolapse, and edge dissection with higher sensitivity than IVUS.[35–37] OCT is of specific benefit in visualizing stent apposition when there are overlapping metallic stents

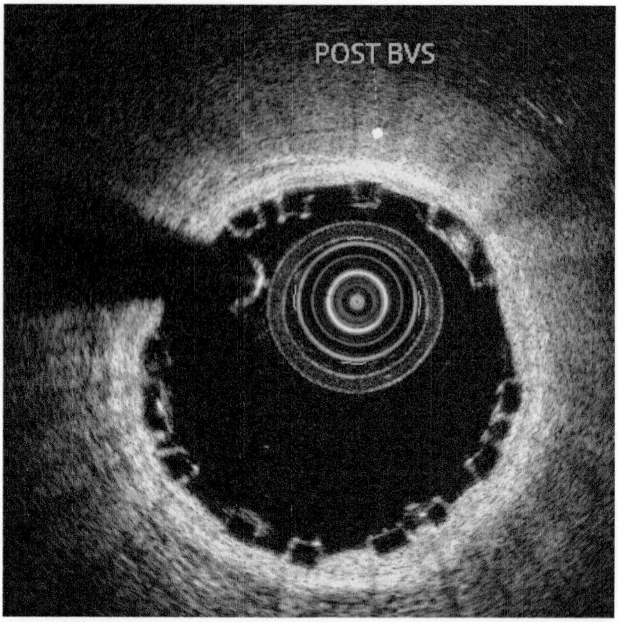

Figure 16.7 OCT of BVS.

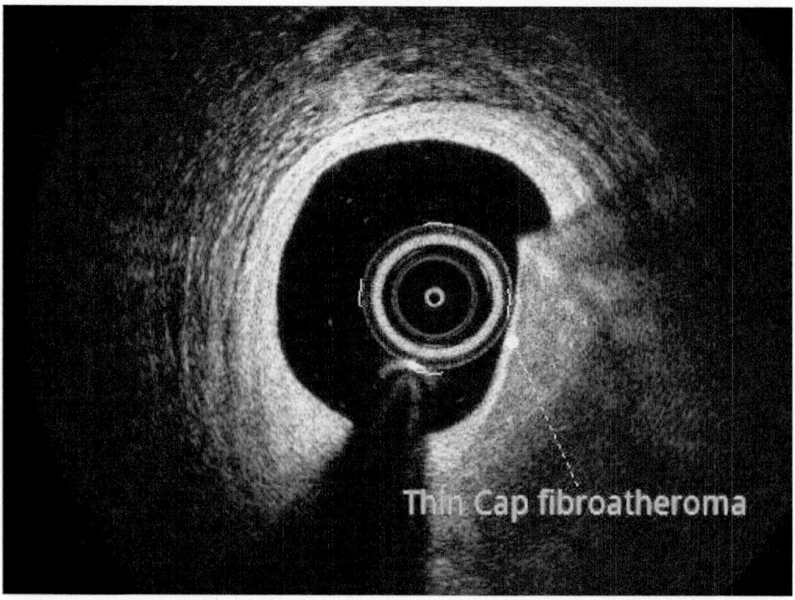

Figure 16.8 Thin cap Fibro atheroma.

(Figure 16.6).[37,38]. A dissection flap is seen as a linear rim of tissue that is clearly away from the vessel wall (Figure 16.8).[38–41] In some studies, stent strut malapposition appears to correlate with poor endothelization of the stent and may be a risk factor for late stent thrombosis.

In-stent restenosis (Figure 16.6) can be picked up easily on imaging by IVUS and OCT; however OCT is better than IVUS to identify a Biovascular scaffold (BVS) (Figure 16.7) as its struts look distinctly different from that of a conventional stent on OCT.

Conclusion

IVUS and OCT as intracoronary imaging tools can be done safely and accurately through the radial route and provide similar wealth of information as an alternative to transfemoral route, but with shorter recovery time, diminished bleeding risk, and lack of severe access-site complications.

References

1. Garrone P, Biondi-Zoccai G, Salvetti I, Sina N, Sheiban I, Stella PR, Agostoni P. Quantitative coronary angiography in the current era: principles and applications. *J Interv Cardiol.* 2009;22:527–36.
2. Mintz GS, Nissen SE, Anderson WD, Bailey SR, Erbel R, Fitzgerald PJ, Rosenfield K, Siegel RJ, Tuzcu EM, Yock PG. ACC Clinical Expert Consensus Document on standards for the acquisition, measurement and reporting of intravascular ultrasound studies: a report of the ACC Task Force on Clinical Expert Consensus Documents. *J Am Coll Cardiol.* 2001;37:1478–92.
3. Jang IK, Tearney GJ, MacNeill B, et al. In vivo characterization of coronary atherosclerotic plaque by use of optical coherence tomography. *Circulation.* 2005; 111:1551–5.
4. Yabusita H, Bouma BE, Houser SL, et al. Characterization of human atherosclerosis by optical coherence tomography. *Circulation.* 2002; 106:1640–5.
5. McDaniel MC, Eshtehardi P, Sawaya FJ, Douglas JS Jr., Samady H. Contemporary clinical applications of coronary intravascular ultrasound. *JACC Cardiovasc Interv.* 2011;4:1155–67.
6. Stone GW, Maehara A, Lansky AJ, et al. A prospective natural-history study of coronary atherosclerosis. *N Engl J Med.* 2011;364:226–35.

7. Levine GN, Bates ER, Blankenship JC, et al. 2011 ACCF/AHA/SCAI Guideline for Percutaneous Coronary Intervention: executive summary: a report of the American College of Cardiology Foundation/American Heart Association Task Force on Practice Guidelines and the Society for Cardiovascular Angiography and Interventions. *Circulation.* 2011;124:2574–609.
8. Pijls NH, Sels JW. Functional measurement of coronary stenosis. *J Am Coll Cardiol.* 2012;59:1045–57.
9. Kang SJ, Lee JY, Ahn JM, et al. Validation of intravascular ultrasoundderived parameters with fractional flow reserve for assessment of coronary stenosis severity. *Circ Cardiovasc Interv.* 2011;4:65–71.
10. Ben-Dor I, Torguson R, Gaglia MA Jr., et al. Correlation between fractional flow reserve and intravascular ultrasound lumen area in intermediate coronary artery stenosis. *EuroIntervention.* 2011;7:225–33.
11. Lee CH, Tai BC, Soon CY, et al. New set of intravascular ultrasoundderived anatomic criteria for defining functionally significant stenoses in small coronary arteries (results from Intravascular Ultrasound Diagnostic Evaluation of Atherosclerosis in Singapore [IDEAS] study). *Am J Cardiol.* 2010;105:1378–84.
12. Briguori C, Anzuini A, Airoldi F, et al. Intravascular ultrasound criteria for the assessment of the functional significance of intermediate coronary artery stenoses and comparison with fractional flow reserve. *Am J Cardiol.* 2001;87:136–41.
13. Leesar MA, Masden R, Jasti V. Physiological and intravascular ultrasound assessment of an ambiguous left main coronary artery stenosis. *Catheter Cardiovasc Interv.* 2004;62:349–57.
14. Jasti V, Ivan E, Yalamanchili V, Wongpraparut N, Leesar MA. Correlations between fractional flow reserve and intravascular ultrasound in patients with an ambiguous left main coronary artery stenosis. *Circulation.* 2004;110:2831–36.
15. de la Torre Hernandez JM, Herna´ndez Hernandez F, Alfonso F, et al., for the LITRO Study Group. Prospective application of pre-defined intravascular ultrasound criteria for assessment of intermediate left main coronary artery lesions: results from the multicenter LITRO study. *J Am Coll Cardiol.* 2011;58:351–58.
16. Fassa AA, Wagatsuma K, Higano ST, et al. Intravascular ultrasoundguided treatment for angiographically indeterminate left main coronary artery disease: a long-term follow-up study. *J Am Coll Cardiol.* 2005;45:204–11.
17. Smith SC Jr., Feldman TE, Hirshfeld JW Jr., et al. ACC/AHA/SCAI 2005 guideline update for percutaneous coronary intervention—summary article: a report of the American College of Cardiology/American Heart Association Task Force on Practice Guidelines (ACC/AHA/SCAI Writing Committee to Update 2001 Guidelines for Percutaneous Coronary Intervention). *J Am Coll Cardiol.* 2006;47:216–35.
18. Kang SJ, Mintz GS, Kim WJ, et al. Preintervention angiographic and intravascular ultrasound predictors for side branch compromise after a single-stent crossover technique. *Am J Cardiol.* 2011;107:1787–93.
19. Muhammad KI, Lombardi WL, Christofferson R, Whitlow PL. Subintimal guidewire tracking during successful percutaneous therapy for chronic coronary total occlusions: insights from an intravascular ultrasound analysis. Catheter

Cardiovasc Interv. 2012 Jan 12;79(1):43–8. doi: 10.1002/ccd.23139. Epub 2011 Jun 6. PMID: 21542105.

20. Raffel OC, Akasaka T, Jang IK. Cardiac optical coherence tomography. *Heart.* 2008;94:1200–10.
21. Tearney GJ, Waxman S, Shishkov M, et al. Three-dimensional coronary artery microscopy by intracoronary optical frequency domain imaging. *J Am Coll Cardiol Img.* 2008;1:752–61.
22. Barlis P, Schmitt JM. Current and future developments in intracoronary optical coherence tomography imaging. *EuroIntervention.* 2009;4:529–34.
23. Kume T, Akasaka T, Kawamoto T, et al. Assessment of coronary arterial thrombus by optical coherence tomography. *Am J Cardiol.* 2006;97:1713–7.
24. Kubo T, Imanishi T, Takarada S, et al. Assessment of culprit lesion morphology in acute myocardial infarction: ability of optical coherence tomography compared with intravascular ultrasound and coronary angioscopy. *J Am Coll Cardiol.* 2007;50:933–9.
25. Tanimoto T, Imanishi T, Tanaka A, et al. Various types of plaque disruption in culprit coronary artery visualized by optical coherence tomography in a patient with unstable angina. *Circ J.* 2009;73:187–9.
26. Jang I-K, Bouma BE, Kang DH, et al. Visualization of coronary atherosclerotic plaques in patients using optical coherence tomography: comparison with intravascular ultrasound. *J Am Coll Cardiol.* 2002;39:604–9.
27. Glagov S, Weisenberg E, Zarins CK, Stankunavicius R, Olettis GJ. Compensatory enlargement of human atherosclerotic coronary arteries. *N Engl J Med.* 1987;316:1371–75.
28. Narula J, Strauss HW. The popcorn plaques. *Nat Med.* 2007;13 :532–34.
29. Nicholls SJ, Hsu A, Wolski K. Intravascular ultrasound-derived measures of coronary atherosclerotic plaque burden and clinical outcome. *J Am Coll Cardiol.* 2010;55:2399–07.
30. Stone GW, Maehara A, Lansky AJ. PROSPECT investigators a prospective natural-history study of coronary atherosclerosis. *N Engl J Med.* 2011;364:226–35.
31. Calvert PA, Obaid DR, O'Sullivan M. Association between IVUS findings and adverse outcomes in patients with coronary artery disease: the VIVA (VH-IVUS in Vulnerable Atherosclerosis) study. *J Am Coll Cardiol Img.* 2011;4:894–901.
32. Suter MJ, Nadkarni SK, Weisz G, Tanaka A, Bouma BE, Tearney GJ. Intravascular optical imaging technologies for investigating the coronary artery. *J Am Coll Cardiol Img.* 2011;4:1022–39.
33. Gonzalo N, Escaned J, Alfonso F, et al. Morphometric assessment of coronary stenosis relevance with optical coherence tomography: a comparison with fractional flow reserve and intravascular ultrasound. *J Am Coll Cardiol.* 2012;59:1080–89.
34. Yonetsu T, Kakuta T, Lee T, et al. Impact of plaque morphology on creatine kinase-MB elevation in patients with elective stent implantation. *Int J Cardiol.* 2011;146:80–5.

38\. Bouma BE, Tearney GJ, Yabushita H, et al. Evaluation of intracoronary stenting by intravascular optical coherence tomography. *Heart.* 2003;89:317–20.

35\. Jang IK, Tearney G, Bouma B. Visualization of tissue prolapse between coronary stent struts by optical coherence tomography: comparison with intravascular ultrasound. *Circulation.* 2001;104:2754.

36. Tanigawa J, Barlis P, Dimopoulos K, Di Mario C. Optical coherence tomography to assess malapposition in overlapping drug-eluting stents. *EuroIntervention.* 2008;3:580–83.
37. Rath PC, Reddy K, Agarwal MK, Purohit BV, Deb T, Reddy AM Optical coherence tomography guided PCI - initial experience at Apollo Health City, Jubilee Hills, Hyderabad. *Indian Heart J.* 2014;66(1):31–7.
38. Prati F, Regar E, Mintz GS, Arbustini E, Di Mario C, Jang IK, Akasaka T, Costa M, Guagliumi G, Grube E, Ozaki Y, Pinto F, Serruys PW; Expert's OCT Review Document. Expert review document on methodology, terminology, and clinical applications of optical coherence tomography: physical principles, methodology of image acquisition, and clinical application for assessment of coronary arteries and atherosclerosis. *Eur Heart J.* 2010; 31:401–15.
39. Prati F, Guagliumi G, Mintz GS, Costa M, Regar E, Akasaka T, Barlis P, Tearney GJ, Jang IK, Arbustini E, Bezerra HG, Ozaki Y, Bruining N, Dudek D, Radu M, Erglis A, Motreff P, Alfonso F, Toutouzas K, Gonzalo N, Tamburino C, Adriaenssens T, Pinto F, Serruys PW, Di Mario C. for the Expert's OCT Review Document. Expert review document part 2: methodology, terminology and clinical applications of optical coherence tomography for the assessment of interventional proceduresa. *Eur Heart J.* 2012.
40. Gonzalo N, Serruys PW, Okamura T, et al. Optical coherence tomography assessment of the acute effects of stent implantation on the native vessel wall: a systematic quantitative approach. *Heart.* 2009; 95:1913–9.
41. Cook S, Wenaweser P, Togni M, et al. Incomplete stent apposition and very late stent thrombosis after drug-eluting stent implantation. *Circulation.* 2007;115:2426–34.
42. Dash and Daggubati, An Update on Clinical Applications of Intravascular Ultrasound *J Cardiovasc Dis Diagn.* 2015;3:5.
43. Regar E, Ligthart J, Bruining N, van Soest G, The diagnostic value of intracoronary optical coherence tomography. *Herz.* 2011;36:417–29.
44. Koganti S, Kotecha T, Rakhit RD. Choice of intracoronary imaging: when to use intravascular ultrasound or optical coherence tomography. *Interv Cardiol.* 2016;11(1):11–16.

17 (i)
Transradial Access Site Practice and Outcomes in Patients with Acute Coronary Syndromes

Zaid Alirhayim and Mamas A. Mamas

Introduction

Rupture of an atherosclerotic plaque with subsequent intraluminal thrombosis is the usual inciting event in an acute coronary syndrome (ACS), resulting in impaired epicardial blood flow and myocardial perfusion with consequent myocardial ischaemia or infarction.[1] Primary percutaneous coronary intervention (PPCI) is the reperfusion therapy of choice in patients presenting with ST elevation myocardial infarction (STEMI). Similarly, in patients with non-ST elevation myocardial infarction (NSTEMI), an invasive strategy (coronary angiography with an intention to proceed to revascularization) is considered to be one of the mainstays of therapy and has been shown to reduce mortality and rates of re-infarction. To complement the invasive strategy in ACS management, the clinician must also choose appropriate adjunctive antithrombotic drugs in order to optimize angiographic and clinical outcomes. Akin to walking a tightrope, a balance must be struck between efficacy and bleeding risks. Such decisions are often complex and prone to vary greatly between patients and even temporally within the same patient.

Mortality rates after STEMI have improved remarkably over the past two decades, largely due to PPCI and the widespread uptake of medical therapy[2] With the application of nationwide initiatives, patients experiencing a STEMI anywhere in the United States can now expect to receive PPCI reperfusion in less than 90 min.[3] Improvements in the design and drug delivery platforms of contemporary drug eluting stents have resulted in reduced rates of stent thrombosis.[4] Despite these improvements in care, mortality continues to be high, with STEMI being associated with a higher risk of short-term mortality, and NSTEMI associated with a higher risk of long-term mortality.[5] Major bleeding appears to be an important driver of mortality in patients with ACS, especially in the first 30 days post PCI. In the OASIS five trials of more than 20,000 patients with ACS, approximately one in six of all deaths within the first 30 days occurred in patients who experienced bleeding.[6] Often overlooked in this early period is that the daily risk of bleeding events exceeds that of ischaemic events.[1] While definitions of major bleeding differ, it is apparent that regardless of the definition used, major bleeding magnifies the risk of adverse clinical events and mortality in patients with ACS. Major bleeding can be directly harmful owing to hypoxemia, hypotension, and the resulting adaptive changes, as well as indirectly owing to blood transfusions and potential interruption of dual antiplatelet therapy (DAPT) leading to stent thrombosis and MI.[7] A meta-analysis of 42 studies including over half a million patients found that major bleeding was independently associated with a threefold increase in mortality and major adverse cardiac events (MACE), with a mortality signal that was sustained even a year following the bleed.[8] Bleeding complications can be classified into non-access site bleeding (e.g. intracranial, gastrointestinal, retroperitoneal, etc.) and access-site bleeding, both of which have a similar prevalence of ~10%.

Non-access site bleeding is associated with a significantly worse outcome with a 4-fold increase in mortality, while access site bleeding confers a 1.7-fold increase in mortality compared to patients without a bleeding event.[9] In addition to decreased survival, major bleeding post PCI is associated with an increased length of hospital stay and financial costs.[10] Around half of all major bleeding events[11–14] encountered during PCI are derived from the access site. One of the earliest pieces of evidence that a change in access practice may be associated with a reduction in major bleeding and a decreased risk of mortality was derived from the Mortality benefit Of Reduced Transfusion after percutaneous coronary intervention via the Arm or Leg (MORTAL) study in British Columbia, a retrospective registry of 38,872 procedures undertaken in 32,822 patients that showed that transradial access was associated with a halving of the transfusion rate and a reduction in 30-day and 1-year mortality.[15]

Randomized Controlled Trials

Whilst registry data provide important insights into access site choice and clinical outcomes in unselected cohorts undergoing PCI, there are important limitations particularly related to selection bias in which higher-risk PCIs are undertaken through the femoral artery. Randomized controlled trials (RCTs) overcome such limitations around unmeasured confounders and selection bias and so provide important insight into access site-related outcomes, albeit in highly selected and lower-risk cohorts. In this section, we will review the current randomized clinical trials pertaining to transradial intervention (TRI) versus transfemoral intervention (TFI) in ACS. Specifically, these trials include RIVAL, RIFLE-STEACS, STEMI-RADIAL and the MATRIX study.

Published in 2011, the RadIal Versus femorAL access for coronary intervention (RIVAL) trial was the first large study comparing TRI versus TFI in patients with ACS. In this trial, 7,021 patients with ACS undergoing PPCI were randomized to TRI versus TFI. At 30 days, there was no statistical difference in the primary composite outcome of death, MI, stroke or non-CABG-related major bleeding between the two arms of the trial (3.7% versus 4.0%, $p = 0.50$, [CI 0.72–1.17]). The TRI group demonstrated significantly fewer vascular complications with regards to haematomas (1.2% versus 3.0%, $p < 0.0001$, [CI 0.28–0.57]) and pseudoaneurysms needing closure (0.2% versus 0.65%, $p = 0.006$, [CI 0.13–0.71]. While RIVAL showed no difference overall in the primary outcome between the two arms, it is important to mention that in patients with STEMI, there was a significant benefit in the primary outcome when using the radial approach (HR 0.60, $p = 0.026$, [CI 0.38–0.94]). This benefit was not observed in patients with NSTEMI. One criticism of RIVAL was the relatively low overall bleeding rates compared to 'real world' bleeding rates, a finding attributed to the restrictive definition of major bleeding employed in the trial. A post hoc analysis showed significantly less bleeding in the TRA arm when the less restrictive ACUITY trial major bleeding definition was applied. While this difference may be hypothesis generating, it validates the speculation that the bleeding definition contributed to the surprising results of the trial given the low incidence of major bleeding in the TFA group. Interestingly, the investigators also found a significant interaction between the primary outcome and high-volume radial centres (HR 0.49, p = 0.015, [CI 0.28–0.87]), suggesting that the benefit of TRI over TFI was mainly seen in high-volume centres.

While RIVAL did show benefit in the subgroup of patients with STEMI, it did not find a difference in the overall primary outcome for the general ACS population. The subsequent RIFLE-STEACS (Radial Versus Femoral Randomized Investigation in ST-Elevation Acute Coronary Syndrome) specifically addressed the association between access site and outcomes in the STEMI population.[16] In RIFLE-STEACS, 1,001 patients with acute STEMI undergoing primary/rescue PCI were randomized to TRI versus TFI. The primary endpoint was the 30-day rate of net adverse clinical events (NACEs), defined as a composite of cardiac death, stroke, MI, TLR, and bleeding. Unlike in RIVAL, the definition of bleeding was less restrictive, including types 2, 3, and 5 of the BARC classification. The primary endpoint of 30-day MACEs occurred in 13.6% in the radial arm versus 21.0% in the femoral arm (p = 0.003). In particular, compared with femoral, radial access was associated with significantly lower rates of cardiac mortality (5.2% versus 9.2%, p = 0.020), bleeding (7.8% versus 12.2%, p = 0.026), and shorter hospital stay. Unlike RIVAL, RIFLE-STEACS did not exclude patients with cardiogenic shock, with 8% of all patients in RIFLE-STEACS requiring IABP (intra-aortic balloon pump) support. Indeed, in this nearly all comers study, the selection criteria were less stringent and also included patients with failed thrombolysis. These factors were thought to be relevant towards the relatively high 30-day cardiac mortality rate of 7.2% compared to the 2.9% rate reported in the HORIZONS-AMI trial. On the basis of RIVAL and RIFLE-STEACS, considerable randomized evidence had now accumulated to show the potential of radial access in reducing access-site bleeding complications and mortality in patients with STEMI. The magnitude of the benefit of TRI based on these trials was significant: a 44% reduction in the RIVAL STEMI substudy and a 60% reduction in RIFLE STEACS with a pooled RR for 30-day mortality = 0.50 [95% CI 0.33–0.76]. Around the same time, the results of the STEMI-RADIAL trial were published, providing further evidence favouring TRI in STEMI. In STEMI-RADIAL, 707 patients presenting with STEMI undergoing PPCI were randomized to either TRI or TFI.

The primary endpoint of 30-day bleeding and access site complications was significantly reduced in the TRA arm as compared with the TFA arm (1.4% versus 7.2%, p = 0.0001).[17] This was driven predominantly by a reduction in large haematomas >15% (0.6% versus 5.3%) and haemoglobin drop ≥3 g/dl (0.9% versus 2.8%). The incidence of gastrointestinal bleeding (0.3% versus 1.1%) and vascular complications (0.3% versus 0.8%) was also numerically lower in the TRA arm. Reduced bleeding also resulted in net adverse clinical events (NACE) at 30 days being significantly lower with TRI compared to TFI (4.6% versus 11.0%, p = 0.0028). MACE rates at 30 days were similar (3.5% versus 4.2%, p = 0.7). The results of this trial were similar to the RIVAL and RIFLE-STEACS trials in demonstrating that TRI was superior to TFI in reducing access site bleeding complications in patients undergoing PPCI for STEMI. Furthermore, contrast use and length of ICU stay were also found to be lower with TRI. In this trial, the majority of benefit was driven by a reduction in large haematomas. Nevertheless, further clarification was warranted regarding whether the benefits of TRA seen in these three trials persisted in patients receiving contemporary anticoagulation, specifically oral thienopyridines and bivalirudin. This formed the basis for the MATRIX trial.

The MATRIX Access trial (Minimizing Adverse Haemorrhagic Events by TRansradial Access Site and Systemic Implementation of angioX) was a large randomized multicentre trial comparing TRA versus TFA in 8,404 patients presenting with ACS.[18] MATRIX found that in patients with ACS undergoing PCI, TRI as compared with TFI reduced net adverse clinical events, through a reduction in major bleeding and all-cause mortality. In total, 410 (9.8%) patients with radial access had net adverse clinical events compared with 486 (11.7%) patients with femoral access (0.83, 95% CI 0.73–0.96; p = 0.0092). The difference was driven by BARC major bleeding unrelated to CABG (1.6% versus 2.3%, RR 0.67, 95% CI 0.49–0.92; p = 0.013) and all-cause mortality (1.6% versus 2.2%, RR 0.72, 95% CI 0.53–0.99; p = 0.045). Overall, the results of MATRIX seemed to show that the benefit of TRI compared with TFI is similar across patients with ACS, though the magnitude of such benefit was more modest than previously reported in STEMI patients, in the range of six fewer fatal events for every 1,000 treated patients.

Radial Access and Operator Experience

One observation from the above trials is that proficiency with the transradial technique is required to realize its maximal benefits over the transfemoral approach. Operator experience varied significantly in the RIVAL trial; indeed, a significant reduction in the primary outcome was seen only in the highest tertile PCI volume group (hazard ratio, 0.49; 95% CI, 0.28–0.87; p = 0.015). This benefit was not realized in intermediate or low-volume centres. All participating interventional cardiologists in RIFLE-STEACS were high-volume operators (>150 PCIs/year) and had adequate expertise in both approaches, meeting minimal proficiency criteria of >50% interventional cases by radial approach per year. Similarly, in the MATRIX study, operators were required to have done most of their procedures transradially (>50%) and to have done at least 75 TRIs in the previous year. In both RIFLE-STEACS and MATRIX, the access site crossover rates (considered a useful indicator of radial proficiency) were low, at 4.7% and 5.7%, respectively. In the RIVAL trial, crossover rates varied with operator experience: 4.4% in the highest tertile group, as opposed to 9.7% in the intermediate tertile and 8% in the lowest tertile. The length of the learning curve for TRI is debatable, but patients with ACS, especially STEMI, present a particularly challenging population.

Adoption of TRA

TRA is the default and first-line method of performing invasive cardiac catheterization procedures in many European centres. This is reflected in the strong endorsement of the European Society of Cardiology guidelines which give a level IA recommendation for the transradial approach for PCI in patients with ACS.[19] In the US, TRA has gained much popularity with a 13-fold increase in adoption of TRI.[20] Nevertheless, the current adoption rate for TRI in the US remains low, with only 28% of PCIs being performed transradially based on data from the NCDR (National Cardiovascular Data Registry) Cath PCI registry.[21] A number of factors may explain this finding. To begin with, most interventionalists in the US have limited TRA experience.[22] For interventionalists who are well away from fellowship training, the transition from TFA to TRA in the

STEMI setting is a long-term process requiring practice and time. In one regional STEMI registry, several hundred PCI cases treated over a three-year time frame were deemed necessary to make TRI the more prevalent access site in the acute setting of STEMI treatment.[23] In the US, 44% of operators perform less than the minimum average of 50 PCI annually recommended by professional guidelines. It is this same group that is least likely to perform TRI and most likely to perform emergency PCI or PPCI for STEMI.[24] Indeed this is a well described paradox, with the patients most likely to develop access site complications from TFA being the group least likely to receive TRA.[25] As more US-based interventional fellowship programmes adopt TRA, this trend will hopefully change over time. Furthermore, as the country's healthcare system moves towards a value-based system, educational and training opportunities led by the Society of Cardiovascular Angiography and Interventions (SCAI) such as transition for VALUE are meant to highlight the clinical and economic advantages of TRA and to guide TRA adoption.[26] Another reason cited for physician reluctance to use TRA in the STEMI setting is the concern that it could lead to longer door to balloon times. In experienced operators, this has not been found to be true, with similar door to balloon times reported between TRI and TFI in RIFLE-STEACS. Nevertheless, the focus on door-to-balloon time for primary PCI may discourage operators from attempting TRA given concern that it could prolong door-to-balloon time even though it may lead to improved outcomes.[27] In an interesting analysis, it was calculated that a physician would need to introduce a substantial delay of more than 20 min through performing TRI compared with TFI in order to neutralize the mortality benefit of TRA in STEMI.[28] Such findings have important implications for operators reluctant to transition to TRA in STEMI. For Tips for Transradial Primary Angioplasty in Acute Myocardial Infarction, please refer to page 236, Chapter 10.

Despite the benefits of TRA, concerns have been raised regarding the higher radiation dose received by patients and operators. While this was initially attributed to low operator volume in a RIVAL substudy,[29] it was not true of MATRIX which required operators to have completed >75 TRI in the year before the trial. In the radiation sub-study (RAD-MATRIX), TRA was associated with greater radiation to the operator and the patient. Operator equivalent dose at the thorax was significantly higher with radial than femoral access (77 μSv [IQR:40–112] versus 41 μSv [IQR:23–59], $p = 0.02$).[30] These small differences in increased patient radiation exposure are likely negligible and likely to be significantly outweighed by the mortality benefit of TRI.[31] Nevertheless, the findings of RAD-MATRIX suggest that it is imperative that radial operators need to remain vigilant about reducing their own radiation exposure.

In a national UK cohort, it was found that TFI independently increased a patient's odds of sustaining a RPH (retroperitoneal haemorrhage) over 20-fold when compared to TRI. Indeed, the decreased incidence of RPH in the UK has been at least partially credited to the transition to TRA.[32] Another benefit of TRA over TFA, investigated in the AKI MATRIX study, found that among patients with ACS who underwent PCI, TRI was significantly associated with a reduced occurrence of AKI compared with TFI. These findings were consistent across pre-defined patient subgroups and were attributed to a reduction in bleeding events, reduction in embolization in the renal circulation (by avoiding aortic traversal) and the need for less transfusion.[33]

The NSTEMI Population

The benefits of TRI in the NSTEMI population have sometimes been called into question, partially due to a lack of published randomized data (Bates, 2016[34]). The two main clinical trials comparing access site selection in NSTEMI patients—RIVAL and MATRIX—were both underpowered to study differences in outcomes in NSTEMI specifically. In RIVAL, similar rates of the primary outcome in NSTEMI patients were seen in the radial (3.8%) and femoral (3.5%) groups with a trend towards higher mortality risk in those allocated to TRA (1.25% versus 1.66%; $p = 0.082$). In the MATRIX trial, TRI was associated with a significant 28% relative risk reduction in all-cause mortality and a 15% relative risk reduction for MACE, although this effect did not meet the pre-specified alpha level of 2.5%.A pooled meta-analysis of studies including randomized comparisons between TRI and TFI in NSTEMI patients found that in the 125, 463 subjects analysed, no significant difference was found in the incidence of short-term all-cause mortality between TRA and TFA (odds ratio [OR] 0.78, 95% CI 0.57–1.07, $p = 0.12$).[36] Nevertheless, TRI was associated with significant reduction in major bleeding (OR 0.52, 95% CI 0.36–0.73, $p = 0.0002$), access-site bleeding (OR 0.41, 95% CI 0.22–0.78, $p = 0.007$), and the need for blood transfusions (OR 0.61, 95% CI 0.41–0.91, $p = 0.02$). Furthermore, the 1-year mortality was significantly lower in TRI (OR 0.72, 95% CI 0.55–0.95, $p = 0.02$).

Similar findings were reported in a large British registry of 439,947 patients, which found that TRA was independently associated with a reduction in bleeding (OR: 0.35, $p < 0.001$), access site complications (OR: 0.19; $p < 0.001$) and MACE (OR: 0.72, $p < 0.001$).[37]

TRA in Cardiogenic Shock

While there is a dearth of data guiding access site selection in ACS with cardiogenic shock, observational studies have suggested that TRI may be associated with favourable outcomes even in higher risk patients undergoing PCI and requiring intra-aortic balloon pump (IABP). In a retrospective study of STEMI patients receiving IABP support during PPCI, TFI had a higher unadjusted rate of NACE when compared with TRI (57.4 versus 36.6%, $p < 0.01$), mainly due to a greater incidence of access-related bleedings (18.7 versus 6.3%, $p < .01$).[38] Analysis of the BCIS registry data of close to 8,000 patients presenting in cardiogenic shock showed that TRI was associated with a 44% reduction in 30-day mortality and 63% reduction in major bleeding compared to TFI, although this was only observed in experienced radial centres.[39]

Conclusion

Bleeding complications represent an important cause of morbidity and mortality therapy after PCI for ACS indications, with access-site related bleeding complications contributing up to half of all major bleeding complications recorded during PCI. TRA has been recommended as a class 1A indication for ACS in international guidelines and represents best current practice. TRI has gained widespread adoption in many international centres and continues to gain momentum, particularly in the US. The accumulating evidence of its value in reducing bleeding complications and mortality rate is robust in the STEMI population, with benefits also seen in the NSTEMI population. While certain barriers to adoption continue to exist, a number of educational programmes and value-based initiatives have shown promise towards overcoming these challenges.

References

1. Giustino G, Mehran R, Dangas GD, et al. Characterization of the average daily ischemic and bleeding risk after primary PCI for STEMI. *Journal of the American College of Cardiology*. 2017;*70*(15):1846–57.
2. Johansson S, Rosengren A, Young K, Jennings E. Mortality and morbidity trends after the first year in survivors of acute myocardial infarction: a systematic review. *BMC Cardiovascular Disorders*. 2017;*17*(1):53.
3. Krumholz HM, Herrin J, Miller LE, et al. Improvements in door-to-balloon time in the United States, 2005 to 2010. *Circulation*. 2011;*124*(9):1038–45.
4. Kang S-H, Chae I-H, Park J-J, et al. Stent thrombosis with drug-eluting stents and bioresorbable scaffolds: evidence from a network meta-analysis of 147 trials. *JACC: Cardiovascular Interventions*. 2016;*9*(12):1203–12.
5. Chan MY, Sun JL, Newby LK, et al. Long-term mortality of patients undergoing cardiac catheterization for ST-elevation and non-ST-elevation myocardial infarction. *Circulation*. 2009;*119*(24):3110–17.
6. Budaj A, Eikelboom JW, Mehta SR, et al. Improving clinical outcomes by reducing bleeding in patients with non-ST-elevation acute coronary syndromes. *European Heart Journal*. 2009;*30*(6):655–61.
7. De Silva K, Myat A, Cotton J, James S, Gershlick A, Stone GW. Bleeding associated with the management of acute coronary syndromes. *Heart*. 2017;*103*(7): 546–62.
8. Kwok CS, Rao SV, Myint PK, et al. Major bleeding after percutaneous coronary intervention and risk of subsequent mortality: a systematic review and meta-analysis. *Open Heart*. 2014;Feb 13;1(1):e000021. doi: 10.1136/openhrt-2013-000021. PMID: 25332786; PMCID: PMC4195929.
9. Kwok CS, Khan MA, Rao SV, et al. Access and non–access site bleeding after percutaneous coronary intervention and risk of subsequent mortality and major adverse cardiovascular events. *Systematic Review and Meta-Analysis*. Circulation: Cardiovascular Interventions 2015-04-01 8(4): e001645 https://doi.org/10.1161/CIRCINTERVENTIONS.114.001645.
10. Ewen EF, Zhao L, Kolm P, et al. Determining the in-hospital cost of bleeding in patients undergoing percutaneous coronary intervention. *Journal of Interventional Cardiology*. 2009;*22*(3):266–73.
11. Marso SP, Amin AP, House JA, et al. Association between use of bleeding avoidance strategies and risk of periprocedural bleeding among patients undergoing percutaneous coronary intervention. *JAMA*. 2010;*303*(21):2156–64.

12. Patel MR, Jneid H, Derdeyn CP, et al. Arteriotomy closure devices for cardiovascular procedures: a scientific statement from the American Heart Association. *Circulation*. 2010;*122*(18):1882–93.
13. Shahzad A, Kemp I, Mars C, et al. Unfractionated heparin versus bivalirudin in primary percutaneous coronary intervention (HEAT-PPCI): an open-label, single centre, randomised controlled trial. *The Lancet*. 2014;*384*(9957):1849–58.
14. Erlinge D, Omerovic E, Fröbert O, et al. Bivalirudin versus heparin monotherapy in myocardial infarction. *New England Journal of Medicine*. 2017;*377*(12):1132–42.
15. Chase AJ, Fretz EB, Warburton WP, et al. Association of the arterial access site at angioplasty with transfusion and mortality: the M.O.R.T.A.L study (Mortality benefit Of Reduced Transfusion after percutaneous coronary intervention via the Arm or Leg). *Heart*. 2008;*94*(8):1019–25.
16. Romagnoli E, Biondi-Zoccai G, Sciahbasi A, et al. Radial versus femoral randomized investigation in ST-segment elevation acute coronary syndrome: the RIFLE-STEACS (Radial Versus Femoral Randomized Investigation in ST-Elevation Acute Coronary Syndrome) study. *Journal of the American College of Cardiology*. 2012;*60*(24):2481–89.
17. Bernat I, Horak D, Stasek J, et al. ST-segment elevation myocardial infarction treated by radial or femoral approach in a multicenter randomized clinical trial: the STEMI-RADIAL trial. *Journal of the American College of Cardiology*. 2014;*63*(10):964–72.
18. Valgimigli M, Gagnor A, Calabró P, et al. Radial versus femoral access in patients with acute coronary syndromes undergoing invasive management: a randomised multicentre trial. *The Lancet*. 2015;*385*(9986):2465–76.
19. Windecker S, Kolh P, Alfonso F, et al. 2014 ESC/EACTS Guidelines on myocardial revascularizationThe Task Force on Myocardial Revascularization of the European Society of Cardiology (ESC) and the European Association for Cardio-Thoracic Surgery (EACTS)Developed with the special contribution of the European Association of Percutaneous Cardiovascular Interventions (EAPCI). *European Heart Journal*. 2014;*35*(37):2541–19.
20. Feldman DN, Swaminathan RV, Kaltenbach LA, et al. Adoption of radial access and comparison of outcomes to femoral access in percutaneous coronary intervention. An updated report from the national cardiovascular data registry (2007–2012). *Circulation*. 2013;*127*(23):2295–306.
21. Shamim S, Tang F, Safley D, Jones P, Spertus JA, Baklanov D. Patient versus physician variation in use of transradial percutaneous coronary intervention. *American Journal of Cardiology*. 2017;*119*(12):1937–41.
22. Rao SV, Ou F-S, Wang TY, et al. Trends in the prevalence and outcomes of radial and femoral approaches to percutaneous coronary intervention: a report from the National Cardiovascular Data Registry. *JACC: Cardiovascular Interventions*. 2008;*1*(4):379–86.
23. Valgimigli M, Saia F, Guastaroba P, et al. Transradial versus transfemoral intervention for acute myocardial infarction: a propensity score-adjusted and -matched analysis from the REAL (REgistro regionale AngiopLastiche

dell'Emilia-Romagna) multicenter registry. *JACC: Cardiovascular Interventions.* 2012;*5*(1):23–35.

24. Fanaroff AC, Zakroysky P, Dai D, et al. Outcomes of PCI in relation to procedural characteristics and operator volumes in the United States. *Journal of the American College of Cardiology*. 2017;*69*(24):2913–24.
25. Wimmer NJ, Resnic FS, Mauri L, et al. Risk-treatment paradox in the selection of transradial access for percutaneous coronary intervention. *Journal of the American Heart Association*. 2013;*2*(3):e000174.
26. Shroff A. SCAI launches educational initiative as nation shifts to value-based healthcare. [https://scai.org/scai-launches-educational-initiative-nation-shifts-value-based-healthcare]. 2017.
27. Yeh RW, Kirtane AJ, Rao SV. Incentivizing transradial access for primary percutaneous coronary intervention while maintaining timely reperfusion. *JAMA Cardiology*. 2017;*2*(10):1057–58.
28. Wimmer NJ, Cohen DJ, Wasfy JH, Rathore SS, Mauri L, Yeh RW. Delay in reperfusion with transradial percutaneous coronary intervention for ST-elevation myocardial infarction: Might some delays be acceptable? *American Heart Journal*. 2014;*168*(1):103–109.
29. Jolly SS, Cairns J, Niemela K, et al. Effect of radial versus femoral access on radiation dose and the importance of procedural volume: a substudy of the multicenter randomized RIVAL trial. *JACC: Cardiovascular Interventions*. 2013;*6*(3):258–66.
30. Sciahbasi A, Frigoli E, Sarandrea A, et al. Radiation exposure and vascular access in acute coronary syndromes: the RAD-matrix trial. *Journal of the American College of Cardiology*. 2017;*69*(20):2530–537.
31. Kleiman NS, Kleiman NJ. At arm's length: radiation safety during radial percutaneous coronary intervention*. *Journal of the American College of Cardiology*. 2017;*69*(20):2538–41.
32. Kwok CS, Kontopantelis E, Kinnaird T, et al. Retroperitoneal hemorrhage after percutaneous coronary intervention: incidence, determinants, and outcomes as recorded by the British Cardiovascular Intervention Society. *Circulation: Cardiovascular Interventions*. 2018;*11*(2):e005866.
33. Andò G, Cortese B, Russo F, et al. Acute kidney injury after radial or femoral access for invasive acute coronary syndrome management: AKI-MATRIX. *Journal of the American College of Cardiology*. 2017;*69*(21):2592–603.
34. Bates ER, Tamis Holland JE, Bittl JA, O'Gara PT, Levine GN, PCI Strategies in patients with ST segment Elevation Myocardial Infarction and Multivessel Coronary Artery Disease *J Am Coll Cardiol*. 2016 Sep 6;*68*(10);1066–81. doi:10.1016/j.jacc.2016.05.086.PMID:17585512.
35. Ferrante G, Rao SV, Jüni P, et al. Radial versus femoral access for coronary interventions across the entire spectrum of patients with coronary artery disease: a meta-analysis of randomized trials. *JACC: Cardiovascular Interventions*. 2016;*9*(14):1419–34.
36. Bavishi C, Panwar SR, Dangas GD, et al. Meta-analysis of radial versus femoral access for percutaneous coronary interventions in non-ST-segment elevation acute coronary syndrome. *The American Journal of Cardiology*. 2016;*117*(2):172–78.

37. Ratib K, Mamas MA, Anderson SG, et al. Access site practice and procedural outcomes in relation to clinical presentation in 439,947 patients undergoing percutaneous coronary intervention in the United Kingdom. *JACC: Cardiovascular Interventions*. 2015;*8*(1, Part A):20–9.
38. Romagnoli E, De Vita M, Burzotta F, et al. Radial versus femoral approach comparison in percutaneous coronary intervention with intraaortic balloon pump support: the RADIAL PUMP UP Registry. *American Heart Journal*. 2013;*166*(6):1019–26.
39. Mamas MA, Anderson SG, Ratib K, et al. Arterial access site utilization in cardiogenic shock in the United Kingdom: is radial access feasible? *American Heart Journal*. 2014;*167*(6):900–908.

17 (ii)

(Corollary to Chapter 17) Study Update

The SAFARI-STEMI Study and Editorial Comment

Yashasvi Chugh, Sunita Chugh, and Sanjay Kumar Chugh

SAFARI-STEMI Study

A recent trial comparing radial Vs femoral access for primary percutaneous coronary intervention (PCI) in ST-Segment Elevation Myocardial Infarction (STEMI) was published in the Journal of American Medical Association (JAMA) Cardiology; The Safety and Efficacy of Femoral Access vs Radial Access in ST-Segment Elevation Myocardial Infarction, The SAFARI-STEMI Randomized Clinical Trial by Michel Le May, George Wells, Derek So, et al Published online in JAMA Cardiol January 2, 2020. doi: https://doi.org/10.1001/jamacardio.2019.4852.

This was a multicenter randomized clinical trial which enrolled patients of STEMI for Primary PCI performed in 1082 of 1136 patients (95.2%) in the transradial group Vs. 1109 of 1156 patients (95.9%) in the transfemoral group. The study was stopped prematurely following a futility analysis, as the 30-day all-cause mortality (17 [1.5%] vs 15 [1.3%] patients) or other clinical end points of re-infarction (1.8% vs 1.6%; RR, 1.07; 95% CI, 0.57-2.00; P=.83), stroke (1.0% vs 0.4%; RR, 2.24; 95% CI, 0.78-6.42; P=.12), and bleeding (1.4% vs 2.0%; RR, 0.71; 95% CI, 0.38-1.33; P=.28) did not show significant difference between the two groups.

In response this study, an editorial comment, a critique of the paper (voted 74:26 by audience, in favour of the author(SKC) debating against principal investigator of SAFARI-STEMI, Dr Le May, at Transcatheter Therapeutics, 2018, SanDiego) has been inserted here.

Editorial Comment on the SAFARI STEMI Study

The superiority of transradial over transfemoral access for primary angioplasty in STEMI still remains unchallenged, even after the SAFARI - STEMI study.

Why the SAFARI STEMI Study?

The results of the major randomized controlled trials (RCTs) which established the superiority of transradial (TR) percutaneous coronary intervention (PCI) over transfemoral (TF) PCI in ST elevation myocardial infarction (STEMI) [1,2] in terms of bleeding, major adverse cardiac events (MACE) and mortality were attributed by some[3] to high doses of Heparin and GP IIb/IIIa inhibitors over bivalirudin. The SAFARI STEMI[4] study was therefore designed to assess outcomes based on 'access- site alone'[1]; akin to comparing bottles (and not the contents) for differences; after emptying their precious contents!

Hence unlike the seminal studies[1,2], not only was bivalirudin the preferred anticoagulant for PCI; higher bleeding risk (HBR) patients (oral anticoagulant use, post-fibrinolysis patients requiring rescue PCI) were excluded; so were Post-coronary artery bypass graft patients, which are challenging transradially! It was thus not a real-world population either.

Upto 8% of the study population in the TR Vs.TF RCTs, were patients requiring rescue PCI that had a higher mortality (20% with failed Vs. 4% with successful rescue PTCA, p=0.03)[5]; further, bleeding was higher[6] with TF compared to TR PCI in patients on un-interrupted warfarin therapy; and, 90-day mortality was higher in post-CABG patients with STEMI with a bypass graft as culprit (hazard ratio: 1.9, 95% confidence interval: 1.08 - 3.33, p = 0.025)[7]. These categories of patients were however conveniently *excluded* from the SAFARI STEMI study, thus making it a low-risk study population. In addition, a lower proportion of high- risk patients of diabetes mellitus, chronic obstructive pulmonary disease, chronic kidney disease and Killip class 2-4 heart failure further contributed to the proportionately lower mortality in the study (1.3% Vs. 1.5%) Vs. (2.7% Vs.4.7%; for TR Vs. TF access respectively), compared to other RCTs on STEMI[1,2]. No surprise therefore that a mortality difference between TR and TF access was not perceptible in this low -risk study population which led to the data surveillance monitoring board (DSMB) stopping the study prematurely when only half the planned number of patients had been enrolled because they considered the study 'futile' with regard to showing a difference in mortality. The study thus had a power of only 50% and was thus inadequately powered for any conclusions.

Since HBR worsens the outcomes with TF access, by increasing the risk of femoral complications; in order to contain the bleeding risk and obviate the need for bailout GP IIb/IIIa inhibitors; bivalirudin, vascular closure devices (VCDs), and thrombo-aspiration[6] (38.8 vs 42.9% patients in TR vs. TF groups) were used liberally at much higher cost as per design of the study, despite lack of evidence for benefit with the latter.

Nevertheless, the superiority of TR PCI conclusively established in conventional meta-analysis[1] and trial sequential analysis (TSA)[2] of the seminal TR Vs.TF RCTs, with regard to access-site bleeding, major bleeding and MACE remains unchanged post- the SAFARI STEMI study because of serious flaws in the underpowered latter study, as discussed above.

Mortality Benefit with TR PCI in STEMI

Although not powered for mortality, a pooled analysis showed a consistent reduction in mortality across 7 TR Vs.TF trials of STEMI, with low risk of bias [2].

Not only was the SAFARI STEMI under-powered for mortality, it was also severely flawed and did not reflect a real world population of patients.

A TSA[2] of the seminal trials conclusively established a significant reduction in mortality with TR PCI in STEMI at 5% & 1% α errors.

Conclusion

The superiority of TR PCI over TF primary angioplasty in STEMI is conclusively established[8]. TR PCI in STEMI is associated with lower risk of mortality [2.7% vs. 4.7%; odds ratio [OR]:0.55, 95% confidence interval [CI]: 0.40-0.76; $p<0.001$], major bleeding [1.4% vs. 2.9%; OR: 0.51, 95%CI: 0.31-0.85; $p=0.01$], access-site bleeding [2.1% vs. 5.6%; OR: 0.35, 95%CI: 0.25 - 0.50; and MACE [4.6% vs. 6.8%; OR: 0.64, 95%CI: 0.49 - 0.83;

p<0.001][2]. (For Tips for Transradial Primary Angioplasty in Acute Myocardial Infarction, please refer to page 236, Chapter 10)

The study does highlight that though bivalirudin, VCDs, and thrombo-aspiration can be used at a higher cost to contain bleeding risk with TF PCI in STEMI; the same does not seem justified over the use of TR PCI with low –cost heparin and bailout GP2b3a inhibitors in STEMI.

Nevertheless, VCDs and meticulous care to TF access may be considered appropriate for wide-bore access for structural interventions and left ventricular mechanical support devices.

References

1. Karrowni W, Vyas A, Giacomino B, et al. Radial versus femoral access for primary percutaneous interventions in ST-segment elevation myocardial infarction patients: a meta-analysis of randomized controlled trials. JACC: Cardiovascular Interventions, 6:8, 2013:814–23.
2. Giuseppe Andò and Davide Capodanno. Radial Access Reduces Mortality in Patients With Acute Coronary Syndromes Results From an Updated Trial Sequential Analysis of Randomized Trials. JACC: Cardiovascular Interventions Volume 9, Issue Issue 7, 2016.
3. MS Lee, M Wolfe and M Stone, TRI Vs TFI in ACS, JACC Cardiovascular Interventions 6:11,1149-52;2013.
4. Michel Le May, George Wells, Derek So, et al. Safety and Efficacy of Femoral Access vs Radial Access in ST-Segment Elevation Myocardial Infarction, The SAFARI-STEMI Randomized Clinical Trial.JAMA Cardiol. Published online January 2, 2020. doi: https://doi.org/10.1001/jamacardio.2019.4852.
5. Philippe Gabriel Steg, Laurent Francois, Bernard Iung, Dominique Himbert, Pierre Aubry, et al. Long-term clinical outcomes after rescue angioplasty are not different from those of successful thrombolysis for acute myocardial infarction. European Heart Journal, Volume 26, Issue 18, September 2005, Pages 1831–1837).
6. Baker NC, O'Connell EW, Htun WW, et al. Safety of coronary angiography and percutaneous coronary intervention via the radial versus femoral route in patients on uninterrupted oral anticoagulation with warfarin. Am Heart J. 2014;168:537-44.
7. Bavry AA, Kumbhani DJ, Bhatt DL. Role of adjunctive thrombectomy and embolic protection devices in acute myocardial infarction: a comprehensive meta-analysis of randomized trials. European Heart Journal. 2008;29(24):2989–3001.
8. Yashasvi Chugh, Sunita Chugh, Sanjay Kumar Chugh, Post-the SAFARI STEMI study: Is there still a debate on radial vs. femoral access in STEMI?, Indian Heart Journal, Volume 72, Issue 5, 2020, Pages 466–468, ISSN 0019-4832, https://doi.org/10.1016/j.ihj.2020.08.006.(https://www.sciencedirect.com/science/article/pii/S0019483220301905)

18(i)

Transradial Access in the Elderly

Justin Paul Gnanaraj and N. Nilavan

Elderly and Coronary Artery Disease

Advancement in health care system worldwide has improved average life expectancy, and we find more and more of population surviving beyond 70s, 80s, and 90s, at the cost of increasing morbidity. Elderly population are predisposed to atherosclerosis because of cardiac risk factors like diabetes, hypertension, and age. Age is a major cardiovascular risk factor for coronary artery disease (CAD), and it is the most common cause of death in elderly.[1] Elderly patients also have complex comorbidities of other systems like renal, hepatic, pulmonary, and nervous system, which have significant impact on the disease process, therapeutics, and management.

As a result, we find more and more of the elderly patients seeking medical attention with complex cardiac problems, which need to be addressed with special care. It's the duty of the interventional cardiologist to provide effective care to the elderly so that they have a good quality of life. Rao et al. showed that 25% of all percutaneous coronary interventions (PCIs) are performed in age >75 years and 12% of all PCIs are performed in >80 years.[2] One of the important parts in percutaneous procedure is arterial access, as elderly have vascular abnormalities that cause difficulty during percutaneous procedure when compared with young population.

Elderly often have vascular abnormalities related to atherosclerosis, tortuosity, obstructions, aneurysms, and calcifications of the aorta, neck vessels, forearm vessels, iliac arteries, and femoral arteries. They have lower lean body mass, subnormal metabolism, abnormal drug response, and associated vascular friability. All these lead to an increased incidence of vascular and bleeding complications in these populations whatever may be the access route. The vascular and bleeding complications are ultimately responsible for the increased in-hospital mortality and morbidity in the elderly. Data show that patients older than 70 years are at an increased risk for access site haematoma, gastrointestinal bleeding, and a higher mortality at three-year follow-up.[3] Upper extremity complications associated with the transradial approach include perforations, forearm haematomas, compartment syndromes, radial artery occlusion, and palmar ischaemia.

Even though there is a higher burden of coronary artery disease in the elderly, gaps in research for appropriate therapies are significant, leading to lack of proper guidelines for therapy in the elderly.[4] Transradial access for elderly has been one such area, where there is a paucity of clinical data in the elderly.

Transradial compared to transfemoral is associated with a significant decrease in vascular complications. Transradial approach in patients aged 75 years and older has been shown to have a high success rate and lower major and minor complication rates.[5] However, what really happens in the real world is that the elderly, who stand to benefit most, are less often given the benefit of radial approach. We can call this an elderly transradial paradox. The reason for underutilization is due to obstacle in the operator's mind or lack of operator skill or social factors.[6]

DATA SO FAR—Summary of Studies of TRI in the Elderly

Data from a Canadian registry showed a threefold increase in the use of transradial approach in nonagenarians from 2004 to 2014.[7]

One of the earliest prospective studies evaluating radial access in elderly was the OCTOPLUS study, which showed that transradial approach was associated with a significant decrease in access site haematoma and other vascular complications in 377 patients above the age of 80 years.[8] Procedural success, fluoroscopy time, and utilization of contrast media were equivalent with both approaches. The elderly population has proven to be a consistently vulnerable group not only in the more immediate vascular complications but also in major adverse cardiac events weeks to months post-procedure. The OCTOPLUS study also showed that the primary endpoint of death, acute myocardial infarction, stroke, and major bleeding at 30 days was similar in both the approaches.[8]

Transradial approach makes the elderly population have early ambulation and shorter in hospital stay, who would otherwise suffer from prolonged immobilization and increased venous thromboembolism risk in transfemoral approach. Gao et al. showed that transradial approach is an independent negative predictor for vascular complications in 279 octogenarians.

The Cardio-ARSIF registry showed that femoral access was associated with a twofold increase in mortality compared to radial access in a group of 418 nonagenarians[9] and transfemoral approach was found to be an independent factor of in-hospital mortality. Daniel et al. from the London Heart Attack Group showed that radial access compared to femoral access was one of the two multivariate predictors of improved survival after primary PCI for STEMI in a group of 1,051 octogenarian patients. They further showed that the risk reduction associated with radial access was more marked in octogenarians with STEMI PCI compared to those younger than 80 years [42% versus 16%][10] in spite of lower radial access in octogenarians [18% versus 24%]. They also found that radial access, glycoprotein (GP) II/IIIa inhibition and drug-eluting stents (DES) use were associated with improved all-cause mortality.

Lee et al. showed that in 1,945 octogenarian's trans-femoral access for PCI in acute myocardial infarction was a significant predictor of in-hospital mortality.[11]

There are concerns that radial approach by leading to prolongation of time to arterial access, and door-to-balloon time, may not be an ideal strategy for primary angioplasty where "time is muscle", and delays lead to increased myocardial damage. However, Secco et al., in a study of 283 patients with STEMI above 75 years, showed that time to arterial puncture and balloon inflation time was significantly shorter and door-to-balloon time was non-significantly shorter with transradial approach, suggesting the efficacy of this approach in STEMI patients without cardiogenic shock at presentation.[12]

Door-to-balloon time was 103.1 ± 58.4 min in the TRA group compared with 110.3 ± 62.4 min in the TFA group (P = NS). Time to arterial puncture was 10.6 ± 4.1 min in the TRA group compared with 12.1 ± 4.5 min in the TFA group ($P < 0.01$) (For further details, please refer to Chapter 10, page 241, and Figure 10.9a).

Summary of Studies of TRI in the Elderly

Study	Population	Number	Results	P value
OCTOPLUS Study	Above 80 years	377	TRA PCI had lower vascular complications compared with TFA (1.6% versus 6.5%)	0.03
London Heart attack Group	Above 80 years	1,051	1. Radial access Primary PCI predictor of reduced bleeding event (OR 0.20,95% CI 0.10–0.77) 2. Radial access Primary PCI independent predictor of improved survival (HR 0.58, 95% CI 0.28–0.98)	0.002
CARDIO-ARSIF Registry	Above 90 years	418	Femoral access independent predictor of mortality (OR 2.07, 95% CI 1.62–2.64) in Primary PCI.	<0.001
Secco et al.[12]	Above 75 years	283	1. Door-to-balloon time was 103.1 ± 58.4 min in the TRA group compared with 110.3 ± 62.4 min in the TFA group 2. Time to arterial puncture was 10.6 ± 4.1 min in the TRA group compared with 12.1 ± 4.5 min in the TFA group	NS <0.01
KAMIR Registry[11]	Above 80 years	1,945	Trans radial approach predictor of lower in hospital mortality	Odds Ratio: 0.355

Though there are few studies which have showed that transradial approach have higher crossover rate to alternate access, it is mainly related to operator expertise.

A recent worldwide practice survey showed that right radial artery access is used in 90% and LRA is used in 10% of cases.[6] Regarding the side of radial approach, there are few studies that are in favour of left radial artery approach. OPERA study found that LRA approach was associated with lower radiation dose,[13] and PREVAIL study found that LRA approach was associated with short procedure time.[14] But Freixa et al.[15]and Pristipino[16] did not find any significant difference in procedure time and radiation dose between the two groups. So, at present, there is not sufficient strong evidence to recommend LRA approach over RRA approach. For further details please refer to Chapter 10, pages 143–144, 194–195, 214, 238, 262; and Chapter -11, 'Radial Access for Transradial Procedures: Right versus Left'.

TR band and Radiostop are the two devices commonly used for haemostatic control in transradial approach which requires immediate sheath removal. Rathore et al. compared the efficacy of these devices in 790 elderly patients. It showed that both devices were effective in achieving haemostasis. TR band device produced little discomfort and pain where as Radiostop device took shorter time to achieve haemostasis.[17] Alternatively, a hemostatic bandage may be used. (Please refer to Chapter 10, Pages 278–280, Figures 10.19a-g).

One of the main problems with transradial approach is radial artery spasm and occlusion. Two most important risk factors responsible are larger sheath and smaller radial artery size. Predictors for small artery diameter are women, smaller wrist circumference, and South Asian patients.[18] Downsizing and miniaturizing coronary interventional material and equipment such as thin-walled catheters, sheathless catheters, anchor wire, and balloon-assisted tracking will help in reducing arterial occlusion.[19] Please see Chapter 19, Complications of Transradial Access: Management and Prevention, pages 417–432.

Summary

Coronary artery disease is the leading cause of death in elderly population. Elderly population are unique in relation to their vascular anatomy, and it's important to provide an appropriate site for vascular access for coronary intervention. Despite a proven decrease in vascular complications in elderly by radial access, there is still unwillingness for many operators to adopt TR catheterization into their practices, likely due to concerns about technical challenges, prolonged procedural and fluoroscopy times and contrast usage.

However, clinical data shows that benefits of transradial access for cardiac interventions outweigh the potential concerns, particularly in elderly population. Radial access is compatible with complex coronary interventions and primary PCI for STEMI in the elderly. All access site complications and bleeding complications are reduced by radial access in elderly. Recent data are encouraging as there is a slow increase in use of radial access in the elderly.

It's our responsibility to provide efficient care, use the clinical evidence, and overcome the hesitancy in our mind to improve the quality of life in elderly population undergoing coronary intervention.

References

1. Kung HC, Hoyert DL, Xu J, et al. Division of vital statistics. deaths: final data for 2005. National vital statistics reports. *Natl Vital Stat Rep.* 2008;56:1–120.
2. Rao SV, et al. Trends in the prevalence and outcomes of radial and femoral approaches to percutaneous coronary intervention: a report from the National Cardiovascular Data Registry. *JACC Cardiovasc Interv.* 2008;1(4):379–86.
3. Bagur R, Bertrand OF, Rodes-Cabau J, et al. Comparison of outcomes in patients > or = 70 years versus <70 years after transradial coronary stenting with maximal antiplatelet therapy for acute coronary syndrome. *Am J Cardiol.* 2009;104(5):624–29.
4. Alexander KP, Newby LK, Cannon CP, et al. Acute coronary care in the elderly, part I: non-ST-segment-elevation acute coronary syndromes: a scientific statement for healthcare professionals from the American Heart Association Council on Clinical Cardiology: in collaboration with the Society of Ger. *Circulation.* 2007;115:2549–69.
5. Achenbach S, Ropers D, Kallert L, et al. Transradial versus transfemoral approach for coronary angiography and intervention in patients above 75 years of age. *Catheter Cardiovasc Interv.* 2008;72(5):629–35.
6. Bertrand OF, Rao SV, Panchoy S, et al. Transradial approach for coronary angiography and interventions: results of the first international transradial practice survey. *JACC Cardiovasc Interv.* 2010;3:1022–31.
7. Spagnoli V, de Hemptinne Q. Percutaneous coronary intervention in nonagenarians: prevalence, indications, vascular approach and mortality at 3 months. *J Cardiovasc Dis Diagn.* 2016, 4:2.
8. Louvard Y, Benamer H, Garot P, et al. Comparison of transradial and transfemoral approaches for coronary angiography and angioplasty in octogenarians (the OCTOPLUS study). *Am J Cardiol.* 2004;94(9):1177–80.
9. Gérard Helft, Jean-Louis Georges, Xavier Mouranche, et al. for e-MUST and CARDIO-ARSIF Registries. Outcomes of primary percutaneous coronary interventions in nonagenarians with acute myocardial infarction, *Int J Cardiol.* 2015;192:24–29. DOI:https://doi.org/10.1016/j.ijcard.2015.04.227IF
10. Bromage DI, Jones DA, Rathod KS, et al. Outcome of 1051 Octogenarian Patients With ST-Segment Elevation Myocardial Infarction Treated With Primary Percutaneous Coronary Intervention: Observational Cohort From the London

Heart Attack Group. J Am Heart Assoc. 2016 Jun 27;5(6):e003027. doi: 10.1161/JAHA.115.003027. PMID: 27353606; PMCID: PMC4937253.
11. Lee, et al. Comparison of transradial and transfemoral coronary intervention in octogenarians with acute myocardial infarction. *Int J Cardiol.* 2016;202:419–24.
12. Secco GG, Marinucci L, Uguccioni L. Transradial versus transfemoral approach for primary percutaneous coronary interventions in elderly patients. *J Invasive Cardiol.* 2013;25(5):254–56.
13. Dominici M, Diletti R, Milici C, et al. Operator exposure to x-ray in left and right radial access during percutaneous coronary procedures: OPERA randomized study. *Heart.* 2013;99:480–84.
14. Pelliccia F, Trani C, Biondi-Zoccai GG, et al. Comparison of the feasibility and effectiveness of transradial coronary angiography via right versus left radial artery approaches (from the PREVAIL STUDY). *Am J Cardiol.* 2012;110:771–75.
15. Freixa X, Trilla M, Feldman M, Jimenez M, Betriu A, Masotti M. Right versus left transradial approach for coronary catheterization in octogenarian patients. *Catheter Cardiovasc Intev.* 2012;80:267–72.
16. Pristipino C. Radial artery catheterization and radiological exposure. *Eur Heart J.* 2008;29:2316–17.
17. Rathore S, Stables RH, Pauriah M, et al. A randomized comparison of TR band and radiostop hemostatic compression devices after percutaneous transradial coronary intervention. *Catheter Cardiovasc Interv.* 2010;76:660–67.
18. Kotowycz MA, Johnston KW, Ivanov J, et al. Predictors of radial artery size in patients undergoing cardiac catheterization: insights from the Good Radial Artery Size Prediction (GRASP) study. *Can J Cardiol.* 2014;30:211–16.
19. Kiemeneij F, Yoshimachi F, Matsukage T, et al. Focus on maximal miniaturization of transradial coronary access materials and techniques by the Slender Club Japan and Europe: an overview and classification. *Catheter Cardiovasc Interv.* 2010;76:660–67.

18(ii)

Transradial Approach in Women

A Safe and Useful Alternative to the Transfemoral Approach

Justin Paul Gnanaraj and Jeff Redleene

Introduction

Vascular access complications are common after transfemoral percutaneous coronary intervention and diagnostic coronary angiography and include hematoma, arterial access site bleeding, retroperitoneal hemorrhage & pseudoaneurysm formation[1].They extend the hospital stay, result in transfusion of blood products, often also necessitating interruption of antiplatelet medications & peripheral vascular procedures that have their own risks. Increased risk of death occurs in patients with increasing severity of bleeding following PCI [2](fig 1). Steps to decrease bleeding and vascular complication rates in patients undergoing PCI and coronary angiography which include moving to default radial access.

Women & Transradial PCI

Bleeding is the most important and common complication of PCI. Bleeding is directly related to mortality. Women are at high risk of bleeding and access site complications following PCI when compared to men[1,3-5]. Though radial access PCI has been shown to reduce vascular and bleeding complications after PCI, women are less often offered radial access during PCI. Radial artery access is technically more challenging in women because women have smaller radial arteries than men. Saito et al found that 20% of men and 40% of women have internal diameter of radial artery smaller than the external diameter of a 6 Fr sheath[6]. They also have a greater rate of radial artery spasm[6] (Please refer to Table 6.1, Chapter 6, "Role of Colour Doppler Ultrasound in Transradial Interventions" for further details.), resulting in failure of procedure & crossover to femoral approach[7]. Women tend to be shorter than men. It has been shown that shorter the person higher the transradial intervention (TRI) failure.

Further it is noted that, lesser number of women have been enrolled in the trials comparing radial with femoral access[9]. It is known that female sex itself is an independent risk factor for major bleeding and so the use of radial access is warranted for PCI since it reduces this risk of major bleeding.[5,8]

Data on Radial Access in Women so far: SAFE PCI Trial

Three prospective studies have been published showing the comparative data on women undergoing radial access procedures with those undergoing femoral access procedures, and of which only the SAFE PCI trial enrolled only women, while the other two trials published the subgroup data (Figure 18.1).

SAFE PCI trial[9], was a multi-center, prospective, open-label, randomized control trial that compared radial and femoral artery access in women undergoing coronary angiogram with a plan of doing PCI if necessary either electively or after acute myocardial infarction (AMI). The study was terminated early due to lower rates of bleeding and vascular complications.

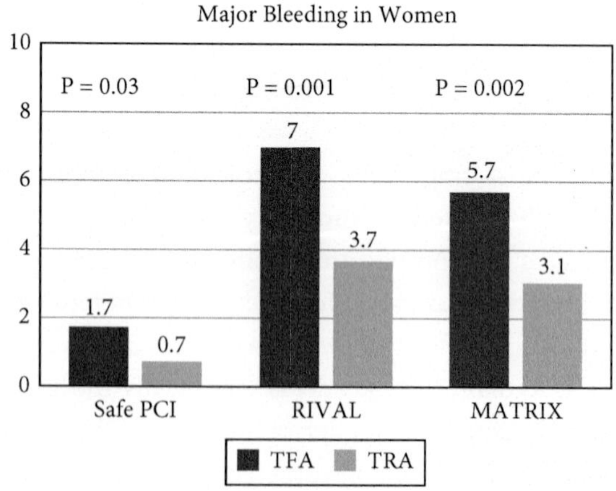

Figure 18.1 Major bleeding with trans femoral vs radial approach in women.

The crossover rate from radial to femoral access in this study was 6.7%. In the PCI subgroup, there was no difference in the rate of access-site complication. However in the entire cohort of patients who underwent coronary angiogram, there was a significant decrease in vascular and bleeding complications using the radial approach[9]. Women had a high rate of cross- over to femoral access, which was attributed to smaller radial artery diameters in women and higher concomitant radial artery spasm.[10,11]

Radial Versus Femoral Access for Coronary Intervention trial[12] was a large trial that randomised 7021 patients with ACS going for coronary angiography and PCI to radial vs femoral access and showed that radial access significantly reduced, major vascular complications, without any difference in the primary composite outcome[12]. This trial had a prespecified subgroup of 1861 women. A comparison of outcomes in the women subgroup was done with the 5,160 men enrolled in the trial. Women were twice as likely to require a crossover to alternate access compared to men (11.1% in women & 6.3% in men). Radial artery spasm was the commonest reason for this (9.5% in women vs. 3.3% in men; $p < 0.001$). PCI was equally successful in men & women, irrespective of the access site. However, major vascular complications rates were higher in women (4.7% vs. 1.7%; $p < 0.0001$) irrespective of the access site. Female sex itself was an independent risk factor of major vascular complications, with a hazard ratio of 2.4. Radial access was seen to prevent more vascular complications in women than in men. The number needed to treat (NNT) to prevent one vascular complication is 33 in women, while 49 for women.

MATRIX Study

MATRIX study was a prospective study of radial versus femoral access in 8084 patients with ACS of whom 2232 were women. The recently published subgroup analysis of 1071 radial access and 1161 femoral access in women showed that radial access significantly reduced the composite end point of death, MI and stroke9% vs 12% (P=0.019) and access site bleeding [3% vs 6% [P = 0.0016). Transradial approach was found better than transfemoral approach in women in all outcomes (Please see Chapter 19).[13]

Radial Access in Women: Unresolved Issues

The available studies do have certain limitations. Most of the studies so far, were not powered to assess differences between sexes & randomization was not stratified according to sex.

RIVAL and MATRIX data were from sub-group analysis, though RIVAL was a pre-specified sub group analysis. SAFE PCI study did not include women, and it had to be terminated prematurely and it was not powered enough to show benefit of either approach during PCI. Safety and Efficacy of Femoral Access Versus Radial for Primary Percutaneous Coronary Intervention in ST-Elevation Myocardial Infarction trial [SAFARI STEMI] study [15,16] randomized men & women presenting with STEMI to radial versus femoral access. (Please refer to Chapter 17(ii) for the SAFARI STEMI Study and Editorial Comments)

Bivalirudin is a direct thrombin inhibitor, which has been shown to decrease bleeding risk in patients undergoing PCI[14].

In SAFARI STEMI[15] study bivalirudin was used as the anticoagulant. Please see Chapter 17(ii), Corollary to Chapter 17: SAFARI STEMI study update and editorial comment" pages 399–402, for further details.

The available data on radial access in reducing vascular complications in women undergoing PCI & coronary angiography & PCI comes from experienced radial access operators (please see Chapter 10, pages 230–238, for further details). It is important to remember that data from several studies support that, if performed by experienced operators, radial approach is superior to the femoral approach[12]. The results may not be applicable to operators who are not well versed with radial access.

Conclusion

Even though transradial access remains technically challenging in women with a higher failure rate, it reduces the vascular and bleeding complications. The benefit is observed more in women than observed in men. The use of ultrasound to assess and choose the appropriate forearm artery (please see Chapter 6), the choice of low profile sheaths, appropriate puncture techniques, and medications is likely to improve the success rate of trans-radial access in women and thus reduce the morbidity and mortality of PCI in women.

References

1. Moscucci M., Foa K.A.A., Cannon C.P., *et al. (2003) Predictors of major bleeding in acute coronary syndromes: the Global Registry of Acute Coronary Events. Eur Heart J* **24**:1815–1823.
2. *Mehran R., Pocock S., Nikolsky E., et al.* (2011) Impact of bleeding on mortality after percutaneous coronary intervention: results from a patient-level pooled analysis of the REPLACE-2 (Randomized Evaluation of PCI Linking Angiomax to Reduced Clinical Events), ACUITY (Acute Catheterization and Urgent Intervention Triage Strategy), and HORIZONS-AMI (Harmonizing Outcomes With Revascularization and Stents in Acute Myocardial Infarction) trials. J Am CollCardiolIntv **4**:654–664.
3. *Lansky A.J., Hochman J.S., Ward P.A., et al.* (2005) Percutaneous coronary intervention and adjunctive pharmacotherapy in women: a statement of healthcare professionals from the American Heart Association. Circulation **111**:940–953.
4. Doyle B.J., Ting H.H., Bell M.R., *et al. (2008) Major femoral bleeding complications after percutaneous coronary intervention: incidence, predictors, and impact on long-term survival among 17, 901 patients treated at Mayo Clinic from 1994 to 2005.J Am CollCardiolIntv* **1**:202–209.
5. *Mrdovic I., Savic L., Asanin M., et al.* (2013) Sex-related analysis of short-and long-term clinical outcomes and bleeding among patients treated with primary percutaneous coronary intervention: an evaluation of the RISK-PCI data. Can J Cardiol**29**:1097–1103.
6. *Saito S., Ikei H., Hosokawa G., Tanaka S.* (1999) Influence of the ratio between radial artery inner diameter and sheath outer diameter on radial artery flow after transradial coronary intervention. Catheter CardiovascInterv **46**:173–178.
7. *Dehghani P., Mohammad A., Bajaj R., et al.* (2009) Mechanism and predictors of failed transradial approach for percutaneous coronary interventions. J Am CollCardiolIntv 2:1057–1064.
8. Pristipino C, Pelliccia F, Granatelli A, et al. Comparison of access-related bleeding complications in women versus men undergoing percutaneous coronary catheterization using the radial versus femoral artery. Am J Cardiol 2007;99: 1216–21.
9. *Rao S.V., Hess C.N., Barham B.*, al. (2014) A registry-based randomized trial comparing radial and femoral approaches in women undergoing percutaneous coronary intervention: the SAFE-PCI for Women (Study of Access Site for Enhancement of PCI for Women) trial. J Am CollCardiol Intv7:857–867.
10. *Chugh1 S, Chugh Y.* Transradial PCI in Women: Zeroing in on Crossovers. JACC Cardiovasc Interv. 2015 Apr 20;8(4):638. doi: 10.1016/j.jcin.2014.12.230. PMID: 25907091
11. *Connie N. Hess, Mitchell W. Krucoff, Sunil V. Rao.* Reply: Transradial PCI in Women: Zeroing in on Crossovers, JACC: Cardiovascular Interventions, Volume 8, Issue 4, 2015, Page 639, ISSN 1936-8798, https://doi.org/10.1016/j.jcin.2015.01.010.
12. *Jolly S.S., Cairns J., Niemela K., et al.* (2011) Radial versus femoral access for coronary angiography and intervention in patients with acute coronary syndromes (RIVAL): a randomised, parallel group, multicentre trial. Lancet **377**:1409–1420.

13. Giuseppe Gargiulo MD, Sara Ariotti MD, Pascal Vranckx MD, PhD, Sergio Leonardi MD, *et al. Impact of Sex on Comparative Outcomes of Radial Versus Femoral Access in Patients With Acute Coronary Syndromes Undergoing Invasive Management: Data From the Randomized MATRIX-Access Trial* J Am Coll Cardiol Intv. 2018 Jan, 11 (1) 36–50.
14. *Stone G.W., McLaurin B.T., Cox D.A., et al. (2006)* Bivalirudin for patients with acute coronary syndromes. N Engl J Med 355:2203–2216.
15. Le May M, Wells G, So D, et al. Safety and Efficacy of Femoral Access vs Radial Access in ST-Segment Elevation Myocardial Infarction: The SAFARI-STEMI Randomized Clinical Trial. *JAMA Cardiol.* 2020;5(2):126–134. doi:10.1001/jamacardio.2019.4852
16. Yashasvi Chugh, Sunita Chugh, Sanjay Kumar Chugh, Post-the SAFARI STEMI study: Is there still a debate on radial vs. femoral access in STEMI?, Indian Heart Journal, Volume 72, Issue 5, 2020, Pages 466–468, ISSN 0019-4832, https://doi.org/10.1016/j.ihj.2020.08.006 (https://www.sciencedirect.com/science/article/pii/S0019483220301905).

19

Complications of Transradial Access: Management and Prevention

Yashasvi Chugh, Sunita Chugh, and Sanjay Kumar Chugh

Background

Complications related to radial artery access are rare in transradial procedures and can be prevented with training and appropriate selection of hardware, minimizing manipulation and exchange of catheters. Training is important before a cardiologist takes on radial procedures independently.

Pre-procedure planning helps minimize access artery spasm and could reduce risk of radial artery occlusion (RAO). The role of colour Doppler ultrasound in pre-procedure assessment of arm arteries has been amply illustrated[1] and by allowing assessment of radial artery diameter (RAD), a near 1:1 sheath:artery size ratio can help minimize spasm in radial artery. It also helps reduce complications such as extravasation while negotiating cubital loops by pre-procedure detection of cubital loops or anomalies, allowing the operator to choose an alternative access, i.e. contralateral radial or ipsilateral ulnar artery. Also, avulsion of radial artery reported with 8F[2–4] can be prevented by knowing the RAD and avoiding large bore sheath and catheters in smaller radials especially radial artery (RA) ≤ 1.7 mm.

Radial Artery Spasm (RAS)

Radial artery spasm (RAS), which is reported to occur in 15–30% of patients after radial artery catheterization,[5,6] is lower when sheath radial artery mismatch is reduced by selecting sheath according to a sheath sizing protocol based on RAD assessed by pre-procedure ultrasound.[1] Radial artery (RA)-sheath mismatch has been shown to be the strongest independent predictor of RAS (OR 4.7, 95% CI: 1.35–16.5, p = 0.009).[7,8] RAS is better prevented than treated. A spasm grading, first proposed by Chugh et al.,[1] is given below. It provides options of treatment and crossover to alternate access based on severity of spasm.

Spasm Grades

Grade-1: Mild pain and spasm, not restricting catheter movement; no pause required and only 1 dose of either or both intra-arterial 5 mg diltiazem and/or 0.5 mg intravenous midazolam given to tackle RAS (Chugh et al.[1]).

Grade-2: Mild pain and spasm, not restricting catheter movement; no pause required but 2 or more additional doses of intra-arterial 5 mg diltiazem and/or 0.5 mg intravenous midazolam given to tackle RAS.

Grade-3: Moderate pain and spasm, restricting catheter movement, necessitating pause required before spasm settles and procedure can be resumed. Even after two additional doses of 5 mg intra-arterial diltiazem and/or 1 mg intravenous midazolam.

Grade-4: Severe pain and spasm disallowing any catheter movement despite repeated intra-arterial diltiazem and intravenous midazolam, necessitating crossover to alternate access.

Risk Factors for RAS

- RA pulse grading ≤2 (OR: 8, 95% CI: 1.8–36.2, p = 0.007)[7,8]
- RA size[1]
- Low body mass index (BMI)
- Female gender (OR: 10.6, 95% CI: 2.2–51.2, p = 0.03)
- Repeated multiple puncture attempts
- Pain
- Diabetes mellitus
- Elderly
- Guide catheter use (OR: 25.8, 95% CI: 6.1–108.5, p<0.001)

RAS is a common complication associated with radial access and is better prevented than treated because spasm begets spasm, and once the vicious cycle of spasm is initiated, often the procedure becomes delayed, as catheter manipulation becomes difficult and procedure failure leading to crossover to alternative access often becomes necessary.

The strategy to prevent RAS begins as soon as the patient walks into the catheterization laboratory as short stature has been found to be associated with smaller RAD, puncture failure and spasm.[7–9] Relation to wrist size is debatable as no relation exists between radial size and wrist size.

Figures 19.1(a–c, c') illustrate how in a short-statured woman, with a 1.4 mm right RA a combination of grade 3 RAS at one end and tortuous right subclavian at the other, combined to cause a 'candy wrapper' effect on a 6F Cordis™ JR 3.5 guide while torquing it for engaging the right coronary artery for angioplasty. The angioplasty had to be completed via the left radial (Figures 19.1 d,e).

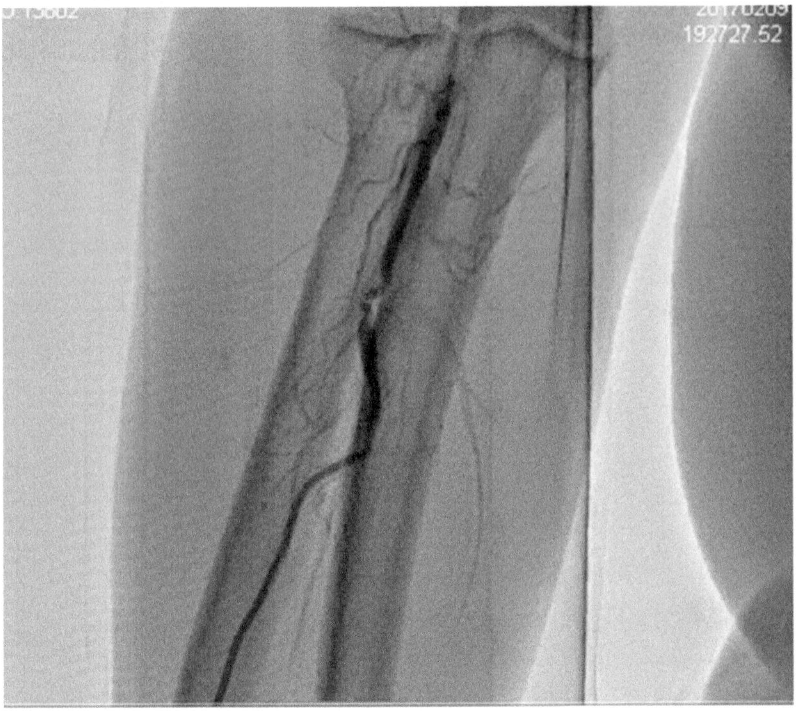

Figure 19.1a Severe spasm (grade 3) in proximal radial artery with a short segment of tortuosity.

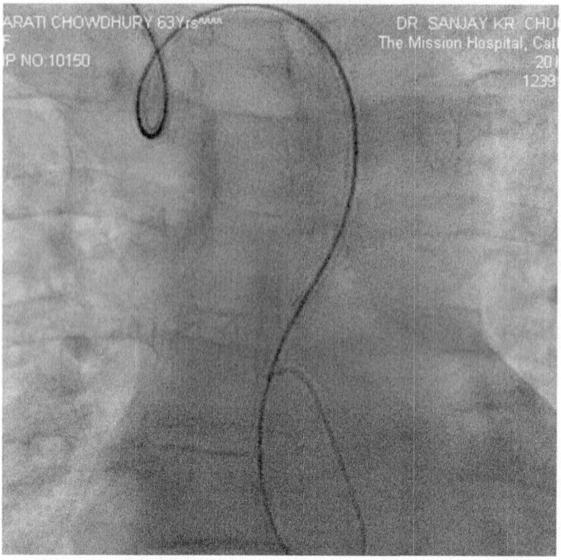

Figure 19.1b Severe subclavian tortuosity and a JR guide being advanced over a 0.035 Dacron angiography guide wire.

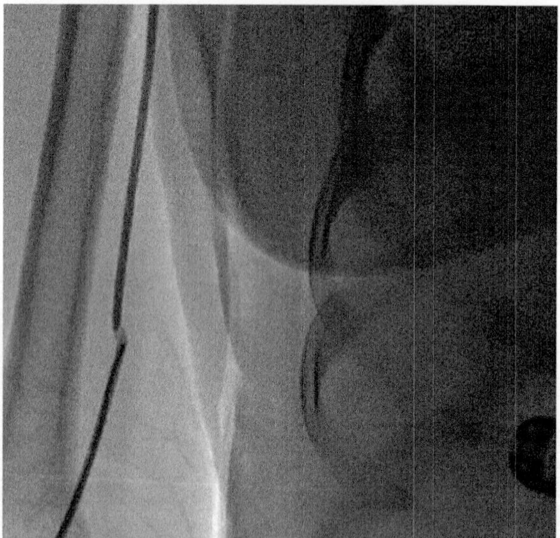

Figure 19.1c A kink in the body of the guide catheter. A consequence of resistance point Please also see figure 19.1c(i).

1. Proximally at the small diameter radial artery with severe spasm in it.
2. Resistance point distally in the tortuous subclavian. As a result, the torque given to the Judkins Right guiding catheter doesn't get transmitted to the catheter tip and instead causes kink in the body of the guide. This has been described by us as the 'candy wrapper effect'.

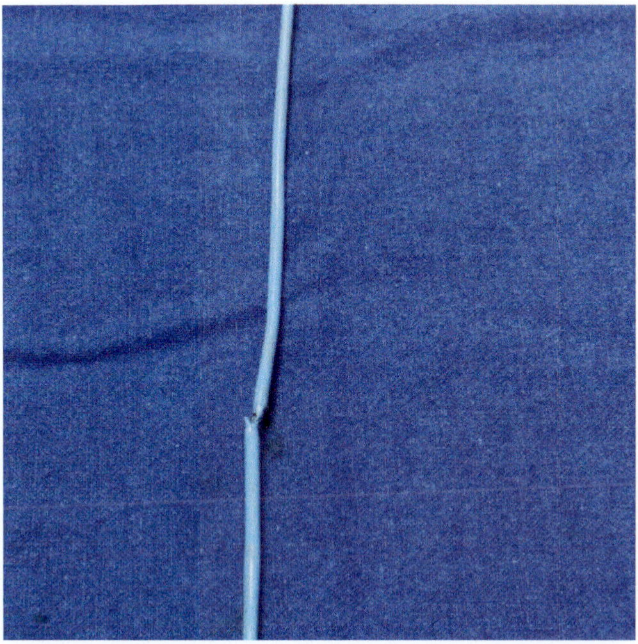

Figure 19.1c(i) Continued

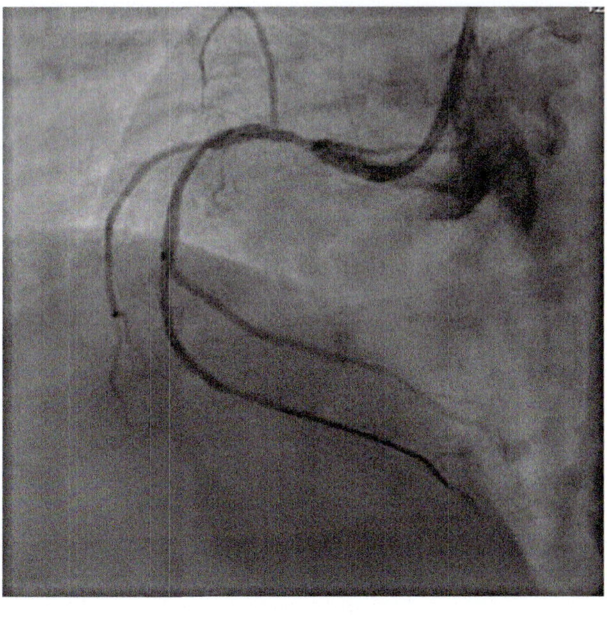

Figure 19.1d Guide catheter hooks the Right Coronary Artery (RCA) using left radial access. The figure shows stent being positioned after pre dilatation.

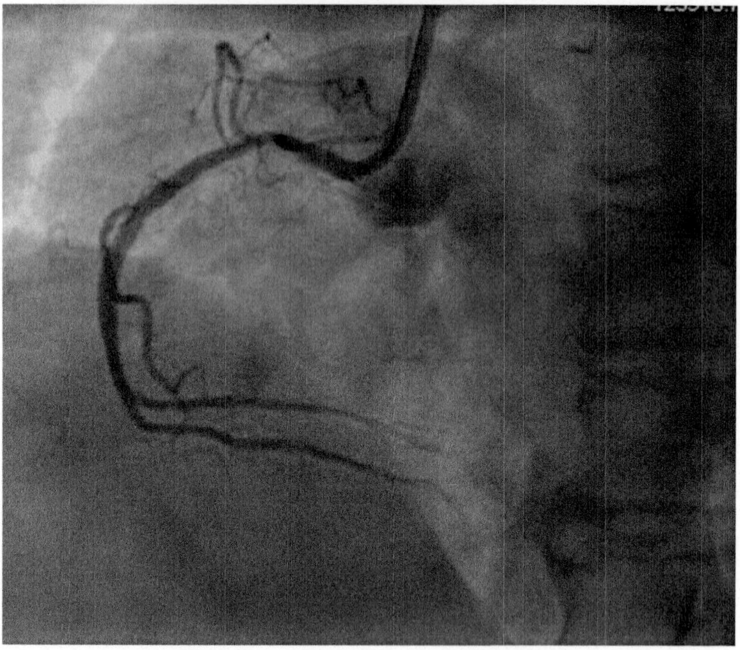

Figure 19.1e Final angiogram shows TIMI 3 flow in RCA.

RAS can be prevented by the use of proper local anaesthesia, appropriate sheath to RA ratio (1:1) avoiding mismatch with radial diameter, as per sheath sizing protocol[1–4] (Please refer to Figure 10.3, Chapter 10.) spasmolytic cocktail[5] use after sheath insertion and with each catheter exchange as well as before sheath removal; shorter hydrophilic arterial sheaths[10] and/or catheters, minimizing catheter exchange and manipulation,[11] and anti-anxiety medication as recommended by both the European Society of Cardiology (ESC) and Society for Cardiovascular Angiography and Interventions (SCAI) guidelines,[12,13] though Astarcioglu and his colleagues found no difference in the occurrence of RAS between midazolam treatment group (20%) and the control group (21.3%).[14] Routine use of spasmolytic cocktail significantly decreases incidence of RAS.[5]

Spasmolytic Cocktail

With the use of spasmolytic cocktail of nitroglycerine and verapamil,[15] RAS decreased from 22% to 8% ($p = 0.02$); in another study, verapamil was found to be more effective than phentolamine (RAS 13.2 versus 23.2%, respectively).[16] Diltiazem is an effective alternative[17] to verapamil. A combination of verapamil and molsidomine has been found to be more effective than either given alone.[18] Intra-arterial nicorandil[19] and nitroprusside have also been used successfully and have been found to be equally effective.

Spasmolytics commonly used include 1–5 mg of intra-arterial injection of verapamil or diltiazem, and/or nitroglycerine.

What to Do when RAS Develops?

1. Sedation and analgesia: injectable midazolam and fentanyl can be injected intravenously in small doses with due caution for those with respiratory disorders and obstructive sleep apnea as the latter can desaturate rapidly with sedation.[20]
2. Intra-arterial diltiazem or verapamil in doses of 3–5 mg, sometimes combined with 50–100 mcg of injectable nitroglycerine and or Inj Nicorandil 2 mg intra-arterially.
3. If occurrence of RA spasm after sheath insertion (Figure 19.2a) limits advancement of a 0.038 or 0.035" angiographic Dacron or Terumo guidewire then in addition to intra-arterial spasmolytic, an angioplasty wire can be used to cross the spasm segment (Figure 19.2b). A 4F diagnostic catheter can track over it. Once the 4F diagnostic catheter reaches the ascending aorta, the angioplasty wire can be changed for a Dacron 0.035" wire and an appropriate 5F guiding can be advanced over it for completing the angioplasty (Figures 19.2a–i).
4. With grade ≥3 or significant spasm:
   (a) Pause for a minute or two
   (b) Downsize catheters to a lower French (F) size
   (c) Use exchange length (260 cm) 0.035" or 0.038" Teflon or glide guide wire for exchange of catheters because with the shorter 180 cm guide wire, the wire often comes back too far into the segment of spasm in the access artery making re-advancement of the guidewire difficult.

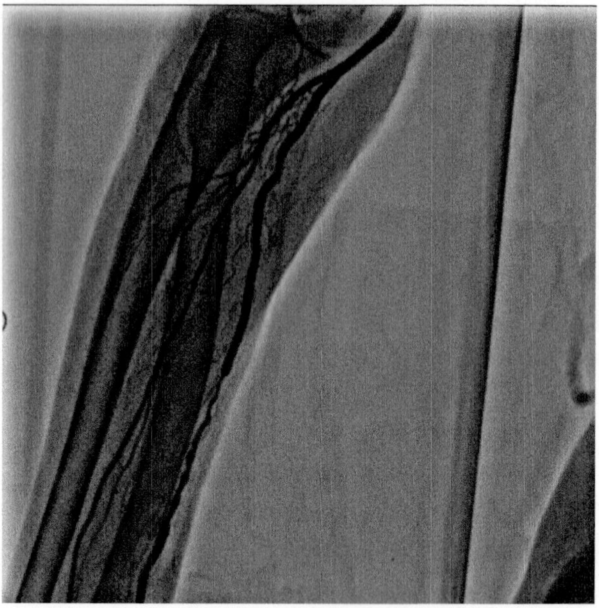

Figure 19.2a A long segment of spasm and disease in the radial artery. Distal trans-radial access used (radial artery punctured in the snuff box).

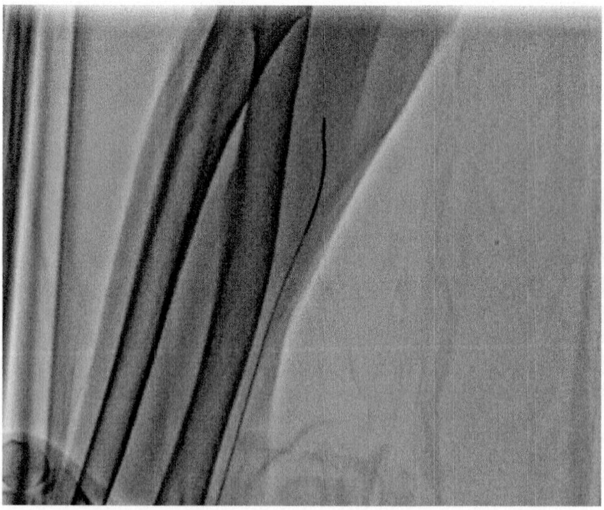

Figure 19.2b Angioplasty wire is advanced through spasm and disease of the radial artery.

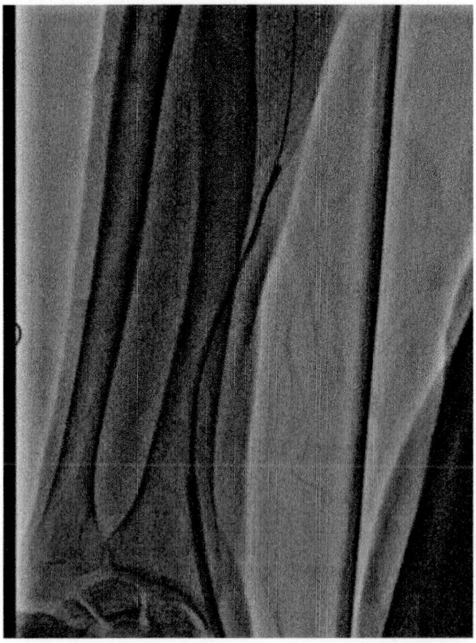

Figure 19.2c 4F diagnostic catheter tracks on the angioplasty wire.

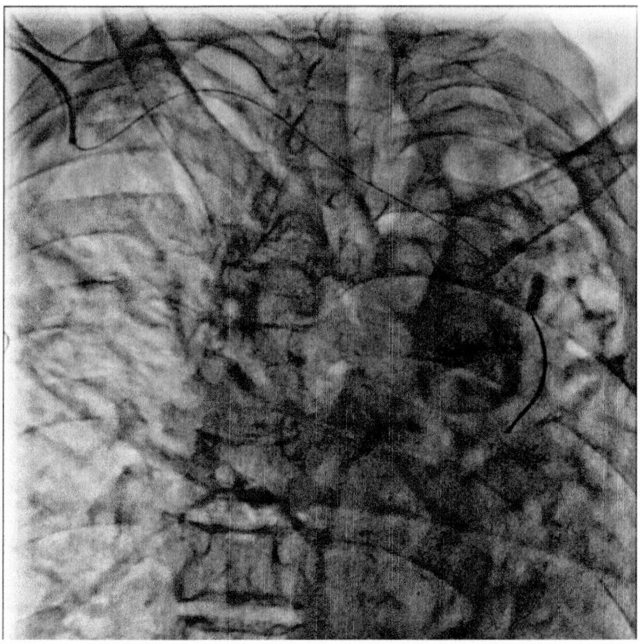

Figure 19.2d The diagnostic catheter and angioplasty wire reach the descending aorta.

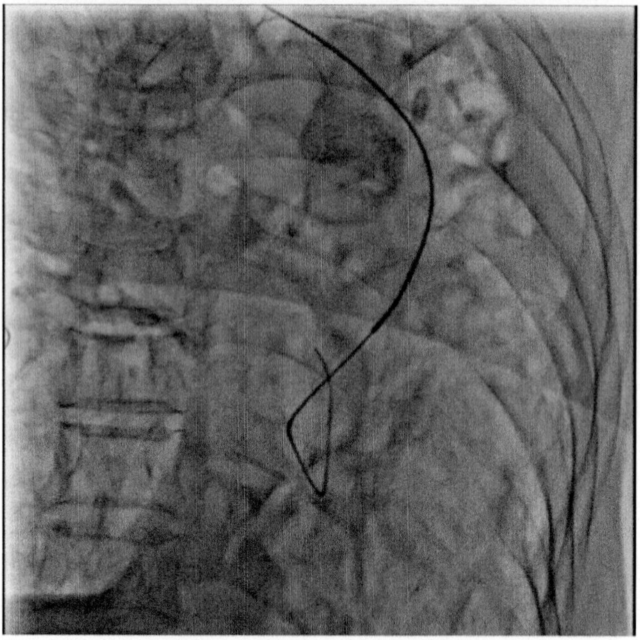

Figure 19.2e Angioplasty wire is exchanged for a Dacron 0.035 angiography guide wire.

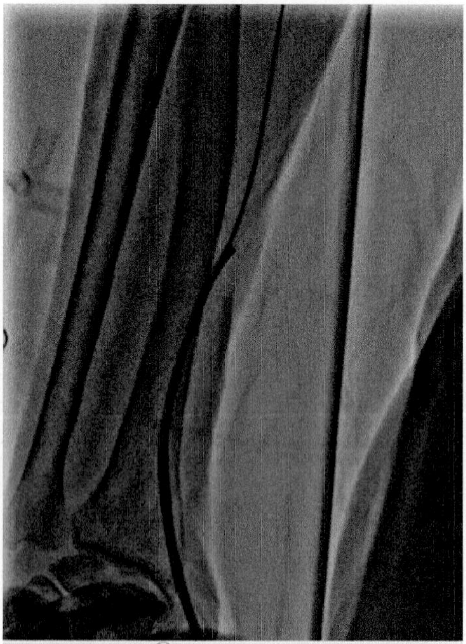

Figure 19.2f 5F, JR guiding catheter now tracks on the 0.035 angiography guide wire.

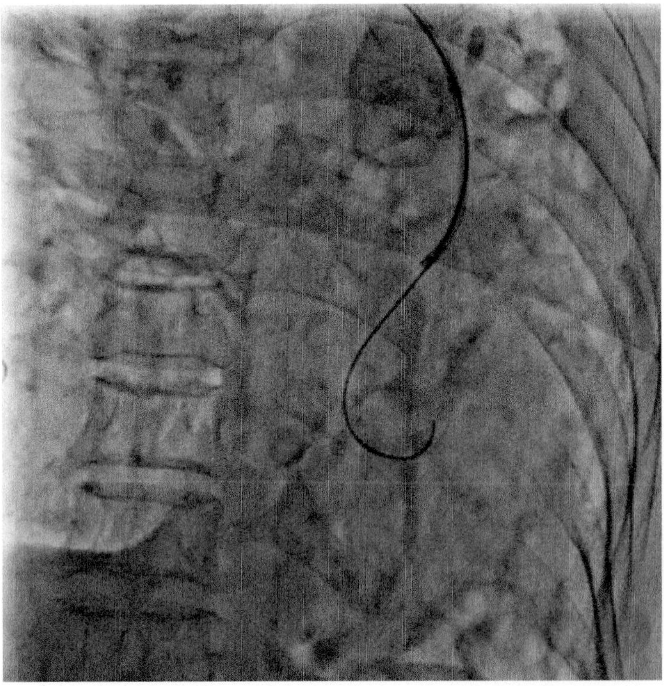

Figure 19.2g The guide catheter reaches the ascending aorta.

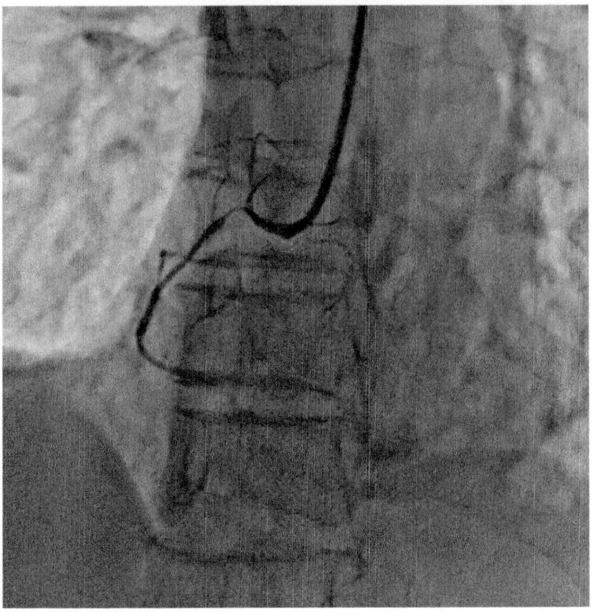

Figure 19.2h The JR guide engages the RCA. Critical stenosis is noted in the proximal RCA.

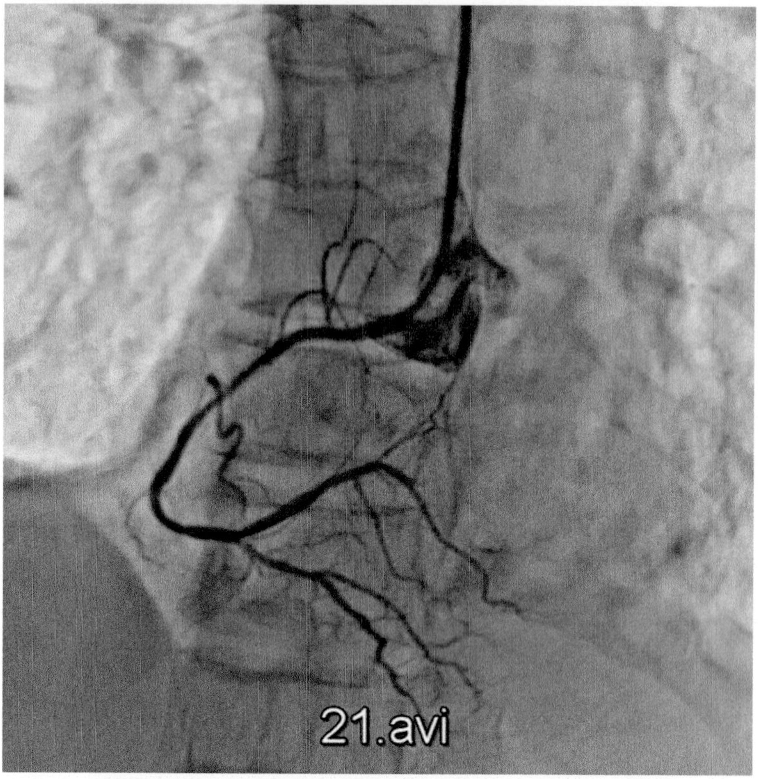

Figure 19.2i Final TIMI 3 flow post successful deployment of stent.

Prevention of RAS:

Use of mild sedative such as midazolam given to patient intravenously in small doses.

Routine use of hydrophilic hardware (5-6Fr short sheath).

Routine use of intra-arterial spasmolytic cocktail after sheath insertion, with each catheter exchange and prior to sheath removal.

Pre-procedure ultrasound to measure RAD to choose sheath size to minimize mismatch between RAD and sheath size preferable for small diameter radials ≤1.7 or when use of large bore ≥ 7F sheath is contemplated.

Prior planning of procedure with appropriate choice of catheter curve size based on aortic root size[19] can help minimize catheter exchanges and radial spasm.

Although rough idea of radial size can be had with palpation of radial pulse before puncture; use of pre-procedure ultrasound of arm arteries (PPUAA), to assess diameter and other abnormalities of radial and ulnar arteries on both sides, the incidence of grade-3-4[1] or significant spasm can be reduced significantly. PPUAA allows selection of the straightest and the biggest artery for access.[1]

Radial Artery Occlusion (RAO)

Post-procedure RAO is reported in 2–18%.[19,20] RAO can be best confirmed by using colour Doppler ultrasound[1] (Figures 19.3a and 19.3b) because clinical exam can be fallacious, although compared to feeling the radial pulse palpating the radial pulse with ulnar compression is a better method of assessing patency.

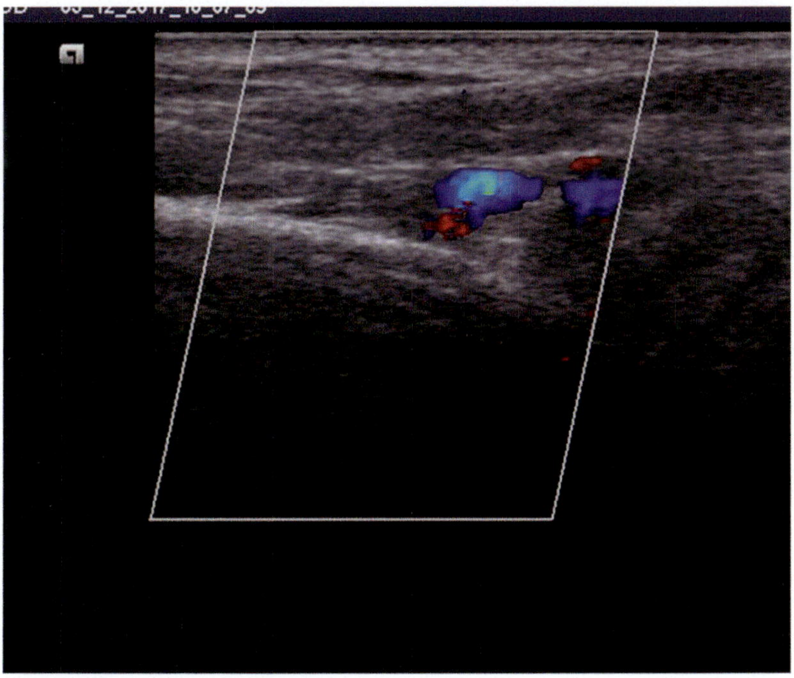

Figure 19.3a Blocked radial artery on colour Doppler.
(Courtesy Dr Sunita Chugh, FMRI, Gurugram)

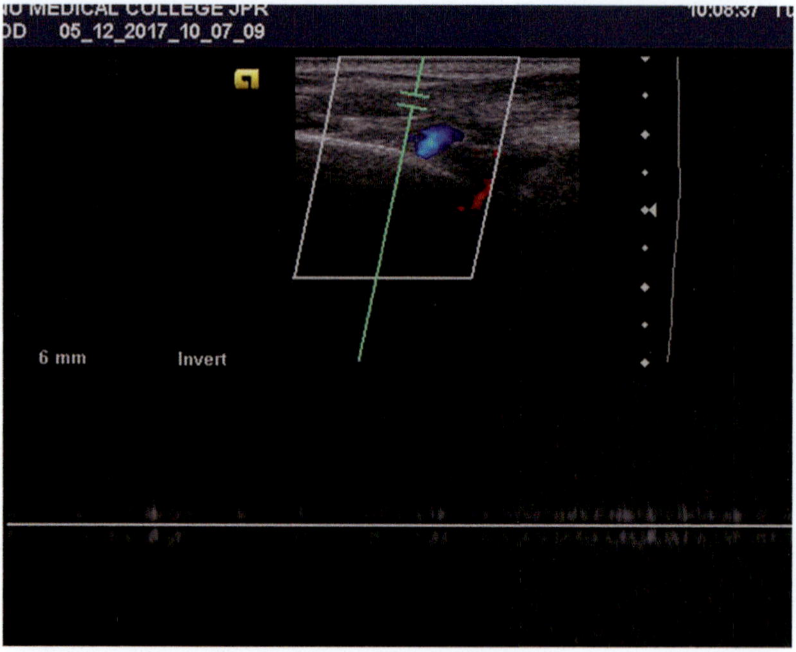

Figure 19.3b Blocked radial artery on pulse Doppler.
(Courtesy Dr Sunita Chugh, FMRI, Gurugram)

The Risk Factors Associated with RAO

1. Inadequate anticoagulation

70 IU/Kg Heparin is recommended in patients undergoing diagnostic catheterization, The incidence of RAO dropped significantly with use of 5,000 IU of heparin compared to 2,000 units of heparin (5.8% versus 2.9%, $p = 0.17$).[21]

2. RA: Sheath size mismatch[22]

The incidence of RAO was 13% versus 4% with a Sheath/Catheter:RA ratio of >1 versus < 1 and RAO was $< 5\%$ with use of 6F but increased with larger sheath sizes.[23]

3. Haemostasis: compression method and time[19,20]

Non-occlusive compression during haemostasis has been shown to reduce RAO.[24–27] Various other factors such as intra-arterial spasmolytic use, number of catheter exchanges, RAS are known to play a role in RA occlusions. Prolonged compression increases risk of RAO.[21]

RAOs have been reported more with a RA diameter ≤1.7 mm versus >1.7 mm[28] and may merit definition as 'small arteries'.[29]

What to Do when RAO Happens?

Spontaneous recanalization occurs within one month in up to 50% cases of RAO.[21] When detected early, additional doses of heparin usually additional 1,000 IU (bolus) and compression of the ulnar for 20 minutes to 1 hour to increase flow through the radial is often enough to re-open the vessel.[1,21] Compression of the ulnar artery for one hour[22] and/or low-molecular-weight heparin. The latter given for four weeks has also been reported in an observational study to completely and partially re-canalize the occluded radial artery in 70% and 20%, respectively, in four weeks.[31]

The incidence of RAO can be minimized to 0.8% with appropriate anticoagulation, proper sheath selection, and avoiding prolonged high-pressure compression following the procedure.[1] A recent meta-analysis found that higher doses of heparin decreased the incidence of RAO (risk ratio 0.36, 95% CI: 0.17–0.76). Compression of ipsilateral ulnar artery for 60 min, reduced the incidence of RAO from 5.9% to 4.1% and 2.9% to 0.8% ($p = 0.03$), respectively, in the low-dose and high-dose heparin group.[32]

There are several case reports of dis-obliteration of RAO with balloon angioplasty; intra-thrombus infusion of abciximab use has also been described.[30]

No significant difference was reported in RAO with bivalirudin compared to heparin (3.5% bivalirudin, 7.0% heparin) 4–8 weeks after the procedure.[33,34]

How to diagnose RAO:

- Assessment of RA patency should be done post-procedure,
  - (i) Clinically by palpating radial artery pulse while compressing the ulnar artery.
  - (ii) Reverse Barbeau test.

(iii) Confirmation of RAO can be done using Colour Doppler ultrasound (Figure 19.3a,b).

How to prevent RAO:

- With adequate anticoagulation.
- With use of patent haemostasis.
- Smaller French size sheaths and catheters.
- Patent haemostasis requires close monitoring to watch for development of forearm haematoma which needs prompt treatment to prevent compartment syndrome.[20]
- Reducing duration of compression of the puncture site after sheath removal post procedure.
- Also, the addition of Tab Rivaroxaban 10mg x daily for 1 week to standard care (RIVARAD trial) reduced RAO by 50% (from 13% to 6.9% (p0.011)).

How to treat RAO:

- Occlude ipsilateral ulnar artery for up to one hour to improve radial artery patency, with additional dose of intravenous unfractionated heparin.
- Asymptomatic RAO requires observation alone as spontaneous recanalization occurs with time.

For symptomatic RAO: anticoagulation is recommended.[20,31] Rarely there can be thromboembolic digital infarct of the thumb or index finger following RA thrombus formation when adequate heparin is not given or sheath is not removed after procedure for prolonged period. This can be prevented by adequate heparinization, prompt removal of radial sheath after the catheterization procedure and practicing non-occlusive haemostasis.

3. Local access bleeding (5%): Local haematomas are usually ecchymoses only (Figure 19.4).

Reasons: Improper device application or device failure.

Prevention: Compression of the radial artery both proximal and distal to the puncture site must be performed because of retrograde flow from the palmar arch collaterals.

Too much pressure can lead to skin necrosis and pressure ulcer at site of radial access (Figure 19.5).

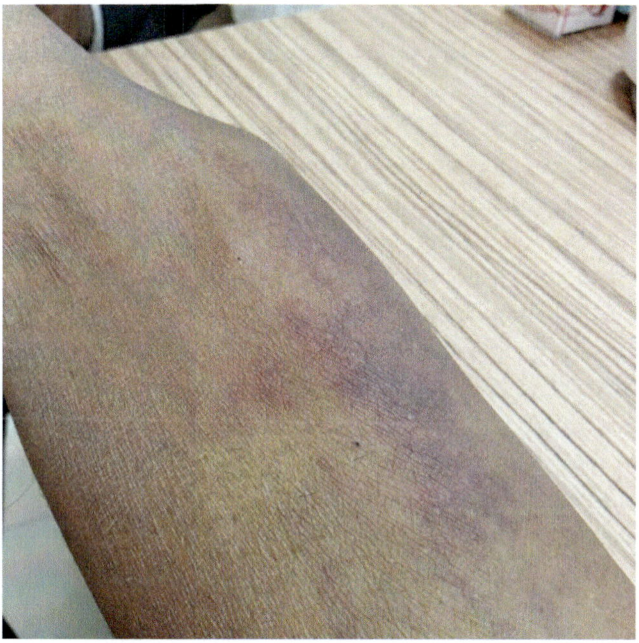

Figure 19.4 Local haematoma (ecchymosis) due to local access bleeding.

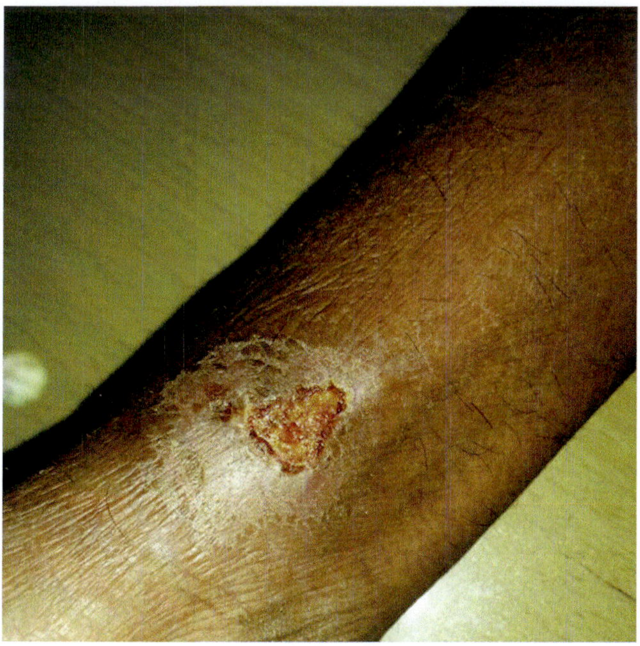

Figure 19.5 Pressure ulcer from excessive pressure at the puncture site.

4. Forearm Haematoma (3 per thousand): Bleeding remote from the access site, with perforation of a small side branch by the guidewire (Figure 19.6a). Extravasation in negotiating a cubital loop or a radial recurrent artery arising from a radial loop may also be responsible. For early detection of forearm haematoma because of bleeding remote from access site, the forearm proximal to access site must be palpated frequently to note for any hardness as compared to the feel at baseline or compared to contralateral forearm. This is important, especially after the haemostatic bandage is loosened or TR band is deflated to achieve non-occlusive haemostasis. Just observing for haematoma is not enough because a visible swelling in forearm is noticed only after significant collection of blood in the forearm has already happened. Early detection of a developing haematoma is crucial to prevent compartment syndrome. Once the haematoma is advanced, it becomes difficult to achieve haemostasis as the radial artery cannot be compressed adequately manually or with device.

(Figure 19.6b) shows a minor remote site bleed from guidewire injury. Haematoma was prevented by early detection and prompt compression.

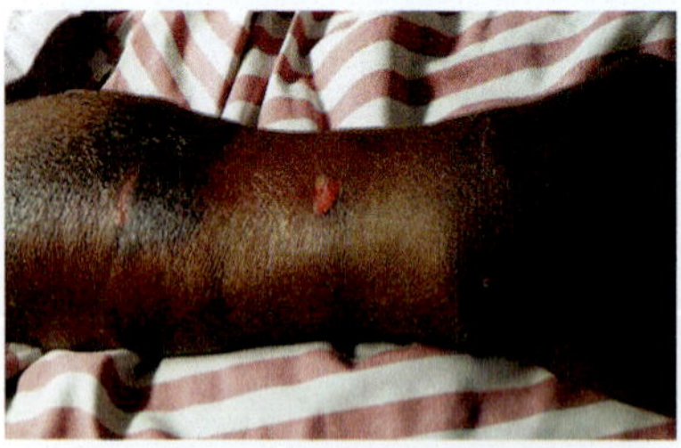

Figure 19.6a Forearm hematoma

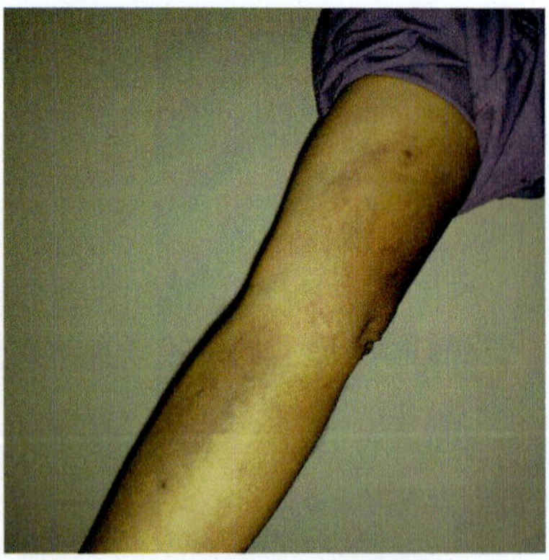

Figure 19.6b Forearm haematoma because of bleeding remote from access site.

Prevention of Forearm Haematoma from Remote Site Bleed

Performing a radial artery check arteriogram when any resistance to guide-wire or catheter insertion is encountered.

Treatment of Forearm Haematoma

Recognition of bleeding from remote site is important as haemostatic pressure must be applied to the area remote from the access site. Constant vigil is required by nursing staff assigned to post-procedure care of patients. As mentioned earlier, palpation of the forearm proximal to access site is mandatory immediately after the bandage or TR band is applied at puncture site and at frequent intervals thereafter to detect development of hardness in the forearm, which denotes development of haematoma from bleeding from remote sites. This is crucial especially after the TR band is deflated or bandage is loosened for non-occlusive haemostasis.

Gauze balls with elastic bandage along the course of the radial artery with compression bandage which selectively compresses the radial and spares the ulnar can be used to achieve haemostasis (Figure 19.7). Adequate hand perfusion is indicated by adequate waveform on SpO2 trace from a saturation probe on the ipsilateral index finger or thumb.

In addition, a sphygmomanometer cuff inflated to above systolic pressure (Figure 19.8) and intermittently deflated every 3 minutes for 10 seconds and then re-inflated helps compress the brachial artery.[7] Alternatively, the latter may be inflated to systolic pressure and then gradually released over a period of two hours.[19]

Sealing of a perforation with a long sheath is also an option, but this is rarely necessary.

Colour Doppler ultrasound can help localize the site of active bleed as well as can be used to confirm haemostasis (Figure 19.9).[19]

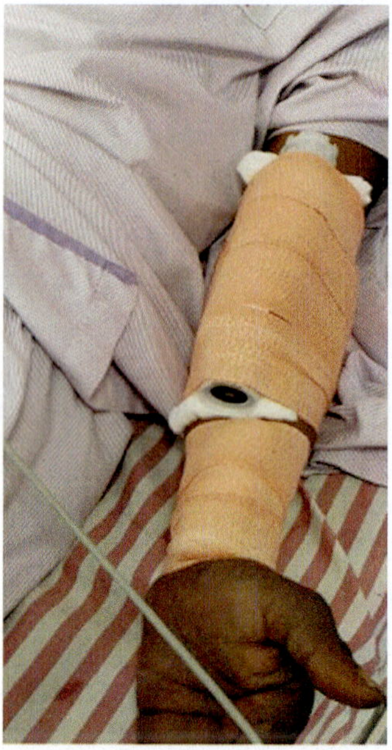

Figure 19.7 How gauze balls with elastic bandage placed along the course of radial artery are used to control bleeding from remote site, as soon as initial development of haematoma is detected.

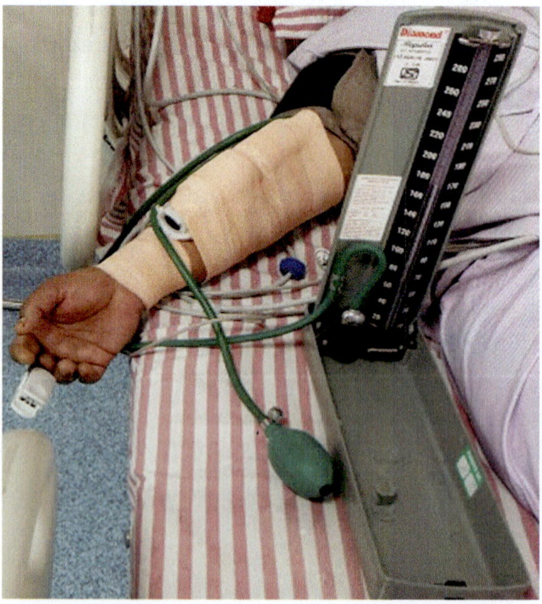

Figure 19.8 A sphygmomanometer cuff is inflated to systolic pressure and deflated intermittently to reduce bleeding remote from access site.

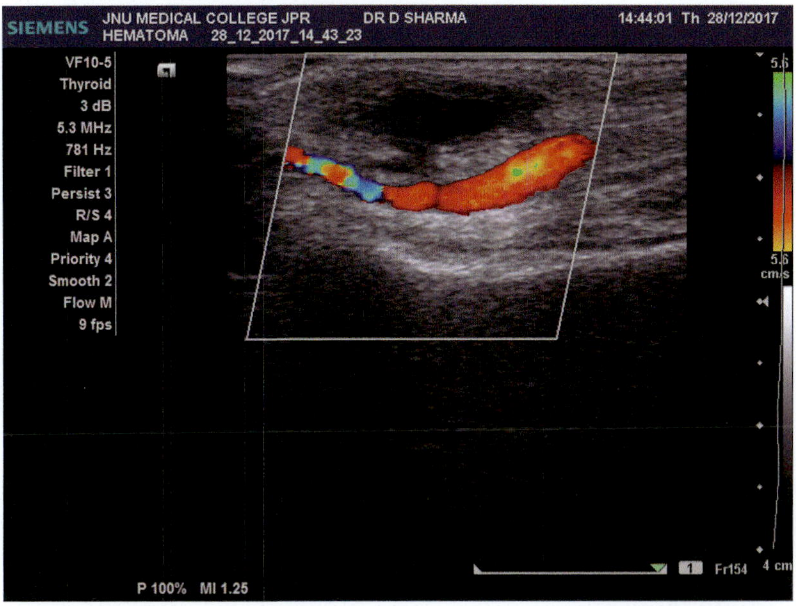

Figure 19.9 Colour Doppler used to confirm haemostasis. A non-communicating haematoma is noted anterior to the radial artery.
(Courtesy Dr Sunita Chugh, FMRI, Gurugram)

If radial artery perforation is detected while advancing a catheter, before doing an angioplasty, the guiding catheter can be advanced and the procedure completed, by which time the perforation usually seals off (Figures 19.10a and 19.10b). Compartment syndrome, the most dreaded complication of radial artery haemorrhage, is extremely rare and should be avoided at all costs by aggressive compression along the course of access artery as described earlier, close monitoring the bleed and, if in doubt, use of colour Doppler ultrasound to confirm that bleeding has stopped. No forearm bleed should be taken lightly for this reason.[19] Prolonged compression can increase the risk of RAO.

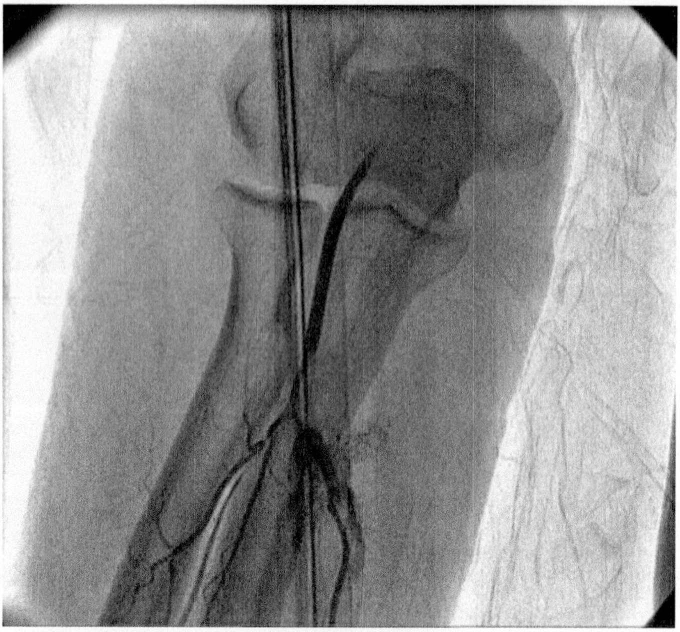

Figure 19.10a Extravasation from perforation in a radial artery.

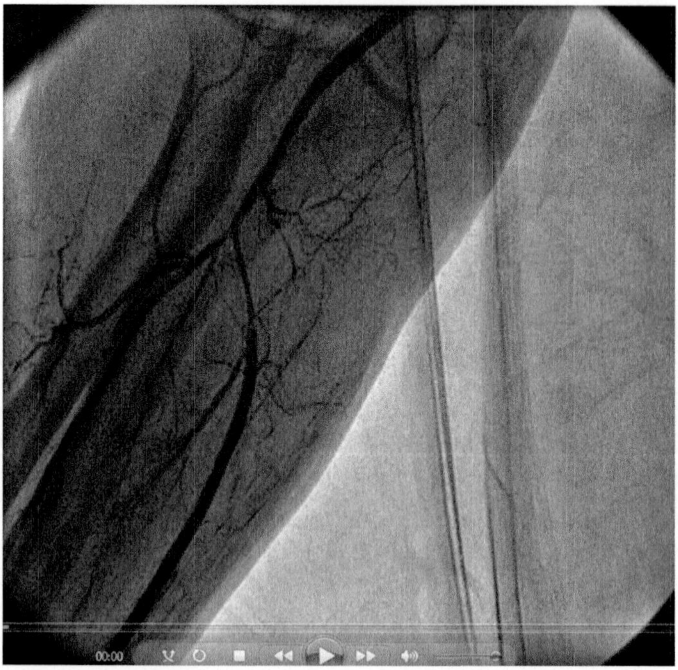

Figure 19.10b Perforation sealed off as seen in a check angiogram done after completion of coronary angioplasty procedure.

Compartment Syndrome of Forearm

In our experience of over 20,000 cases, because of care and vigilance as described earlier, we have not encountered compartment syndrome in any of our cases. Compartment syndrome is potentially life-threatening and anecdotes abound in literature. Hand ischaemia, gangrene are consequences; hence, prompt surgical decompression is urgently required.[35] Untreated, compartment syndrome can be potentially fatal.

Distal radial access can also be associated with complication of extravasation (Figure 19.11a), localized haematoma of dorsum of hand and palm (Figure 19.11b and c) as well as occlusion of distal radial (Figure 19.11d) or radial at wrist consequent to slow flow and flow reversal (Figure 19.11e) in distal radial. A typical bandage used by us for patients with extravasation in distal radial or with evolving haematoma of dorsum of hand or palm is shown in (Figure 19.11f).

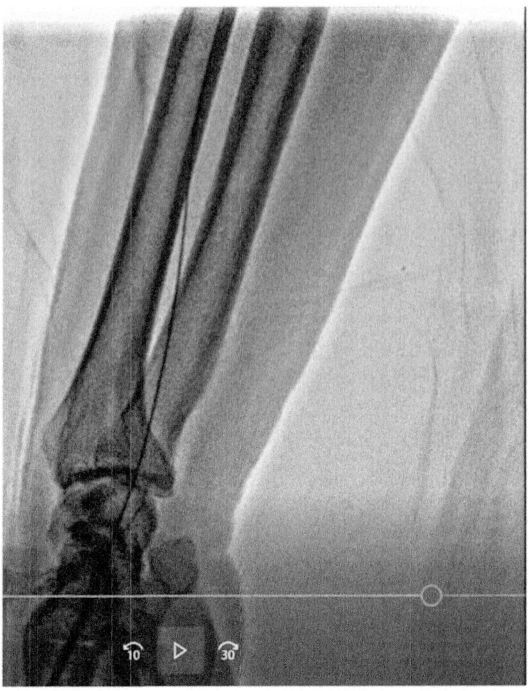

Figure 19.11a Extravasation during distal radial artery access.

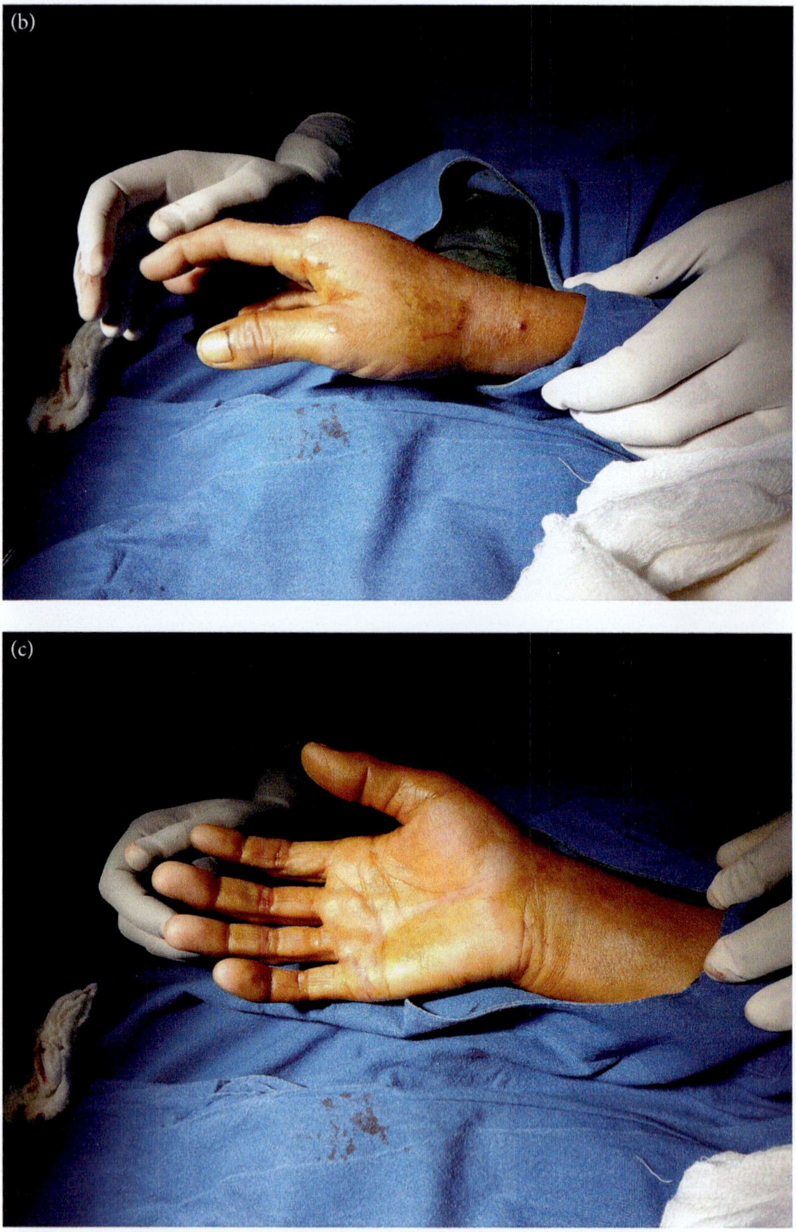

Figure 19.11b and c
Local haematoma of dorsum of hand and palm following distal transradial percutaneous coronary intervention.

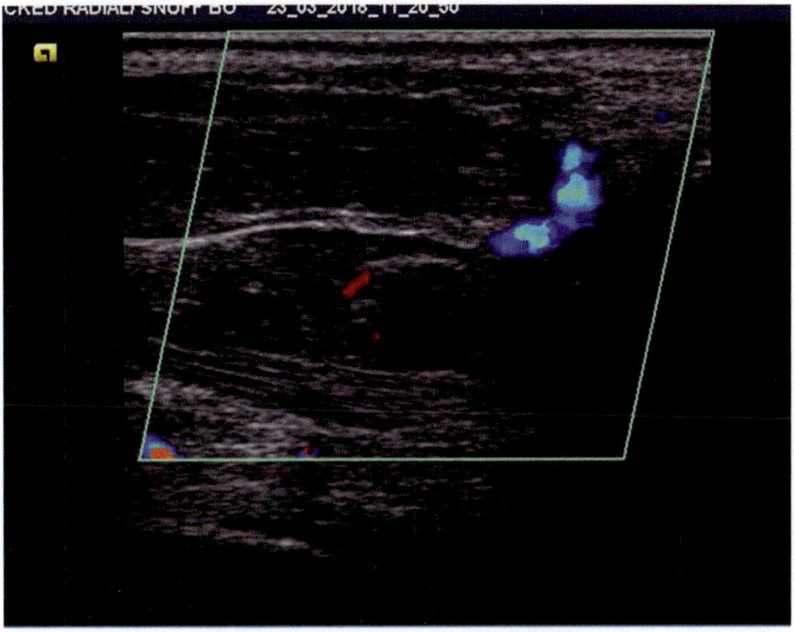

Figure 19.11d Occlusion of distal radial colour Doppler shows flow reversal.
(Courtesy Dr Sunita Chugh, FMRI, Gurugram)

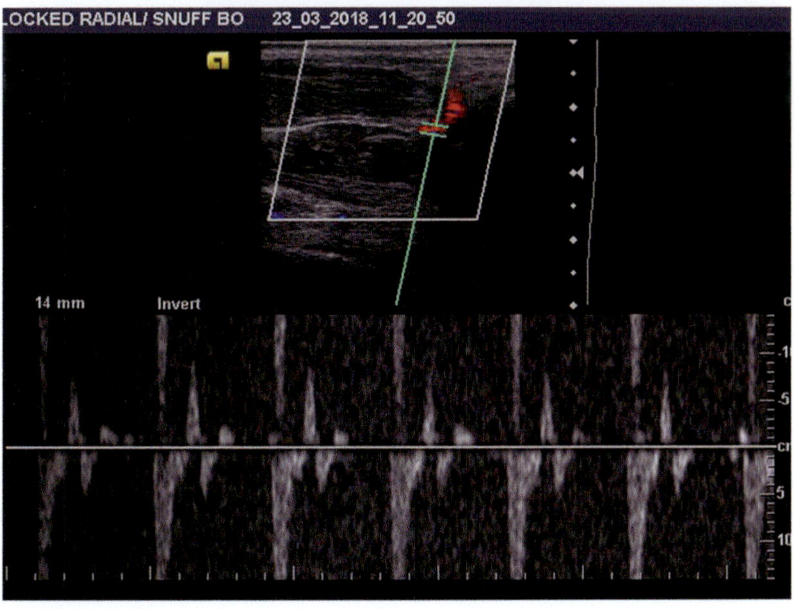

Figure 19.11e Occlusion of distal radial pulse Doppler shows flow reversal.
(Courtesy Dr Sunita Chugh, FMRI, Gurugram)

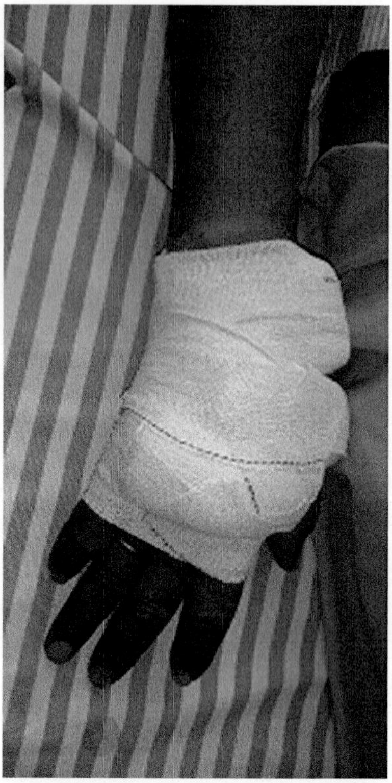

Figure 19.11f A typical bandage used by us for patients with extravasation in distal radial or with evolving haematoma of dorsum of hand or palm.

Miscellaneous Complications

Pseudo-aneurysm formation may rarely occur at the radial artery access site. In the only case that we had (1/14,330 cases), compression for 20 minutes led to occlusion of the pseudo-aneurysm (Figures 19.12a–c). Surgery, if required, is performed under local anaesthesia and is an out-patient procedure.

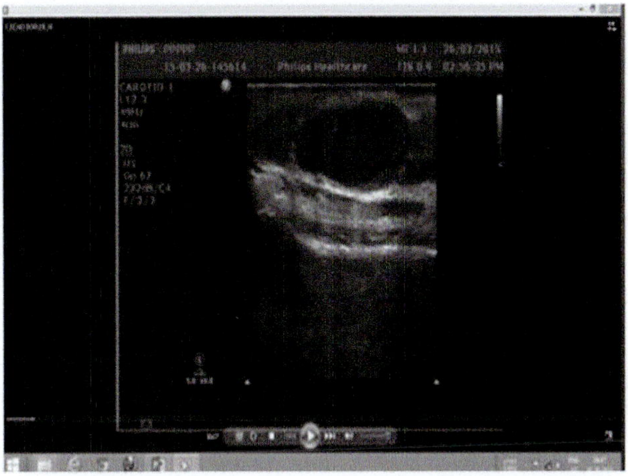

Figure 19.12a Pseudo-aneurysm at radial artery access site (2D ultrasound image). (Courtesy Dr Sunita Chugh, FMRI, Gurugram)

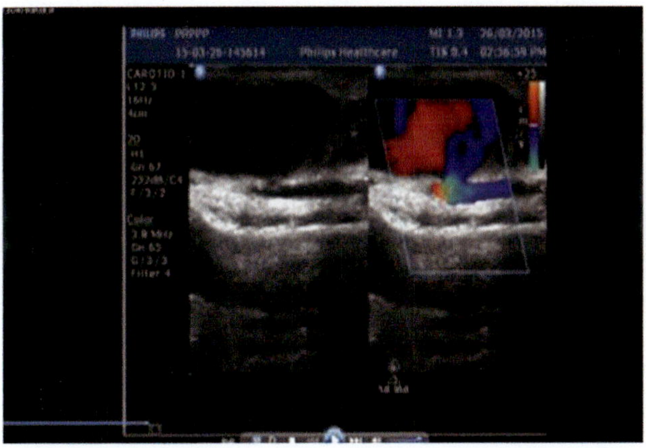

Figure 19.12b Pseudo-aneurysm at radial artery access site, colour flow shows flow from radial artery to pseudo aneurysm. (Courtesy Dr Sunita Chugh, FMRI, Gurugram)

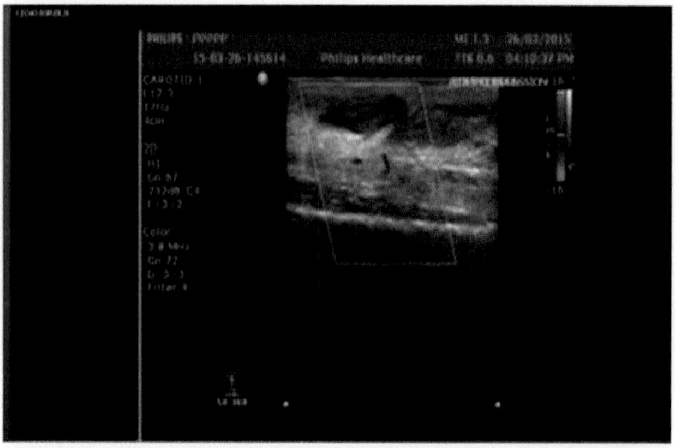

Figure 19.12c Pseudo-aneurysm obliterated after 20 minutes of compression.
(Courtesy Dr Sunita Chugh, FMRI, Gurugram)

References

1. Kumar Chugh S., Chugh S., Chugh Y., Rao S.V. Feasibility and utility of pre-procedural ultrasound imaging of the arm to facilitate transradial coronary diagnostic and interventional procedures (PRIMAFACIE-TRI) Catheter Cardiovasc Interv. 2013;82:64–73.
2. Alkhouli M, Cohen HA, Bashir R. Radial artery avulsion--a rare complication of transradial catheterization. Catheter Cardiovasc Interv. 2015;85(1):E32–4.
3. Dieter RS, Akef A, Wolff M. Eversion endarterectomy complicating radial artery access for left heart catheterization. Catheter Cardiovasc Interv. 2003;58(4):478–80.
4. Arzamendi D, Romeo P, Gosselin G. Radial artery avulsion: a rare complication of percutaneous coronary intervention. Revista espanola de cardiologia. 2011;64(1):62.
5. Ruiz-Salmeron RJ, Mora R, Velez-Gimon M, Ortiz J, Fernandez C, Vidal B, et al. Radial artery spasm in transradial cardiac catheterization. Assessment of factors related to its occurrence, and of its consequences during follow-up. Revista espanola de cardiologia. 2005;58(5):504–11.
6. Sławin J, Kubler P, Szczepański A, Piątek J, Stępkowski M, Reczuch K. Radial artery occlusion after percutaneous coronary interventions—an underestimated issue. Postępy w Kardiologii Interwencyjnej, Advances in Interventional Cardiology. 2013;9(4):353–61.
7. Zencirci E, Degirmencioglu A. Can radial artery pulse grading predict radial artery spasm during transradial approach? Kardiologia polska. 2017;75(4):360–7.
8. Van der Heijden D, van Leeuwen MA, Janssens GN, Hermie J, Lenzen MJ, Ritt MJ, et al. Endothelial dysfunction and the occurrence of radial artery spasm during transradial coronary procedures: the ACRA-Spasm study. EuroIntervention. 2016;12(10):1263–70.

9. Dehghani P, Mohammad A, Bajaj R, Hong T, Suen CM, Shariff W, Chisholm RJ, Kutryk MJ, Fam NP, Cheema AN. Mechanism and predictors of failed transradial approach for percutaneous coronary interventions. JACC Cardiovasc Interv. 2009;2(11):1057–64.
10. Kiemeneij F, Fraser D, Slagboom T, Laarman G, van der Wieken R. Hydrophilic coating aids radial sheath withdrawal and reduces patient discomfort following transradial coronary intervention: a randomized double-blind comparison of coated and uncoated sheaths. Catheter Cardiovasc Interv. 2003;59(2):161–4.
11. SK Chugh. 'Transradial Right or Left?' Indian Heart J 2008(Suppl A)60:1;A 27–35.
12. Hamon M, Pristipino C, Di Mario C, Nolan J, Ludwig J, Tubaro M, et al. Consensus document on the radial approach in percutaneous cardiovascular interventions: position paper by the European Association of Percutaneous Cardiovascular Interventions and Working Groups on Acute Cardiac Care** and Thrombosis of the European Society of Cardiology. EuroIntervention. 2013;8(11):1242–51.
13. Caputo RP, Tremmel JA, Rao S, Gilchrist IC, Pyne C, Pancholy S, et al. Transradial arterial access for coronary and peripheral procedures: executive summary by the Transradial Committee of the SCAI. Catheter Cardiovasc Interv. 2011;78(6):823–39.
14. Astarcioglu MA, Sen T, Kilit C, Durmus HI, Gozubuyuk G, Agus HZ, et al. Procedural sedation during transradial coronary angiography to prevent spasm. Herz. 2016;41(5):435–8.
15. Saito S, Tanaka S, Hiroe Y, et al. Usefulness of hydrophilic coating on arterial sheath introducer in transradial coronary intervention. Cathet Cardiovasc Intervent. 2002;56:328–32.
16. Salmeron R, Mora R, Masotti M, et al. Assessment of the efficacy of phentolamine vs. verapamil. Cathet Cardiovasc Intervent. 2005;66:192–8.
17. Filho JR, Assad JA, Zago AC, et al. Comparative study of the use of dilzem as an antispasmodic drug in coronary angiography via the trans radial approach. Arq Bras Cardiol. 2003;81(1):54–8.
18. Varenne O, Jegou A, Cohen R, et al. Prevention of arterial spasm during percutaneous coronary interventions through radial artery: the SPASM Study. Cathet Cardiovasc Intervent. 2006;68:231–5.
19. Kim SH. Comparative Study of nicorandil and aspasmolytic cocktail in preventing radial artery spasm during trans radial coronary angiography. Intl J Cardiol 2007, 3;120(3):325–30.
20. Chugh SK, Chugh Y, Chugh S. How to tackle complications in radial procedures: Tip and tricks. Indian Heart J. 2015;67(3):275–81.
21. Rashid M, Kwok CS, Pancholy S, Chugh S, Kedev SA, Bernat I, et al. Radial Artery Occlusion After Transradial Interventions: A Systematic Review and Meta-Analysis. J Am Heart Assoc. 2016;5(1).
22. Bernat J, Bertrand OF, Rokyta R, et al. Efficacy and safety of transient ulnar artery compression to recanalize acute radial artery occlusion after transradial catherization. Am J Cardiol. 2011;107 (11):1698–701.
23. S Chugh, Y Chugh. Radial Artery Occlusion: Size and More—How Small is Too Small? The Journal of invasive cardiology 27 (6), E113–E113.

24. Saito S, Ikei H, Hosokawa G, Tanaka S. Influence of the ratio between radial artery inner diameter and sheath outer diameter on radial artery flow after transradial coronary intervention. *Cathet Cardiovasc Intervent* 1999;46:173–8.
25. Sanmartin M, Gomez M, Rumoroso JR, et al. Interruption of Blood Flow During Compression and Radial Artery Occlusion After Transradial Catheterization. *Cathet Cardiovasc Intervent* 2007;70:185–9.
26. Pancholy S, Coppola J, Patel T, Roke-Thomas M. Prevention of radial artery occlusion – Patient hemostasis evaluation trial (PROPHET study): A randomized comparison of traditional versus patency documented hemostasis after transradial catheterization. *Cathet Cardiovasc Intervent* 2008;72:335–40.
27. Pancholy SB. Impact of Two Different Hemostatic Devices on Radial Artery Outcomes after Transradial Catheterization. *J Invasive Cardiol* 2009;21:101–4.
28. Cubero JM, Lombardo J, Pedrosa C, et al. Radial Compressions Guided by Mean Artery Pressure Versus Standard Compression with a Pneumatic Device (RACOMAP). *Cathet Cardiovasc Intervent* 2009;73:467–72.
29. S Chugh, Y Chugh. Radial Artery Occlusion: Size and more—How small is too Small? The Journal of invasive cardiology 27(6), E113, 2015.
30. SK Chugh, S Chugh, Y Chugh. Addressing the challenge of access of small radial and ulnar arteries in transradial and transulnar interventions: insights .... Journal of the American College of Cardiology 12(63), A1671,2014.
31. Zankl AR, Andrassy M, Volz C, et al. Radial artery thrombosis following transradial angiography: incidence and rationale for treatment of symptomatic patients with low molecular weight heparin. Clin Res Cardiol. 2010;99(12):841–7.
32. Pancholy SB. Strategies to Prevent Radial Artery Occlusion After Transradial PCI. Current Cardiology Reports. 2014;16(7):505.
33. Bernat I, Bertrand O, Rokyta R, et al. Efficacy and safety of transient ulnar artery compression to recanalize acute radial artery occlusion after transradial catheterization. Am J Cardiol 2011;107(11):1698–701.
34. Plante S, Cantor WJ, Goldman L, Miner S, Quesnelle A, Ganapathy A, et al. Comparison of bivalirudin versus heparin on radial artery occlusion after transradial catheterization. Catheter Cardiovasc Interv. 2010;76(5):654–8.
35. Tizon- Marcos H, Barbeau GR. Incidence of compartment syndrome of the arm in a large series of transradial approach for coronary procedures. J Interv Cardiol. 2008; 21 (5): 380–4.

20

Radiation Exposure and Stroke Risk: The Radial Approach

Devang S. Parikh and Mladen I. Vidovich

Introduction

Radial cardiac catheterization and intervention has continued its increased implementation worldwide. Benefits of transradial approach (TRA) include decreased bleeding complications, decreased mortality in ST-elevation myocardial infarction (STEMI), decreased cost, and better patient satisfaction as well as overall patient preference. However, there remains concern over radiation exposure and stroke risk with TRA compared to the transfemoral approach (TFA). These concerns have been proposed as slowing the adoption of the radial approach.[1]

Radiation Exposure with Transradial Procedure

Femoral Versus Radial Approach

There has been considerable research devoted towards determining differences in fluoroscopy time and overall radiation exposure when comparing TRA and TFA. To date, the largest prospective randomized control trial reporting radiation dose was the RIVAL trial. Within this trial, 7,021 patients were evaluated. Overall, fluoroscopy times were longer with TRA versus TFA at 9.0 min (6.0–15.0) and 8.3 (5.0–13.0) min, respectively ($p < 0.0001$). The radiation dose, measured in air kerma (AK) was borderline statistically significantly higher with TRA at 1,046 mGy (584–1591) compared to 930 mGy (538–1572) with the TFA ($p = 0.051$). Similarly, the dose area product (DAP) was also slightly higher though not clinically significant with TFA compared to femoral (52.8 Gy-cm^2 vs. 51.2 Gy-cm^2, $p = 0.83$).[2] Nevertheless, when further evaluating these differences, it was noted that the differences were occurring mainly at centers where operators had the least experience. When considering the 'radiation gap' at high-volume centers, the difference was indistinguishable.

Similarly, in a largest-to-date meta-analysis in of radiation exposure associated with TFA based on arterial access site for diagnostic coronary angiography or percutaneous coronary intervention (PCI), Plourde et al. noted that differences in radiation exposure narrowed with operator experience.[3]

While it should be noted that large observational studies, such as the National Cardiovascular Data Registry analysis in the United States, have revealed a measurable increase in fluoroscopy times with a radial approach, the implication of this variable to the actual radiation dose is uncertain.[4] The study identified 818 hospitals participating in the Cath PCI registry between July 2009 and June 2012. Within the three-year study period, the investigators evaluated changes in the implementation of transradial approach for PCI. While the primary outcome measured was bleeding, the study also sought to evaluate secondary endpoints including fluoroscopy time. From their evaluation, the authors were able to demonstrate a difference of 1.3 min between hospitals demonstrating a higher implementation of TRA versus hospitals slow to incorporate TRA. While the difference in time was similar to that noted in the RIVAL trial, the authors did not adjust for patient and procedural characteristics.

It is important to note that fluoroscopy time alone should not be used as a surrogate for radiation dose. Much of the increased fluoroscopy in TRA is to help navigate catheters through the upper extremity vessels or during coronary artery cannulation. However, most of the radiation exposure during a procedure comes from cine-angiography. In PCI performed with TRA, cine-angiography doses have been shown to be largely similar to TFA.[5]

Lastly, while the preponderance of studies prior to RIVAL demonstrated a slightly increased radiation dose with TRA compared to TFA, a minority did demonstrate equal or improved radiation doses. In fact, after RIVAL, a large retrospective, observational study of 20,669 patients was performed in the Swedish SCAAR Registry. Within this study, unadjusted radiation doses were equivalent for patients undergoing coronary angiography (31 Gy-cm^2 for both TRA and TFA, $p = 0.18$) and, importantly, higher with PCI utilizing a TFA (TRA 79 Gy-cm^2 versus TFA 93 Gy-cm^2, $p < 0.001$). After careful, multivariate analysis, the investigators determined that patient and procedure characteristics such as chronic total occlusions, high body mass index, and number of treated lesions were associated more with elevated radiation exposure compared to approach technique.[6]

In summary, the relation between access site and radiation dose is complex (Table 20.1). Variables such as operator experience, patient and procedure characteristics, as well as amount of radiation safety education play a significant role. Fluoroscopy times alone are inadequate measures of overall radiation exposure compared to AK and DAP. While current data reveal an overall absolute increased radiation dose with TRA, this difference is reduced or non-existent with experienced operators in high-volume centers and when adjusted for procedural and patient characteristics. This concept was very elegantly and pragmatically demonstrated by the REVERE trial. In this study, Pancholy et al. sought to compare radiation exposure through not only different access sites but based on operator proficiency in patients undergoing diagnostic coronary angiography. While 1,493 patients were randomized in a 1:1:1 fashion to different access sites between August 2012 and November 2013, operators themselves were similarly categorized. The authors defined operators as low, medium, or high proficiency for TRA based on the number of procedures they had performed (less than 500, 501–999 and greater than 1,000, respectively). The study demonstrated that not only was there no difference between the access sites in radiation exposure as measured by AK and DAP but that the fluoroscopy times were also similar. Moreover, operators with less experience had increased radiation and fluoroscopy time regardless of access site while operators with more experience had lower radiation and fluoroscopy times.[7]

Left Versus Right Radial Access

The majority of TRA worldwide are performed via right radial access (RRA) at greater than 80–90%.[1,8] There are many reasons for the preponderance of RRA including patient positioning, current design, and

Table 20.1 Radiation Exposure Transradial vs. Transfemoral

	Year		Number Patients		DAP (Gycm²)		p-value
			Radial	Femoral	Radial	Femoral	
Achenbach et al.[29]	2008		152	155	37.4	32.0	NS
Brasselet et al.[30]	2008		240	181	80	51.25	< 0.001
Brueck et al.[31]	2009		512	512	41.9	38.2	< 0.034
Geijer et al.[32]	2004		55	114	51.9	54.0	0.038
Kuipers et al.[33]	2012	CAG	138	314	40	44	NS
		PCI	1,212	2,309	72	75	NS
Lange et al.[34]	2006	CAG	92	103	15.1	13.1	< 0.05
		PCI	54	48	46.3	51	NS
Lo et al.[27]	2006		28	31	33.9	31	NS
Neill et al.[35]	2010		965	848	18.37	16.57	< 0.001
Sandborg et al.[16]	2004		60	82	75	47	0.013
REVERE[7]	2015		995	498	27.11	25.37	NS
RADIAL-CABG[11]	2013		63	63	1.29 Gy	1.08 Gy	NS
					Fluoroscopy Time (min)		
Looi et al.[36]	2011		661	340	4.5	4.4	NS
Mercuri et al.[19]	2011		1,764	5,954	5.46	3.82	< 0.001
Lehmann et al.[37]	2011	CAG	624	842	4.1	2.9	0.002
		PCI	290	370	8.9	9.7	NS
Santas et al.[38]	2009		670	335	5.0	4.0	NS
Tayeh et al.[39]	2014		586	214	3.43	3.86	NS
Yigit et al.[9]	2006		75	105	3.9	2.28	< 0.0001
CARAFE[40]	2001		140	70	4.0	3.1	< 0.01
FARMI[41]	2007		57	57	13.0	8.0	<0.01
RIVAL[2]	2011		3,507	3,514	9.3	8.0	< 0.0001
OCEAN RACE[42]	2014		52	51	2.95	3.23	NS
STEMI RADIAL[43]	2014		348	359	7.9	8	NS
TEMPURA[44]	2003		77	72	15.1	16.1	NS

CAG = Coronary angiography; PCI = Percutaneous coronary intervention.

workflow environment in cardiac catheterization laboratories, reduced operator back discomfort with RRA, and overall ease of access to the right wrist. Yet, left radial access (LRA) is inherently less challenging technically when compared to RRA. In fact, when transradial catheterization was initially developed by Lucien Campeau, in 1989, the primary access site was the left radial artery.[9] Predominantly, use of LRA avoids subclavian tortuosity found in elderly, obese, and short-statured patients. Additionally, standard diagnostic and guiding catheters have been designed for the femoral approach and might be more difficult to manipulate from RRA. Given that the left radial artery accesses the ascending aorta in a manner anatomically similar to the femoral artery it could be predicted that LRA compared to RRA might allow for faster procedures.

Part of the debate between LRA and RRA has also been related to overall radiation exposure. Multiple studies have been performed, but conclusions are difficult to surmise given considerable heterogeneity in inclusion criteria, study design, and outcome variables. Equally important, some European and Asian populations may have lower body mass indices compared to North American studies further complicating the analyses. In observational and retrospective studies, operator bias in choosing RRA vs. LRA might have affected the final radiation exposure findings. Lastly, there is a significant difficulty in determining the optimal outcome variable in studies reporting radiation exposure. Many studies have addressed fluoroscopy times, AK or DAP. As elegantly demonstrated in the TALENT trial, during diagnostic angiography, fluoroscopy times, and DAP appeared higher for RRA than LRA. There was no difference between RRA and LRA during PCI.[5] The most striking finding in the TALENT trial is that the RRA-LRA radiation dose differences were most pronounced among trainees and in elderly patients. This is quite consistent with the aforementioned considerations comparing TFA to TRA. It is likely that patient, procedural, and operator characteristics are more important for radiation dose than approach technique of RRA or LRA. While patient radiation exposure is an important variable, measuring operator radiation exposure is equally important. In the previously mentioned REVERE trial, while no significant difference was noted in radiation exposure based on AK or DAP, Pancholy et al. did demonstrate that patients undergoing diagnostic angiography with LRA had higher operator radiation exposure (3 mrem, interquartile range (IQR)2–5 mrem) compared to FA (2 mrem, IQR 2–4 mrem, $p < 0.001$) or RRA (3 mrem, IQR 2–5 mrem, $p < 0.0001$). However, as proficiency increases, the study investigators again noted a significant reduction is operator radiation exposure, as well.[7]

As no final consensus can be adequately reached, there is a clear need for more contemporary studies examining the issue while accounting for procedural, operator, and site characteristics. The TRansradial access site and systemic implementation of angioX-RAdiation Dose (RAD-MATRIX) trial is expected to shed additional light to these important questions.[10] However, a few conclusions can be made after reviewing current available literature: (1) LRA is hardly ever associated with higher radiation exposure than RRA and (2) increased operator experience reduces overall radiation doses and reduces and nearly eliminates the radiation exposure differences between RRA and LRA (Table 20.2).

Table 20.2 Radiation Exposure Right Radial vs. Left Radial

	Year		Patients		DAP (Gycm²)		p-value
			Right Radial	Left Radial	Right Radial	Left Radial	
Hu et al.[45]	2014		700	700	28.0	26.0	NS
Norgaz et al.[46]	2012		500	500	18.9	19.4	NS
Rigattieri et al.[47]	2015	CAG	1,175	289	44.8	35.4	0.003
		PCI	538	155	115	100.9	0.03
OPERA[48]	2013		209	204	73.8	70.1	NS
PREVAIL[20]	2012		304	205	45.6	59.6	< 0.0001
TALENT[5]	2011	CAG	732	735	12.1	10.7	0.004
		PCI	344	344	63.1	53.7	NS
REVERE[7]	2015		497	498	27.7	26.6	NS
					Fluoroscopy Time (min)		
Dominici et al.[49]	2012		420	612	8.18	6.29	0.001
Fernandez-Portales et al.[50]	2006		171	180	8.9	6.13	0.0001
Freixa et al.[51]	2012		50	50	8.9	8.6	NS
Kado et al.[52]	2014		50	50	10.9	10.5	NS
Kanei et al.[53]	2011		98	91	9.2	10.5	NS
Kawashima et al.[54]	2004		205	232	5.0	3.7	<0.001
Santas et al.[38]	2009		335	335	5.0	5.0	NS
CARAFE[40]	2001		70	70	3.8	4.2	< 0.001

CAG = Coronary angiography; PCI = Percutaneous coronary intervention.

Coronary Artery Bypass Graft (CABG) Patients and Radiation

Performing TRA in patients with previous bypass grafting requires considerable skill and expertise. More importantly, patients with prior CABG are underrepresented in previously referenced studies, though limited observational studies have reported TRA as equally safe and feasible to TFA. In 2013, the RADIAL-CABG trial sought to further evaluate these patients. Within a single center, 128 consecutive patients who had previously undergone CABG were prospectively randomized in a 1:1 fashion to TRA or TFA. Investigators evaluated radiation exposure (AK) as one of their primary endpoints and noted no clinically significant difference between the two approaches (1.29 ± 0.67 TRA vs. 1.08 ± 0.54 TFA, $p = 0.06$).[11] Again, while there was increased fluoroscopy time associated with TRA, the significance of this variable remains clinically ambiguous. Overall, similar to standard patients, it appears that procedural, patient, and operator characteristics play a more significant role in radiation dose compared to the access site itself when evaluating those with a prior history of CABG. Similarly, in 2006, Sanmartin et al. retrospectively evaluated 304 diagnostic procedures in patients with prior CABG between January 2001 and December 2004. Amongst these cases, total procedure time (41 min ± 22 vs. 40 min ± 23), fluoroscopy time (15 ± 10 min vs. 18 min ± 13) and dye volume (180 ml ± 64 vs. 192 ml ± 73) were similar between LRA and FA.[12] Currently, many trials exclude patients with prior CABG in the evaluation of radiation exposure and more effort is necessary to prospectively assess any true differences that may exist between access sites in these patients. More importantly, as newer catheters are developed for imaging of bypass grafts in patients undergoing coronary angiography via the radial approach, any real differences may be further mitigated.

Radiation Protection and Education

Regardless of arterial access site considerations, aggressive radiation hygiene is of paramount importance for radial operators. Radial protection boards and radiation protection pads have been shown to reduce radiation to the operator.[13] In fact, patient pelvic lead shielding can further decrease operator radiation exposure as demonstrated by Lange et al. (2012).[14] Operator dose is mainly due to scatter radiation and dedicated radial drapes can further reduce radiation dose to the operator.[13]

Similarly, availability of radiation education and continued quality control in the cardiac catheterization laboratories with radiation dose reporting is needed to maintain the lowest doses possible (ALARA principle—as low as reasonably achievable). It is critical to educate cardiology trainees about radiation safety practices.[15]

Current advances in X-ray technology and modern cardiac catheterization laboratories will make a dramatic impact in radiation dose both to the patient and to the operator. The current prospective software algorithms available on most modern systems may reduce radiation dose by up to 70%.[16] Such dramatic reductions in radiation dose will make the differences between various approaches, including LRA vs. RRA as well as TFA vs. RRA, negligible. Reduction in frame rates to 7.5 per second from current 15 frames per second will further reduce the TRA/TFA radiation gap. In combination with aggressive radiation reduction, continuous meaningful operator radiation education and increased operator experience, radiation dose concerns previously stated in this chapter will become of lesser concern.

Operator Proficiency and Learning Curve

Experienced operators tend to have lower fluoroscopy times and radiation exposures compared to trainees or femoral operators in their early adoption phases of the radial approach. While the precise number of radial procedures needed to achieve proficiency is uncertain, it appears that the number of procedures is around 50.[17] The number of procedures to achieve 'expert' status is likely significantly higher and includes continued procedural experience performed in high-volume centers, as suggested in the RIVAL[18] and REVERE trials.[7]

It is, however, quite important to mention that high radiation exposure femoralists are also high radiation exposure radialists, whereas low exposure femoralists also perform TRA with overall lower doses. Therefore, individual operator practices significantly impact radiation doses with both TFA and TRA.[19]

Cerebrovascular Accident Risk with Transradial Procedures

Femoral Versus Radial

While the reported incidence of cardiovascular accident (CVA) during coronary angiography has varied from as low as 0.1% to 0.4% and as high as 1.4% for PCI, periprocedural CVA is a devastating complication from coronary angiography.[20] Periprocedural CVA is associated with very high mortality, and up to a third of patients will die after PCI-related CVA.[21] The etiology of this complication can occur via dislodgement of debris made up of thrombus, calcific material, or cholesterol particles from atherosclerotic plaque. CVA can also occur through intra-cranial bleeding or embolization of air or thrombus at catheter and guidewire tips themselves.[22] Assessment of CVA associated with TRA has been a heavily researched topic not only because of the increasing popularity and implementation of TRA but also because of manipulation required in the subclavian arteries and especially the right brachiocephalic artery given that the vertebral and carotid arteries emanate from that vessel.

Recently, the MATRIX trial was performed at 78 centers in Europe to evaluate the complications arising from TRA versus TFA approach for invasive management of patients presenting with acute coronary syndrome (ACS). Between 2011 and 2014, the study prospectively randomized 8,404 patients in a 1:1 fashion for either approach. One of the primary measures of the study included 30-day outcomes that evaluated for overall mortality, stroke, and myocardial infarction. The study found that there was no difference between the radial and femoral approach to development of CVA. Additionally, there was an overall less likelihood of bleeding and overall mortality through the TRA.[23] Similarly, in China, a retrospective study recently evaluated 21,242 patients that underwent elective PCI to look for short and medium-term effects comparing TRA and TFA. While almost 86% of patients underwent TRA compared to TFA for PCI, the incidence of in-hospital net adverse clinical events

(NACE), which included stroke, was lower with TRA (1.8% TRA vs. 4.0% TFA, $p < 0.0001$) and one-year major adverse clinical event (MACE), which also included stroke, was equivalent between the two groups (4.7% TRA vs. 4.9% TFA, $p = 0.272$). As has been previously demonstrated, access site complications and bleeding were also higher in the TFA vs. TRA groups (Figure 20.1).[24] In fact, in a retrospective review from a single north Indian institution, Tewari et al. evaluated 26,238 patients where 53.92% cases were performed via TRA. In their review, they noted three patients with transient neurological deficits post coronary angiography in the TFA compared to two in TRA.[25]

Intra-aortic Balloon Pump (IABP) and CVA

The use of IABP has been associated with increased risk of stroke. In a study by Romagnoli et al. where the rates of stroke were compared in patients who had TFA vs. TRA performed along with IABP there was no difference in stroke rates observed. This was a small, underpowered study to compare incidence of stroke, but it further underscores the fact that there is likely no difference in stroke rates between TFA and TRA.[26]

STEMI, TRA, and CVA

TRA has demonstrated marked mortality and bleeding advantages when performed for STEMI when compared to TFA. However, STEMI procedures are frequently performed in patients with significant comorbidities, and the requirement for an expeditious procedure may expose patients to risk of stroke given hypothetical potential for plaque mobilization, air embolism, and overall hypercoagulable state seen with STEMI. In a large meta-analysis analysing TRA in STEMI, there was no difference observed in the rate of stroke between TFA and TRA (OR 1.07, 95% CI 0.45–2.45, $p = 0.87$).[27]

Further highlighting this issue was the 2013 retrospective analysis of the British Cardiovascular Intervention Society registry performed by Nolan et al. Here, researchers evaluated stroke risk when comparing almost 500,000 PCI cases in the UK. Included within the study were

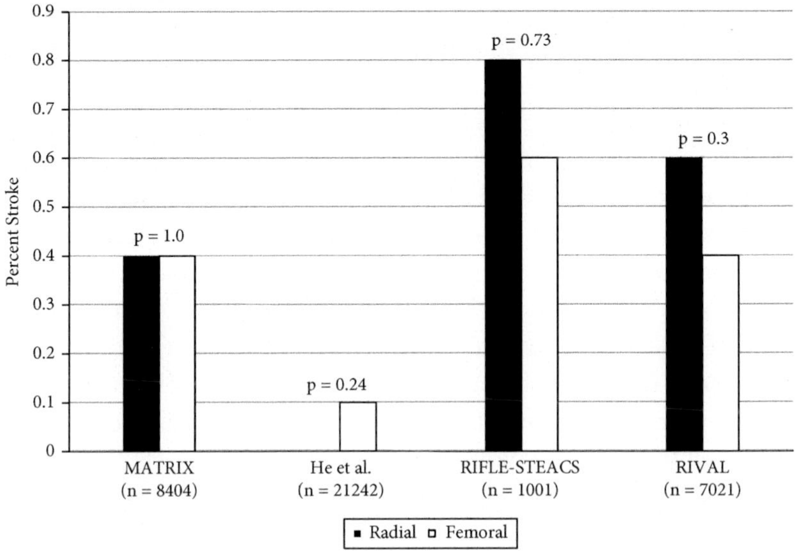

Figure 20.1 Stroke risk radial vs. femoral.

223,476 femoral cases and 124,616 radial cases between January 2006 and December 2010. When evaluating the results, the researchers noted that the rate of stroke complication was 0.11% from both approaches. Though the overall occurrence of stroke increased over the study period from 0.08% to 0.14%, this was thought to be from the increase in PCI for ACS across the country during that same time period (47–61%). In fact, after performing a multivariate analysis of the patients, the risk of stroke was not affected by access site, rather it was age, prior history of stroke, female sex, presence of peripheral vascular disease, use of glycoprotein IIb/IIIa inhibitors, PCI for ACS, and pre-PCI shock.[28]

LRA Versus RRA and CVA

As has been previously discussed, the use of LRA may provide a unique method of utilizing traditional catheters given it approaches the aorta in a manner similar to femoral approach. Particularly in short, obese, and elderly patients, use of LRA may provide a less challenging procedure technically. Any change in the occurrence of stroke, however, would have clear ramifications on choice of approach. Due to these potential implications in practice, many studies have examined the risk of stroke in LRA and RRA. While the retrospective review of the British Cardiovascular Intervention Society registry primarily evaluated femoral versus radial, the researchers also compared stroke complications between left versus right radial artery approaches. Of the 124,616 radial cases performed between January 2006 and December 2010, 96% were by the right radial artery. However, no significant difference was found in stroke complication when comparing a left radial versus right radial approach.[28] Similarly, the TALENT trial in 2011, which prospectively randomized 1,540 patients to RRA versus LLA for PCI, evaluated major vascular complications as one of their primary endpoints. This included stroke and transient ischaemic attack. Of the 770 cases performed through each approach, there was 1 stroke in the RRA group with none in the LLA arm with a $p = 0.31$.[5] It appears that multiple studies show no significant increase in stroke risk when comparing LRA to RRA for coronary angiography. Multiple other factors therefore likely increase stroke risk independent of the approach method utilized.

Previous CABG and Stroke Risk Associated with TRA

To date, the only prospective, randomized control trial that has sought to evaluate stroke risk in the angiography of coronary artery bypass grafts is the RADIAL-CABG trial described earlier. While its primary endpoint was contrast volume, secondary endpoints included major adverse cardiac events incorporating stroke. When comparing secondary outcomes, the researchers noted that one patient in the TFA group had transient numbness in the left arm but no changes were noted on magnetic resonance imaging of the brain. Overall, there was no significant different between TFA and TRA in stroke risk.[11] While no studies have specifically evaluated neurological complications in patients undergoing angiography with a prior history of CABG, it appears likely that access site will not play as significant of a role as other independent risk factors mentioned earlier. Given the low incidence of peri-procedural stroke, the RADIAL-CABG trial was underpowered to detect CVA differences between RRA and LRA.

Summary

The explosive growth of TRA and its worldwide adoption has been occasionally met with challenges. Some of the barriers to 'radial-first approach' have been concern for increased radiation exposure and perceived potential for increased risk of periprocedural stroke. At this time, the radiation exposure is slightly increased with TRA compared to TFA. However, increase in operator experience and education, use of radiation protection, and contemporary X-ray equipment design will likely eliminate this 'radiation gap' in the next several years. The highest quality up-to-date evidence convincingly demonstrates that there is no evidence of increased risk of stroke with TRA compared with TFA.

References

1. Helfrich CD, Tsai TT, Rao SV, Lemon JM, Eugenio EC, Vidovich MI, et al. Perceptions of advantages and barriers to radial-access percutaneous coronary intervention in VA cardiac catheterization laboratories. *Cardiovascular Revascularization Medicine: Including Molecular Interventions.* 2014;15(6–7):329–33. PubMed PMID: 25282521.
2. Jolly SS, Yusuf S, Cairns J, Niemela K, Xavier D, Widimsky P, et al. Radial versus femoral access for coronary angiography and intervention in patients with acute coronary syndromes (RIVAL): a randomised, parallel group, multicentre trial. *The Lancet.* 2011;377(9775):1409–20. PubMed PMID: 21470671. Epub 2011/04/08. eng.
3. Plourde G, Pancholy SB, Nolan J, Jolly S, Rao SV, Amhed I, et al. Radiation exposure in relation to the arterial access site used for diagnostic coronary angiography and percutaneous coronary intervention: a systematic review and meta-analysis. *The Lancet.* 2015;386(10009):2192–203.
4. Bradley SM, Rao SV, Curtis JP, Parzynski CS, Messenger JC, Daugherty SL, et al. Change in hospital-level use of transradial percutaneous coronary intervention and periprocedural outcomes: insights from the national cardiovascular data registry. *Circulation Cardiovascular Quality and Outcomes.* 2014;7(4):550–59. PubMed PMID: 24899678.
5. Sciahbasi A, Romagnoli E, Burzotta F, Trani C, Sarandrea A, Summaria F, et al. Transradial approach (left vs right) and procedural times during percutaneous coronary procedures: TALENT study. *American Heart Journal.* 2011;161(1):172–79. PubMed PMID: 21167351. Epub 2010/12/21.
6. Delewi R, Hoebers LP, Ramunddal T, Henriques JP, Angeras O, Stewart J, et al. Clinical and procedural characteristics associated with higher radiation exposure during percutaneous coronary interventions and coronary

angiography. *Circulation Cardiovascular Interventions*. 2013;6(5):501–6. PubMed PMID: 24065442.

7. Pancholy SB, Joshi P, Shah S, Rao SV, Bertrand OF, Patel TM. Effect of vascular access site choice on radiation exposure during coronary angiography: the REVERE rrial (Randomized Evaluation of Vascular Entry Site and Radiation Exposure). *JACC Cardiovascular Interventions*. 2015;8(9):1189–96. PubMed PMID: 26210808.
8. Bertrand OF, Rao SV, Pancholy S, Jolly SS, Rodes-Cabau J, Larose E, et al. Transradial approach for coronary angiography and interventions: results of the first international transradial practice survey. *JACC Cardiovascular Interventions*. 2010;3(10):1022–31. PubMed PMID: 20965460. Epub 2010/10/23. eng.
9. Yiğit F SA, Erol T, Demircan S, Tekin G, Katircibaşi T, Tekin A, Müderrisoğlu H. An experience on radial versus femoral approach for diagnostic coronary angiography in Turkey. *Anadolu Kardiyoloji Dergisi*. 2006;6(3):229–34. PubMed Central PMCID: 16943106.
10. Sciahbasi A, Calabro P, Sarandrea A, Rigattieri S, Tomassini F, Sardella G, et al. Randomized comparison of operator radiation exposure comparing transradial and transfemoral approach for percutaneous coronary procedures: rationale and design of the minimizing adverse haemorrhagic events by TRansradial access site and systemic implementation of angioX - RAdiation Dose study (RAD-MATRIX). *Cardiovascular Revascularization Medicine: Including Molecular Interventions*. 2014;15(4):209–13. PubMed PMID: 24746599.
11. Michael TT, Alomar M, Papayannis A, Mogabgab O, et al. A randomized comparison of the transradial and transfemoral approaches for coronary artery bypass graft angiography and intervention: the RADIAL-CABG Trial (RADIAL Versus Femoral Access for Coronary Artery Bypass Graft Angiography and Intervention). JACC Cardiovasc Interv. 2013 Nov;6(11):1138–44. doi: 10.1016/j.jcin.2013.08.004. Epub 2013 Oct 16. PMID: 24139930.
12. Sanmartin M, Cuevas D, Moxica J, Valdes M, Esparza J, Baz JA, et al. Transradial cardiac catheterization in patients with coronary bypass grafts: feasibility analysis and comparison with transfemoral approach. *Catheterization and Cardiovascular Interventions: Official Journal of the Society for Cardiac Angiography & Interventions*. 2006;67(4):580–84. PubMed PMID: 16547928.
13. Ertel A, Nadelson J, Shroff AR, Sweis R, Ferrera D, Vidovich MI. Radiation dose reduction during radial cardiac catheterization: evaluation of a dedicated radial angiography absorption shielding drape. *ISRN Cardiology*. 2012;2012:769167. PubMed PMID: 22988525. Pubmed Central PMCID: 3439952.
14. Lange HW, von Boetticher H. Reduction of operator radiation dose by a pelvic lead shield during cardiac catheterization by radial access: comparison with femoral access. *JACC Cardiovascular Interventions*. 2012;5(4):445–49. PubMed PMID: 22516403. Epub 2012/04/21.eng.
15. Kim C, Vasaiwala S, Haque F, Pratap K, Vidovich MI. Radiation safety among cardiology fellows. *The American Journal of Cardiology*. 2010;106(1):125–28. PubMed PMID: 20609659. Epub 2010/07/09. eng.
16. Sandborg M, Fransson SG, Pettersson H. Evaluation of patient-absorbed doses during coronary angiography and intervention by femoral and radial artery access. *European Radiology*. 2004;14(4):653–58. PubMed PMID: 14618362.

17. Hess CN, Peterson ED, Neely ML, Dai D, Hillegass WB, Krucoff MW, et al. The learning curve for transradial percutaneous coronary intervention among operators in the United States: a study from the National Cardiovascular Data Registry. Circulation. 2014 Jun 3;129(22):2277–86. doi:10.1161/CIRCULATIONAHA.113.006356. Epub 2014 Apr 22. PMID: 24756064; PMCID: PMC4048735.
18. Jolly SS, Niemela K, Xavier D, Widimsky P, Budaj A, Valentin V, et al. Design and rationale of the radial versus femoral access for coronary intervention (RIVAL) trial: a randomized comparison of radial versus femoral access for coronary angiography or intervention in patients with acute coronary syndromes. *American Heart Journal*. 2011;161(2):254-60.e1-4. PubMed PMID: 21315206. Epub 2011/02/15. eng.
19. Mercuri M, Mehta S, Xie C, Valettas N, Velianou JL, Natarajan MK. Radial artery access as a predictor of increased radiation exposure during a diagnostic cardiac catheterization procedure. *JACC Cardiovascular Interventions*. 2011;4(3):347–52. PubMed PMID: 21435615. Epub 2011/03/26. eng.
20. Pelliccia F, Trani C, Biondi-Zoccai GG, Nazzaro M, Berni A, Patti G, et al. Comparison of the feasibility and effectiveness of transradial coronary angiography via right versus left radial artery approaches (from the PREVAIL Study). *The American Journal of Cardiology*. 2012;110(6):771–75. PubMed PMID: 22651876.
21. Hoffman SJ, Routledge HC, Lennon RJ, Mustafa MZ, Rihal CS, Gersh BJ, et al. Procedural factors associated with percutaneous coronary intervention-related ischemic stroke. *JACC Cardiovascular Interventions*. 2012;5(2):200–6. PubMed PMID: 22361605.
22. Raposo L, Madeira S, Teles RC, Santos M, Gabriel HM, Goncalves P, et al. Neurologic complications after transradial or transfemoral approach for diagnostic and interventional cardiac catheterization: a propensity score analysis of 16,710 cases from a single centre prospective registry. *Catheterization and Cardiovascular Interventions: Official Journal of the Society for Cardiac Angiography & Interventions*. 2015;86(1):61–70. PubMed PMID: 25676170.
23. Valgimigli M, Gagnor A, Calabró P, Frigoli E, Leonardi S, Zaro T, et al. Radial versus femoral access in patients with acute coronary syndromes undergoing invasive management: a randomised multicentre trial. *The Lancet*. 2015;385(9986):2465–76.
24. He P, Yang Y, Qiao S, Xu B, Yao M, Wu Y, et al. Comparison of short- and medium-term clinical outcomes between transradial approach and transfemoral approach in a high-volume PCI heart center in China. *PloS One*. 2015;10(3):e0118491. PubMed PMID: 25826213. PubMed Central PMCID: 4380354.
25. Tewari S, Sharma N, Kapoor A, Syal SK, Kumar S, Garg N, et al. Comparison of transradial and transfemoral artery approach for percutaneous coronary angiography and angioplasty: a retrospective seven-year experience from a north Indian center. *Indian Heart Journal*. 2013;65(4):378–87. PubMed PMID: 23992998. Pubmed Central PMCID: 3861289.
26. Biondi-Zoccai G, Sciahbasi A, Bodi V, Fernandez-Portales J, Kanei Y, Romagnoli E, et al. Right versus left radial artery access for coronary procedures: an international collaborative systematic review and meta-analysis including 5 randomized trials and 3210 patients. *International Journal of Cardiology*. 2013;166(3):621–26. PubMed PMID: 22192284.

27. Lo TS BA, Hall IR, Hildick-Smith DJ, Nolan J. Percutaneous left and right heart catheterization in fully anticoagulated patients utilizing the radial artery and forearm vein: a two-center experience. *Journal of Interventional Cardiology*. 2006;19(3):258–63. Pubmed Central PMCID: 16724969.
28. Ratib K, Mamas MA, Routledge HC, Ludman PF, Fraser D, Nolan J. Influence of access site choice on incidence of neurologic complications after percutaneous coronary intervention. *American Heart Journal*. 2013;165(3):317–24. PubMed PMID: 23453099.
29. Achenbach S, Ropers D, Kallert L, Turan N, Krahner R, Wolf T, et al. Transradial versus transfemoral approach for coronary angiography and intervention in patients above 75 years of age. *Catheterization and Cardiovascular Interventions: Official Journal of the Society for Cardiac Angiography & Interventions*. 2008;72(5):629–35. PubMed PMID: 18798237.
30. Brasselet C, Blanpain T, Tassan-Mangina S, Deschildre A, Duval S, Vitry F, et al. Comparison of operator radiation exposure with optimized radiation protection devices during coronary angiograms and ad hoc percutaneous coronary interventions by radial and femoral routes. *European Heart Journal*. 2008;29(1):63–70. PubMed PMID: 17999984. Epub 2007/11/15. eng.
31. Brueck M, Bandorski D, Kramer W, Wieczorek M, Holtgen R, Tillmanns H. A randomized comparison of transradial versus transfemoral approach for coronary angiography and angioplasty. *JACC Cardiovascular Interventions*. 2009;2(11):1047–54. PubMed PMID: 19926042. Epub 2009/11/21. eng.
32. Geijer H, Persliden J. Radiation exposure and patient experience during percutaneous coronary intervention using radial and femoral artery access. *European Radiology*. 2004;14(9):1674–80. PubMed PMID: 15103500. Epub 2004/04/23. eng.
33. Kuipers G, Delewi R, Velders XL, Vis MM, van der Schaaf RJ, Koch KT, et al. Radiation exposure during percutaneous coronary interventions and coronary angiograms performed by the radial compared with the femoral route. *JACC Cardiovascular Interventions*. 2012;5(7):752–57. PubMed PMID: 22814780.
34. Lange HW, von Boetticher H. Randomized comparison of operator radiation exposure during coronary angiography and intervention by radial or femoral approach. *Catheterization and Cardiovascular Interventions: Official Journal of the Society for Cardiac Angiography & Interventions*. 2006;67(1):12–6. PubMed PMID: 16331696.
35. Neill J, Douglas H, Richardson G, Chew EW, Walsh S, Hanratty C, et al. Comparison of radiation dose and the effect of operator experience in femoral and radial arterial access for coronary procedures. *The American Journal of Cardiology*. 2010;106(7):936–40. PubMed PMID: 20854953. Epub 2010/09/22. eng.
36. Looi JL, Cave A, El-Jack S. Learning curve in transradial coronary angiography. *The American Journal of Cardiology*. 2011;108(8):1092–95. PubMed PMID: 21798498.
37. Lehmann R, Ehrlich JR, Weber V, de Rosa S, Gotarda MN, Schachinger V, et al. Implementation of the transradial approach for coronary procedures is not associated with an elevated complication rate and elevated radiation patient exposure. *Journal of Interventional Cardiology*. 2011;24(1):56–64. PubMed PMID: 20973820.

38. Santas E BV, Sanchis J, Núñez J, Mainar L, Miñana G, Chorro FJ, Llácer A. The left radial approach in daily practice. A randomized study comparing femoral and right and left radial approaches. *Revista Española de Cardiología*. 2009;62(5):482–90. Pubmed Central PMCID: 19406062.
39. Tayeh O, Ettori F. Coronary angiography safety between radial and femoral access. *The Egyptian Heart Journal*. 2014;66(2):149–54.
40. Louvard Y LT, Allain A, Morice M. Coronary angiography through the radial or the femoral approach: the CARAFE study. *Catheterization and Cardiovascular Interventions*. 2001;52(2):181–87. Pubmed Central PMCID: 11170325.
41. Brasselet C, Tassan S, Nazeyrollas P, Hamon M, Metz D. Randomised comparison of femoral versus radial approach for percutaneous coronary intervention using abciximab in acute myocardial infarction: results of the FARMI trial. *Heart*. 2007;93(12):1556–61. PubMed PMID: 17639099. Pubmed Central PMCID: 2095748.
42. Koltowski L, Filipiak KJ, Kochman J, Pietrasik A, Rdzanek A, Huczek Z, et al. Access for percutaneous coronary intervention in ST segment elevation myocardial infarction: radial vs. femoral--a prospective, randomised clinical trial (OCEAN RACE). *Kardiologia Polska*. 2014;72(7):604–11. PubMed PMID: 24671918.
43. Bernat I, Horak D, Stasek J, Mates M, Pesek J, Ostadal P, et al. ST-segment elevation myocardial infarction treated by radial or femoral approach in a multicenter randomized clinical trial: the STEMI-RADIAL trial. *Journal of the American College of Cardiology*. 2014;63(10):964–72. PubMed PMID: 24211309.
44. Saito S, Tanaka S, Hiroe Y, Miyashita Y, Takahashi S, Tanaka K, et al. Comparative study on transradial approach vs. transfemoral approach in primary stent implantation for patients with acute myocardial infarction: results of the test for myocardial infarction by prospective unicenter randomization for access sites (TEMPURA) trial. *Catheterization and Cardiovascular Interventions: Official Journal of the Society for Cardiac Angiography & Interventions*. 2003;59(1):26–33. PubMed PMID: 12720237.
45. Hu H, Fu Q, Chen W, Wang D, Hua X, Chen B. A prospective randomized comparison of left and right radial approach for percutaneous coronary angiography in Asian populations. *Clinical Interventions in Aging*. 2014;9:963–68. PubMed PMID: 25018624. Pubmed Central PMCID: 4073974.
46. Norgaz T, Gorgulu S, Dagdelen S. A randomized study comparing the effectiveness of right and left radial approach for coronary angiography. *Catheterization and Cardiovascular Interventions: Official Journal of the Society for Cardiac Angiography & Interventions*. 2012;80(2):260–64. PubMed PMID: 22334420.
47. Rigattieri S, Di Russo C, Cera M, Fedele S, Sciahbasi A, Pugliese FR. Patient radiation exposure in right versus left trans-radial approach for coronary procedures. *Cardiovascular Revascularization Medicine: Including Molecular Interventions*. 2015;16(1):15–9. PubMed PMID: 25576274.
48. Dominici M, Diletti R, Milici C, Bock C, Placanica A, D'Alessandro G, et al. Operator exposure to x-ray in left and right radial access during percutaneous coronary procedures: OPERA randomised study. *Heart*. 2013;99(7):480–84. PubMed PMID: 23343690.

49. Dominici M, Diletti R, Milici C, Bock C, Garg S, De Paolis M, et al. Left radial versus right radial approach for coronary artery catheterization: a prospective comparison. *Journal of Interventional Cardiology*. 2012;25(2):203–9. PubMed PMID: 22272568.
50. Fernández-Portales J VR, Carreras R, Jiménez-Candil J, Serrador A, Romaní S. Right versus left radial artery approach for coronary angiography. Differences observed and the learning curve. *Revista Española de Cardiología*. 2006;59(10):1071–74. Pubmed Central PMCID: 17125718.
51. Freixa X, Trilla M, Feldman M, Jimenez M, Betriu A, Masotti M. Right versus left transradial approach for coronary catheterization in octogenarian patients. *Catheterization and Cardiovascular Interventions: Official Journal of the Society for Cardiac Angiography & Interventions*. 2012;80(2):267–72. PubMed PMID: 22422735.
52. Kado H, Patel AM, Suryadevara S, Zenni MM, Box LC, Angiolillo DJ, et al. Operator radiation exposure and physical discomfort during a right versus left radial approach for coronary interventions: a randomized evaluation. *JACC Cardiovascular Interventions*. 2014;7(7):810–16. PubMed PMID: 24954573.
53. Kanei Y, Nakra NC, Liou M, Vales LL, Gowda R, Rosero H, et al. Randomized comparison of transradial coronary angiography via right or left radial artery approaches. *The American Journal of Cardiology*. 2011;107(2):195–97. PubMed PMID: 21129711.
54. Kawashima O, Endoh N, Terashima M, Ito Y, Abe S, Ootomo T, et al. Effectiveness of right or left radial approach for coronary angiography. *Catheterization and Cardiovascular Interventions: Official Journal of the Society for Cardiac Angiography & Interventions*. 2004;61(3):333–37. PubMed PMID: 14988891.

21

Transradial Access: Haemostasis, Anticoagulation, and the Anticoagulated

Shahid Karim and Sanjay Sastry

Post-procedure Haemostasis

Haemostasis following radial artery procedures serves two important functions—the control of bleeding and the maintenance of radial artery patency. The main difference compared to haemostasis of the femoral artery, related largely to the smaller size of the radial, is the use of compression in some form as the main mechanism of achieving haemostasis.

Vascular closure devices commonly used to achieve femoral haemostasis act either by active or passive means. The 'gold standard' for femoral access remains manual compression which is still necessitated in some situations as dictated by the anatomical level of puncture or the presence of underlying femoral vascular disease. However, its use has all but fallen out of fashion due to time constraints placed on healthcare professionals, discomfort experienced by patients as well as lengthy bed rest requirements, and the need to wait for reduction in activated clotting time after percutaneous coronary intervention (PCI). Passive closure devices such as FemoStop™ (St. Jude Medical) do share similarities with radial access closure by achieving haemostasis through mechanical compression over the arteriotomy. Active femoral closure devices such as Angio-Seal or Perclose use either collagen or sutures to seal the arteriotomy. Appelgate et al. found Angio-Seal achieved closure success in 97.1% of femoral access cases of PCI including heparin and GP IIb/IIIa inhibitor therapy and Perclose 94.1%.[1] They found no significant difference in rates of major complication between manual compression, Angio-Seal, or Perclose (1.3%, 1.1%, and 1.0%, respectively).

There are multiple factors influential in the prevention of radial artery occlusion (RAO) following transradial procedures including the provision of anticoagulation, the use of appropriately sized sheaths and the method of haemostasis, amongst others.

Radial Artery Occlusion

Although RAO is often of limited symptomatic significance, it renders the access route obsolete for both further catheterization or for use as an arterial graft during surgery. The possibility of arteriovenous fistula formation is also lost. Dual blood supply via both palmar arch arteries provides backup circulation to the hand in the vast majority of patients; however, 1.5%[2] of patients do not demonstrate adequate dual hand blood supply when tested via means of a Barbeau's test and may be unsuitable for cardiac catheterization via this route (Figures 21.1, 21.2, and 21.3).

Acute RAO is thought to be secondary to interruption of antegrade flow due to the presence of an introducer sheath as well as the endothelial and intimal injuries that occur during its insertion. This environment promotes thrombus formation and luminal flow reduction. When combined with occlusive pressure following a radial access procedure, particularly if for longer than necessary, this can significantly increase the probability of a resultant arterial occlusion.

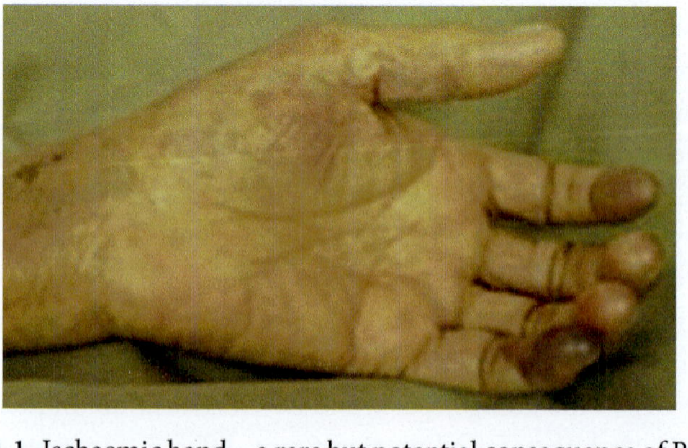

Figure 21.1 Ischaemic hand—a rare but potential consequence of RAO.

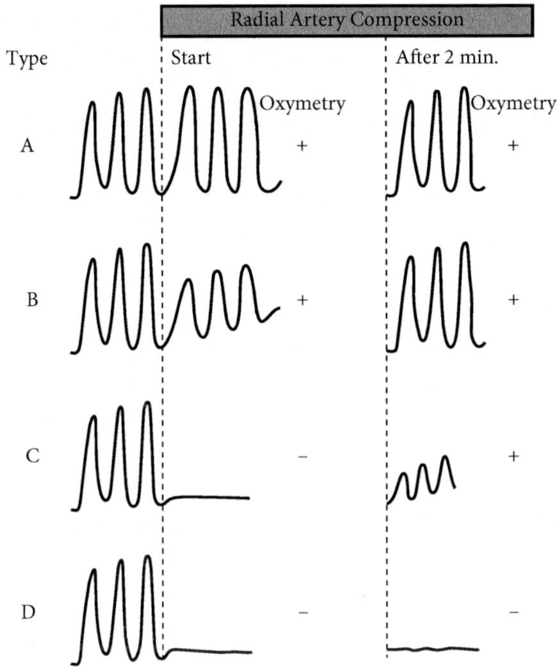

Figure 21.2 Plethysmographic tracings following radial artery compression.

Patent Haemostasis

Patent haemostasis is one of the key methods of reducing the likelihood of RAO. The aim of patent haemostasis is to preserve antegrade flow whilst preventing bleeding from the arteriotomy. Preservation of flow along the radial artery is one of the key methods of maintaining patency after catheterization. Activation of the fibrinolytic pathway is essential in opposing thrombus formation following access and requires flow. A pulse oximeter with plethysmography is placed on the index finger and a compression device fitted over the radial artery puncture site with removal of the sheath. Occlusive pressure is applied to the ulnar artery until loss of the saturation curve. The radial artery compression device is then gradually loosened until the saturation curve returns and bleeding remains halted.

The Prophet study compared conventional and patent haemostasis in 436 consecutive patients undergoing transradial catheterization.[3]

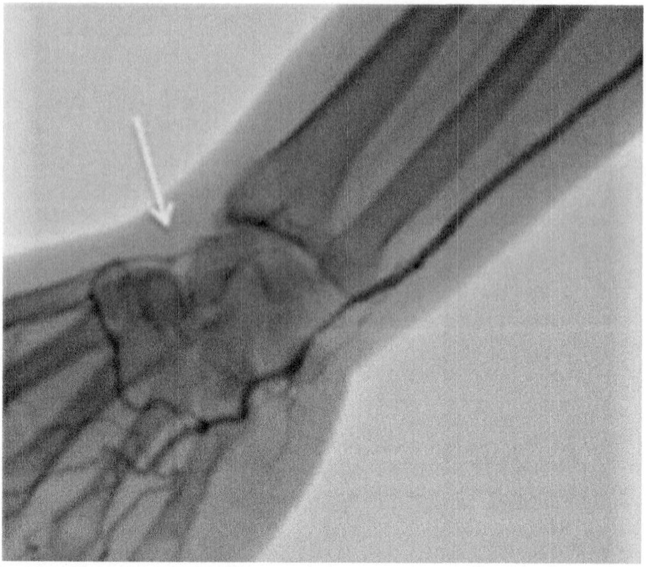

Figure 21.3 RAO post catheterization.

Conventional haemostasis was performed using a Hemoband™ applying a fixed level of pressure over the radial access site for two hours. Patients in the group receiving patent haemostasis had the same band applied but with Barbeau's test performed and the band loosened until radial artery patency was confirmed. The band was then left in place for two hours with an hourly check for continued radial artery patency. Both groups had Barbeau's test repeated after 24 hours and 1-month post procedure to assess on going radial artery patency.

When assessed using the reverse Barbeau's test, 5% of those treated with patent haemostasis demonstrated RAO at 24 hours versus 12% in the group treated with conventional haemostasis. Rates at one month were similarly reduced with 1.8% RAO in the patent haemostasis group versus 7% in the conventional arm.

Sub-group analysis of the patients treated with conventional occlusive compression found that those who developed RAO at 1 month were significantly older (~8 years) and more likely to be female (12.9% female versus 1% male). Interestingly, patients who were heavier (~88 kg versus 68 kg) were significantly less likely to develop RAO at one month, probably as they had larger calibre arteries but this is unclear as the study did not measure radial artery diameters. No patients developed bleeding complications in either arm, as defined by bleeding causing haemodynamic instability or death or requiring transfusion.

The practice of patent haemostasis application is variable across catheter labs. There are likely several reasons for this. Striking the balance between prevention of bleeding and maintenance of patency requires time and input from staff who are adequately trained in both the method as well as action necessary in the event of a complication. Specific training in the technique is required alongside the availability of saturation probes with plethysmography displays which do not feature on many observation machines. We suggest that every catheter lab should make concerted efforts to ensure provision of such machines alongside adequate training in the importance of patent haemostasis and the relevant technical information.

Prophet-II observed 3,000 patients across multiple sites undergoing diagnostic cardiac catheterization via the radial artery route.[4] Patients were assigned either to standard patent haemostasis (all cases received nitroglycerin, verapamil, and heparin) as described earlier with two hours of radial artery compression or to patent haemostasis alongside ipsilateral ulnar artery compression with a cylindrical composite made of a needle cap wrapped in gauze. Plethysmography was used to confirm occlusive pressure on the ulnar artery.

Rates of RAO were significantly reduced with ipsilateral ulnar artery compression immediately (1.5% versus 13.9%), at 24 hours (1.0% versus 4.3%) and at 30 days following the procedure (0.9% versus 3.0%). Thirty-day univariate predictors of RAO included female patients, diabetic status, age, and patients who experienced pain during compression. There was no evidence of significant hand ischaemia despite compression of both arteries—likely due to the continued patency of the radial artery during its compression as well as micro and macro collateralization of the palmar arterial circulation.

Compressive Radial Haemostasis Devices

Several methods of radial artery compression exist. There are more basic methods of compression and more complex systems with variable

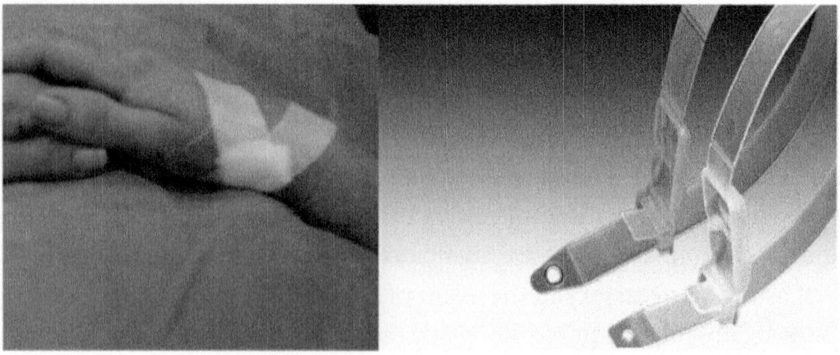

Figure 21.4 Basic compression bandage and Hemoband™.

levels of compression possible. The most basic form of standard compression is performed using sterile gauze over the puncture site held in place with a tight bandage. This method is straightforward to perform; however, it does not allow direct visualization of the puncture site during haemostasis nor does it allow variation in compressive pressure and so patent haemostasis is not guaranteed by any means. The Hemoband™ works in a similar way but includes a zip tie like locking mechanism (Figure 21.4).

There are a number of compression devices available that allow variable compression over the radial artery and are much more able to provide patent haemostasis, some with direct visualization of the puncture site during compression.

TR Band

The TR band is a transparent band with a pneumatic compression system (Figure 21.5). It allows variable and reproducible pressure over the arteriotomy as well as direct visualization of the puncture site. Its straightforward application and pressure management system has led to extensive uptake.

Pancholy compared rates of RAO between the TR band with the Hemoband device in 500 patients undergoing transradial catheterization.[5] Radial artery patency was assessed at 30 and 60 min as well as 24 hours and 30 days post procedure. Of the 250 patients in each

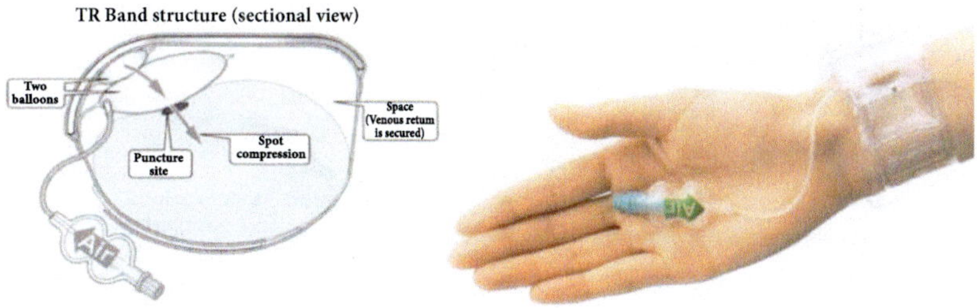

Figure 21.5 TR band (Terumo Interventional Systems).

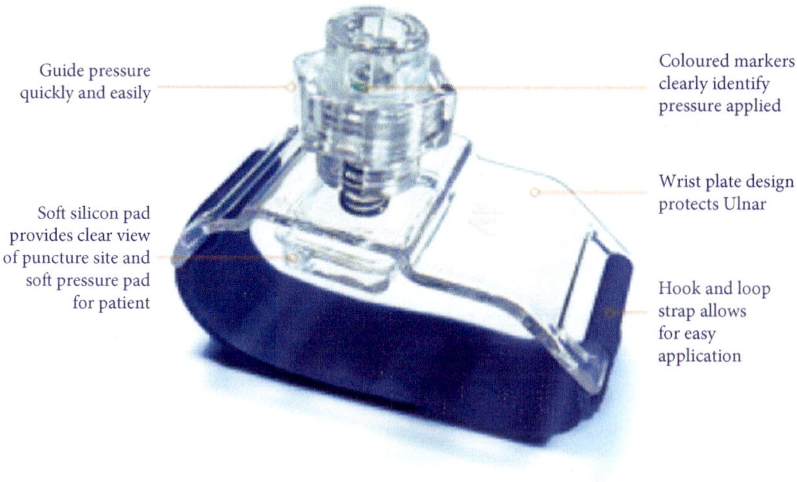
Guide pressure quickly and easily
Soft silicon pad provides clear view of puncture site and soft pressure pad for patient
Coloured markers clearly identify pressure applied
Wrist plate design protects Ulnar
Hook and loop strap allows for easy application

Figure 21.6 Helix compression device (vascular perspectives).

arm, rates of RAO were significantly more frequent at all time-points in the Hemoband group when compared to those receiving TR band haemostasis.

Helix

The Helix device is similar to the TR band (Figure 21.6). It also has a transparent construction with a screw-bolt design to allow variable compression over the radial artery.

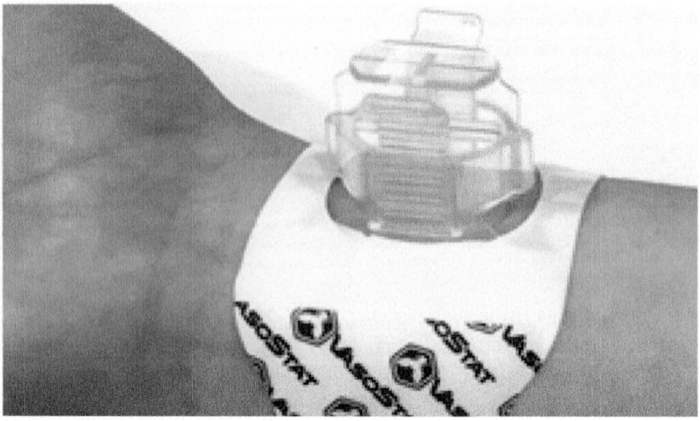

Figure 21.7 VasoStat haemostasis device.

Vasostat

The Vasostat is a relatively new haemostasis device which may be used in a number of sites including radial, brachial and after transpedal procedures (Figure 21.7). The device aims to allow pressure to be applied over a very specific point and uses a ratcheting system to allow variable pressure to be applied. It also has a transparent hub to allow continuous observation of the puncture site.

Kwan et al. used either TR bands or VasoStat devices in 314 patients undergoing retrograde tibial artery access for peripheral vascular interventions and found no significant difference between each in achieving haemostasis or in rates of loss of access site patency.[6]

Devices with Coagulating Factors

QuikClot

The QuikClot device uses a gauze pad impregnated with Kaolin (Figure 21.8). Kaolin is a naturally occurring mineral which activates Factor XII of the coagulation cascade. Originally formulated for military applications it has multiple hospital setting uses. The pad is applied to the access site and held in place with an elasticated bandage.

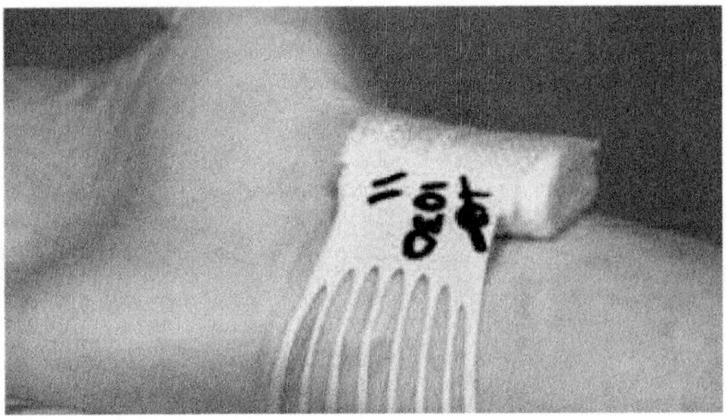

Figure 21.8 QuikClot radial.

Roberts et al. compared haemostasis between TR Band and the QuikClot Radial Pad (applied for 30 or 60 min) with 10 patients in each arm.[7] TR band use was with 10 ml air inflation (3 ml more if unable to provide immediate haemostasis) deflated by 2 ml after 40 min then by 2 ml every 20 min. The QuikClot group had 5 min of manual compression applied after application and then had the bandage left for either 25 or 55 min more before the bandage was removed and the Kaolin dressing left in place until the next morning. No significant differences were noted in rates of RAO (no cases reported).

Chitoclot

The Chitoclot pad is made of Chitosan—a linear polysaccharide made from the shells of shrimp and other crustaceans (Figure 21.9). It has profound haemostatic properties and has been used in military applications. Chitosan enhances platelet aggregation. The Chitoclot radial compression device functions in a similar manner to the Helix device whilst encouraging the formation of fibrin in the tract leading to the arteriotomy, shortening the time needed for compression and so aims to encourage lasting patent haemostasis.

Dai et al. assessed 600 patients after radial catheterization using either the TR band or a Chitosan-based pad for haemostasis.[8] They found a significant reduction in the rates of RAO at 24 hours (11.7% versus 5.4%) and 30 days (10% versus 5%) in those treated with the Chitoclot based

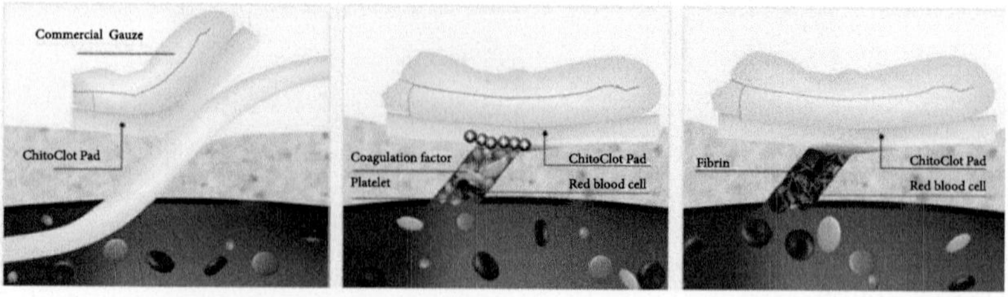

Figure 21.9 ChitoClot pad.

pad. Compression time required was also significantly reduced in the group receiving Chitoclot pad haemostasis.

Anticoagulant Use for Transradial Procedures

Administration of an anticoagulant during radial artery catheterization is associated with lower rates of RAO. In their prospective study, Spaulding et al. found administration of between 2,000 and 3,000 IU of heparin intravenously at the start of the case lead to a reduction in radial occlusion rates from 71% to 24% when compared to no heparin.[9] Precisely, 4.3% of patients receiving 5,000 IU of heparin demonstrated RAO when assessed post-procedure. The series of 415 patients found sex (female) and radial artery diameter (<2.7 mm) to be the most likely predictors of RAO in the groups receiving low-dose or no heparin. Compression of the ulnar artery for 60 min also reduced the incidence of RAO from 5.9% to 4.1% in the group receiving a lower dose of heparin with a reduction from 2.9% to 0.8% in the higher dose heparin group.

There is no significant difference in the rate of RAO following radial angiography between cases with heparin administration via the intra-arterial or intravenous route.[10] The number of patients reporting a burning sensation in the forearm at the time of heparin administration was found by Pancholy to be significantly higher in those receiving heparin via the intra-arterial route. The risk of discomfort can be reduced by haemodilution of heparin before administration if this is still preferred via the intra-arterial route/operator administered.

Although lower doses of heparin such as 50 IU/kg are associated with lower radial artery compression times (RACT),[11] there is no significant increase in risk of bleeding with higher doses such as 5,000 IU and rates of RAO are lower as discussed. This is despite the fact that shorter radial artery compression time itself is associated with a lower likelihood of RAO.

Bivalirudin, a reversible direct thrombin inhibitor, is the predominant antithrombotic agent utilized in radial access procedures in the United States. No significant difference in rates of RAO has been demonstrated over heparin use.[12,13] Given the significant cost difference, we recommend the use of heparin bolus for diagnostic radial access coronary angiography.

Transradial Procedures in Patients on Anticoagulants

An additional advantage of transradial versus transfemoral access is the ability to perform invasive procedures without stopping anticoagulation where required. This is relevant to patients taking anticoagulation for atrial fibrillation (AF), prosthetic heart valves and the prevention or treatment of thromboembolic disease.

The largest group is represented by patients in AF which has increasing incidence and prevalence (2%). The prevalence of AF has doubled in the past decade, and its identification is improved with greater awareness and investigation. Few operators will perform routine femoral access with an INR > 1.5, whilst therapeutic levels of anticoagulation with INR 2–3 are not considered a contraindication to transradial access.

In their prospective study of 50 patients, Helft et al. found radial access for coronary intervention both feasible and safe in patients already taking vitamin K antagonists before the time of the procedure. No bridging therapy was required and average INR at the time of procedure was 2.2 ± 0.6 with a mixture of elective and acute coronary cases.[14]

Gallego-Sanchez et al.'s prospective study included 140 anticoagulated patients with an average INR of 2.4 ± 0.9. Aspirin was taken alongside acenocumarol in 52% of patients and dual antiplatelets (aspirin and clopidogrel) in 16%. No significant differences were found in rates of RAO at 24 hours or one month following catheterization in either the acenocumarol or the group receiving peri-procedural heparin (5,000 units).[15]

Pancholy et al. found rates of RAO to be significantly higher in patients who were anticoagulated with warfarin and did not receive additional heparin when compared with those who were non-anticoagulated and received an additional bolus dose of heparin at the time of coronary angiography.[12]

Routine practice in our institution is to continue anticoagulants in patients undergoing purely diagnostic angiography when using the radial access route. In those patients undergoing PCI who have a low risk of thromboembolism, we hold novel oral anticoagulants (NOAC)s two days pre-procedure and hold warfarin for five days, proceeding once the INR is less than 1.5. In cases where the patient has a significant risk of thromboembolism, the warfarin will be continued or if stopped, intravenous or low-molecular-weight heparin substituted depending on the indication. If warfarin is continued for the procedure, a small dose of heparin (typically 2,500 IU) will be given during the procedure.

References

1. Applegate RJ, Grabarczyk MA, Little WC, et al. Vascular closure devices in patients treated with anticoagulation and IIb/IIIa receptor inhibitors during percutaneous revascularization. *J Am Coll Cardiol.* 2002;40:78–83.
2. Barbeau GR, Arsenault F, Dugas L, Simard S, Lariviere MM. Evaluation of the ulnopalmar arterial arches with pulse oximetry and plethysmography: comparison with the Allen's test in 1010 patients. *Am Heart J.* 2004; 147: 489–93.
3. Pancholy S, Coppola J, Patel T, Roke-Thomas M. Prevention of radial artery occlusion-patent hemostasis evaluation trial (PROPHET study): a randomized comparison of traditional versus patency documented hemostasis after transradial catheterization. *Catheter Cardiovasc Interv.* 2008;72:335–40.
4. Pancholy SB, Bernat I, Bertrand OF, Patel TM. Prevention of radial artery occlusion after transradial catheterization: the PROPHET-II randomized trial. *JACC Cardiovasc Interv.* 2016;9:1992–99.
5. Pancholy SB. Impact of two different hemostatic devices on radial artery outcomes after transradial catheterization. *J Invasive Cardiol.* 2009;21:101–4.
6. Kwan TW, Patel A, Parikh R, Auguste U, Rosero H, Huang Y, Liou M, Ratcliffe J, Puma J. Comparison of TR Band™ and VasoStat™ hemostasis devices following transpedal catheterization for lower extremity revascularization for peripheral arterial disease. *J Interv Cardiol.* 2016;29:424–30.
7. Roberts JS, Niu J, Pastor-Cervantes JA. Comparison of hemostasis times with a kaolin-based hemostatic pad (QuikClot Radial) vs mechanical compression (TR Band) following transradial access: a pilot prospective study. *J Invasive Cardiol.* 2017;29(10):328–34. Epub 2017 Aug 15.

8. Dai N, Xu DC, Peng WH, Wei YD, Xu YW. A comparison of 2 devices for radial artery hemostasis after transradial coronary intervention. *J Cardiovasc Nurs.* 2015;30(3):192–96.
9. Spaulding C, Lefèvre T, Funck F, Thébault B, Chauveau M, Ben Hamda K, Chalet Y, Monségu H, Tsocanakis O, Py A, Guillard N. Left radial approach for coronary angiography: results of a prospective study. *Cathet Cardiovasc Diagn.* 1996;39(4):365–67.
10. Pancholy SB, Shah S, Patel TM. Radial artery access, hemostasis, and radial artery occlusion. *Interv Cardiol Clin.* 2015;4(2):121–25.
11. Schiano P, Barbou F, Chenilleau MC, Louembe J, Monsegu J. Adjusted weight anticoagulation for radial approach in elective coronarography: the AWARE coronarography study. *EuroIntervention.* 2010;6:247–50.
12. Pancholy SB, Ahmed I, Bertrand OF, Patel T. Frequency of radial artery occlusion after transradial access in patients receiving warfarin therapy and undergoing coronary angiography. *Am J Cardiol.* 2014;113:211–14.
13. Plante S, Cantor WJ, Goldman L, Miner S, Quesnelle A, Ganapathy A, Popel A, Bertrand OF. Comparison of bivalirudin versus heparin on radial artery occlusion after transradial catheterization. *Catheter Cardiovasc Interv.* 2010;76:654–58.
14. Helft G, Dambrin G, Zaman A, Le Feuvre C, Barthelemy O, Beygui F, et al. Percutaneous coronary intervention in anticoagulated patients via radial artery access. *Catheter Cardiovasc Interv.* 2009;73(1):44–7.
15. Gallego-Sánchez G, Gallardo-López A, Córdoba-Soriano JG, Gutiérrez-Díez A, Melehi D, Barrionuevo-Sánchez MI, Jiménez-Mazuecos J. Safety of transradial diagnostic cardiac catheterization in patients under oral anticoagulant therapy. *J Cardiol.* 2017;69(3):561–64.

22

Radial Artery Occlusion After Transradial Access

Muhammad Rashid and Mamas A. Mamas

Background

Over the past decade, there has been a global upsurge in use of radial artery for cardiac catheterization and percutaneous coronary intervention (PCI).[1–3] The rapid increase in uptake of transradial access (TRA) is mainly driven by its widely accepted and well-recognized benefits such as reduction in mortality,[4–7] fewer access site and bleeding complication,[2,8–10] early ambulation,[11] and greater patient satisfaction.[12] International guidelines also recommend use of radial approach for coronary intervention in patients with acute coronary syndromes.[13] Whilst TRA has shown efficacy in improving patient outcomes, radial artery occlusion (RAO) is an important complication which may occur following TRA.

RAO is defined as *'loss of radial pulse on palpation subsequently confirmed by doppler ultrasonography or plethysmography'*.

RAO is usually silent, but once occluded, the use of radial artery for any future intervention, as a conduit for coronary artery bypass graft (CABG) or fistula formation is precluded. There is also concern that non-occlusive injuries[14] sustained by the radial artery during TRA may have negative influence on longevity of radial artery patency and reduce the success of future TRA procedures. In this chapter, we sought to review the incidence and mechanisms of radial occlusion following transradial cardiac catheterization and provide an overview of the strategies that can facilitate radial artery patency.

Incidence of RAO

The incidence of RAO varies greatly from <1% up to 30%[15–17] depending upon the timing of assessment of arterial patency and method employed for detection of RAO. Table 22.1 provides an overview of some the key studies reporting the incidence of RAO after TRA. A recent meta-analysis of 66 studies reported a combined incidence of 7.7% in first 24 hours after the procedure which reduced to 5.5% at one-week follow-up.[18]

Table 22.1 Key studies reporting incidence of radial artery occlusion using ultrasound Doppler or Barbeau's test

Study	Timing and method employed for detection of RAO	Results
Chugh et al. (2013)[24]	Early RAO after the procedure and late RAO at 4 weeks using ultrasound Doppler	Early RAO incidence: 0.48% Late RAO incidence: 0.16%
Cubero et al. (2009)[58]	RAO assessment at 24–72 hours using inverse Allen's test and bidirectional Doppler.	Incidence of RAO: 6.5%
Dharma et al. (2014)[63]	RAO assessment at 24 hours using ultrasound duplex	Incidence of RAO: 9.9%
Garg et al. (2015)[44]	RAO assessment 1 day after the procedure using US.	Incidence of RAO: 15.2%.
Honda et al. (2012)[43]	RAO assessment at 24 hours with US.	Incidence of RAO: 10.4%
Nagai et al. (1999)[23]	RAO assessment at early (1–8 days) and late (37–182 days) using US.	Early undetectable flow confirmed on US 9%. Late RAO = 3%.
Pancholy et al. (2008)[15]	RAO assessment at 24 hours and 30 days using plethysmography.	Incidence of RAO at 24 hours: 8.7% Incidence of RAO at 30 days: 4.5%
Pancholy et al. (2014)[68]	RAO assessment at 24 hours and 30 days using plethysmography.	Incidence of early RAO: 11.9% Incidence of late RAO: 7.4%.
Politi et al. (2011)[51]	RAO assessment at 24 hours using the Barbeau's test.	Incidence of RAO: 5%
Sanmartin et al. (2007)[16]	RAO assessment at 7 days with pulse oximeter and plethysmograph.	Absent pulsation: 4.4% Absent radial flow (True RAO): 10.5%.
Schiano et al. (2010)[69]	RAO assessment at 24 hours using US Doppler.	Incidence of RAO: 0%.

Interestingly, the incidence of RAO was much higher at 8.8% in patients requiring diagnostic coronary angiogram, whereas it was only 4.5% in patients undergoing PCI which is likely due to the judicious use of antithrombotics in patients undergoing PCI.

Clinical Presentation

RAO is usually a silent complication of transradial intervention. Anastomoses of radial and ulnar arteries form superficial and deep palmar arches supplying blood to hand. Due to this collateral circulation, occlusion of one artery very rarely results in hand ischaemia. Furthermore, there is growing evidence now to suggest that another artery, the interosseous artery, may also contribute to the circulation of hand providing added protection against hand ischaemia.[19] Patients may complain of pain at the puncture site or in the forearm on movement due to underlying stenosis of radial artery. A minority of patients may have absent palmar blush representative of reduce blood flow in the radial artery. Critical hand ischaemia is exceedingly rare despite millions of procedures being undertaken via TRA.[20,21] On clinical examination, patients may have a very weak or absent radial pulse. However, a weak or absent radial pulse does not always constitute a diagnosis of RAO as an occluded radial artery may be palpable due to recruitment of retrograde filling from collaterals. Therefore, diagnosis of RAO should be made using a more objective method of assessment such as Barbeau's test or duplex ultrasonography as discussed later in the chapter.

Finally, as RAO is usually asymptomatic, the long-term course of patients with RAO remains unclear. HANGAR (HANd Grip test After tRansradial percutaneous coronary procedures) study evaluated the force of small muscle of hands in patients with prolonged RAO at 30 days.[22] The investigators performed hand grip and thumb and finger pinch tests in patients with RAO diagnosis confirmed on ultrasound. There was no effect of RAO on the hand grip strength or thumb and forefinger pinch at 30 days. More interestingly, TRA itself was associated with significant reduction in hand muscle strength a day after the procedure, but it returned to baseline in all patients at 30 days. In another study to evaluate the clinical course of RAO, Nagai et al. performed serial ultrasonic assessment of patients undergoing TRA over a period of three months.[23] They found that rate of acute RAO was 9% but 60% of these patients had recanalization of radial artery at three-month follow-up. A recent meta-analysis[18] of 66 studies showed that rates of RAO reduce significantly 7.7% at 24 hours to 5.5% at >1-week follow-up supporting the hypothesis that RAO may recanalize due to activation of innate tissue plasminogen and urokinase facilitating the resolution of thrombus. In conclusion, RAO alone is unlikely to have any significant impact on function of hand owing to excellent collateral circulation. Furthermore, a considerable proportion of RAO recanalizes without any long-term sequel.

Assessment of Radial Artery Patency

An objective assessment of radial artery patency should be an integral part of any TRA to ensure that there is adequate collateral circulation of hand present before the procedure. Additionally, pre-assessment will also aid in identifying patients who may be at risk of developing radial occlusion and prevent any potential vascular complication. In PRIMAFACIE-TRI registry, pre-procedural ultrasonic assessment of radial artery improved procedural success and reduced vascular complication such as arterial spasm.[24] Despite these obvious benefits, the idea of pre-assessment remains elusive amongst majority of operators. On the other end, post-procedural assessment of radial artery is mainly focused to determine radial artery patency. We will now explore various methods described in literature to assess the patency of radial artery.

a. Modified Allen's Test

Modified Allen's test (MAT) is a simple but rather crude method to assess the circulation of hand at the bedside. MAT is conducted by asking the patient to make a fist for approximately 30 seconds and then occluding both the radial and ulnar artery simultaneously by applying manual pressure with fingers. Patient is then asked to open the fist and pressure is selectively released over the ulnar artery whilst compressing the radial artery. Full blushing of hand should ensue within 10–12 seconds if there is sufficient blood flow through ulnar artery suggesting intact collateral circulation via ulnar artery. Similarly, patency of radial artery can be assessed by reverse Allen's test during which same method is repeated whist compressing the ulnar instead of radial artery. Although MAT can easily be performed at bedside without the need for any specialist equipment, MAT is a very subjective method to assess for radial artery patency, and several factors such as hyperextension of wrist, presence of interosseous artery, inadequate occlusive pressure, and lack of consensus over time required for return of maximal palmar blush can lead to false interpretation of MAT. Due to these limitations, MAT is not considered a reliable method to assess hand circulation.

b. Barbeau's Test

Barbeau developed a more objective way of assessing the collateral hand circulation by combining the use of pulse oximetry and digital plethysmography. Pulse oximetry uses simple principle of tissue hypoxia in an event of cessation of blood supply and is measured by recording changes in the oxygen saturation levels, whereas digital plethysmography is recorded by placing a sensor at the thumb and plethysmography tracings are captured in a waveform. A change in waveform pattern or complete disappearance will be suggestive of underlying arterial occlusion.[25] In Barbeau's test, pulse oximetry and plethysmography tracing are obtained simultaneously whilst manually occluding the radial artery. In the absence of collateral circulation, i.e. occlusion of ulnar artery, there will be damping of plethysmographic wave form and pulse oximetry.[26] Similarly, radial artery patency can be demonstrated by repeating the same method whilst manually occluding the ulnar artery at the wrist. Absence of plethysmographic waveform and pulse oximetry will be indicative of RAO. Reverse Barbeau's test provides a more subjective and reliable technique to assess the patency of radial artery.

c. Duplex Ultrasonography

Duplex ultrasound is a gold standard method to assess the radial artery patency. It provides accurate and detailed information about the anatomical structure, size, and blood flow through the radial artery. When compared with other method of assessment such MAT, a vast majority of patients who have abnormal MAT actually have been demonstrated to have patent radial artery using duplex ultrasonography.[27,28] However, use of ultrasound in practice is limited due to lack of equipment in the catheter lab, operator training and time constraints.

In conclusion, despite its inconclusive results, MAT is still being used by a vast majority of radial operators.[3] However, duplex ultrasound and reverse Barbeau's test are recommended methods of assessment of radial artery blood flow status.[29] Ultrasound has an added advantage of providing detailed information about vascular anatomy of hand.

Mechanism of RAO

RAO can be detected as early as immediately after the procedure or chronic occlusion may be diagnosed at subsequent follow-up after TRA. Acute thrombus formation mainly accounts for development of RAO. Cannulation and instrumentation during TRA causes endothelial damage exposing the highly thrombogenic tissue which acts as a precursor for expression of procoagulation factors such as tissue factor (TF) and van Willebrand factor (vWF), platelet activation and adhesion, increased thrombin generation and ultimately leading to thrombus formation. The stasis of blood whilst achieving haemostasis along with thrombus formation creates a highly favourable environment for clot stabilization and arterial occlusion. More recently, retrieval of organized thrombus from occluded radial artery[30] as well as presence of thrombus in radial artery on vascular ultrasound and angiography[31,32] further supports the hypothesis that acute thrombosis plays a key role in occlusion of radial artery.

TRA is also responsible for negative impact on arterial wall structure and function. Vascular endothelium is the first layer of arterial wall which comes into contact with sheaths and catheters and likely to suffer from structural and functional injuries. Endothelium also plays a key role in maintaining vascular tone by releasing various mediators in response to vascular injury.[33] The structural damage to endothelial is likely to initiate thrombotic process as discussed earlier; however, TRA is also thought to be responsible for introduction of functional changes in vascular endothelium. For instance, recent work has been focused around investigating changes in flow-mediated dilatation (FMD) as a marker for endothelial dysfunction. FMD is a non-invasive ultrasound method used to assess

NO-mediated endothelial function by measuring the changes in blood flow within the blood vessel.[34] Studies assessing the changes in FMD in setting of using 6Fr TR PCI systems illustrated a significant reduction in FMD.[35,36] Similarly, Heiss et al. demonstrated a significant reduction in FMD when using 5Fr TR PCI system. More interestingly, studies evaluating the effects of large size (6Fr) PCI system showed a greater reduction and longer recovery time in FMD compared to smaller (5Fr) PCI systems reinforcing the theory that large catheter size cause greater trauma to radial artery. Burstein[35] and Dawson[36] also showed that vascular injury during TR catheterization is extended to the vascular smooth muscle cell function of the arterial wall by demonstrating an impaired vasodilatory response of radial artery to glyceral trinitrate (GTN).

Another important aspect of vascular injury is the direct trauma caused to intima and media of vessel wall from sheath insertion and catheter manipulation. Several studies have used advance imaging modalities such as intravascular ultrasound (IVUS) and optical coherence tomography (OCT) to study the acute injuries to arterial wall during TRA.[14,37,38] An OCT guided serial analysis of radial wall post TR cardiac catheterization using 6Fr catheter systems revealed 76.1% acute intimal tears and 35.6% medial dissection in radial artery.[14] Similarly, another study performed serial IVUS on 100 patients undergoing TR cardiac catheterization and found a significant proportion of patient developed intimal and medial thickening after the procedure.[37] Finally, histological examinations of radial artery used as CABG conduit also confirmed previous TRA accounts for development of intimal thickening, medial calcification, adventitial inflammation, and necrosis.[39]

These data suggest that TRA may introduce significant structural and functional changes in the radial artery. The endothelial dysfunction and intimal hyperplasia may persist long term, resulting in significant stenosis. These patterns of radial injury have important implications particularly in patient requiring future procedures for revascularization. In one large series of 812 patients undergoing repeated TRA, the failure rates of procedure due to access increased proportionately to number of attempts particularly in women. Procedure failure rates were 3.5% and 7.9% at the second attempt in men and women, respectively, which increased to 30% and 50% at the fifth attempt.[40] In conclusion, radial occlusion and non-occlusive injuries to vessel wall increases procedure failure rates and limit

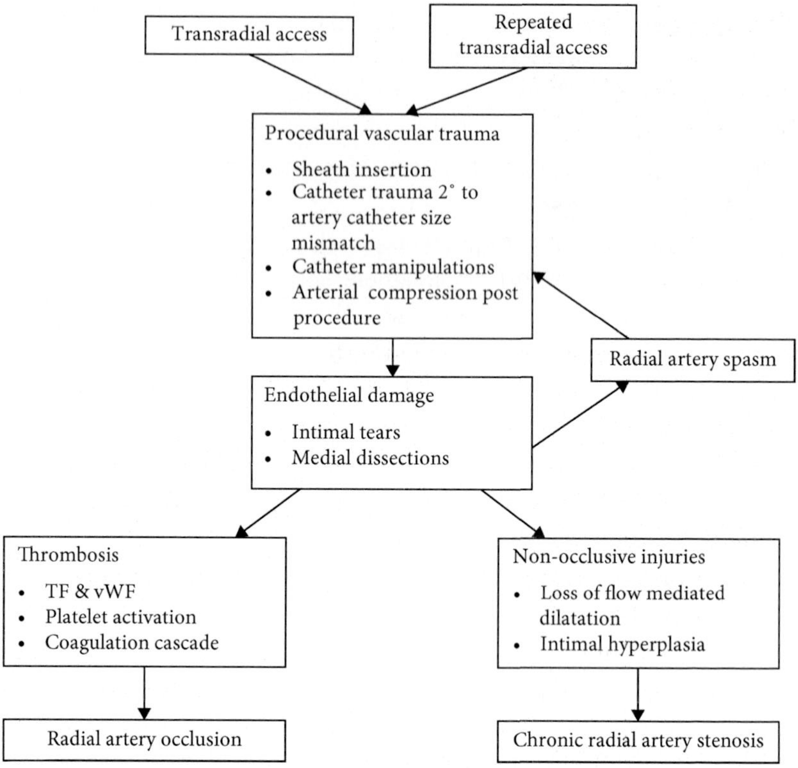

Figure 22.1 Various patterns of injuries leading to radial artery occlusion following TR cardiac catheterization. TF: tissue factor; VWF: von wilibrond factor

use of radial artery in future interventions. Figure 22.1 illustrates the some of the key radial wall injuries sustained during TRA.

Predictors of RAO

Researchers have investigated various patient's baseline characteristics and procedural variables using statistical models to predict RAO. Table 22.2 provides an overview of some of the landmark studies investigating the predictors of RAO and summary of their findings.

Patient's baseline characteristics such as gender, age, body mass index (BMI), and hyperlipidaemia have been shown to predict RAO.[41–44]

Table 22.2 Predictors of radial artery occlusion

Study ID	Study Description	Predictors of RAO (Patient's characteristics)	Predictors of RAO (Procedural Variables)
Aykan et al. (2015)[41]	Patients undergoing radial artery catheterization who were randomized to 2,500 IU or 5,000 IU heparin.	Male (p = 0.008), age (p = 0.950), body mass index (p = 0.838), hypertension(p=0.035), dyslipidemia (p = 0.034	Fluoroscopy time (p = 0.893), procedure time (p = 0.659), sheath removal time (p = 0.001), heparin group (p = 0.010).
Buturak et al. (2013)[42]	Patients undergoing first transradial coronary procedure.		Sheath-to-artery ratio >1 (p<0.001).
Cubero et al. (2009)[58]	Patients undergoing transradial coronary angiography were randomized to pneumatic compression guided by mean arterial pressure or standard compression.	Univariate predictors of RAO: ex-or active smoker p = 0.04, absence antiaggregant p = 0.04	Multivariate predictors of RAO: presence of RA flow after procedures HR 0.06 (0.01–0.2), total haematoma HR 3.7 (1.2–11.0), standard pneumatic compression HR 18.8 (3.8–92.2).
Dharma et al. (2014)[63]	Patients undergoing transradial catheterization were randomized to receive either nitroglycerin (500mcg) or placebo.		Multivariate predictors of RAO: Duration of haemostasis >4 hours OR 3.11(1.66–5.82), Intra-arterial nitroglycerin use OR 0.62(0.44–0.87).
Garg et al. (2015)[44]	Patients who undergoing PCI or adhoc PCI via transradial access.	Female gender OR 0.75 (0.19–2.93), diabetes OR 0.74 (0.22–2.51), BMI 0.91 (0.83–1.56),	Radial artery size ≤2.5mm OR 40.54 (9.91–165.81), radial artery peak systolic velocity OR 0.94 (0.90–1.00), radial artery diameter to sheath ratio <1 OR 0.89 (0.16–5.06).
Honda et al. (2012)[43]	Prospective study of 500 consecutive patients undergoing transradial coronary procedure.	Pretreatment with statin medications OR 0.501 (0.255–0.985).	Outer diameter of sheath OR 5.24 (1.21–22.8),

(continued)

Table 22.2 Continued

Study ID	Study Description	Predictors of RAO (Patient's characteristics)	Predictors of RAO (Procedural Variables)
Pancholy et al. (2008)[15]	Patients from PROPHET study undergoing transradial catheterization who were randomized to conventional pressure application or pressure application confirming radial artery patency using Barbeau's test.	Patient weight ($p=<0.05$),	Patency ($p \leq 0.05$).
Pancholy et al. (2011)[70]	Patients undergoing transradial catheterization who had 2 or 6 hours of haemostatic compression.		Duration of compression ($p = 0.037$)
Pancholy et al. (2012)[71]	Patients undergoing transradial catheterization and were randomized to Seldinger and modified Seldinger technique.	Diabetes OR 11 (3–38),	Patent radial artery during haemostasis OR 0.03 (0.004–0.28), heparin OR 0.45 (0.13–1.54).
Plante et al. (2010)[57]	Patients underwent transradial catheterization and received heparin or bivalirudin.	Patient body weight OR 2.78 (1.08–8.00),	Bivalirudin OR 0.45 (0.11–2.06), procedure ≤20 minutes OR 7.52 (1.57–36.0).
Politi et al. (2011)[51]	Patients underwent transradial catheterization and were randomized to QuikClot, short compression or conventional compression.		Heparin OR 0.70 (0.49–0.99).
Uhlemann et al. (2012)[72]	Patients with transradial cardiac catheterization who had 5 Fr and 6 Fr sheath.	Female sex OR 2.36 (1.50–3.73), peripheral arterial occlusive disease OR 2.04 (1.02–4.22), age OR 0.96 (0.94–0.98).	6 Fr sheath OR 2.68 (1.56–4.59).

Elderly patients with smaller BMI are likely to have smaller calcified arteries and hence are at an increased risk of developing radial artery spasm (RAS) and vascular complications following TRA. For example, 1 kilogram (kg) increase in patient's weight reduces the possibility of RAO by 5.6%.[15] Similarly, female gender has been associated with increased risk of developing RAS.[44] As discussed already, development of RAS increases the risk of endothelial damage and intimal tears following TRA. Hyperlipidaemia is recognized risk factor for development of atherosclerosis. In a study of 500 patients, Honda et al. reported that lack of statin treatment increase the risk of occlusive complication in patients undergoing TRA.[43] This concept is novel and needs further studies to show if baseline atherosclerotic changes in vessel wall are responsible for RAO.

Procedural variables associated with RAO have been subject of more rigorous investigation lately as they are thought to be modifiable factors. Radial artery diameter and its association with sheath size,[23,24,45,46] use of anticoagulation,[41,47–49] patent haemostasis, and duration of radial artery compression[16,50,51] have been identified as important procedural variables predicting RAO.

Radial Artery and Sheath Size

Radial artery internal luminal diameter and introducer sheath/catheter outer diameter mismatch (sheath outer diameter > artery inner diameter) has been associated with increased risk of reduce blood flow in the radial artery[52] and higher RAS and RAO rates.[23,38] The average diameter of a radial artery is reported to be around 2.5 mm–3.0 mm,[53] whereas the internal diameter of a radial artery is been reported to be around 2.5 mm.[14,23,38,52] In GRASP (Good Radial Artery Size Prediction) study, male sex, wrist circumference, and non-south-Asian ancestry were shown to be independent predictors of radial artery diameter.[54] Table 22.3 illustrates a summary of variation in diameter of radial artery amongst different population cohorts. The industrial standards for the outer diameter of a 5Fr, 6Fr, 7Fr, and 8 Fr introducer sheath are typically around 2.28 mm, 2.52 mm, 2.85 mm, and 3.22 mm, respectively.[55] Although an average sized artery of 2.5 mm will be able to accommodate a 6 Fr sheath of 2.52 mm due to inherent elasticity of the vessel wall, but

Table 22.3 Reported diameter of radial artery in different cohorts

Study	Ethnicity	Mean diameter	Male	Female
Aykan et al. (2015)[41]	Turkish	2.62 ± 0.45 mm	2.73 ± 0.39 mm	2.15 ± 0.35 mm
Garg et al. (2015)[44]	Indian	2.8 ± 0.4 mm	2.8 ± 0.4 mm	2.4 ± 0.4 mm
Chugh et al. (2014)[24]	Indian	1.9 ± 1.1 mm	1.9 ± 1.1 mm	1.7 ± 0.29 mm
Kotowycz et al. (2013)[54]	Caucasian	2.44 ± 0.60 mm	2.59 ± 0.57 mm	1.91 ± 0.55 mm
Baumann et al. (2015)[73]	Caucasian	3.03 ± 0.57 mm	3.2 ± 0.56 mm	2.7 ± 0.45 mm
Loh et al. (2007)[74]	Chinese	2.45 ± 0.54 mm	NA	NA
Ashraf et al. (2010)[75]	Pakistani	2.3 ± 0.4 mm	2.3 ± 0.39 mm	2.11 ± 0.29 mm
Saito et al. (1999)[52]	Japanese	NA	3.10 ± 0.60 mm	2.80 ± 0.60 mm

it is easy to imagine that an oversized sheath in a relatively small radial artery is likely to result in an arterial-sheath mismatch causing endothelial damage and reduction in blood flow through radial artery. This will be further exacerbated in an event of development of RAS causing more trauma to the vessel wall. Consequently, blood stasis and acute endothelial damage will trigger the thrombotic process leading to RAO. In a very early study of Japanese patients, Saito et al. observed a significant reduction of blood flow through the artery with increasing Fr size of introducer sheath. More importantly, the incidence of reduction in radial blood flow was significantly reduced in patients when radial artery inner diameter to sheath outer diameter ratio was greater than 1.0.[52] Similar observation were made by many other investigators that artery-sheath mismatch predicts poor outcomes in RAO.[23,42,43,45,56]

Anticoagulation

Radial artery injury and blood stasis in radial artery creates a hypercoagulable state within the artery. Therefore, many operators routinely use anti-thrombotic such as heparin or bivalirudin to minimize the risk of RAO. The evidence for use of heparin came from a very early study in which 71% of the patients developed asymptomatic RAO receiving no heparin at all. This reduced to 24% and 4.3% when given 2,000–3,000 units or 5,000 units of heparin, respectively.[47] In another study, Plante et al. tested the effectiveness of heparin versus bivalirudin in preventing RAO in patients undergoing diagnostic coronary angiography or diagnostic coronary angiography ± ad hoc PCI.[57] They concluded that heparin or bivalirudin were similarly efficacious in preventing RAO but preferred heparin due to its low cost. Current expert guidelines from Society of Cardiac Angiography and Interventions (SCAI) advocate using 3,000–5,000 units of heparin in patients undergoing routine coronary angiography.[29] There is no randomized data on superiority of heparin or bivalirudin in preventing RAO and their use is usually dictated by operator preferences, costs and local protocols.

Patent Haemostasis

As discussed earlier, no-flow state in the radial artery provides the nidus for arterial occlusion generating the hypothesis that anterograde flow through radial artery whilst achieving haemostasis may predict RAO. Sanmartin et al. observed that patient with no blood flow through radial artery during compression are likely to develop RAO.[16] These findings were subsequently confirmed in a randomized trial where patients were randomly assigned to conventional pressure application for haemostasis versus pressure application whilst maintaining radial artery patency (just enough pressure to allow anterograde blood flow through radial artery) using Barbeau's test.[15] There was 59% reduction in RAO at 24 hours increasing to an impressive 75% reduction at 30 days in patients assigned to patent haemostasis arm. In logistic regression analysis, patent haemostasis was found to be a strong predictor of RAO. Compression devices such as TR band (Terumo Medical Corporation, Somerset, NJ) which allow patent haemostasis have also been found to significantly reduce the incidence of RAO.[50,58] Furthermore, compression duration is also an important predictor of RAO as longer compression time promotes blood stasis and arterial damage as described earlier. A recent meta-analysis showed that shorter duration of compression of 15 minutes favours better RAO outcomes compared to longer compression times of 2 hours.[18] However, there may be a trade off with bleeding complication with such a short compression and one must be careful to allow time for appropriate haemostasis.

Strategies to Minimize Radial Injury

Radial artery undergoes significant structural remodelling due to TRA in addition to evident arterial occlusion leading to progressive narrowing of the artery. Preventative strategies to minimize the remodelling in radial artery may assist in preserving radial artery for future interventions.

At molecular level, number of medications has shown promising results in improving endothelial dysfunction.[59,60] One such agent is trimetazidine (TMZ) which has been reported to have novel properties to reduce intimal hyperplasia and protect endothelium in vascular injury.[61] In one study, patients were randomly assigned to receive TMZ after going TR catheterization using 5Fr sheaths.[62] At 10 weeks, patients receiving TMZ had full recovery of FMD reflecting positive impact of TMZ on endothelial dysfunction incurred following TRA. Another observational study reported pretreatment with statin reduces radial occlusion by modulating intimal hyperplasia.[43] The exact mechanism by which statin influence radial occlusion is not clear, but statin are known to have pleiotropic actions that modulate endothelial function and thrombogenesis. Finally, a very recent large randomized study used a novel pharmacological approach of administering 500 mcg of nitroglycerin into radial artery post procedure.[63] A significant reduction in RAO rates was observed in patients receiving nitroglycerine compared to placebo arm. They hypothesized that vasodilatory effect of nitroglycerine helps in minimizing the intimal inflammation and intimal hyperplasia in the radial artery.

Radial artery diameter and more importantly artery to sheath diameter ratio[52] has been associated with increased risk of radial injury and arterial occlusion. This attracted interventionists to move towards using smaller sheaths and guide catheters in performing TRI to prevent vascular complications such as RAO. For instance, a meta-analysis of 18 studies using conventional catheter systems illustrated 0% RAO rates with 4Fr catheter systems increasing to 11.1% with 8Fr catheter systems.[18] One disadvantage of smaller Fr guide catheters is limited back-up support. Furthermore, use of instruments for complex PCI such as rotational atherectomy, treatment of bifurcation lesions, with some 2 stent strategies; and use of bulkier devices for PCI often require larger size catheters. Sheathless guide catheter systems provide one potential means for maintaining the size of guide catheters and minimizing the injury to radial artery. The outer diameter of sheathless guides is typically 2Fr smaller than conventional catheter systems. For instance, the outer diameter of 6.5Fr sheathless guide is usually equivalent to external diameter of 4.5Fr conventional introducer sheath. Thus, sheathless guides may provide an attractive alternative to conventional catheter systems in performing complex transradial coronary interventions and minimizing RAO. In an effort to further reduce the size of conventional sheath, Terumo (Tokyo, Japan) developed a glide sheath slender (GSS) system dedicated for TRA. GSS has hydrophilic coated outer thin wall with an external diameter approximately one Fr smaller than the corresponding conventional system and offering the same internal diameter. For example, 6Fr GSS has an internal diameter of 2.22 mm whereas the outer diameter has been reduced from 2.63 mm to 2.45 mm which is similar to outer diameter of 5Fr. There is small risk of increased sheath kinking due to very delicate outer sheath wall which can be tackled by handling the system with care and using a small skin incision before sheath insertion.

Another strategy to minimize the artery-sheath diameter mismatch is to predict the radial artery diameter which will enable the operator to make appropriate selection of equipment or switch the access to contralateral artery. Ultrasonic imaging of radial artery provides very important information about anatomical course of radial artery. In one large prospective registry, use of pre-procedure ultrasound significantly improved procedure success rate and reduced the incidence of RAO[24] In RAUST trial, feasibility of using real time ultrasound was evaluated to gain TRA.[64] Although this study was not powered to capture vascular complications such as RAO, there was significant reduction in incidence of RAS and puncture attempts with use of ultrasound, both of which have been associated with increased risk of vascular injury. In conclusion, use of ultrasound provides useful information about radial anatomy which

Table 22.4 Preventative strategies to minimize radial injury

Mechanism of prevention	Study details		Results
Pharmacological	Park et al. (2010)[62]	Patients undergoing transradial catheterization using a 5Fr sheath were randomly assigned to the TMZ group or the control group.	TMZ therapy after transradial catheterisation reduces the endothelial dysfunction of the radial artery by improving FMD.
	Honda et al. (2010)[43]	Multivariable analysis of consecutive patients undergoing transradial PCI.	Pretreatment with statin medications reduces the risk of radial artery occlusion.
	Dharma et al. (2014)[63]	Patients undergoing transradial catheterization were randomized to receive either nitroglycerin (500mcg) or placebo.	The use of nitroglycerin as compared to placebo reduces the risk of the radial artery occlusion [8.3% vs. 11.7%; OR 0.62 95% confidence interval (CI) 0.44–0.87.
Use of smaller sheaths	Rashid et al. (2016)[18]	Pooled meta-analysis of 18 studies	One study with 4Fr catheter system 0% RAO rates, 6 studies with 5Fr catheter system 5% RAO rates, 8 studies with 6Fr catheter systems 11.6% RAO rates.
Use of Sheathless guides	Rashid et al. (2016)[18]	Pooled meta-analysis of 10 studies	2 studies with 3Fr sheathless guides 0% RAO rates, 1 study with 4Fr sheathless gudie 2% RAO rates, 5 studies with 6.5 Fr sheathless guide 0.7% RAO rates.
Patent Haemostasis	Sanmartin et al. (2007)[16]	Prospective analysis of 275 consecutive patients undergoing transradial catheterization	Absence of radial flow during compression was strong predictor of RAO (OR 5 6.7; 95%CI: 1.95–22.9)
	Pancholy et al. (2008)[15]	Patients from PROPHET study undergoing transradial catheterization who were randomized to conventional pressure application or pressure application confirming radial artery patency using Barbeau's test.	59% reduction in acute radial artery occlusion by using patent haemostasis at 24 hours. 75% reduction in chronic radial artery occlusion by using patent haemostasis at 30 days.

Table 22.4 Continued

Mechanism of prevention	Study details		Results
	Cubero et al. (2009)[58]	Patients undergoing transradial coronary angiography were randomized to pneumatic compression guided by mean arterial pressure or standard compression.	Study was suspended after analysing the results of 50% of the scheduled patients. Radial artery compression guided by mean arterial pressure resulted in 10-fold reduction in the rate of RAO (1.2% versus 12.0%, P = 0.0001).
Anticoagulation	Spaulding et al. (1996)[47]	Prospective analysis of 415 consecutive patients undergoing transradial catheterization with no heparin or 2,000–3,000 units of heparin or 5,000 units heparin administrated during the procedure.	71% of patients receiving no heparin, 24% of patients receiving 2,000–3,000 U of heparin, and 4.3% of patients receiving 5,000 U of heparin developed RAO.
Shorter compression time	Politi et al. (2011)[51]	Patients underwent transradial catheterization and were randomized to QuikClot, short compression (15 minutes) or conventional compression (2 hours).	RAO rates where doubled in patients treated with conventional 2 hours of compression times.

in conjunction with appropriate selection of catheter system may help greatly in minimizing the radial injury.

Appropriate and effective use of anticoagulation helps in preventing thrombotic complications during TRA as discussed earlier. Low-molecular-weight heparin (LMWH) is preferred choice of anticoagulation across many centres in the world due to its low cost. Current expert opinion recommends 3,000–5,000 units of unfractionated heparin for patients undergoing TR catheterization to prevent thrombotic complications.[29] Patent haemostasis in conjunction with appropriate anticoagulation allows sustained flow through radial artery and prevents thrombus formation. Patent haemostasis is usually applied after the procedure by withdrawing the sheath 2–3 cm and applying the compression device. The device is then inflated to allow the removal of the sheath from radial artery. Compression device is then slowly deflated whilst closely observing for the arterial bleeding from the skin site entry at which point the small amount of air is injected again in the compression device to stop the bleeding. To confirm patent haemostasis (antegrade blood through radial artery) reverse Barbeau's test should be performed as described earlier.

RAS is another frequently encountered vascular complication during TRA. It is logical to conclude that occurrence of RAS will result in significant reduction in arterial internal diameter predisposing the artery to increase risk of injury during cannulation, catheter exchange and manipulation. Use of hydrophilic sheaths,[65] pharmacological agents such as verapamil and nitroglycerin[66] reduce incidence of RAS and help in minimizing radial injury. Table 22.4 describes few essential preventative strategies to minimize radial injury.

Treatment

Occlusion of radial artery is usually quiescent and hence often overlooked in clinical practice. Once a patient is detected to have RAO, it is usually managed conservatively with close observation as in some cases it recanalizes due to activation of primary fibrinolysis. When RAO is encountered after the procedure, compression of ipsilateral ulnar artery may help restoring the patency of radial artery by increasing the retrograde flow through radial artery.[49] This technique requires transient compression of ipsilateral ulnar artery for one hour which will promote reopening of radial artery by increasing the high velocity blood through radial artery. Subcutaneous LMWH may also assist in dissolution of acute thrombus. Zankl et al.[67] demonstrated successful treatment of symptomatic RAO with administration of subcutaneous LMWH for four weeks.

In case of chronic occlusion, successful recanalization of radial artery can be performed percutaneously using antegrade approach from brachial artery or retrogradely from distal radial artery. This may require considerable experience as there is risk of embolization of thrombus.

Conclusion

The radial artery has become the default access site choice across the world for PCI due to the significant mortality benefits and associated reduction in major bleeding complications observed with its use in high risk patient cohorts. Recent data suggest that radial artery injury and occlusion is not an infrequent occurrence and may limit the radial artery as an access site for future PCI procedures. Minimization of radial injury and prevention of occlusion should be integral part of all procedures taken through radial artery. Pre-procedure ultrasound may help in access and appropriate selection. Pharmacological agents such as TMZ and nitroglycerine, small Fr size catheter systems, appropriate anticoagulation in the form of 3,000–5,000 units of unfractionated Heparin, or Tab Rivaroxaban 10mg x daily for 1 week (RIVARAD trial); patent haemostasis, and shorter compression times have proven to reduce vascular trauma and occlusion rates.

References

1. Mamas MA, Nolan J, de Belder MA, Zaman A, Kinnaird T, Curzen N, Kwok CS, Buchan I, Ludman P and Kontopantelis E. Changes in arterial access site and association with mortality in the United Kingdom: observations from a national percutaneous coronary intervention database. *Circulation*. 2016;133:1655–1667. Originally published11 Mar 2016 https://doi.org/10.1161/CIRCULATION AHA.115.018083.
2. Jolly SS, Yusuf S, Cairns J, Niemela K, Xavier D, Widimsky P, Budaj A, Niemela M, Valentin V, Lewis BS, Avezum A, Steg PG, Rao SV, Gao P, Afzal R, Joyner CD, Chrolavicius S and Mehta SR. Radial versus femoral access for coronary angiography and intervention in patients with acute coronary syndromes (RIVAL): a randomised, parallel group, multicentre trial. *Lancet*. 2011;377:1409–20.
3. Bertrand OF, Rao SV, Pancholy S, Jolly SS, Rodes-Cabau J, Larose E, Costerousse O, Hamon M and Mann T. Transradial approach for coronary angiography and interventions: results of the first international transradial practice survey. *JACC Cardiovasc Interv*. 2010;3:1022–31.
4. Ratib K, Mamas MA, Anderson SG, Bhatia G, Routledge H, De Belder M, Ludman PF, Fraser D and Nolan J. Access site practice and procedural outcomes in relation to clinical presentation in 439,947 patients undergoing percutaneous coronary intervention in the United kingdom. *JACC Cardiovasc Interv*. 2015;8:20–9.

5. Valgimigli M, Gagnor A, Calabro P, Frigoli E, Leonardi S, Zaro T, Rubartelli P, Briguori C, Ando G, Repetto A, Limbruno U, Cortese B, Sganzerla P, Lupi A, Galli M, Colangelo S, Ierna S, Ausiello A, Presbitero P, Sardella G, Varbella F, Esposito G, Santarelli A, Tresoldi S, Nazzaro M, Zingarelli A, de Cesare N, Rigattieri S, Tosi P, Palmieri C, Brugaletta S, Rao SV, Heg D, Rothenbuhler M, Vranckx P and Juni P. Radial versus femoral access in patients with acute coronary syndromes undergoing invasive management: a randomised multicentre trial. *Lancet.* 2015;385:2465–76.
6. Baklanov DV, Kaltenbach LA, Marso SP, Subherwal SS, Feldman DN, Garratt KN, Curtis JP, Messenger JC and Rao SV. The prevalence and outcomes of transradial percutaneous coronary intervention for ST-segment elevation myocardial infarction: analysis from the National Cardiovascular Data Registry (2007 to 2011). *J Am Coll Cardiol.* 2013;61:420–6.
7. Chase AJ, Fretz EB, Warburton WP, Klinke WP, Carere RG, Pi D, Berry B and Hilton JD. Association of the arterial access site at angioplasty with transfusion and mortality: the M.O.R.T.A.L study (Mortality benefit Of Reduced Transfusion after percutaneous coronary intervention via the Arm or Leg). *Heart.* 2008;94:1019–25.
8. Mamas MA, Anderson SG, Carr M, Ratib K, Buchan I, Sirker A, Fraser DG, Hildick-Smith D, de Belder M, Ludman PF and Nolan J. Baseline bleeding risk and arterial access site practice in relation to procedural outcomes after percutaneous coronary intervention. *J Am Coll Cardiol.* 2014;64:1554–64.
9. Jolly SS, Amlani S, Hamon M, Yusuf S and Mehta SR. Radial versus femoral access for coronary angiography or intervention and the impact on major bleeding and ischemic events: a systematic review and meta-analysis of randomized trials. *Am Heart J.* 2009;157:132–40.
10. Mehta SR, Jolly SS, Cairns J, Niemela K, Rao SV, Cheema AN, Steg PG, Cantor WJ, Dzavik V, Budaj A, Rokoss M, Valentin V, Gao P and Yusuf S. Effects of radial versus femoral artery access in patients with acute coronary syndromes with or without ST-segment elevation. *J Am Coll Cardiol.* 2012;60:2490–9.
11. Brasselet C, Tassan S, Nazeyrollas P, Hamon M and Metz D. Randomised comparison of femoral versus radial approach for percutaneous coronary intervention using abciximab in acute myocardial infarction: results of the FARMI trial. *Heart.* 2007;93:1556–61.
12. Nathan S and Rao SV. Radial versus femoral access for percutaneous coronary intervention: implications for vascular complications and bleeding. *Curr Cardiol Rep.* 2012;14:502–9.
13. Roffi M, Patrono C, Collet JP, Mueller C, Valgimigli M, Andreotti F, Bax JJ, Borger MA, Brotons C, Chew DP, Gencer B, Hasenfuss G, Kjeldsen K, Lancellotti P, Landmesser U, Mehilli J, Mukherjee D, Storey RF, Windecker S, Baumgartner H, Gaemperli O, Achenbach S, Agewall S, Badimon L, Baigent C, Bueno H, Bugiardini R, Carerj S, Casselman F, Cuisset T, Erol C, Fitzsimons D, Halle M, Hamm C, Hildick-Smith D, Huber K, Iliodromitis E, James S, Lewis BS, Lip GY, Piepoli MF, Richter D, Rosemann T, Sechtem U, Steg PG, Vrints C and Luis Zamorano J. 2015 ESC guidelines for the management of acute coronary syndromes in patients presenting without persistent ST-segment elevation: Task Force for the Management of Acute Coronary Syndromes in Patients Presenting

without Persistent ST-Segment Elevation of the European Society of Cardiology (ESC). *Eur Heart J*. 2016;37:267–315.

14. Yonetsu T, Kakuta T, Lee T, Takayama K, Kakita K, Iwamoto T, Kawaguchi N, Takahashi K, Yamamoto G, Iesaka Y, Fujiwara H and Isobe M. Assessment of acute injuries and chronic intimal thickening of the radial artery after transradial coronary intervention by optical coherence tomography. *Eur Heart J*. 2010;31:1608–15.
15. Pancholy S, Coppola J, Patel T and Roke-Thomas M. Prevention of radial artery occlusion—patent hemostasis evaluation trial (PROPHET study): a randomized comparison of traditional versus patency documented hemostasis after transradial catheterization. *Catheter Cardiovasc Interv*. 2008;72:335–40.
16. Sanmartin M, Gomez M, Rumoroso JR, Sadaba M, Martinez M, Baz JA and Iniguez A. Interruption ofblood flow during compression and radial artery occlusion after transradial catheterization. *Catheter Cardiovasc Interv*. 2007;70:185–9.
17. Stella P, Kiemeneij F, Laarman G, Odekerken D, Slagboom T and Van der Wieken R. Incidence and outcome of radial artery occlusion following transradial artery coronary angioplasty. *Catheter Cardiovasc Diag*. 1997;40:156–8.
18. Rashid M, Kwok CS, Pancholy S, Chugh S, Kedev SA, Bernat I, Ratib K, Large A, Fraser D, Nolan J and Mamas MA. Radial artery occlusion after transradial interventions: a systematic review and meta-analysis. *J Am Heart Assoc*. 2016;Jan 25;5(1):e002686.doi: 10.1161/JAHA.115.002686
19. Haerle M, Tonagel F and Schaller HE. Collateral arterial pathways in the forearm. *Surg Radiol Anat: SRA*. 2004;26:208–11.
20. Rhyne D and Mann T. Hand ischemia resulting from a transradial intervention: successful management with radial artery angioplasty. *Catheter Cardiovasc Interv*. 2010;76:383–6.
21. Ayan M, Smer A, Azzouz M, Abuzaid A and Mooss A. Hand ischemia after transradial coronary angiography: resulting in right ring finger amputation. *Cardiovasc Revasc Med*. 2015;16:367–9.
22. Sciahbasi A, Rigattieri S, Sarandrea A, Cera M, Di Russo C, Fedele S, Romano S, Penco M and Rocco Pugliese F. Radial artery occlusion and hand strength after percutaneous coronary procedures: results of the HANGAR study. *Catheter Cardiovasc Interv*. 2016 Apr;87(5):868–74. doi: 10.1002/ccd.26142. Epub 2015 Aug 13
23. Nagai S, Abe S, Sato T, Hozawa K, Yuki K, Hanashima K and Tomoike H. Ultrasonic assessment of vascular complications in coronary angiography and angioplasty after transradial approach. *Am J Cardiol*. 1999;83:180–6.
24. Chugh SK, Chugh S, Chugh Y and Rao SV. Feasibility and utility of pre-procedure ultrasound imaging of the arm to facilitate transradial coronary diagnostic and interventional procedures (PRIMAFACIE-TRI). *Catheter Cardiovasc Interv*. 2013;82:64–73.
25. Fronek A and King D. An objective sequential compression test to evaluate the patency of the radial and ulnar arteries. *J Vasc Surg*. 1985;2:450–2.
26. Barbeau GR, Arsenault F, Dugas L, Simard S and Lariviere MM. Evaluation of the ulnopalmar arterial arches with pulse oximetry and plethysmography: comparison with the Allen's test in 1010 patients. *Am Heart J*. 2004;147:489–93.

27. Abu-Omar Y, Mussa S, Anastasiadis K, Steel S, Hands L and Taggart DP. Duplex ultrasonography predicts safety of radial artery harvest in the presence of an abnormal Allen test. *Ann Thorac Surg*. 2004;77:116–9.
28. Hosono M, Suehiro S, Shibata T, Sasaki Y, Kumano H and Kinoshita H. Duplex scanning to assess radial artery suitability for coronary artery bypass grafting. *Jpn J Thorac Cardiovasc Surg*. 2000;48:217–21.
29. Rao SV, Tremmel JA, Gilchrist IC, Shah PB, Gulati R, Shroff AR, Crisco V, Woody W, Zoghbi G, Duffy PL, Sanghvi K, Krucoff MW, Pyne CT, Skelding KA, Patel T and Pancholy SB. Best practices for transradial angiography and intervention: a consensus statement from the society for cardiovascular angiography and intervention's transradial working group. *Catheter Cardiovasc Interv*. 2014;83:228–36.
30. Pancholy SB. Transradial access in an occluded radial artery: new technique. *J Invasive Cardiol*. 2007;19:541–4.
31. Kim KS, Park HS, Jang WI and Park JH. Thrombotic occlusion of the radial artery as a complication of the transradial coronary intervention. *J Cardiovasc Ultrasound*. 2010;18:31.
32. Babunashvili A and Dundua D. Recanalization and reuse of early occluded radial artery within 6 days after previous transradial diagnostic procedure. *Catheter Cardiovasc Interv*. 2011;77:530–6.
33. Ramcharan KS, Lip GY, Stonelake PS and Blann AD. The endotheliome: a new concept in vascular biology. *Thromb Res*. 2011;128:1–7.
34. Charakida M, Masi S, Luscher TF, Kastelein JJ and Deanfield JE. Assessment of atherosclerosis: the role of flow-mediated dilatation. *Eur Heart J*. 2010;31:2854–61.
35. Burstein JM, Gidrewicz D, Hutchison SJ, Holmes K, Jolly S and Cantor WJ. Impact of radial artery cannulation for coronary angiography and angioplasty on radial artery function. *Am J Cardiol*. 2007;99:457–9.
36. Dawson EA, Rathore S, Cable NT, Wright DJ, Morris JL and Green DJ. Impact of catheter insertion using the radial approach on vasodilatation in humans. *Clin Sci (London, England: 1979)*. 2010;118:633–40.
37. Wakeyama T, Ogawa H, Iida H, Takaki A, Iwami T, Mochizuki M and Tanaka T. Intima-media thickening of the radial artery after transradial intervention. An intravascular ultrasound study. *J Am Coll Cardiol*. 2003;41:1109–14.
38. Buturak A, Tekturk BM, Degirmencioglu A, Ulus S, Surgit O, Ariturk C, Zencirci E and Gorgulu S. Transradial catheterization may decrease the radial artery luminal diameter and impair the vasodilatation response in the access site at late term: an observational study. *Heart Vessels*. 2016 Apr;31(4):482–9. doi: 10.1007/s00380-015-0640-x.
39. Staniloae CS, Mody KP, Sanghvi K, Mindrescu C, Coppola JT, Antonescu CR, Shah S and Patel T. Histopathologic changes of the radial artery wall secondary to transradial catheterization. *Vasc Health Risk Manag*. 2009;5:527–32.
40. Sakai H, Ikeda S, Harada T, Yonashiro S, Ozumi K, Ohe H, Ochiai M, Miyahara Y and Kohno S. Limitations of successive transradial approach in the same arm: the Japanese experience. *Catheter Cardiovasc Interv*. 2001;54:204–8.
41. Aykan AC, Gokdeniz T, Gul I, Kalaycioglu E, Cetin M, Hatem E, Cavusoglu IG, Karabay CY, Guler A, Aykan DA and Yildiz M. Comparison of low dose versus

standard dose heparin for radial approach in elective coronary angiography? *Int J Cardiol.* 2015;187:389–92.

42. Buturak A, Gorgulu S, Norgaz T, Voyvoda N, Sahingoz Y, Degirmencioglu A and Dagdelen S. The long-term incidence and predictors of radial artery occlusion following a transradial coronary procedure. *Cardiol J.* 2014;21:350–6.
43. Honda T, Fujimoto K, Miyao Y, Koga H and Hirata Y. Access site-related complications after transradial catheterization can be reduced with smaller sheath size and statins. *Cardiovasc Interv Ther.* 2012;27:174–80.
44. Garg N, Madan BK, Khanna R, Sinha A, Kapoor A, Tewari S, Kumar S and Goel PK. Incidence and predictors of radial artery occlusion after transradial coronary angioplasty: Doppler-guided follow-up study. *J Invasive Cardiol.* 2015;27:106–12.
45. Yoo BS, Yoon J, Ko JY, Kim JY, Lee SH, Hwang SO and Choe KH. Anatomical consideration of the radial artery for transradial coronary procedures: arterial diameter, branching anomaly and vessel tortuosity. *Int J Cardiol.* 2005;101:421–7.
46. Zhou YJ, Zhao YX, Cao Z, Fu XH, Nie B, Liu YY, Guo YH, Cheng WJ and Jia DA. [Incidence and risk factors of acute radial artery occlusion following transradial percutaneous coronary intervention]. *Zhonghua yi xue za zhi.* 2007;87:1531–4.
47. Spaulding C, Lefevre T, Funck F, Thebault B, Chauveau M, Ben Hamda K, Chalet Y, Monsegu H, Tsocanakis O, Py A, Guillard N and Weber S. Left radial approach for coronary angiography: results of a prospective study. *Catheter Cardiovasc Diag.* 1996;39:365–70.
48. Hahalis G, Xathopoulou I, Tsigkas G, Almpanis G, Christodoulou I, Grapsas N, Davlouros P, Koniari I, Deftereos S, Raisakis K, Christopoulou G, Giannopoulos G, Kounis N, Pyrgakis V and Alexopoulos D. A comparison of low versus standard heparin dose for prevention of forearm artery occlusion after 5 French coronary angiography. *Int J Cardiol.* 2015;187:404–10.
49. Bernat I, Bertrand OF, Rokyta R, Kacer M, Pesek J, Koza J, Smid M, Bruhova H, Sterbakova G, Stepankova L and Costerousse O. Efficacy and safety of transient ulnar artery compression to recanalize acute radial artery occlusion after transradial catheterization. *Am J Cardiol.* 2011;107:1698–701.
50. Pancholy SB. Impact of two different hemostatic devices on radial artery outcomes after transradial catheterization. *J Invasive Cardiol.* 2009;21:101–4.
51. Politi L, Aprile A, Paganelli C, Amato A, Zoccai GB, Sgura F, Monopoli D, Rossi R, Modena MG and Sangiorgi GM. Randomized clinical trial on short-time compression with Kaolin-filled pad: a new strategy to avoid early bleeding and subacute radial artery occlusion after percutaneous coronary intervention. *J Interv Cardiol.* 2011;24:65–72.
52. Saito S, Ikei H, Hosokawa G and Tanaka S. Influence of the ratio between radial artery inner diameter and sheath outer diameter on radial artery flow after transradial coronary intervention. *Catheter Cardiovasc Interv.* 1999;46:173–8.
53. Gellman H, Botte MJ, Shankwiler J and Gelberman RH. Arterial patterns of the deep and superficial palmar arches. *Clin Orthop Relat Res.* 2001Feb;(383):41–6.doi10.1097/00003086-200102000-00007.
54. Kotowycz MA, Johnston KW, Ivanov J, Asif N, Almoghairi AM, Choudhury A, Nagy CD, Sibbald M, Chan W, Seidelin PH, Barolet AW, Overgaard CB and Dzavik V. Predictors of radial artery size in patients undergoing cardiac

catheterization: insights from the Good Radial Artery Size Prediction (GRASP) study. *Can J Cardiol.* 2014;30:211–6.

55. From AM, Gulati R, Prasad A and Rihal CS. Sheathless transradial intervention using standard guide catheters. *Catheter Cardiovasc Interv.* 2010;76:911–6.
56. Dahm JB, Vogelgesang D, Hummel A, Staudt A, Volzke H and Felix SB. A randomized trial of 5 vs. 6 French transradial percutaneous coronary interventions. *Catheter Cardiovasc Interv.* 2002;57:172–6.
57. Plante S, Cantor WJ, Goldman L, Miner S, Quesnelle A, Ganapathy A, Popel A and Bertrand OF. Comparison of bivalirudin versus heparin on radial artery occlusion after transradial catheterization. *Catheter Cardiovasc Interv.* 2010;76:654–8.
58. Cubero JM, Lombardo J, Pedrosa C, Diaz-Bejarano D, Sanchez B, Fernandez V, Gomez C, Vazquez R, Molano FJ and Pastor LF. Radial compression guided by mean artery pressure versus standard compression with a pneumatic device (RACOMAP). *Catheter Cardiovasc Interv.* 2009;73:467–72.
59. Vita JA, Yeung AC, Winniford M, Hodgson JM, Treasure CB, Klein JL, Werns S, Kern M, Plotkin D, Shih WJ, Mitchel Y and Ganz P. Effect of cholesterol-lowering therapy on coronary endothelial vasomotor function in patients with coronary artery disease. *Circulation.* 2000;102:846–51.
60. Boger RH, Bode-Boger SM, Szuba A, Tsao PS, Chan JR, Tangphao O, Blaschke TF and Cooke JP. Asymmetric dimethylarginine (ADMA): a novel risk factor for endothelial dysfunction: its role in hypercholesterolemia. *Circulation.* 1998;98:1842–7.
61. Mamas MA, Fraser DG, Ratib K, Fath-Ordoubadi F, El-Omar M, Nolan J and Neyses L. Minimising radial injury: prevention is better than cure. *EuroIntervention.* 2014;10:824–32.
62. Park KH, Park WJ, Kim MK, Park DW, Park JH, Kim HS and Cho GY. Effects of trimetazidine on endothelial dysfunction after sheath injury of radial artery. *Am J Cardiol.* 2010;105:1723–7.
63. Dharma S, Kedev S, Patel T, Kiemeneij F and Gilchrist IC. A novel approach to reduce radial artery occlusion after transradial catheterization: postprocedural/prehemostasis intra-arterial nitroglycerin. *Catheter Cardiovasc Interv.* 2015;85:818–25.
64. Seto AH, Roberts JS, Abu-Fadel MS, Czak SJ, Latif F, Jain SP, Raza JA, Mangla A, Panagopoulos G, Patel PM, Kern MJ and Lasic Z. Real-time ultrasound guidance facilitates transradial access: RAUST (Radial Artery access with Ultrasound Trial). *JACC Cardiovasc Interv.* 2015;8:283–91.
65. Rathore S, Stables RH, Pauriah M, Hakeem A, Mills JD, Palmer ND, Perry RA and Morris JL. Impact of length and hydrophilic coating of the introducer sheath on radial artery spasm during transradial coronary intervention: a randomized study. *JACC Cardiovasc Interv.* 2010;3:475–83.
66. Kwok CS, Rashid M, Fraser D, Nolan J and Mamas M. Intra-arterial vasodilators to prevent radial artery spasm: a systematic review and pooled analysis of clinical studies. *Cardiovasc Revasc Med.* 2015;16:484–90.
67. Zankl AR, Andrassy M, Volz C, Ivandic B, Krumsdorf U, Katus HA and Blessing E. Radial artery thrombosis following transradial coronary angiography: incidence

and rationale for treatment of symptomatic patients with low-molecular-weight heparins. *Clin Res Cardiol.* 2010;99:841–7.

68. Pancholy SB, Ahmed I, Bertrand OF and Patel T. Frequency of radial artery occlusion after transradial access in patients receiving warfarin therapy and undergoing coronary angiography. *Am J Cardiol.* 2014;113:211–4.
69. Schiano P, Barbou F, Chenilleau MC, Louembe J and Monsegu J. Adjusted weight anticoagulation for radial approach in elective coronarography: the AWARE coronarography study. *EuroIntervention.* 2010;6:247–50.
70. Pancholy SB and Patel TM. Effect of duration of hemostatic compression on radial artery occlusion after transradial access. *Catheter Cardiovasc Interv.* 2012;79:78–81.
71. Pancholy SB, Sanghvi KA and Patel TM. Radial artery access technique evaluation trial: randomized comparison of Seldinger versus modified Seldinger technique for arterial access for transradial catheterization. *Catheter Cardiovasc Interv.* 2012;80:288–91.
72. Uhlemann M, Mobius-Winkler S, Mende M, Eitel I, Fuernau G, Sandri M, Adams V, Thiele H, Linke A, Schuler G and Gielen S. The Leipzig prospective vascular ultrasound registry in radial artery catheterization: impact of sheath size on vascular complications. *JACC Cardiovasc Interv.* 2012;5:36–43.
73. Baumann F and Roberts JS. Real time intraprocedural ultrasound measurements of the radial and ulnar arteries in 565 consecutive patients undergoing cardiac catheterization and/or percutaneous coronary intervention via the wrist: understanding anatomy and anomalies may improve access success. *J Interv Cardiol.* 2015;28:574–82.
74. Loh YJ, Nakao M, Tan WD, Lim CH, Tan YS and Chua YL. Factors influencing radial artery size. *Asian Cardiovasc Thorac Ann.* 2007;15:324–6.
75. Ashraf T, Panhwar Z, Habib S, Memon MA, Shamsi F and Arif J. Size of radial and ulnar artery in local population. *JPMA J Pak Med Assoc.* 2010;60:817–9.

23

Moving to Forearm Access

Yashasvi Chugh, Sunita Chugh, and Sanjay Kumar Chugh

Conventionally, the right radial artery is the preferred access for most radial operators because of ease and comfort of operating from the right side of the patient. The right ulnar has been used for access instead of radial, as default by few and as alternate access in select situations by some operators. However, there is a growing consensus towards forearm access using the biggest and straightest artery of the forearm (radial or ulnar, right or left), which could minimize the risk of procedure failure and patient discomfort arising out of maneuvers through loops and anomalies or through very small access arteries.

The ulnar artery is not always bigger than the radial and equally, one, or both radial arteries could be larger than the ulnar in a patient.[1] Table 23.1 and Figures 23.1 and 23.2 show radial and ulnar artery size[1] according to gender and side (n = 2,344) in an Indian cohort of patients. Figures 23.3 and 23.4 show distribution of difference in size of radial and ulnar on the right and left side in the same cohort.

Since post-procedure access artery occlusion occurs more often in smaller access arteries (≤1.7 versus > 1.7 mm[2,3]), choosing an access artery in the forearm with the largest diameter based upon pre-procedure ultrasound assessment of the four forearm arteries[1] would be a preferred strategy.

Systematic Review and Meta-analysis of Transradial Versus Transulnar Studies

A recent meta-analysis[4] of six studies with nearly 4,800 patients showed that neither ulnar access was associated with increase in fluoroscopy time, contrast load, or access time, nor was there significant difference in the risk of major adverse cardiovascular events, defined as myocardial infarction (MI), stroke, urgent target vessel revascularization (TVR), or death, among patients treated with the transulnar versus transradial approach. Access-site failure was more than twice as high among patients undergoing percutaneous coronary intervention (PCI) via the ulnar artery (OR 2.63; 95% CI 2.07–3.34). Complications associated with access,

Table 23.1 Showing radial and ulnar artery size[1] according to gender and side (n = 2,344)[1]

Size of radial and ulnar artery on the two sides		Mean diameter (mm)
Left radial artery		
Male	1.8	0.29
Female	1.7	0.26
Left ulnar artery		
Male	1.8	0.30
Female	1.7	0.3
Right radial artery		
Male	1.9	1.12
Female	1.7	0.29
Right ulnar artery		
Male	1.8	0.30
Female	1.6	0.28

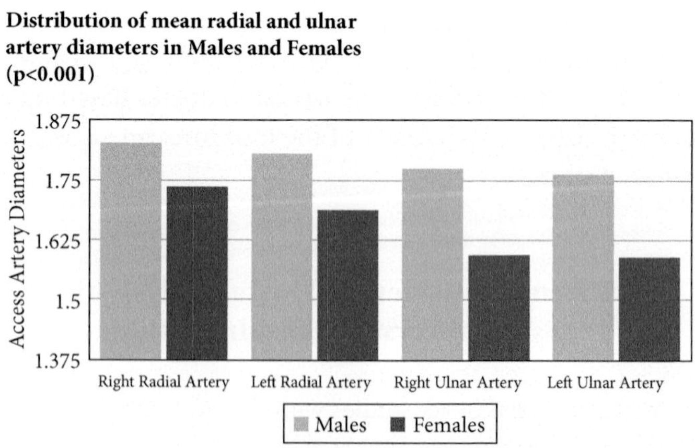

Figure 23.1 Radial and ulnar artery size in males and females.

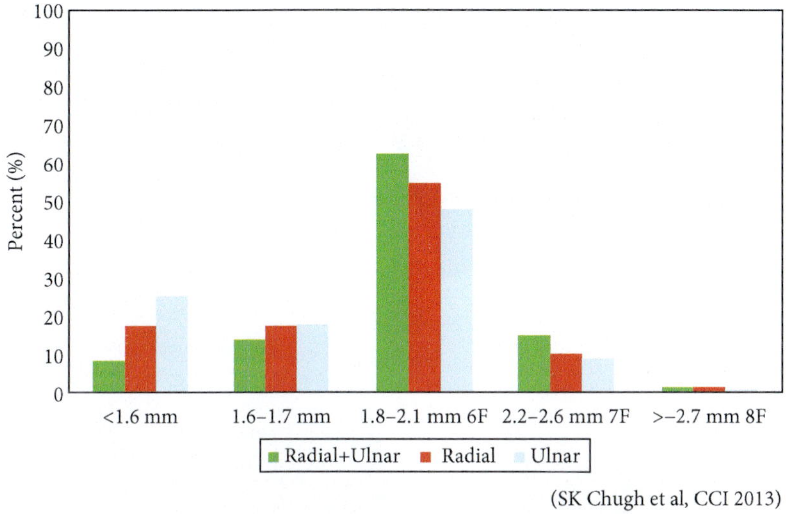

Figure 23.2 Distribution of mean radial and ulnar artery sizes.[1]

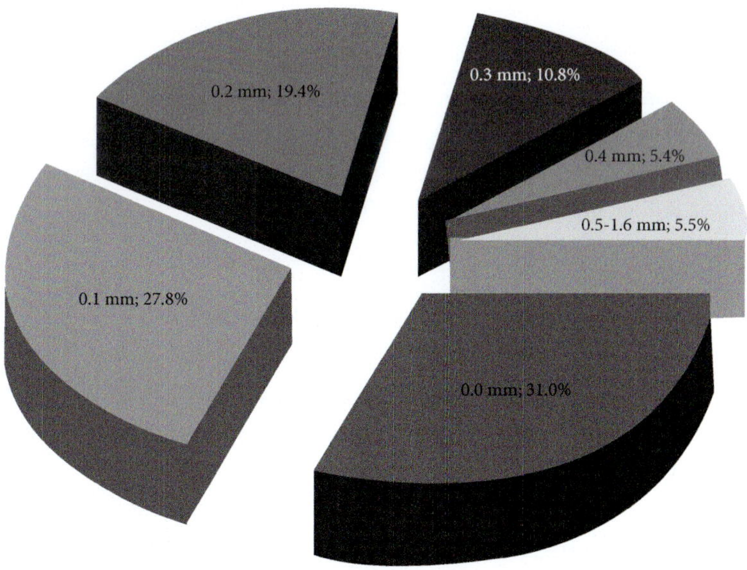

Figure 23.3 Distribution of difference in size between corresponding right and left radial arteries in the patients (n = 2,344).[1]

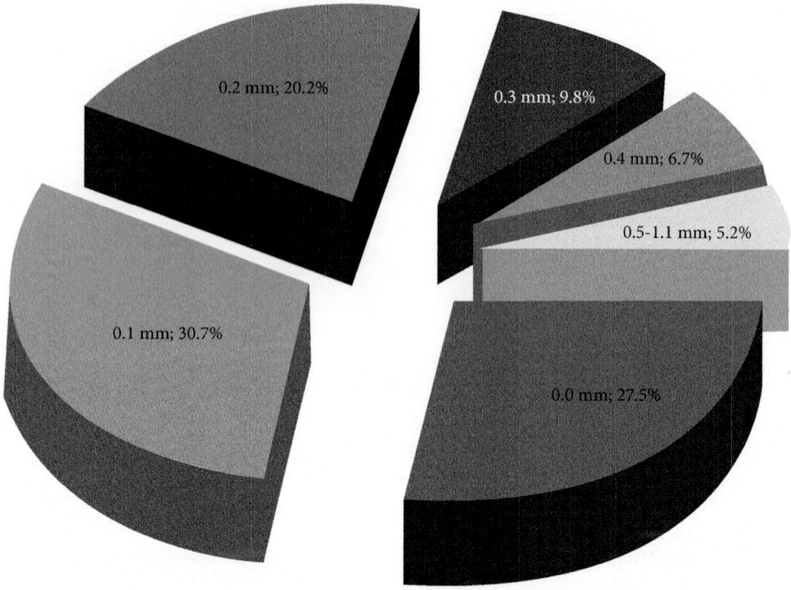

Figure 23.4 Distribution of difference in size between corresponding right and left ulnar arteries in the patients (n = 2,344).[1]

including haematoma formation, pseudo-aneurysm, and arterio-venous fistulae formation, were investigated in five trials in a total of 2,744 patients, with significantly more complications noted in the trans-ulnar group (RR 3.58; CI 2.67–4.79, $P < 0.00001$).

Ajmer Ulnar Artery (AJULAR Study)

Ajmer Ulnar Artery (AJULAR) intervention working group study did not show non-inferiority of ulnar access for large haematomas, when compared to radial access.

By using a protocol of converting to left ulnar access if access through right ulnar failed, they supported the shift of the current paradigm towards interventions through forearm arteries.[5–7]

AJULAR study did not show non-inferiority of ulnar access for large haematomas, when compared to radial access.

The ulnar (which is anatomically deeper) is often harder to compress and the use of compression bandages, as used in AJULAR study, can often lead to large haematomas. Use of manual compression following sheath removal when activated clotting time is <160 seconds for transulnar procedures[1] may lead to a lower incidence of haematomas and may have helped conclusively establish its non-inferiority to transradial access in this regard too. Of course, higher ulnar occlusion on this account was shown in AJULAR study.

Again, in AJULAR study, although a 5-hour compression of the radial access site using a bandage could have contributed to a high radial artery occlusion (RAO) rate as well, it would be hard to conclude the precise rate of access artery occlusion in the absence of ultrasound Doppler use. Shorter compression times have been shown to reduce RAO (risk ratio 0.28, 95% CI 0.05–1.50).[8] Arterial patency testing by palpation alone has inherent limitations; ulnar arteries can be difficult to palpate because of their deeper course compared with the radials. Furthermore, if the clinician palpating the access artery simultaneously does not also occlude the collateralizing forearm artery (radial for ulnar and vice-versa) to prevent its filling through the palmar arch (as is done for reverse Allen's test), the findings can be misinterpreted.

Pre-procedure Ultrasound of Forearm Arteries for Moving to Forearm Access

Pre-procedure Allen's and Barbeau's tests (or testing of dual circulation of the hand) have been found to be unreliable.[9]

In situations with an asymptomatic occlusion of the ulnar artery from a prior translunar procedure, the ipsilateral radial artery pulse is usually well felt (due to an adequate pulse volume from collateral filling through the palmar arch) which may lead an unsuspecting radial operator to intervene through it, potentially putting the patient's hand at risk for vascular compromise if the hand lacks adequate collateralization.

Manual occlusion of ulnar to assess the radial has its fallacies in diagnosing RAO and vice versa for ulnar artery occlusion (UAO). Only colour Doppler ultrasound is reliable in this situation and is far more accurate.

Since Allen's and/or Barbeau's and reverse Allen's and/or reverse Barbeau's testing have limitations,[9] in the absence of a better test to assess adequacy of hand collateralizations, a pre-procedure ultrasound assessment of forearm arteries[7,8] would not only help identify the largest straightest forearm artery for access, it would also establish patency of its corresponding collateralizing artery to avoid inadvertent trans-radial procedures in patients with occluded ulnar arteries, or vice-versa.

Even though data are available for interventions in such situations,[10,11] they are scant and lack validation in randomized multicentre trials; hence, current recommendations advocate avoiding these cases in the interest of patient safety.

Recent Transradial Versus Transulnar Meta-analysis

A recent meta-analysis of 7 randomized controlled trials,[12] with 5721 patients (n= 2874 transulnar (TUA) and n= 2847 transradial (TRA)) found no difference in outcomes between transradial and transulnar access. While bleeding was lower in the TUA group compared with TRA (4.9% vs. 8.5%, OR 0.55, 95% CI [0.33, 0.93]; P = 0.02); there was no difference in access-site complications and large hematoma, procedural time (MD 1.34 min, 95% CI [−1.31, 3.99]; P = 0.32) or fluoroscopy time (MD 0.29 min, 95% CI [−0.33, 0.91]; P = 0.36), access-site cross-over (9.4% vs. 4.1%, OR 1.92, 95% CI [0.91, 4.06]; P = 0.09), access-site complications (12.7% vs. 13%, OR 0.97, 95% CI [0.79, 1.19]; P = 0.75), vasospasm (8.1% vs. 9%, OR 0.83, 95% CI [0.54, 1.27]; P = 0.38), or risk of major adverse cardiovascular and cerebrovascular events (MACCE) (3.05% vs. 3.32%, OR 0.9, 95% CI [0.65, 1.25]; P = 0.53), between TUA and TRA groups.[12]

Therefore, a paradigm shift to 'forearm access' with the equivalent use of radial (including distal radial) or ulnar access is the way to go, with priority of crossing over to an alternate forearm access site to complete the procedure, should the first route of access fail. The same also requires an accurate test of patency of the collateralizing artery using colour Doppler USG.[13]

References

1. Chugh SK, Chugh S, Chugh Y, Rao SV. Feasibility and utility of pre-procedural ultrasound imaging of the arm to facilitate transradial coronary diagnostic and interventional procedures (PRIMAFACIE-TRI). *Catheter Cardiovasc Interv.* 2013;82:64–73.
2. Chugh S, Chugh Y. Radial artery occlusion: size and more—how small is too small? *J Invasive Cardiol.* 2015;27(6):E113.
3. Chugh SK, Chugh S, Chugh Y. Addressing the challenge of access of small radial and ulnar arteries in transradial and transulnar interventions: insights. *J Am College Cardiol.* 2014;12(63):A1671.
4. Fernandez R, Zaky F, Ekmejian A, Curtis E, Lee A. Safety and efficacy of ulnar artery approach for percutaneous cardiac catheterization: Systematic review and meta-analysis. Catheter Cardiovasc Interv. 2018 Jun;91(7):1273–80. doi: 10.1002/ccd.27479. Epub 2018 Feb 1. PMID: 29388387.
5. Gokhroo R, Kishor K, Bhanwar R, Bisht D, Gupta S, Avinash A. Ulnar artery interventions non inferior to radial approach: Ajmer Ulnar Artery (AJULAR) intervention working group study results. *J Invasive Cardiol.* 2016;28:1–8.
6. Sawlani N, Rao SV, Bhatt DL. A call for comprehensive forearm access? *J Invasive Cardiol.* 2016;28:8–9.
7. Chugh SK, Chugh Y, Chugh S. Overcoming the challenge of transradial interventions in women: insights from a color Doppler study. *J Am Coll Cardiol.* 2014;64:B240.
8. Rashid M, Kwok CS, Pancholy S, Chugh S, Kedev SA, Bernat I, Ratib K, Large A, Fraser D, Nolan J, Mamas MA. Radial artery occlusion after transradial interventions: a systematic review and meta-analysis. *J Am Heart Assoc.* 2016;5:e002686.
9. Gilchrist IC. Is the Allen's test accurate for patients considered for transradial coronary angiography? *J Am Coll Cardiol.* 2006;48:1283–8.
10. Kedev S, Zafirovska B, Dharma S, Petkoska D. Safety and feasibility of transulnar catheterization when ipsilateral radial access is not available. *Catheter Cardiovasc Interv.* 2014;83:E51–60.
11. Kwan TW, Ratcliffe JA, Chaudhry M, et al. Transulnar catheterization in patients with ipsilateral radial artery occlusion. *Catheter Cardiovasc Interv.* 2013;82:E849–55.
12. Ramy Sedhom, Michael Megaly, Bishoy Abraham, Jon C. George, et al. Transulnar versus transradial access for coronary angiography and percutaneous coronary intervention: A meta-analysis of randomized controlled trials, *Cardiovascular Revascularization Medicine*, 2020, ISSN 1553 8389, https://doi.org/10.1016/j.carrev.2020.11.001.(https://www.sciencedirect.com/science/article/pii/S1553838920306746)
13. Chugh Y, Chugh S, Chugh S. A paradigm shift toward forearm arterial access requires establishing preprocedure adequacy of hand collateralization or patency of collateralizing forearm arteries. *J Invasive Cardiol.* 2016;28(4):E42–3.

24
Transulnar Interventions

M.A. Azeez Asad, B. Dixit, and P.C. Rath

Introduction

The transradial approach (TRA) for coronary angiography and interventions has gained popularity over the years and has emerged as an alternative to transfemoral coronary procedures. TRA is not feasible in a subset of patients due to aberrations such as undersized artery, radial loops, and arterial spasm may impede successful catheterization or require switch to a femoral approach.[1,2] Still, the safety and feasibility of the radial approach has led to an interest to consider transulnar access (TUA) for cardiac catheterization. However, transulnar approach is still in its nascent stage, being utilized infrequently by interventionalists. The advantages and complication rates for this procedure appear comparable to those for the TRA. Similar to TRA, the TUA is associated with less vascular complications, shorter hospital stay, lesser patient discomfort and lower mortality compared to the transfemoral access (TFA).[3–5] Anatomical anomalies like a loop or vasospasm are less frequent in the ulnar artery compared to the radial artery. The technical success rate is 95–96% through transulnar route comparable to that of TRA and has been demonstrated to be adequate for performing procedures of varying degrees of complexity.[6–8] However use of the TUA access site may spare the radial artery for use as a conduit for coronary artery bypass surgery, for repeat coronary procedures, and for haemodialysis access for chronic kidney disease patients in future.[9,10]

Feasibility of Transulnar Procedures

The transulnar approach was first described by Terashima et al. in a preliminary study of nine patients in 2001 (Figure 24.1). They also

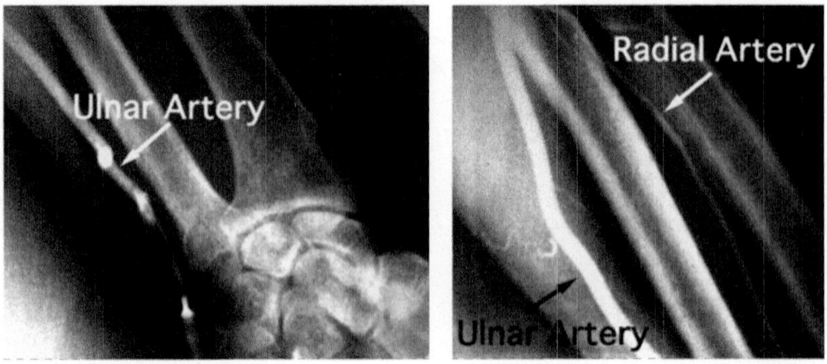

Figure 24.1 The left panel shows the angiograph obtained immediately after injection of contrast media from the left ulnar artery. The right panel shows the angiograph of the left forearm obtained in patient who had weak radial pulsation.[3]

demonstrated excellent ulnar artery patency and freedom from local complications.[3] The transulnar versus transradial artery approach for coronary angioplasty: the PCVI-CUBA study[11] prospectively randomized 413 patients with a normal Allen's test to undergo coronary angiography with or without percutaneous coronary intervention (PCI) through the transradial and transulnar approaches. The two methods had similar success rate (96% versus 93%), PCI success (96% versus 95%), and asymptomatic access site occlusion (5% versus 6%) rates. Procedural time and major adverse cardiovascular events (MACE) were also similar in both arms of the study.[11]

Gokhroo et al. reported their experience using a TUA site for cardiac catheterization, supporting the ulnar artery as a feasible site for both coronary angiography and PCI. Their AJmer ULnar ARtery (AJULAR) intervention working group study is a prospective, open label, observational study that analysed 410 patients who underwent coronary angiography and PCI, if necessary, through the TUA approach. A single, experienced, transradial operator without previous transulnar training performed all procedures. The findings were compared with a retrospective cohort of transradial access angiography patients at the same centre. The study results support TUA catheterization as a safe and feasible approach for angiography and PCI. Of the 410 study patients, only 9 required alternative access. The overall bleeding rate was similar to the TRA group. However, with TUA more attempts were required until successful puncture was achieved.[12]

In our own study published in 2005 in *Indian Heart Journal*, we reported on the safety and feasibility of TUA for coronary angiography and PCI. A total of 100 patients underwent diagnostic angiography (n = 64) and PCIs (n = 36) through transulnar approach. The patients' age ranged from 40 to 70 years, and male-to-female ratio was 7.3:1. The procedure was successful in 95 (95%) patients and unsuccessful in 5 (4 diagnostic and 1 percutaneous coronary intervention). The procedure was done through right ulnar artery in all except one patient in whom it was done through left ulnar artery. The total procedure time ranged between 25 and 45 min. Among the cases of PCIs, single-vessel angioplasty was performed in 23 (65.7%) patients, double vessel in 11 (31.4%) patients and triple vessel in 1 (3%) patient. Complications such as local haematoma, ulnar artery perforation and reversible paraesthesia occurred in one patient each, thus concluding that TUA is a safe and easy alternative technique to perform diagnostic and therapeutic coronary interventions.[13]

Deshmukh et al. studied 30 day and 1-year outcomes in patients undergoing transulnar coronary angiography and interventions. They observed no residual deficits from vascular or neurological complications associated with the index procedure and an overall MACE rate of 3.4%. They concluded that transulnar approach appears to be safe and effective for coronary angiography and complex coronary interventions.[14]

Please refer to Chapter 23 for a recently published meta-analysis of 7 randomized controlled trials comparing TUA with TRA which showed no difference in outcomes between the two groups.

Applied Anatomy

In the forearm, ulnar artery is larger in caliber than the radial artery (Figure 24.2). This makes it less spasm-prone and easily accessible with fewer complications. The ulnar nerve lies on the medial side of lower two-third of the artery and the palmar cutaneous branch of nerve descends on lower part of vessel to the palm of the hand.[15] It crosses the flexor retinaculum lateral to ulnar nerve and Pisiform bone.

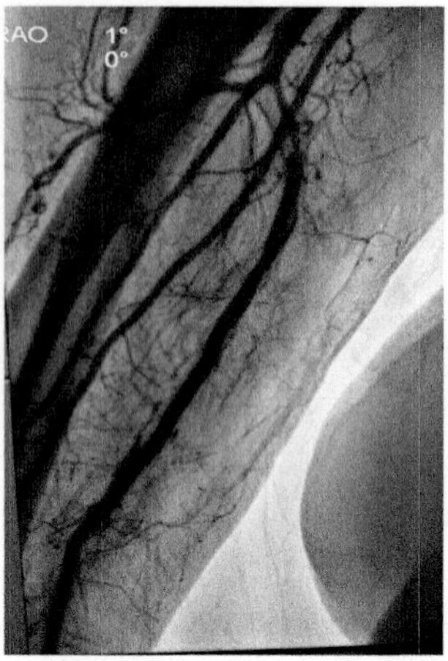

Figure 24.2 Arteriogram through the introducer sheath showing a large sized ulnar artery compared to the radial artery.

Chugh et al. demonstrated comparable size of the ulnar and radial arteries using a preprocedural ultrasound in 2,344 patients (Table 24.1); radial [mean 1.9 mm (male); 1.7 mm (female)] and ulnar artery size [mean 1.8 mm (male); 1.6 mm (female)].[16] Anatomic variations in radial artery were found in 9.6% of patients with failure to cannulate in 3.5%.[17]

Table 24.1 Radial and ulnar artery size according to sex and side (n = 2,344)

Size of radial and ulnar artery on the two sides	**Mean diameter (mm)**
Left radial artery	
Male	1.8 _0.29
Female	1.7 _0.26
Left ulnar artery	
Male	1.8 _0.30
Female	1.7 _0.3
Right radial artery	
Male	1.9 _1.12
Female	1.7 _0.29
Right ulnar artery	
Male	1.8 _0.30
Female	1.6 _0.28

Allen's and Inverse Allen's Test

Traditionally, the Allen's test is performed as follows: while the patient holds his arm flexed and elevated, both radial and ulnar arteries are compressed for about 10 seconds (Figure 24.3). Then, the arm is extended, ulnar compression stops, and the time for palmar skin discolouration to return to normal is recorded. If the time exceeds 10 seconds, then the ulnar circulation support of the hand is considered inadequate. Inverse Allen's test refers to the same test, but looking at radial artery patency, where compression of the radial artery is performed instead of the ulnar. Radial collateral circulation support of the hand is considered adequate when the time of the inverse Allen's test is under 10 seconds.[3] Additionally, ulnar circulation is determined as dominant if Allen's test time is shorter than inverse Allen's.

However, in a study of 1,000 consecutive patients undergoing cardiac catheterization, Benit et al. found only 73% had normal modified Allen's test.[18]

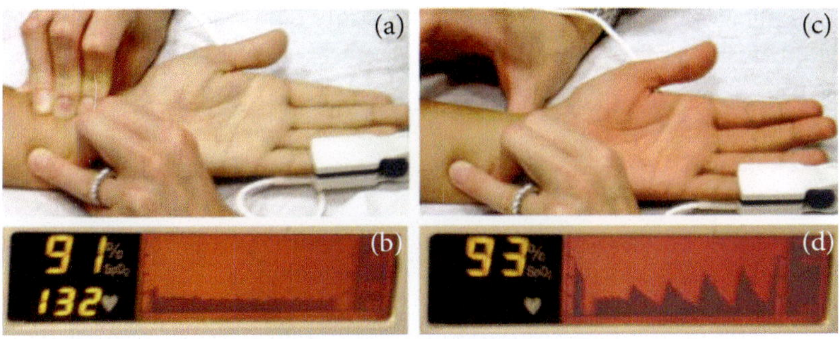

Figure 24.3 Description of the inverse modified Allen's test. (A) Compression of the radial and ulnar arteries. (B) Peripheral oxygen saturation curve of the fifth finger during compression of the radial and ulnar arteries. (C) Release of the radial artery. (D) Peripheral oxygen saturation curve of the fifth finger after release of the radial artery.[19]

Transulnar Catheterization Without Allen's Test

Conventionally, Allen's test has been used to demonstrate the integrity of the palmar arch with some case reports on critical hand ischaemia following transradial coronary intervention. Romagnoli et al. challenged the notion that traditional or plethysmography form of Allen's test should be mandatory before transradial or TUA. They report performing a number of cases in which both radial and ulnar arteries of the same wrist were subsequently or concomitantly accessed during the same procedure, without performing any kind of Allen's test before the procedure without any clinical evidence of hand ischaemia or ensuing complication (Figure 24.1), thus suggesting that even placing two arterial sheaths in the same wrist can be safely done in selected cases and by skilled operators. They acknowledge the reality of risk of hand ischaemia as being extremely rare and postulate that the presence of a rich collateral system and the presence of interosseous branches in several patients allow even concomitant radial and ulnar occlusion (Figure 24.4).[20,21]

Andrade et al. reported the data of a prospective registry involving 62 unselected patients submitted to coronary procedures through the TUA without previous evaluation of the integrity of the deep palmar arch by an Allen's test.[21] The rate of asymptomatic occlusion of the ulnar artery was 3%, without any ischaemic complication. Based on these observations and the lack of outcome data, the performance of Allen's test is not considered absolutely necessary when using TUA.

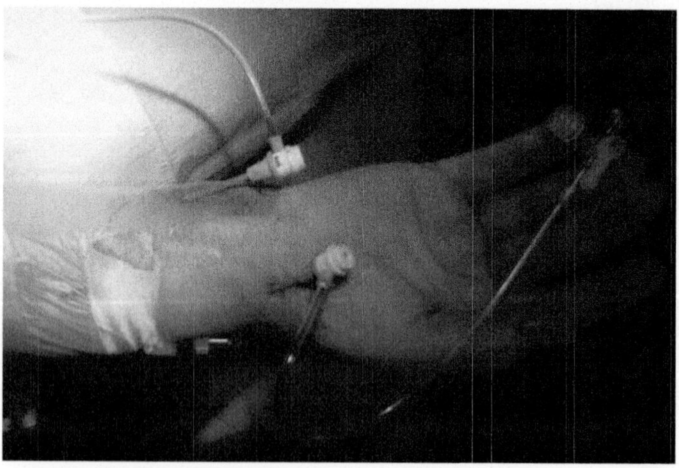

Figure 24.4 A case of simultaneous radial and ulnar access in a 76-year-old woman with non-ST-elevation acute coronary syndrome, undergoing urgent coronary angiography.[21]

TUA Following Failure of TRA

Successful ipsilateral transulnar catheterization can be achieved in patients with documented occlusion of the radial artery and after failure of transradial catheterization. The major reasons for failed TRA include radial loops (Figure 24.5), high take off of radial artery, radial artery spasm (Figure 24.6), radial dissection, or hypoplastic radial artery. In a large single-centre prospective registry of effectiveness and safety, 476 consecutive patients underwent transulnar catheterization. A subgroup analysis was done in 240 patients with documented ipsilateral radial artery occlusion. Procedural success was 97% with a crossover rate of 3% to TFA. Hand ischaemia was not observed in any patient on day 1 after procedure and on 1-month follow-up. None of the patients showed ulnar nerve injury.[22]

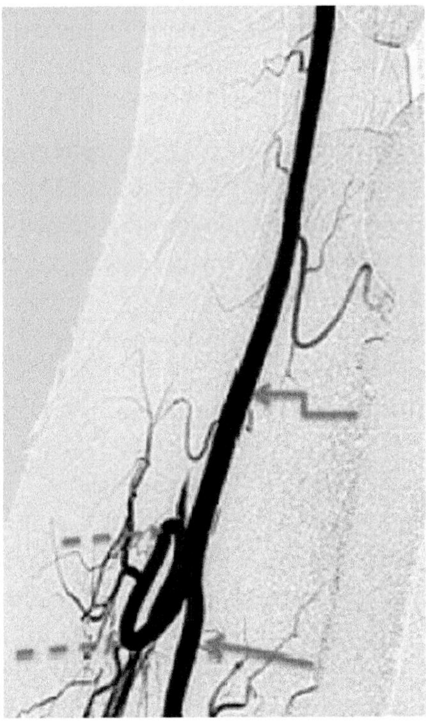

Figure 24.5 Radial loop. Complete radial artery loop resulted in crossover to ulnar approach. Radial loop (dashed arrows), ulnar artery (continuous arrow), and brachial artery (curved arrow).[25]

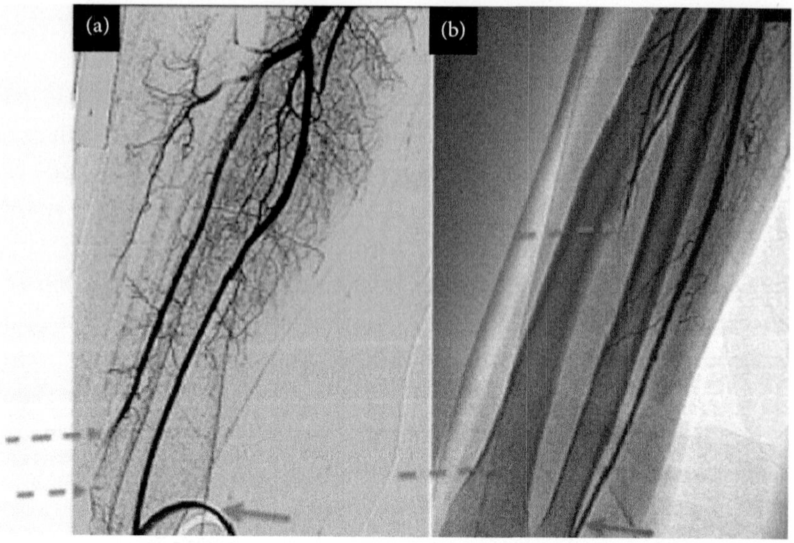

Figure 24.6 Showing spasm in radial artery (dashed arrows) in both left and right panel; Continuous arrow shows ulnar artery.

Slogoff et al. reporting on the safety of radial artery cannulation in cardiovascular surgery patients described a subset of 22 patients who underwent ipsilateral ulnar artery cannulation after numerous failed attempts at radial artery cannulation. No patient experienced ulnar artery occlusion or symptoms/signs of hand ischaemia.[23]

Technique of Transulnar Catheterization

Puncture of Access Artery

The technique for transulnar catheterization is similar to TRA. Ulnar artery is first palpated and inverse Allen's test maybe done to assess patency of radial artery and palmar arch. Once patency is assured then wrist is hyperextended by keeping a gauze roll below it. Local anesthesia with 2–5 ml of lignocaine is administered. To puncture the artery a radial puncture needle or 20G Jelco utilizing the Seldinger technique is used. The artery lies proximal and lateral to pisiform bone and care should be taken to avoid injuring the ulnar nerve which lies medial to the artery.

After puncture is done and free flow of blood is achieved, a 0.025 hydrophilic wire (Terumo) is taken to cannulate the artery. A 0.014" PTCA wire may be utilized in patients with difficulty. Over the wire, a 5F or 6F radial sheath (Terumo/Cordis) is inserted (Figure 24.7). A 7F sheath maybe inserted for complex coronary interventions or imaging provided the access artery diameter is more than 2.2 mm.

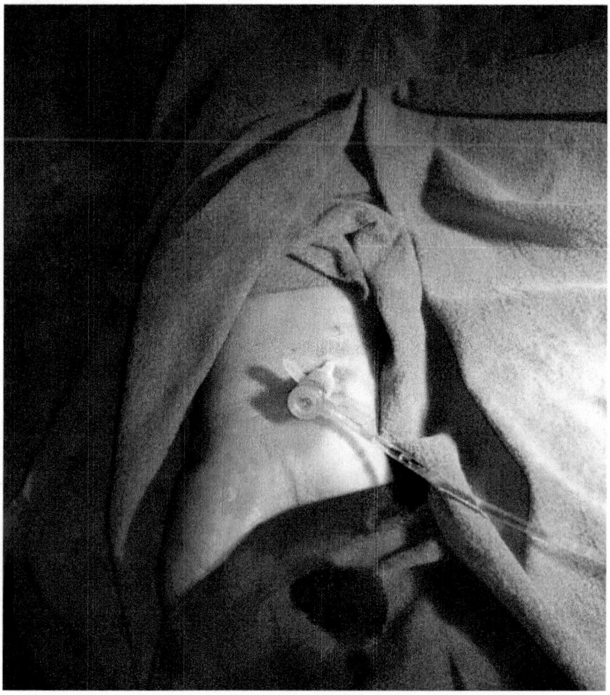

Figure 24.7 Sheath introducer inserted into the right ulnar artery.

Prevention of Access Artery Spasm

- Appropriate sizing of sheath and catheters; ideally less than 1.1:1 with ratio of sheath to artery diameter is chosen.
- After access is achieved, a spasmolytic cocktail (200 μg of nitroglycerine, 5 mg of diltiazem, 2,500 IU of unfractionated heparin) is given intra-arterially. Caution to be exercised in patients prone to hypotension such as severe aortic stenosis.
- Minimize catheter manipulations and exchanges.

- Avoid reuse of sheaths and catheters.
- Repeat use of diltiazem or nitroglycerine if arterial spasm encountered.

Choice of Coronary Diagnostic and Guide Catheters

Diagnostic Procedures

In general, 5F catheters are utilized for coronary diagnostic procedures.

For right ulnar diagnostic coronary angiography, TIG (Terumo) catheter is used as a universal catheter that can engage both left and right coronary arteries as well as used for ventriculography.

In rare cases of anomalies of coronary ostia, other catheters like Amplatz curve, Multipurpose curve, etc. can be used.

In patients with large aortic roots, Judkins catheters—Judkins right (JR) and Judkins left (JL)—can be used to selectively engage the respective coronary ostia.

For left ulnar access, JR and JL are the preferred catheters.

TUA for PCI

In most cases of PCI, 6F guiding catheters are used.

For left coronary PCI-extra back up guides for medium length or long length left main coronary artery (LMCA) and JL for short length LMCA is preferred.

For PCI to RCA, a JR guide is the initial preference. For shepherd hook type of right coronary artery (RCA), internal mammary artery (IMA) catheters can be used.

7F guiding catheters with extra back up are preferred for complex coronary interventions with bulky devices.

TUA for Primary PCI

TRA in primary and rescue angioplasty may be beneficial compared to the femoral access due to the lesser incidence of vascular complications.

Limbruno et al. have reported on 13 patients undergoing primary angioplasty performed using the transulnar approach. Ulnar access was obtained in 10 patients; sheath insertion time ranged from 2 to 5 min, time from arterial puncture to vessel recanalization ranged from 21 to 36 min. Primary angioplasty was successful in all patients. At 30-day echo colour Doppler, all ulnar arteries were patent and with a physiologic pattern of flow.

TUA Success Rates

Success rates of transulnar catheterization have varied depending on the operator experience. The learning curve is slightly longer than the femoral and radial approach. As the artery is deep seated and lies below the tendons, hyperextension and abduction makes the pulsations more forceful and cannulation easy. As the ulnar artery is larger than the radial artery in majority, the success rate is expected to be higher.[19] The success rate has varied from 64% to 95%.[3,24] In the study by Vassilev D et al. the success rate was lowest i.e. 64% and the main reason for this cited was inability to introduce the wire despite good blood flow.[24] If the puncture is made at an angle that is more vertical, the wire will hit the wall and may not enter the artery due to its stiffness which can be overcome by using a 0.014" PTCA wire whose tip is very soft. Use of this technique can increase the success rate to 95%.[3] It only takes 1–2 attempts in majority to cannulate the artery. Successful puncture in first attempt is seen in 64–72% and 86% in second attempt and almost all at 3rd attempt.[3,19] On Average it takes about 2–5 minutes to insert the sheath after beginning the procedure making it feasible to perform primary PCI where time is a concern.[24]

In our study mentioned earlier, out of 100 transulnar cases, 64 were for diagnostic coronary angiography and 36 underwent PCI procedures. Right ulnar artery was used in 99 cases, whereas left ulnar was used in 1 case. In five cases, the procedure was unsuccessful (four during diagnostic and one during PCI) and was completed via femoral approach. The reason was inability to puncture in three patients, and inability to negotiate guidewire due to stenosis at origin of ulnar artery in one patient and due to spasm in another case. The ulnar artery was cannulated within three attempts. In majority of cases (80%), we used a 6F sheath. All the PCI cases were performed

Table 24.2 Details of interventional procedures

Indication	
Recent MI	: 16
Unstable angina	: 6
Stable angina	: 128
Primary PCI	: 2
No. of vessels undergoing PCI	
Single-vessel disease	: 23
Double-vessel disease	: 11
Triple-vessel disease	: 1
Vessels treated	
Left anterior descending	: 23
Left circumflex	: 12
Right coronary artery	: 11
Ramus intermedius	: 2
Anti-platelet/Anti-coagulant used	
Aspirin and clopidogrel	: All
Enoxaparin	: All
Gp IIb / IIIa inhibitor (eptifibatide)	: 7

MI: myocardial infarction; PCI: percutaneous coronary intervention
Gp: glycoprotein.

via a 6F sheath. The procedure time for performing PCI ranged from 25 to 45 min. Details of intervention procedure are given in Table 24.2.

PCI was performed in 35 out of 36 cases attempted. In one patient, it was unsuccessful due to failure to puncture. Majority of cases were of single-vessel angioplasty (65.7%), two-vessel angioplasty in 31.4%, and three-vessel angioplasty in one patient. The procedure was elective in 34 patients and emergency in 2 patients (primary PCI).[13]

Complications After Transulnar Catheterization

The chief purpose to crossover to transulnar approach whenever transradial access fails is to decrease the expected local vascular complications of TFA. Vascular complications are easily diagnosed by an

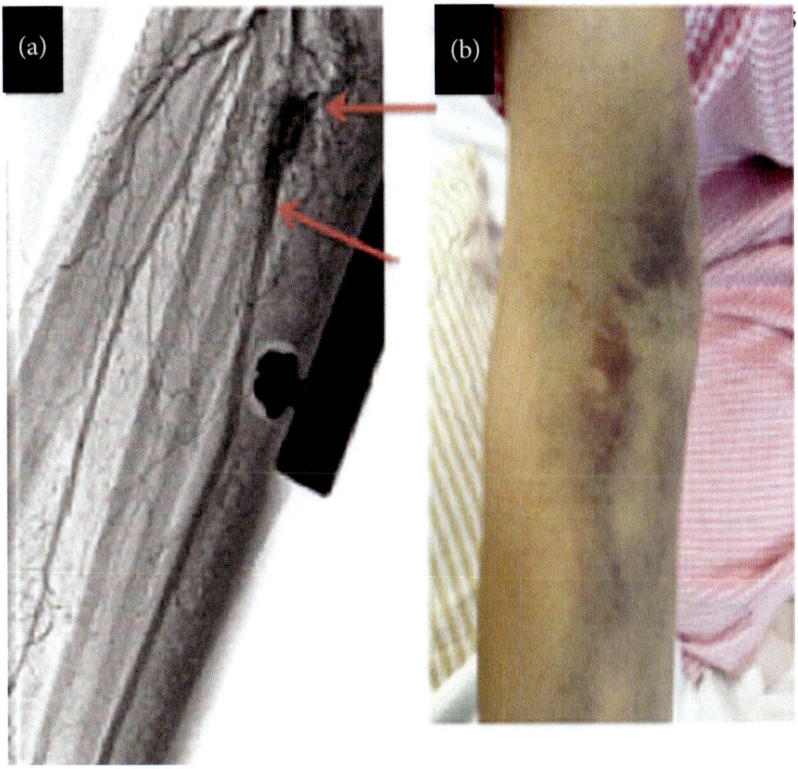

Figure 24.8 Ulnar artery perforation and superficial haematoma: (a) localized ulnar artery perforation and (b) consequent superficial haematoma.[25]

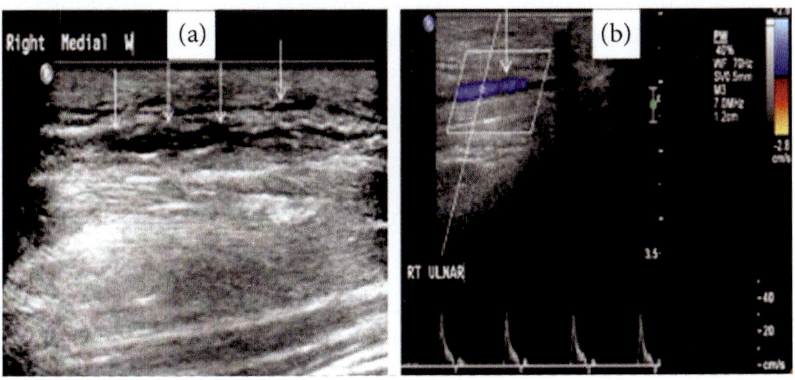

Figure 24.9 Duplex scan after ulnar artery perforation: (a): Grey scale ultrasound image of right wrist demonstrating diffuse subcutaneous hypo echoic haemorrhage (white arrow). (b): Longitudinal colour Doppler image of the right wrist demonstrating normal antegrade flow in ulnar artery with no stenosis or pseudoaneurysm.[25]

ultrasonographic study (Figures 24.8 and 24.9).[25] In our study of hundred patients undergoing transulnar catheterization, complications of subcutaneous haematoma, ulnar artery perforation, and reversible paranesthesia occurred in one patient each amounting to one percentage each.[13]

In another study involving 45 patients, complications after TUA have included minor ones like transient numbness and non-significant haematoma in 15.5% and 13.3%, and one patient with ulnar artery perforation, respectively.[25] None of the patients experienced major bleeding requiring blood transfusion. All local vascular complications including perforation were managed conservatively. Seven patients (15.5%) experienced pain and transient numbness during ulnar cannulation. All improved after a short time with no permanent neurological damage.

Conclusions

Use of TUA in the modern era of interventional cardiology opens an alternate route to heart and coronary arteries. The procedure is simple, safe, and technically feasible with fewer complications. Simple modifications like use of appropriate sized sheaths, adequate spasmolytic therapy, use of hydrophilic or PTCA wires to gain access and minimizing catheter exchanges can lead to increased success rate. This approach also leads to sparing of the radial artery which can be used for future procedures or as a conduit during subsequent revascularization. Thus, transulnar approach is a safe and useful alternative approach for performing routine diagnostic and complex interventional coronary procedures.

References

1. Agostoni P, Biondi-Zoccai GG, de Benedictis ML, et al. Radial versus femoral approach for percutaneous coronary diagnostic and interventional procedures; systematic overview and meta-analysis of randomized trials. *J Am CollCardiol.* 2004;44:349–56.
2. Jolly SS, Amlani S, Hamon M, et al. Radial versus femoral access for coronary angiography or intervention and the impact on major bleeding and ischemic events: a systematic review and metaanalysis of randomized trials. *Am Heart J.* 2009;157:132–140.

3. Terashima M, Meguro T, Takeda H, et al. Percutaneous ulnar artery approach for coronary angiography: a preliminary report in nine patients. *Catheter Cardiovasc Interv.* 2001;53:410–14.
4. Roberts EB, Palmer N, Perry RA. Transulnar access for coronary angiography and intervention: an early review to guide research and clinical practice. *J Invasive Cardiol.* 2007;19:83–7.
5. Mangin L, Bertr OF, De La Rochellie 're R, et al. The transulnar approach for coronary intervention: a safe alternative to transradial approach in selected patients. *J Invasive Cardiol.* 2005;17:77–79.
6. Limbruno U, Rossini R, De Carlo M, et al. Percutaneous ulnar artery approach for primary coronary angioplasty: safety and feasibility. *Catheter Cardiovasc Interv.* 2004;61:56–59.
7. Deftereos S, Giannopoulos G, Tousoulis D, et al. Sheathless transulnar versus standard femoral arterial access for percutaneous coronary intervention on bifurcation lesions. *Int J Cardiol.* 2011;149:398–400.
8. Deftereos S, Giannopoulos G, Tousoulis D, et al. Feasibility and safety of transulnar access for performing rotational atherectomy. *Int J Cardiol.* 2011;147:285–86.
9. Lanspa TJ, Williams MA, Heirigs RL. Effectiveness of ulnar artery catheterization after failed attempt to cannulate a radial artery. *Am J Cardiol.* 2005;95:1529–30.
10. Bertrand OF, Rao SV, Pancholy S, et al. Transradial approach for coronary angiography and interventions: results of the First international transradial practice survey. *J Am Coll Cardiol Cardiovasc Interv.* 2010;3:1022–31.
11. Aptecar E, Pernes JM, Chabane-Chaouch M, et al. Transulnar versus transradial artery approach for coronary angioplasty: the PCVI-CUBA study. *Catheter Cardiovasc Interv.* 2006;67:711–20.
12. Gokhroo R, Bisht D, Padmanabhan D, et al. Feasibility of ulnar artery for cardiac catheterization: AJmer ULnar ARtery (AJULAR) catheterization study. *Catheter Cardiovasc Interv.* 2015;86:42–48.Gokhroo et al. intervention: case reports and anatomic considerations. *Catheter Cardiovasc Interv.* 2002;55:93–6.
13. Rath PC, Purohit BV, Navasundi GB, Sitaram, Reddy AM. Coronary angiogram and intervention through transulnar approach. *Indian Heart J.* 2005;57(4):324–6.
14. Deshmukh AR, Kaushik M, Aboeata A, et al. Efficacy and safety of transulnar coronary angiography and interventions—a single center experience. *Cathet. Cardiovasc. Intervent.* 2014;83:E26–31. doi: 10.1002/ccd.24989
15. Vogelzang RL. Arteriography of the hand and wrist. *Hand Clin.* 1991;7:63–86.
16. Chugh SK, Chugh S, Chugh Y, Rao SV. Feasibility and utility of pre-procedure ultrasound imaging of the arm to facilitate transradial coronary diagnostic and interventional procedures. *Catheter Cardiovasc Interv.* 2013;82(1):64–73. doi: 10.1002/ccd.24585. Epub 2013 Feb 26.
17. Yokoyama N, Takeshita S, Ochiai M, Koyama Y, Hoshino S, Isshiki T, et al. Anatomic variations of the radial artery in patients undergoing transradial coronary intervention. *Catheter Cardiovasc Interv.* 2000;49:357–62.
18. Benit E, Vranckx P, Jaspers L, Jackmaert R, Poelmans C, Coninx R. Frequency of a positive modified Allen's test in 1,000 consecutive patients undergoing cardiac catheterization. *Cathet Cardiovasc Diagn.* 1996;38:352–54.

19. Limbruno U, Rossini R, De Carlo M, et al. Percutaneous ulnar artery approach for primary coronary angioplasty: safety and feasibility. *Catheter Cardiovasc Interv.* 2004;61:56–9.
20. Romagnoli E, Sangiorgi G. Transradial access without preliminary Allen test—letter of comment on Rhyne et al. *Catheter Cardiovasc Interv.* 2011;78:662–63.
21. De Andrade PB, Tebet M, Andrade M, Mattos L, Labrunie A. Performance of coronary procedures through the transulnar access without assessment of the integrity of the deep palmar arch. J Interv Cardiol. 2008 Dec;21(6):562–5. doi: 10.1111/j.1540-8183.2008.00388.x. Epub 2008 Aug 13. PMID: 18705634.
22. Kedev, S., Zafirovska, B., Dharma, S. et al. Safety and feasibility of transulnar catheterization when ipsilateral radial access is not available. *Catheter Cardiovasc Interv.* 2014;83:E51–E60.
23. Slogoff S, Keats AS, Arlund C. On the safety of radial artery cannulation. *Anesthesiology.* 1983;59:42–47.
24. Vassilev D, Smilkova D, Gil R. Ulnar artery as access site for cardiac catheterization: anatomical considerations. *J Interv Cardiol.* 2008;21:56–60.
25. Sallam M, Al-Riyami A, et al. Procedural and clinical utility of transulnar approach for coronary procedures following failure of radial route: single centre experience. *J Saudi Heart Assoc.* 2014;26(3):138–44.

25

Slender Percutaneous Coronary Interventions by Transradial Approach

Giovanni Amoroso

Definition and Rationale

Since its first introduction in the early 1990s, transradial approach (TRA) has demonstrated such clear clinical advantages upon transfemoral approach, that now-a-days it has been endorsed by the international guidelines as the default access for percutaneous coronary interventions (PCI).[1] However, while the femoral artery can easily accommodate sizable introducers and guiding catheters, as its internal diameter ranges between 5 and 7 millimeter, the radial artery, on the other hand, can present compatibility issues. The diameter of the radial artery can be roughly estimated by the wrist circumference, as a linear correlation exists between these two parameters. Ultrasound is, however, a more precise and practical way to assess radial diameter before the puncture. It turns out that internal diameter of most radial arteries rarely exceeds 2.5 mm. In addition to that, the occurrence of a hypoplastic radial artery (<2 mm) ranges between 5% and 10% of cases. Usually, people of Asian descent, elderly, and females are those with smaller radial arteries.[2] When investigators plotted the distribution of radial artery diameters against the external diameter of arterial sheaths, it became clear that 20–40% of the patients would have a radial artery smaller than a 6French (F) introducer (Figure 25.1).[3] A mismatch between the inner diameter of the radial artery and the outer diameter of the introducer, with an arterial/introducer ratio of <1, is responsible for patient's discomfort and possibly procedural failure, arterial spasm and radial artery occlusion (RAO).[4] Now that feasibility, safety, and efficacy of TRA PCI have been granted, RAO is the last remaining drawback of TRA PCI: albeit not life-threatening, RAO could be

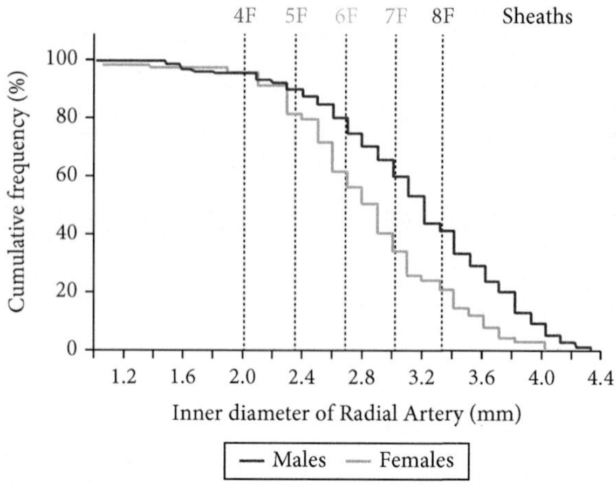

Figure 25.1 Introducer vs. Radial Artery Inner Diameter: approximately 20% of males and 40% of females have an arterial/introducer ratio <1 if a conventional 6F introducer is utilized. This percentage drastically diminishes with smaller introducers.

responsible for deficits of various kind and degree, both in the motoric as the sensorial sphere (so-called 'upper extremity dysfunction'), as well as the impossibility to perform repeated procedures by the same approach.[5]

In order to avoid that, it would be an essential achievement to downsize introducers and devices, possibly down to an external diameter that would fit any radial artery, so that successful and uneventful TRA PCI could be undertaken also in patients with small radial anatomy. Even if not considering the issue of small anatomy, to downsize would minimize the incidence of RAO, by reducing the entry hole and the subsequent trauma to the arterial wall, and, in terms, the time to haemostasis, also in patients with radial arteries of normal caliber. Presently, it will be referred to those TRA PCIs, in which downsizing is referred to as 'Slender' PCIs. We grant the introduction of this term to a group of innovative Japanese colleagues who, more than 10 years ago, joined their efforts in the Slender Club Japan, with the goal of promoting the development of downsized materials and techniques, by both interventional cardiologists and device companies.[6] Usually, it will be referred to as Slender PCI, in case the guiding catheters are smaller than 6F, which is the most accepted and most commonly used size. In order to do that, 'Slender' interventionalists will often, although not necessarily, make use of dedicated devices (balloons and stents, among others). More generally, any procedure, in which efforts are undertaken to reduce radial artery trauma, patient's discomfort, and clinical complications, can be righteously called a Slender PCI. In the last few years, the popularity of 'Slender' transradial interventions has spread from Japan to Europe, where a Slender Club Europe has been instituted,[7] and has also found favour in many other countries where TRA is the dominant approach for PCI.

Five (and Four) French PCI

The easiest and simplest way to perform Slender PCI would be to downsize from 6 to 5F. An important premise is needed. When reporting the size of a guiding catheter we commonly refer to the outer diameter, while, for an introducer, we generally refer to the inner diameter. By doing that, the compatibility between the (outer diameter) of the guiding catheter, and the (inner) diameter of the introducer is immediately evident. For this reason, we usually refer to 6 and 5F introducers, although the more correct term should be 6F-compatible and 5F compatible. Because one French is 1/3 of a millimeter, 6F convert to approximately 2 mm, while 5F to 1.67 mm. In fact, for having the real outer diameter of the introducer, which is the one that matters for the interaction with the radial artery, the thickness of its wall has to be added up to the reported French size. Conventional 6F introducers have, accordingly, an external diameter varying from 2.62 to 2.81 mm, depending on the manufacturers. Conventional 5F introducers, instead, have an external diameter between 2.29 and 2.50 mm (Figure 25.2). Downsizing from 6 to 5F will therefore give a reduction of around 20%, and of 50%, respectively, in outer diameter and area. If these changes might be considered trivial by the most, and therefore not worth the efforts to downsize, one should not forget that the distribution slope of (internal) radial artery diameters is at its steepest between 2.5 and 3 mm. With other words, just to downsize from 6 to 5F, introducers would reduce the chance of arterial-introducer mismatch by almost 50%. Researchers have shown that, by working with 5F guiding catheters the incidence of RAO can be significantly reduced (from 5.9% to 1.1%), at no cost for reduced procedural success (92.9% to

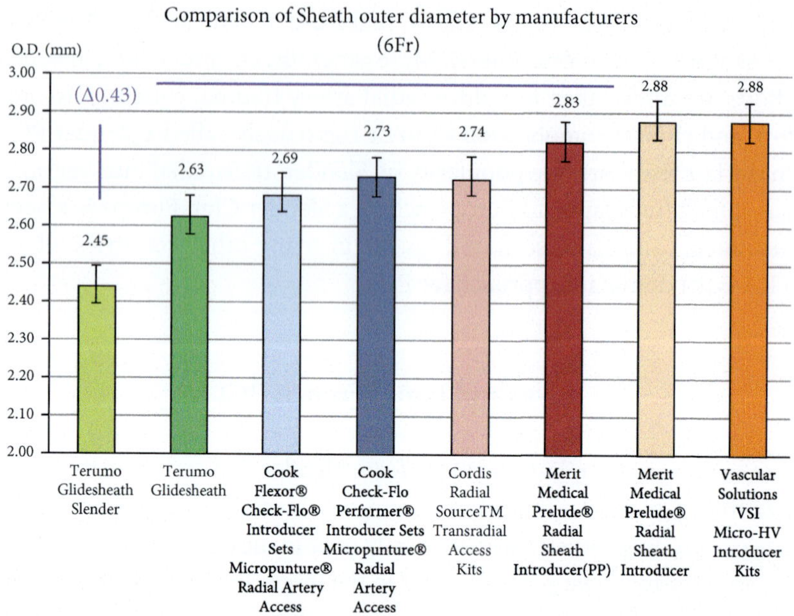

Figure 25.2 Comparison of 6F Sheath Outer Diameter by Manufacturers: the external diameter of a 6F introducer can vary from 2.45 mm (GlideSheath Slender Terumo) to 2.88 (Merit Medical).

95.4%).[8] 5F-based procedures are also associated with the use of less contrast medium, shorter haemostasis, and hospital-stay,[9] which are all additional advantages of a Slender approach. Coronary interventions with smaller catheters present three major technical challenges; reduced catheter support, reduced vessel opacification, and device incompatibility. Let's consider the first issue. The catheter support is less with 5F guiding catheters compared to those with a bigger size: this applies also for more aggressive shapes such as Extra Back-up or Amplatz curves. This is due to the fact that the shaft of the guiding catheter loses rigidity together with size. On the other hand, its flexibility is increased. The limitation in 'passive' support can be overcome by gently advancing the guiding catheter a few centimeters into the coronary artery, while pulling onto the wire or the balloon (so-called 'deep intubation'). Care has to be taken in order to avoid coronary dissections, induced by interaction with the tip of the guiding catheter: hence, it is not advised to advance the guiding onto the coronary wire only. Deep intubation will provide 'active' support to the system, at an extend that is comparable with the 'passive' support given by the rigidity of bigger catheters. The second aspect to consider is poorer visualization by angiography: this is the result of less powerful contrast injections, due to the high viscosity of the contrast dye versus the reduced lumen of the catheter. The presence of any device into the guiding will magnify this effect, in a smaller more than in a bigger catheter. This issue can be solved by using a contrast medium with lower viscosity and/or by means of an automated power injector: with the latter injection's pressures and volume can be customized according to any special need.[10–12] Finally, device incompatibility with 5F guiding catheters has been a reason in the past for avoiding downsizing. If this was true for the first coronary devices, which were bulky, and required at least 6F guiding catheters to be utilized, now-a-days, several years after the first Slender experiences, most conventional devices have evolved to 5F compatibility (Table 25.1). This result has been achieved largely by the efforts of manufacturers to downsize device's profile, as well as to the increased inner diameter of current 5F guiding catheters (0.058"). This means that most of contemporary PCI procedures can be successfully accomplished

Table 25.1 List of devices with 5F compatibility

Devices	5F compatiblility	Product	Manufacturer(s)
Rx balloons	Yes		All
OTW ballons	Yes		All
Drug-eluting stents	Yes		All
IVUS Probes	Electronic	Eagle Eye Platinum	Volcano
OCT catheters	Some	Fastview	Terumo
FFR wires/catheters	Yes		All
Covered Stents	Single Layer	Papyrus	Biotronik
Bioabsorbable Scaffolds	Only ≤3.0		All
Aspiration Catheters	Some	Pronto LP	Vascular Solution
Rota BURR	Only 1.25 mm		Boston Scientific
Microcatheters	Yes		All
Extension catheters	Some	Guidion	IMDS

by 5F. Only a few exceptions would remain, such as complex CTOs, vein graft interventions, left main bifurcations, during which larger guiding catheters might be advised, in order to allow the simultaneous use of multiple devices. The risk of arterial-introducer mismatch would be even less likely with catheters smaller than 5F. Coronary angiography can be, indeed, successfully performed by 4F and in selected cases, even by 3F diagnostic catheters. Radial artery trauma and incidence of RAO are, by this, reduced to their minimum. Unfortunately, once excluded the diagnostic procedures, the spectrum of coronary interventions that are feasible by means of 4F systems is still quite limited, and, therefore, should be reserved for highly-selected cases.[13]

Sheathless PCI

One feasible option to avoid radial arterial/introducer mismatch, at no cost for device compatibility, is to cannulate the radial artery without the use of an arterial sheath: the so-called 'Sheathless' technique. After puncturing the radial artery, the guiding catheter will be introduced and advanced over a long and tapered dilator, which will be retrieved just before engaging the coronary ostia. By removing the introducer from the equation, the factual outer diameter of the whole set (catheter + introducer in case of conventional procedures, only the catheter in case of sheathless procedures) can be decreased by one, up to two French sizes (i.e. the thickness of the introducer). For this reason, for instance, it will be referred to a 5F sheathless procedure as a 'virtual' 3F procedure (Figure 25.3): 'virtual' indicates the size of the guiding (plus introducer) one could use, and have an entry hole of the same diameter in the radial artery. Sheathless 6 and 7F PCI procedures allow achieving a significant reduction in radial artery trauma, without the need to change PCI strategy, or recur to any dedicated Slender device, and have been successfully utilized in various settings.[14] Indeed, because of the lack of an introducer, to exchange catheters, if needed, would be more cumbersome; but the difficulty has been resolved with the Cordis 'Railway sheathless system'. Further, navigation of sheathless catheters throughout the vasculature of the arm is smoother than with conventional catheters: this is because the tapered profile of the whole device (wire, dilator and guiding catheter)

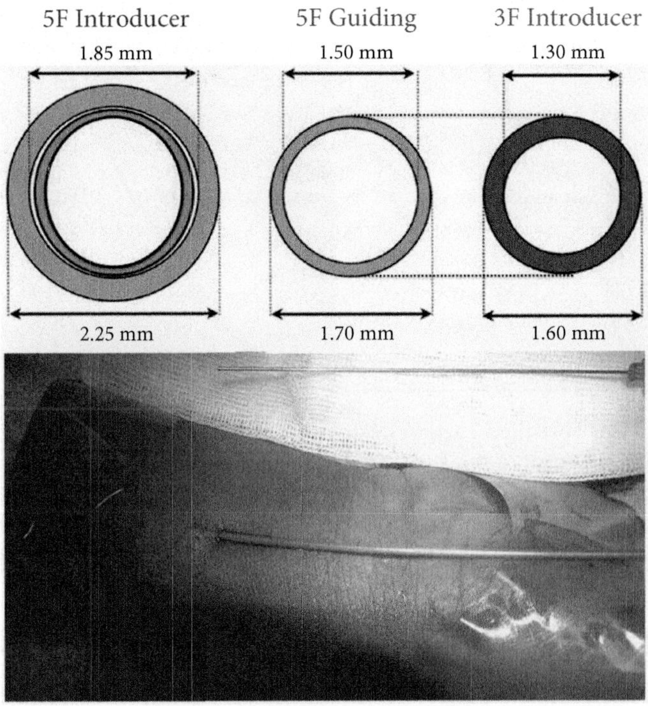

Figure 25.3 Sheathless 5F ('virtual' 3F) guiding catheter (Medikit Japan). Upper panel: a sheathless 5F guiding catheter has approximately the same external diameter (1.7 mm) as a 3F introducer. This explains why it will also be called 'virtual' 3F system. Lower panel: direct introduction of the same guiding into the radial artery, without the need for an introducer.

can prevent, in case of tortuous or small anatomy, the tip of the guiding catheter to scratch alongside the inner vessel wall, so-called 'razor' effect (Figure 25.4). 'Razor' effect has been ascribed, as much as arterial/introducer mismatch, to be responsible for radial artery trauma and its spasm, as well as subsequent occlusion. Sheathless 5F PCI (manufactured by Medikit Japan) will allow to reduce the entry hole's diameter and trauma, to its minimum: the external diameter of these special guiding catheters is of 1.75 mm, which is compatible with virtually any (even hypoplastic) radial artery. Proper haemostasis after sheathless 5F PCI can often be achieved in less than an hour, and without aggressive compression: this is also relevant to minimize the risk of RAO. As it concerns the internal

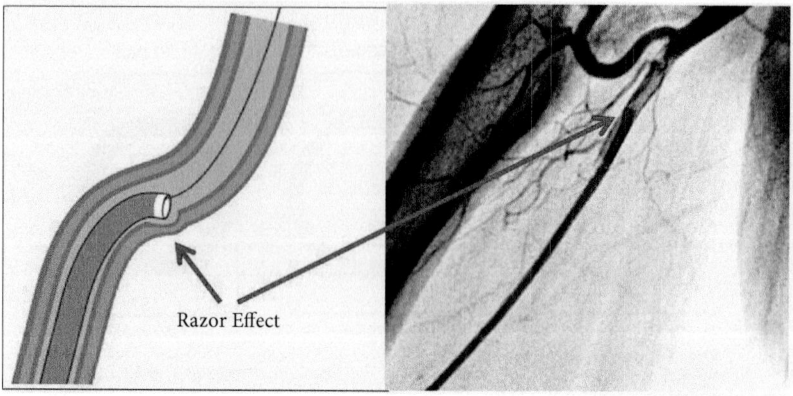

Figure 25.4 So-called 'razor' effect. The tip of the guiding catheter scrapes on the arterial wall (left panel), causing a dissection of the radial artery (right panel).

lumen diameter of this catheter, the same advantages (contrast reduction) and challenges (catheter support and device compatibility) of conventional 5F PCI will apply. Dedicated kits for sheathless PCI include a long-tapered dilator, a compatible guiding catheter and, in some cases, a puncture kit. An alternative way, in order to perform sheathless technique with conventional catheters, is by inflating a small coronary balloon at the tip, and uses it as a sort of dilator to introduce the guiding onto a coronary wire: so-called 'balloon-assisted tracking technique (BAT)'. Very recently, a universal dilator has also become available in Europe and US, which, as with the Cordis 'Railway sheathless system™', allows turning any guiding catheter into a sheathless one. Safety and feasibility of the 5F Sheathless technique has been confirmed in different settings.[15–17] Very recently the V3 registry, named after 'virtual' 3F, has tested its safety and efficacy in a broader and larger subset of patients: in a population of 260 patients with 361 lesions (half of which type B2 or C), procedural success was 99.2%, with only two failures, both in CTO procedures. No adverse events were reported and RAO incidence was 0.4%.[18]

Slender Introducers

Another pragmatic option to reduce arterial/sheath mismatch, without the need to go sheathless, is to use the Slender sheaths called Glidesheath Slender (GSS). These newly-developed arterial sheaths have a wall thickness of 0.12 mm, instead of the 0.20–0.30 mm of the conventional ones: this means that the 'factual' diameter of the sheath + guiding set is reduced by almost one French size.[19] Slender introducers are available in 5, 6, and 7F size. Because this Slender introducer (manufactured by Terumo Japan) has a much thinner wall layer, particular care should be taken not to damage or kink it during introduction and manipulation. The recently published RAP and BEAT study reported excellent feasibility and safety with 6F Slender introducers.[20] The incidence of RAO, though, came close but did not outperform that of conventional 5F sheaths (3.4 versus 1.7%, respectively), which, in fact, have the same outer diameter. Another study demonstrated that, even when the outer diameter was presumably the same (6.5F Sheathless guiding versus Glidesheath Slender), the sheathless procedures offered significant better outcomes in terms of RAO/radial spasm (RAS).[21] These evidences suggest that the traumatic process leading to RAO could be multifactorial, rather than strictly linked to the diameter of the entry hole. We already suggested that sheathless catheters could be of advantage in providing a smoother navigation and preventing vascular trauma, proximal to the puncture site. A bigger catheter could also compromise the physiological laminar flow into the radial artery, particularly in a smaller vessel, and, in that way, promote thrombosis in the artery. Hence, a procedure performed by a 5F guiding catheter and a Slender sheath remains the second-best way (after sheathless) to undertake proper Slender PCIs.

Slender Devices

When the inner lumen of the guiding catheter diminishes, compatibility of devices becomes an issue. With 5F Guiding Catheters, it is possible to undertake most PCI procedures (Table 25.1). Some interventional techniques, however, such as kissing balloon technique or crushing stent technique, require extra lumen for the multiple devices utilized.

To overcome this limitation, devices themselves have to be downsized. The list of devices with 5F compatibility, a feature which once was considered the quality mark for being Slender, is updated by the day, and many of these products have been incorporated in daily routine, in such a way that they no longer need to be identified as Slender. As the bar is moving further to smaller, a few outstanding devices exist which still deserve this recognition. One of them is an ultra-thin angioplasty balloon (manufactured by Kaneka Japan), which can be advanced onto a 0.010" guidewire, instead of the standard 0.014". In this way the entire thickness of the system is thinner, crossing profile of the balloon is smaller, and two balloons of this kind can be accommodated in a 5F guiding catheter, then making kissing balloon technique possible.[22] Another innovative device, specifically developed Systems for Slender PCI, is de Slender Integrated Delivery System (IDS) (manufactured by Svelte Medical USA): this stent delivery system incorporates the coronary wire directly onto the shaft of the balloon. Because no internal lumen for the guidewire is needed, the

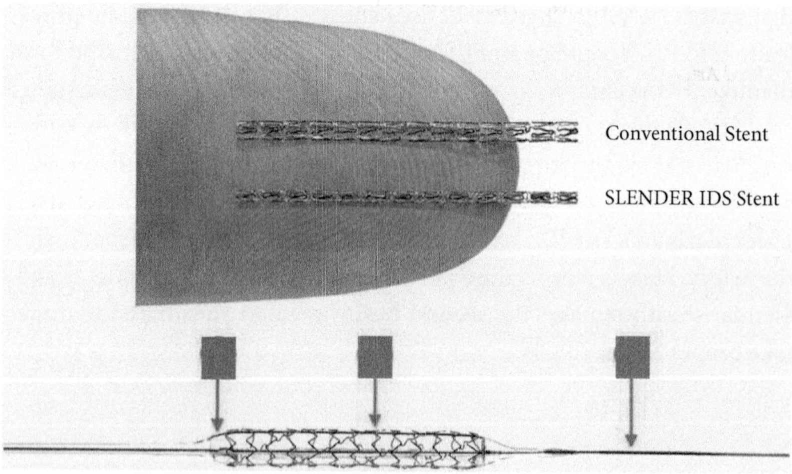

Figure 25.5 Slender IDS Stent (Svelte Medical USA). Upper panel: when crimped onto the balloon this sirolimus-eluting stent has the lowest crossing profile (0.031") available. Lower panel: the delivery system consists of a semi-compliant balloon (1), a cobalt-chromium (81 micron) Sirolimus-Eluting stent (2), and a 0.014" wire (Asahi Japan), directly soldered onto the tip of the balloon.

crossing profile of the whole system is reduced to the lowest currently available (0.031"). The Slender IDS system mounts a Sirolimus Eluting Stent with thin cobalt-chromium struts, which can be implanted not only by 5F Guiding catheters but even 4F diagnostic catheters (Figure 25.5). Moreover, this device allows crushing stenting technique both by 5F and 6F guiding catheters. Safety and feasibility in selected cohort of patients have been demonstrated[23]; results in broader real-life populations are expected soon.

(Left) Distal TRA

The definition of Slender can be applied also to an innovative puncture technique, where the distal, instead of the 'conventional', radial artery is cannulated. The radial artery is then punctured in the anatomical snuffbox, on the dorsal side of the wrist, exactly where it emerges from the floor

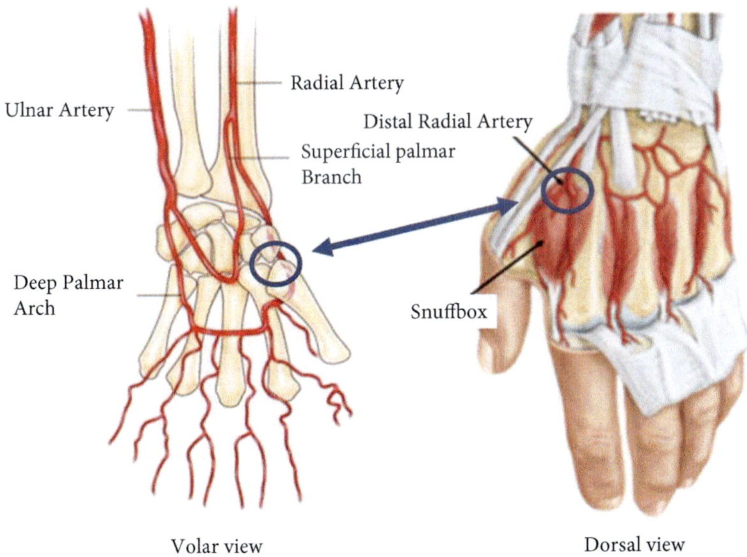

Figure 25.6 Left distal radial approach. Left panel: volar view of the left hand. Right panel: dorsal view of the left hand. The distal radial artery (blue circle) lays in the anatomical snuffbox, between the anastomosis of the superficial and deep palmar arches.

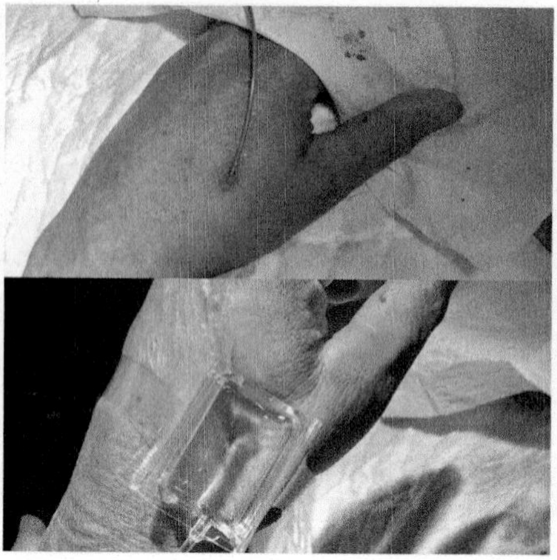

Figure 25.7 Left distal radial approach. Upper panel: 'virtual' 3F PCI performed by left Distal Transradial Approach. Lower panel: compression achieved by TR Band, 8 cc, one hour.

formed by the scaphoid and trapezium bones: this also means that the puncture will take place between the anastomosis with the deep and the superficial palmar arches (Figure 25.6). Distal TRA is preferably practiced by left approach: for doing this, the hand of the patient can be positioned onto their abdomen, with the elbow slightly bent towards the right side. For the operator and the patient himself, this means the same comfort as for conventional right TRA, but right-handed patients (the majority) would prefer not to be treated by their dominant hand. Because the puncture site lays between two anastomotic systems (deep and superficial palmar arches), the chance of RAO is less frequent and, even when it occurs, limited to a much shorter segment of the artery. Besides, distal TRA offers the interesting opportunity to re-canalize occluded proximal radial arteries after previous interventions. Compression can be achieved as for conventional TRA technique but is usually shorter and leaves the motility of the wrist unrestricted. As the distal radial artery is smaller than in its proximal part, the use of sheathless catheters or Slender introducers should be recommended (Figure 25.7). The feasibility and safety of this technique have been recently demonstrated,[24] after preliminary reports of other pioneering operators.

References

1. Steg PG, James SK, Atar D, Badano LP, et al. Task Force on the management of ST-segment elevation acute myocardial infarction of the European Society of Cardiology (ESC). ESC Guidelines for the management of acute myocardial infarction in patients presenting with ST-segment elevation. Eur Heart J. 2012 Oct;33(20):2569–619. doi: 10.1093/eurheartj/ehs215. Epub 2012 Aug 24. PMID: 22922416.
2. Kotowycz MA, Johnston KW, Ivanov J, Asif N, Almoghairi AM, Choudhury A, Nagy CD, Sibbald M, Chan W, Seidelin PH, Barolet AW, Overgaard CB, Džavík V. Predictors of radial artery size in patients undergoing cardiac catheterization: insights from the Good Radial Artery Size Prediction (GRASP) study. *Can J Cardiol.* 2014;30(2):211–6.
3. Saito S, Ikei H, Hosokawa G, Tanaka S. Influence of the ratio between radial artery inner diameter and sheath outer diameter on radial artery flow after transradial coronary intervention. *Catheter Cardiovasc Interv.* 1999;46:173–8.
4. Gwon HC, Doh JH, Choi JH, et al. A 5Fr catheter approach reduces patient discomfort during transradial coronary intervention compared with a 6Fr approach: a prospective randomized study. *J Interv Cardiol.* 2006;19:141–7.
5. Zwaan EM, Koopman AG, Holtzer CA, Zijlstra F, Ritt MJ, Amoroso G, Moerman E, Kofflard MJ, IJsselmuiden AA. Revealing the impact of local access-site complications and upper extremity dysfunction post transradial percutaneous coronary procedures. *Neth Heart J.* 2015;23(11):514–24.
6. Ikari Y, Matsukage T, Yoshimachi F, Masutani M, Saito S. Transradial and slender percutaneous coronary intervention: less invasive strategy in PCI. *Cardiovasc Interv Ther.* 2010;25(2):60–4.
7. Kiemeneij F, Yoshimachi F, Matsukage T, Amoroso G, Fraser D, Claessen BE, Saito S. Focus on maximal miniaturisation of transradial coronary access materials and techniques by the Slender Club Japan and Europe: an overview and classification. *EuroIntervention.* 2015;10(10):1178–86.
8. Dahm JB, Vogelgesang D, Hummel A, Staudt A, Volzke H, Felix SB. A randomized trial of 5 vs. 6 French transradial percutaneous coronary interventions. *Catheter Cardiovasc Interv.* 2002;57:172–6.
9. Grossman PM, Gurm HS, McNamara R, Lalonde T, Changezi H, Share D, Smith DE, Chetcuti SJ, Moscucci M. Blue Cross Blue Shield of Michigan Cardiovascular Consortium (BMC2). Percutaneous coronary intervention complications and guide catheter size: bigger is not better. *JACC Cardiovasc Interv.* 2009;2(7):636–44.
10. Lefevre T, Morice MC, Bonan R, Dumas P, Louvard Y, Karrillon G, Loubeyre C, Piechaud JF. Coronary angiography using 4 or 6 French diagnostic catheters: a prospective, randomized study. *J Invasive Cardiol.* 2001;13(10):674–7.
11. Kaluski E, Moussa ID, Heuser RR, et al. Automated contrast injectors for angiography: devices, methodology, and safety. *Catheter Cardiovasc Interv.* 2009;74:459–64.
12. Chahoud G, Khoukaz S, El-Shafei A, et al., Randomized comparison of coronary angiography using 4F catheters: 4F manual versus "Acisted" power injection technique. *Catheter Cardiovasc Interv.* 2001;53:221–4.

13. Takeshita S, Tanaka S, Saito S. Coronary intervention with 4-French catheters. *Catheter Cardiovasc Interv*. 2010;75:735–9.
14. Mamas M, D'Souza S, Hendry C, Ali R, Iles-Smith H, Palmer K, El-Omar M, Fath-Ordoubadi F, Neyses L, Fraser DG. Use of the sheathless guide catheter during routine transradial percutaneous coronary intervention: a feasibility study. *Catheter Cardiovasc Interv*. 2010;75(4):596–602.
15. Yoshimachi F, Torii S, Naito T. A novel percutaneous coronary intervention technique for chronic total occlusion: contralateral angiography with a single guiding catheter. *Catheter Cardiovasc Interv*. 2016;87(6):E229–32.
16. Takeshita S, Saito S. Transradial coronary intervention using a novel 5-Fr sheathless guiding catheter. *Catheter Cardiovasc Interv*. 2009;74:862–5.
17. Amoroso G, van Dullemen A, Westgeest P, van Duinen M. "Virtual" 3 Fr transradial coronary stenting with the 5 Fr Meito Masamune sheathless guiding catheter: feasibility and safety in an outpatient setting. *J Invasive Cardiol*. 2016;28(3):109–14.
18. Yoshimachi F, Takagawa Y, Terai H, Takahashi A, Shimada Y, Katsuki T, Tohara S, Ueno H, Takada M, Shiode N, Yamada K, Kinoshita N, Honda T, Asano H, Takeshita S, Koiwa H, Shin T, Masutani M, Matsukage T, Saito S, Ikari Y. The V3 Registry Investigators. A prospective multicenter study using a virtual 3 Fr percutaneous coronary intervention system: the V3 registry. *J Invasive Cardiol*. 2017;29(1):16–23.
19. Yoshimachi F, Kiemeneij F, Masutani M, Matsukage T, Takahashi A, Ikari Y. Safety and feasibility of the new 5 Fr Glidesheath Slender. *Cardiovasc Interv Ther*. 2016;31(1):38–41.
20. Aminian A, Saito S, Takahashi A, Bernat I, Jobe RL, Kajiya T, Gilchrist IC, Louvard Y, Kiemeneij F, Van Royen N, Yamazaki S, Matsukage T, Rao SV. Comparison of a new slender 6 Fr sheath with a standard 5 Fr sheath for transradial coronary angiography and intervention: RAP and BEAT (Radial Artery Patency and Bleeding, Efficacy, Adverse evenT), a randomised multicentre trial. *EuroIntervention*. 2017;13(5):e549–56.
21. Matsukage T, Masutani M, Yoshimachi F, Takahashi A, Katsuki T, Saito S, Terai H, Katahira Y, Uehara Y, Tohara S, Ohba Y, Shinohara S, Asano H, Matsumura T, Hata T, Ikari Y. PIKACHU Registry Investigators. A prospective multicenter registry of 0.010- inch guidewire and compatible system for chronic total occlusion: the PIKACHU registry. *Catheter Cardiovasc Interv*. 2010;75:1006–12.
22. Horie K, Tada N, Isawa T, Matsumoto T, Taguri M, Kato S, Honda T, Ootomo T, Inoue N. A randomized comparison of incidence of radial artery occlusion and symptomatic radial artery spasm associated with elective transradial coronary intervention using 6.5-fr sheathless Eaucath guiding catheter vs. 6.0-Fr Glidesheath Slender. *EuroIntervention*. 2017. pii: EIJ-D-17-00239. doi: 10.4244/EIJ-D-17-00239.
23. Verheye S, Khattab AA, Carrie D, Stella P, Slagboom T, Bartunek J, Onuma Y, Serruys PW. Direct implantation of rapamycin-eluting stents with bioresorbable drug carrier technology utilising the Svelte coronary stent-on-a-wire: the DIRECT II study. *EuroIntervention*. 2016;12(5):e615–22.
24. Kiemeneij F. Left distal transradial access in the anatomical snuffbox for coronary angiography (ldTRA) and interventions (ldTRI). *Eurointervention* 2017; 13(7):851–7.

26

Distal Radial Access for Transradial Interventions

Shobhit Piplani, Yashasvi Chugh, Sunita Chugh, and Sanjay Kumar Chugh

Background

Since the first transradial coronary angiography in 1988 and the first transradial angioplasty in 1994,[1,2] radial artery access for coronary procedures has gained immense popularity following publication of randomized studies and meta-analyses[3–5] which showed significant reduction in risk of bleeding, death, and myocardial infarction.[6,7]

Transradial access (TRA) has conventionally been described as percutaneous access to the radial artery (RA) at a level higher than the anatomical snuff box.[8] The major challenges of radial access have been haemostasis and radial artery occlusion (RAO). Haemostasis following standard transradial procedure has been done initially using innovative clamps and recently using RA haemostatic devices including pneumatic devices (TR Band™ Terumo). Non-occlusive haemostasis or patent haemostasis has been reported to reduce RAO significantly.[9] Cotton gauze-ball or bandage-roll with elastic bandage is also commonly used successfully, although no published data are available on this method of haemostasis. With prolonged cannulation of RA,[10–12] rate of occlusion of RA has been reported to be as high as 40%.

Saito et al. have reported reduction in flow in RA around the sheath when the RA sheath size mismatch is >1.[13] However, because the distal blood flow in the superficial palmar arch is likely to be preserved if access is done in the distal radial artery (DRA) in the region of snuff box, it was speculated that RAO may be reduced.

Further, with conventional RA access at the wrist, haematoma of the forearm[14] is a known complication, which can of progress to the dreaded complication of compartment syndrome. This too was expected to be less with distal radial access.

Although remote haematomas from guide-wire tip perforation of radial perforators is a possibility, most major bleeds occur because of failure to compress the puncture site adequately, especially when through and through puncture of the RA in the forearm is done using a needle with cannula as with Jelco™ or with the introducer needle provided with the introducer sheath[Terumo™]. Another major reason for haematomas following bleed from puncture site is the practice of patent haemostasis which requires reduction of compression pressure to allow antegrade flow in radial artery. At this time, close monitoring with frequent palpation of forearm, rather than inspection is warranted[14] for early detection and prevention of development of haematoma from bleeding into forearm.

The practice of patent haemostasis with conventional radial access therefore requires close monitoring by staff, because uncontrolled bleed in the forearm can rapidly lead to compartment syndrome[15]; which if untreated can lead to hand ischaemia, gangrene, and fatality.

However, with DRA access in the anatomical snuff box, haemostasis is easier due to less soft tissue. The, probability of forearm haematoma is also less, except that arising out of remote site bleeding from wire tip perforation of a RA perforator or branch in forearm. Thus, unlike with conventional radial access at the wrist, patients who have trans–distal-radial procedure would require less intensive monitoring because patent haemostasis is not required.

The area requiring anaesthetization being small in the region of snuff box with less soft tissue, pain perception of the patient related to access was also expected to be low, theoretically.

In addition, another hypothetical theoretical advantage of distal radial access was the preservation of the radial artery to be used as conduit for coronary bypass or arteriovenous fistula for haemodialysis or for repeat transradial procedures.

In the first large study on distal radial access,[16] puncture failures were reported to be very low (2.3 versus 4% for DRA access versus RA access), and so was radial artery occlusion (0.3% for RA and DRA occlusion and 0.1% RA occlusion with DRA access). Puncture time after 50 cases was 50 seconds per case; same as puncture time for RA access at wrist. The radial artery size in forearm was 2.7 mm and 2.4 mm at the snuff box. These arteries are larger than that reported from India in an Indian population.[17]

A 90% puncture success was reported in another small study of 52 patients.[18] Kiemeneij et al., reported on feasibility of left radial through distal radial access from anatomical snuffbox in a small series.[19] The technique is challenging because even with case selection, failure rate was high. In a study of 118 patients, only 70 (59.3%) were considered suitable for left DRA access and there were 8 procedure failures (11.4%) requiring crossover to alternate access.

Distal Radial Artery Access

DRA access can be done at one of the two sites:

1. RA for distal assess is cannulated in distal 1/3 of radial artery located in anatomical snuff box which is on dorsal surface of hand.
2. Puncture can be done on the dorsum at the vertex of angle between extensor pollicis longus and metacarpal bone.

Puncture at the vertex between extensor pollicis longus and metacarpal bone is difficult and has more failures.

Puncture Technique

The same puncture needles and sheaths as described in chapter on '*Tips and tricks for transradial interventions*' for forearm radial access are used for distal radial access.

The patient's hand muscles must be relaxed for successful puncture. Prior sedation often helps in relaxing the patient's hand in anxious patients. Puncture of distal radial artery is illustrated in Figures 26.1(a), 26.1(b), and 26.1(d). Figure 26.1(c) shows a superficial anomalous

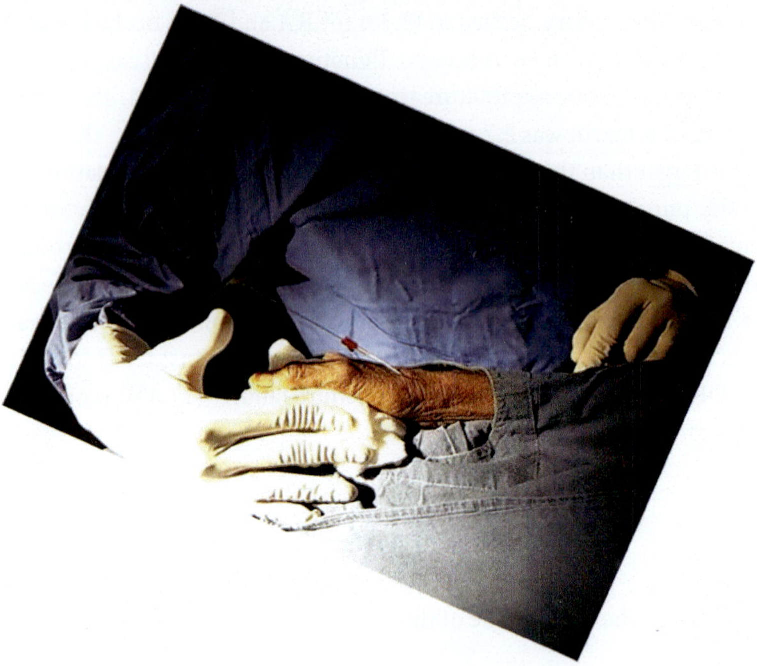

Figure 26.1a Ideal hand – position for DRRA is 30° short of full pronation at the wrist with 15°extension at the wrist. The extent of wrist extension and ulnar flexion were varied per operator discretion, to optimize palpability of the DRA. Bunch of cotton gauze is used to maintain the hand position.

radial artery traversing the roof of the snuffbox which was encountered in 3/264 consecutive patients. Figure 26.1(e) shows a 6F Radial sheath (Terumo) inserted in radial artery (RAD 1.5 mm) at snuffbox in a 63-year-old patient with rheumatoid arthritis and bony deformities at the wrist (Figure 26.1(f)), who presented with acute coronary syndrome and successfully underwent two-vessel angioplasty to both left anterior descending artery and left circumflex artery through DRA access (Figures 26.1(g)–26.1(t)). Figure 26.1(u) illustrates use of angioplasty wire to facilitate puncture, when there is difficulty in inserting the sheath wire. A sheath can then track over the angioplasty wire (Figure 26.1(v)). Alternatively, the Jelco venous cannula can be pushed into the radial artery over the angioplasty wire, which is then removed and subsequently the sheath wire can be introduced, over which the sheath tracks.

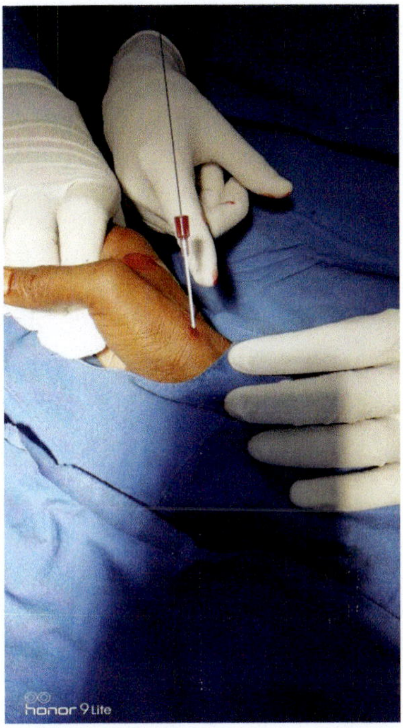

Figure 26.1b Assistant holds hand of patient in 30 degree short of full pronation and 15 degree extension of wrist for DRA puncture.

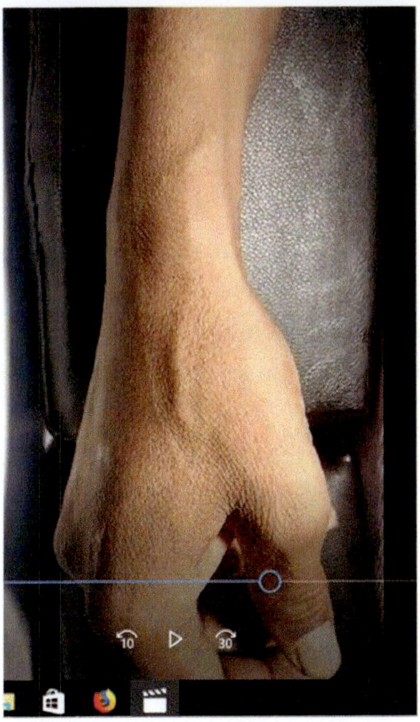

Figure 26.1c Superficial anomalous radial artery traversing the roof of the snuffbox at its lateral border.

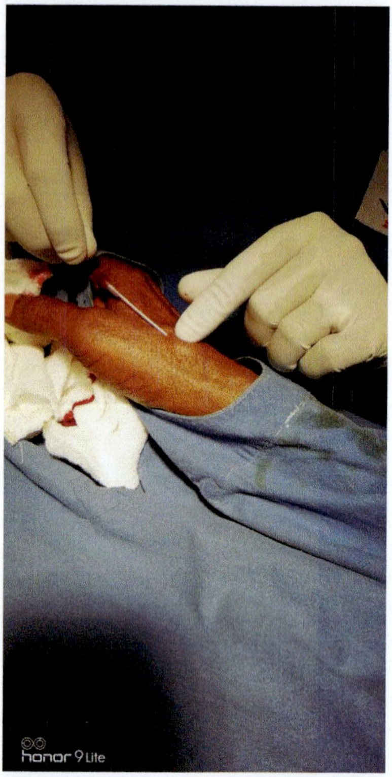

Figure 26.1d Technique of puncturing the artery; Terumo sheathed needle inserted in superficial anomalous distal radial on lateral border of anatomical snuffbox.

The Boundaries of the Anatomical Snuffbox

Anteriorly-Abductor Pollicis longus and Extensor Pollicis Brevis; Posteriorly-Extensor Pollicis longus; Base of triangle-Styloid process of Radius.

A radial sheath is inserted into a radial artery at the snuff box (Figure 26.2).

After gaining access, the same spasmolytics and unfractionated heparin are injected intra-arterially into the RA, as with conventional forearm radial access. The author's experience[20] was presented as an invited faculty lecture at the TransCatheter Therapeutics meeting in San Diego, CA in 2018 and is presented below (the DATA STAR study).

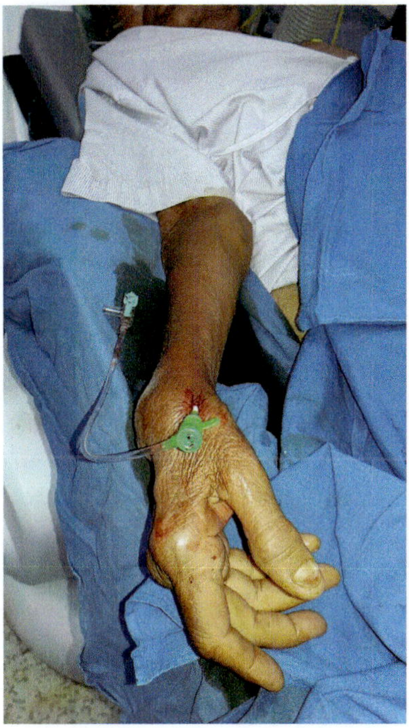

Figure 26.1e 6F Radial sheath (Terumo) inserted in radial artery at snuffbox in a 63-year-old patient with rheumatoid arthritis. Patient underwent successful primary angioplasty to right coronary artery through the anatomical snuff box (DRRA). Note the deformity in the wrist. Patient's RAD was 1.5 mm.

DATA STUDY: The Distal Radial versus Transradial Access Registry: The D.A.T.A STAR Study)[20] was a retrospective analysis of single-centre, single-operator registry of consecutive DRA versus consecutive RA (conventional forearm RA at wrist) access in 545 patients. The study showed that unlike what was suggested by early registry data or believed theoretically, DRA access at anatomical snuffbox takes more time, fails more often and has similar RAO rates as conventional RA access at the wrist; of course the mean RA diameter in the study was 1.63 ± 0.27 mm, hence this was a population with smaller diameter radial arteries. Forearm haematomas did not occur with distal radial access; hand haematomas were easily managed and there was no compartment syndrome.

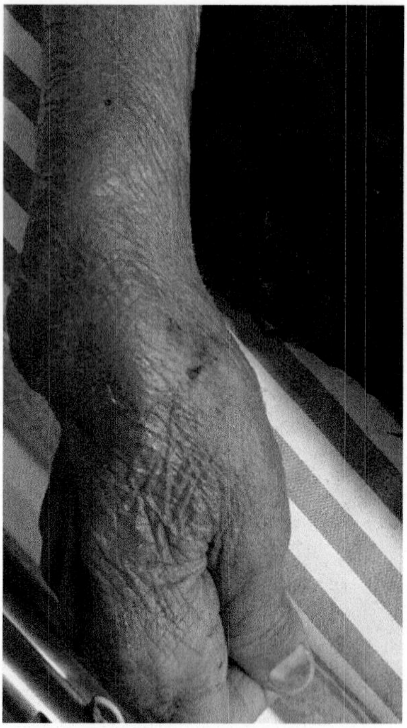

Figure 26.1f Bony deformities at wrist of same patient.

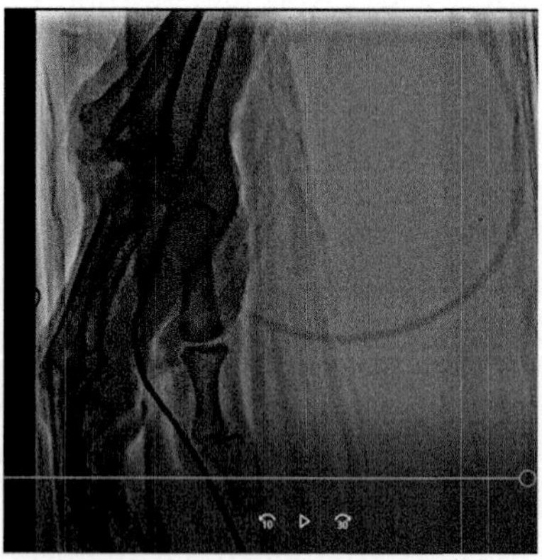

Figure 26.1g 6F sheath inserted via DRRA.

(h) (i)

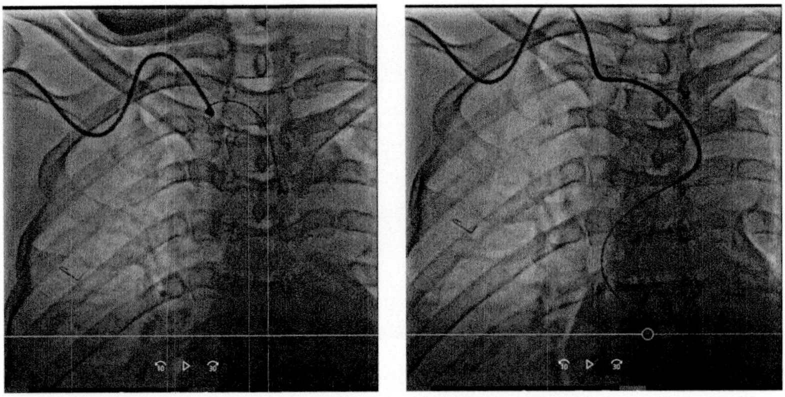

Figure 26.1h and i
Negotiating subclavian tortuosity with help of big breath.

(j) (k)

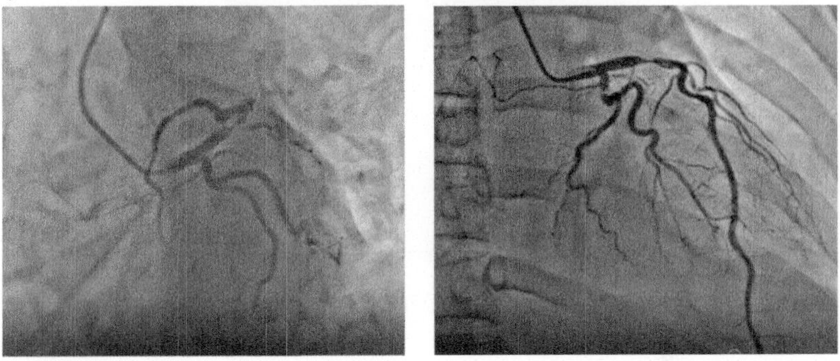

Figure 26.1j and k
Left coronary angiogram with proximal left anterior descending artery (LAD) and left circumflex artery (LCX) lesions.

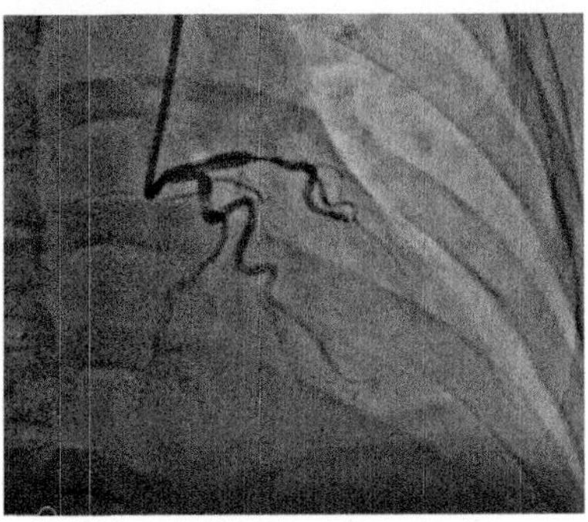

Figure 26.1l Wire crosses LAD lesion.

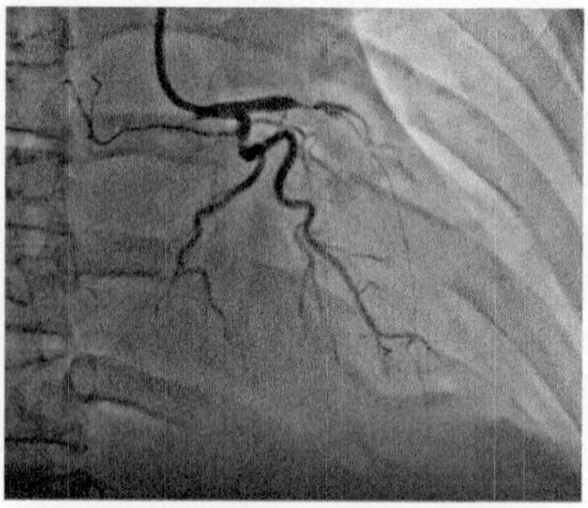

Figure 26.1m LAD lesion pre-dilatation.

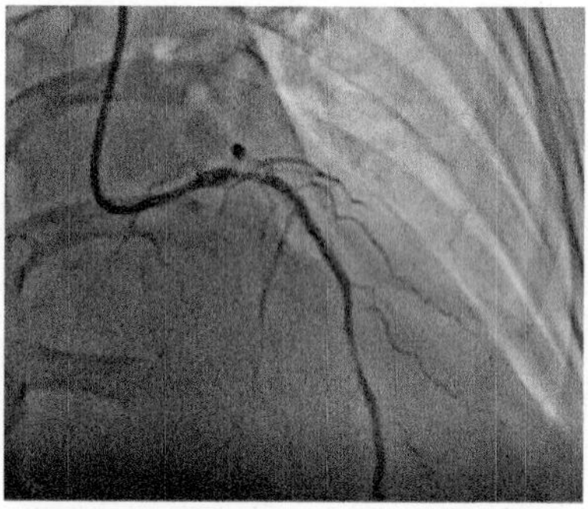

Figure 26.1n Stent in position at LAD lesion.

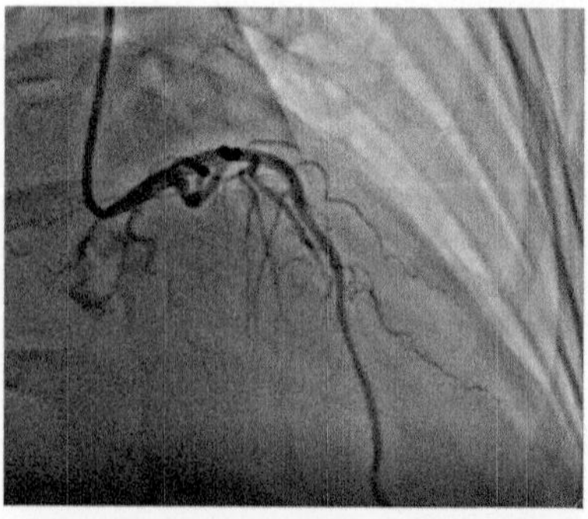

Figure 26.1o Final TIMI 3 flow in LAD after post-dilatation.

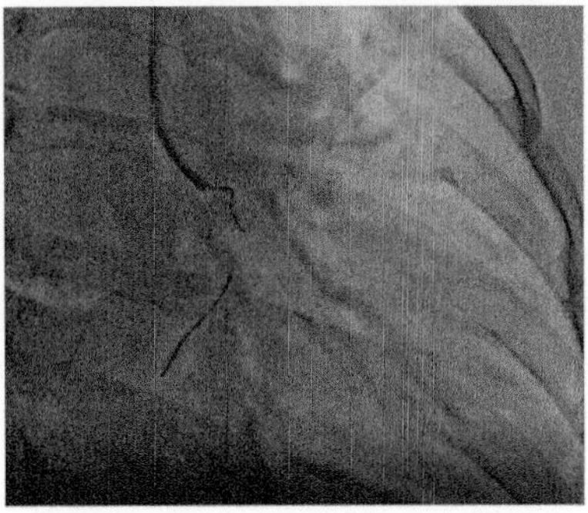

Figure 26.1p A buddy wire is inserted in LCX to stabilize the guiding catheter while a second wire crosses the lesion in proximal LCX into an obtuse marginal.

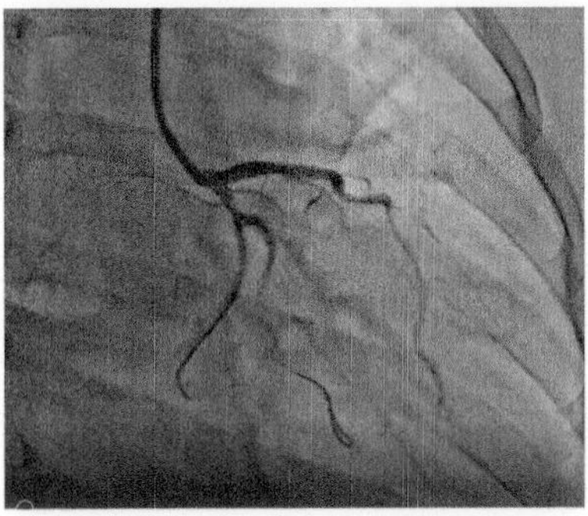

Figure 26.1q After pre-dilatation of LCX lesion.

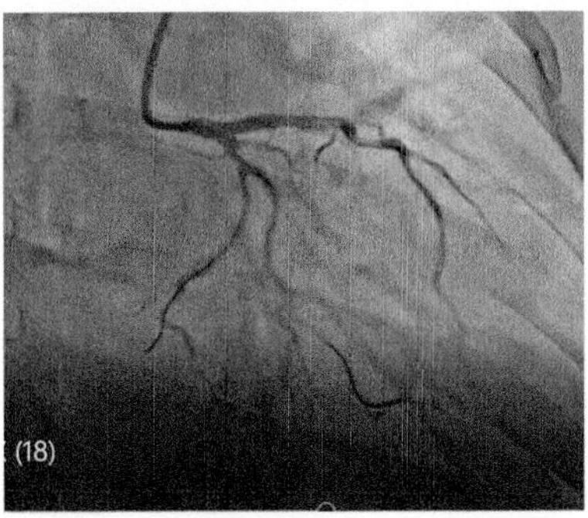

Figure 26.1r Stent in position in LCX lesion.

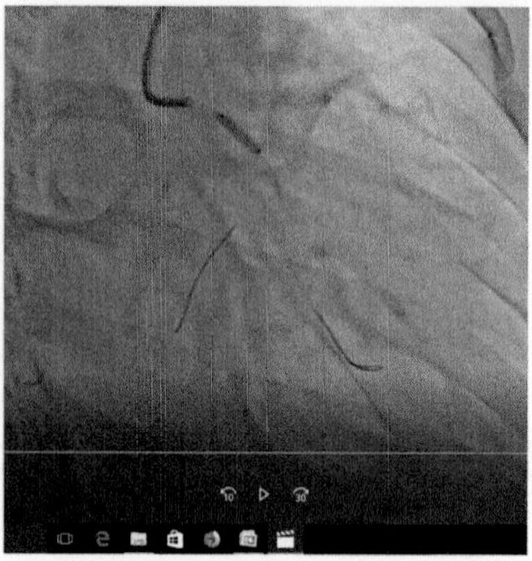

Figure 26.1s Stent deployed in LCX.

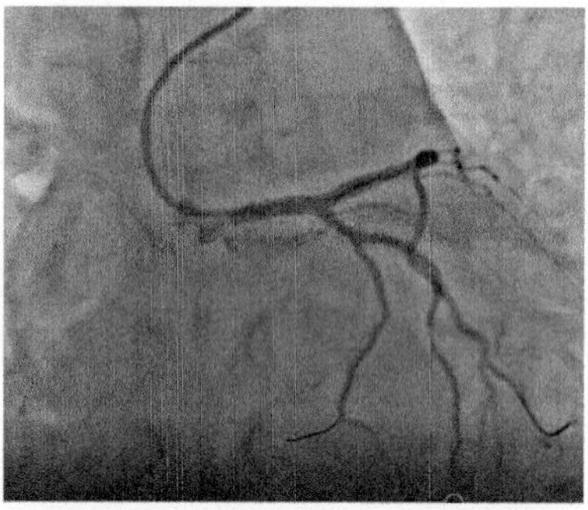

Figure 26.1t Final TIMI3 flow in both LAD and LCX.

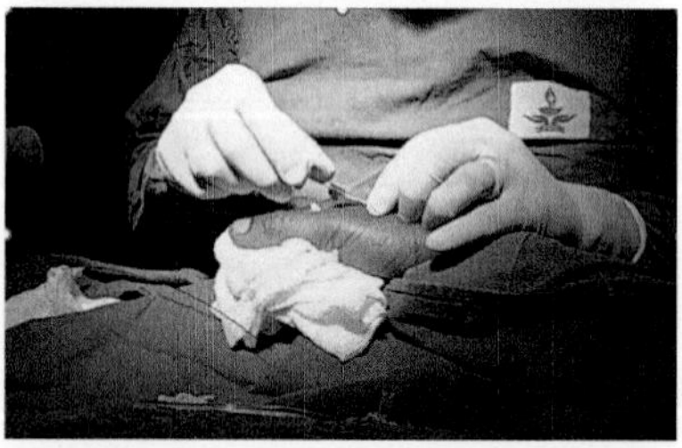

Figure 26.1u PTCA wire introduced through cannula of over the needle cannula system (Jelco™ venous cannula 20-gauge venipuncture catheter needle) because the sheath wire could not be inserted.

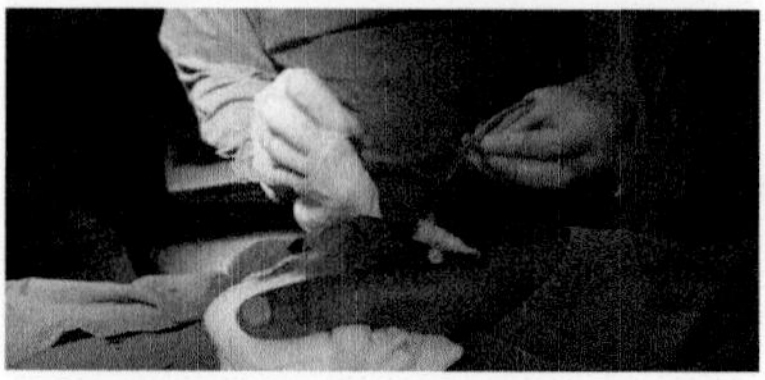

Figure 26.1v 6F Sheath then tracks over the 0.014" angioplasty wire.

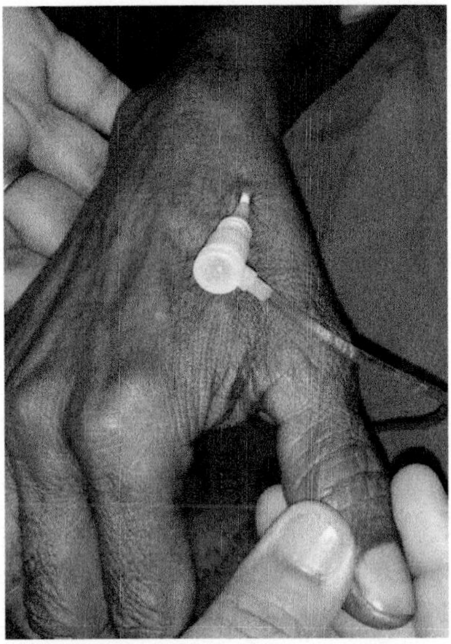

Figure 26.2 Anatomical landmarks for anatomical snuff box: Posteriorly: Extensor Pollicis longus; Anteriorly: Abductor Pollicis longus and Extensor Pollicis Brevis; Base of triangle: Styloid process of Radius. Radial sheath is inserted in radial artery which traverses the floor of the snuff box.

A total of 545 consecutive patients were prospectively enrolled in this single-centre, single-operator registry. Consecutive 282 patients were assigned to standard right radial access (RRA) over a 5 month period, and the following 263 patients were subsequently enrolled in distal right radial access (DRA access group) (Figure 26.3) over the subsequent 5 month period. Patient clinical and procedural characteristics are shown in Tables 26.1 and 26.2 and were comparable in the two groups, except that there were more smokers (70.9% versus 59.3%, $p = 0.005$) and less RA anomalies (4.9% versus 10.6%, $p = 0.013$) in the RA group.

The primary endpoint was puncture success; the secondary endpoints were puncture time, RA occlusion at days 1 and 30 (on ultrasound) and access-site complications. All patients had pre-procedure ultrasound of forearm arteries prior to enrollment, for baseline artery dimensions and presence of anatomical anomalies. Ultrasound of forearm arteries was performed with 2D-colour Doppler using a linear probe using standard protocol, as described in the chapter on 'Role of colour Doppler ultrasound in transradial interventions' Diameters of distal radial arteries

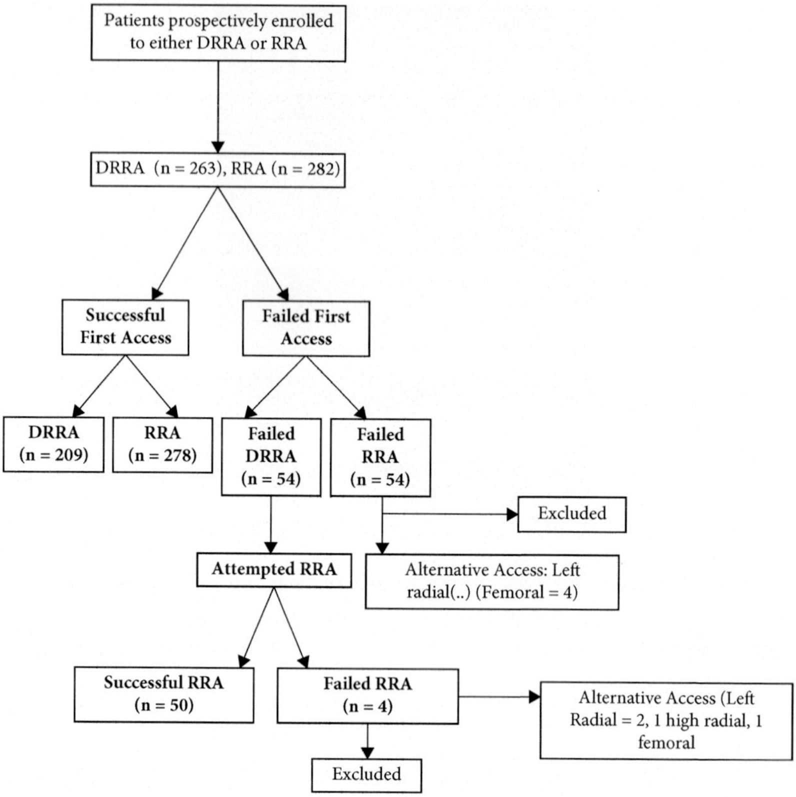

Figure 26.3 Study design.[20]

were not measured owing to its well-known limitations in small-diameter radial arteries(<2.0mm); nor was ultrasound—guided puncture used, because of lack of convincing data on its superiority over blind-puncture of distal radial arteries[20] at the time.

Puncture Time

Puncture time (intra-procedural) was defined as the time taken from first contact of puncture needle with skin to successful cannulation of the access artery with uninterrupted smooth passage of full length of the sheath wire. Secondary endpoint of puncture time was significantly higher in patients with distal right radial access compared with RRA (2.1 min ± 1.4 versus 1.0 min ± 0.45, $p < 0.00001$).

Table 26.1 Patient clinical characteristics[20]

	GROUP 1 (Radial, n = 282)	GROUP 2 (distal radial, n = 263)	P VALUE
PATIENT DEMOGRAPHICS			
AGE	53.79 ± 12.94	55.13 ± 11.94	NS
Male/female	84/198(29.7%/70.3%)	79/184(30%/70%)	NS
Weight(kg)	67.60 ± 9.74	64.01 ± 9.02	NS
Height(cm)	169.25 ± 6.99	169.39 ± 7.52	NS
BMI	23.66 ± 3.61	22.33 ± 3.089	NS
Cigarette Smoker	200(70.9%)	156(59.3%)	0.005
COPD	52(18.4%)	36(13.6%)	NS
Hypertension	34(12%)	32(12.1%)	NS
Diabetes Mellitus	37(13.1%)	37(14%)	NS
Heart Failure with EF<40	44(15.6%)	49(18.8%)	NS
Haemodynamic status			
Unstable	45(15.9%)	61(23.1%)	0.06

Puncture Failure

Puncture success (intra-procedural): Puncture success was defined by us as the ability of the operator to successfully cannulate the access artery.

The radial sheath could not be inserted full length because the sheath wire was in a distal branch of radial (n = 5; no bleed back in 3, extravasation in 2); or because of calcification (n = 2; with RA stenosis in 1 case).

On multivariate analysis, the primary endpoint of puncture success was significantly lower with distal right radial access (79.5% versus 98.5%, $p<0.0001$). RRA had 13.4 ± 7.8 OR of puncture success versus DRA. Risk of puncture failure was higher in patients with RAD < 1.6 mm versus ≥ 1.6 mm in the distal right radial access ($p < 0.0001$) and RRA (p = NS) groups (Table 25.3). All patients who had puncture success had procedure success; though. in 8 cases, the procedure was completed using alternative access ('crossover'). See later under 'crossover' and Figure 26.3.

On multivariate analysis (n = 263), DRA puncture failure was related to RA diameter ($p < 0.0001$) and BMI ($p < 0.04$); smaller diameter radials had higher puncture failure. A composite endpoint of haematoma,

Table 26.2 Procedure-related characteristics[20]

	GROUP 1 (Radial, n = 282)	GROUP 2 (distal radial, n = 63)	p Value
Previous procedure using same access Forearm Ultrasound	70 (24.8%)	61(23.1%)	0.56
PPUAA	282 (100%)	263 (100%) NS	
RA size (mm) (mean ± SD)	1.59 ± 0.27	1.62 ± 0.26	0.948
RA size, Males	1.63 ± 0.27	1.66 ± 0.27	0.26
RA size, Females	1.46 ± 0.22	1.51 ± 0.21	0.17
Vascular Anomalies Intimal Thickness	0 (0%)	2 (0.8%)	0.18
Parallel Radial Artery	6 (2.1%)	13 (4.9%)	
Radial Artery Loop	1 (0.4%)	1 (0.4%)	
Accessory Radial Artery	1 (0.4%)	0 (0%)	
Occluded Artery	1 (0.4%)	3 (1.1%)	
Primary Access			
Success	278 (98.5%)	209 (79.4%)	p<0.0001
Unsuccessful	4 (1.5%)	54 (20.6%)	p<0.0001
Puncture time(min)	1.17 ± 0.8	2.08 ± 0.9	0.0001
Sheath (F)			
5 F	156	107	
6 F	172	102	0.41
Coronary Angiogram	236	152	
PCI (Single vessel)	79	45	
PCI (Two vessel)	2	1	
Radial artery spasm	3 (0.9%)	3 (1.4%)	0.3
PTCA(PAMI)	11	11	NS
POST-PROCEDURE			
Vascular Access Site			
Complications	2 (0.6%)	4 (1.9%)	0.16
Non Vascular Access Site Complications	0 (0%)	3 (1.4%)	0.031

Table 26.2 *Continued*

	GROUP 1 (Radial, n = 282)	GROUP 2 (distal radial, n = 63)	p Value
Radial Artery Occlusion			
Day 1	8 (2.4%)	5 (2.4%)	0.97
Day 30	7 (2.1%)	6 (2.9%)	0.58
Distal Radial Artery Occlusion			
Day 1	8 (2.4%)	5 (2.4%)	0.93
Day 30	5 (1.5%)	6 (2.8%)	0.28

PPUAA = Pre-procedure ultrasound of arm arteries. RA = Radial, RAD = radial artery diameter F = French size of sheath. CAG = Coronary angiogram, PTCA = angioplasty, PAMI = Primary angioplasty in acute myocardial infarction.

non-vascular access site complications and RAO and DRAO was higher in the <1.6 mm DRRA and RRA sub-groups (p < 0.001) (Table 26.3).

After excluding patients with poorly palpable distal radial artery, the puncture failure rate of distal right radial artery in the DATA study was 11.3%; compared to 10% reported in other studies with a selected study patient population which included only those patients with a well-palpable distal radial artery. Another major reason for higher DRRA puncture failure in this population was the smaller diameter of radial arteries (mean RAD 1.63 ± 0.27 mm) versus that reported in other study populations[18,21–24] (mean RAD > 2.1mm); distal radial arteries[18,21,22,25] being even smaller. In addition, anatomical challenges of angulation and tortuosities of distal radial artery may also have contributed to increased risk of puncture failure and time, with DRA compared to conventional radial access which is devoid of such anatomical challenges.

Haemostasis

Manual haemostasis is possible but not usually feasible. We used pre-defined sizes of cotton bandage roll (Figures 26.4a–c) and elastic bandage (Figures 26.4d–e) for haemostasis (Figures 26.4f–j) for both DRA access (as described under haemostasis previously) and RRA

Table 26.3 Outcomes in patients with radial artery diameters <1.6 mm versus ≥ 1.6mm

	Radial Artery Diameter <1.6 mm	**Radial Artery Diameter ≥1.6mm**	**p Value**
DRRA Group	(n = 148)	(n = 61)	
Puncture Success (%)	77.5%	89.8 %	0.0001
Puncture Time (min)	2.02 + 1.43	2.19 + 1.43	0.48
Vascular Access Site Complications	4 (1.7%)	0 (0%)	0.21
Non Vascular Access Site Complications	3 (1.4%)	0 (0%)	0.21
Radial Artery Occlusion			
Day 1	4 (2.7%)	1 (1.6%)	0.34
Day 30	6 (4.1%)	0 (0%)	0.11
Distal Radial Artery Occlusion			
Day 1	5 (2.1%)	0 (0%)	0.16
Day 30	5 (2.1%)	1 (1.6%)	0.71
Composite Secondary Endpoint *	16 (10.8%)	1 (1.6%)	0.001
RRA Group	(n = 239)	(n = 89)	
Puncture Success (%)	96%	100%	<0.05
Puncture Time (min)	1.20 + 0.82	0.76 + 0.34	0.05
Vascular Access Site Complications	1 (0.7%)	1 (1.6%)	0.51
Non Vascular Access Site Complications	0 (0%)	0 (0%)	0.42
Radial Artery Occlusion			
Day 1	7 (2.9%)	1 (1.1%)	0.64
Day 30	6 (2.5%)	1 (1.1%)	0.44
Distal Radial Artery Occlusion			
Day 1	5 (2.1%)	1 (1.1%)	0.56
Day 30	4 (1.7%)	1 (1.1%)	0.49
Composite Secondary Endpoint *	13 (5.4%)	3 (3.3%)	0.001

(please see under 'haemostasis' in chapter on 'tips and tricks for TRI') groups. The bandage was loosened at 1hour and removed after ≥12 hours as pre-defined and as per our usual practice. No other haemostatic device was used. Non-occlusive haemostasis was not done in any of the cases. The bandage was removed day after procedure.

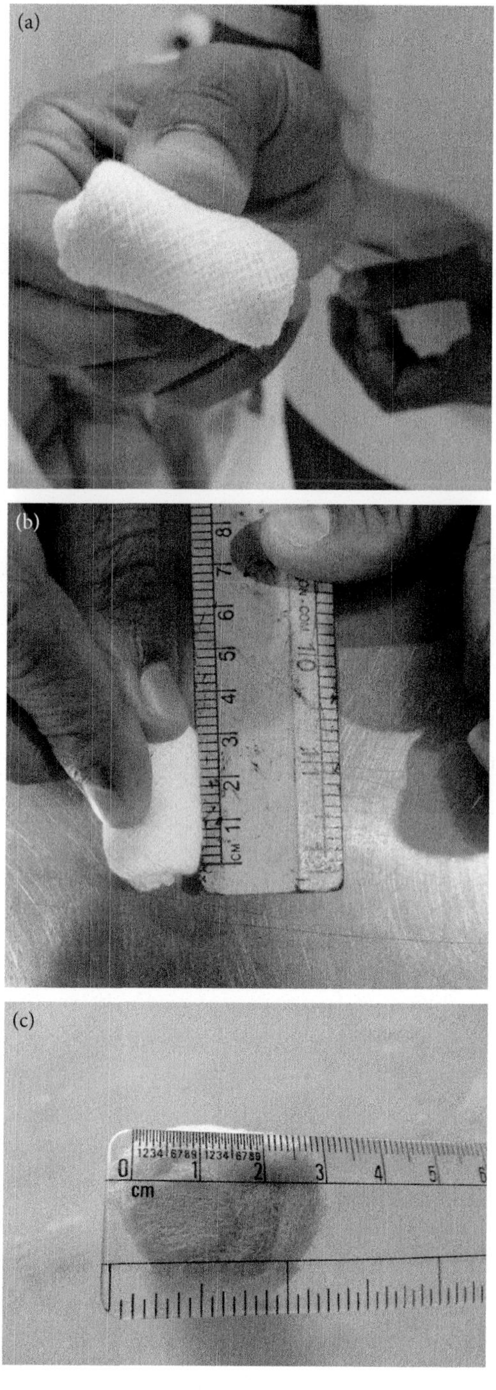

Figure 26.4(a–c)
Pre-defined sizes (diameter and length) of cotton bandage roll for haemostasis for DRRA.

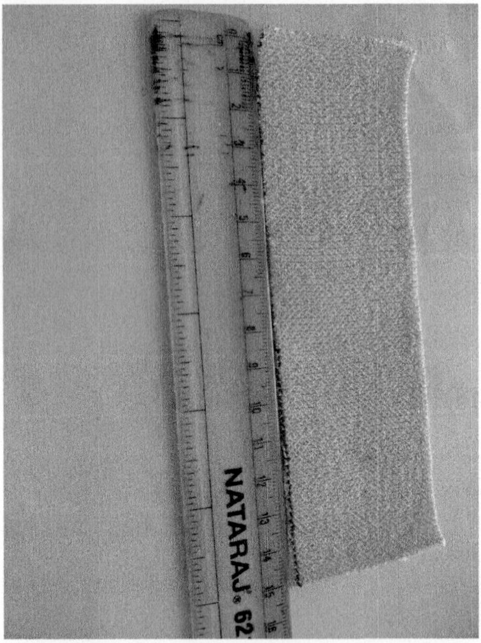

Figure 26.4d Pre-defined sizes (diameter and length) of elastic bandage for haemostasis for DRRA.

Consequence of RA anomalies on procedures (DATA STAR study, n = 545)

- Monophasic Flow
- Monophasic flow n = 6 In one case angioplasty was done through the same right radial. In the remaining, alternative access was used.
- Intimal Thickness
- Intimal thickness was found in 3; of these 2 were densely calcific radials and ulnars bilaterally and required alternate access after DRA access failed; 1 from left radial and femoral in the other.
- Parallel Radial and Ulnar Normal bifurcation of brachial artery into radial and ulnar arteries occurs usually at the cubital fossa. A variation in the location of brachial artery to a higher, more proximal location in arm or axilla is referred to by us as 'Parallel radial and ulnar'.[17]

Out of 545 cases, 19 (3.4%) had 'parallel' radial and ulnar with RAD 1.1–2.5 mm, and 2/545 (0.3%) had bilateral 'parallel' radial and ulnar.

All of these patients underwent successful 5F CAG via DRA access. However, in three patients with RAD <1.6 mm requiring angioplasty, alternate access site (1 DLRA, 1femoraL, 1 by high RA puncture (Figures 26.5a–l)) was necessary because of narrow radial artery origin in 3/19 (15.8%) (Type 3 bifurcation) which did not accommodate a 6F guiding catheter.

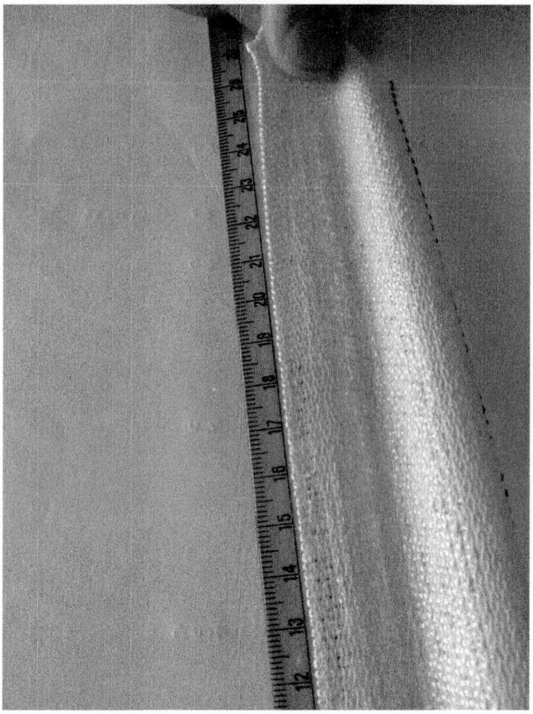

Figure 26.4e Length of stretched elastic bandage: increased by 20% from baseline.

Follow-up Post-DRR Access

In 3 patients with 1.1 mm radial diameter, the RA occluded on follow-up at day 1 (all had ≥ grade 3 spasm); DRA access and RRA were patent in remaining 16 patients at 30 days.

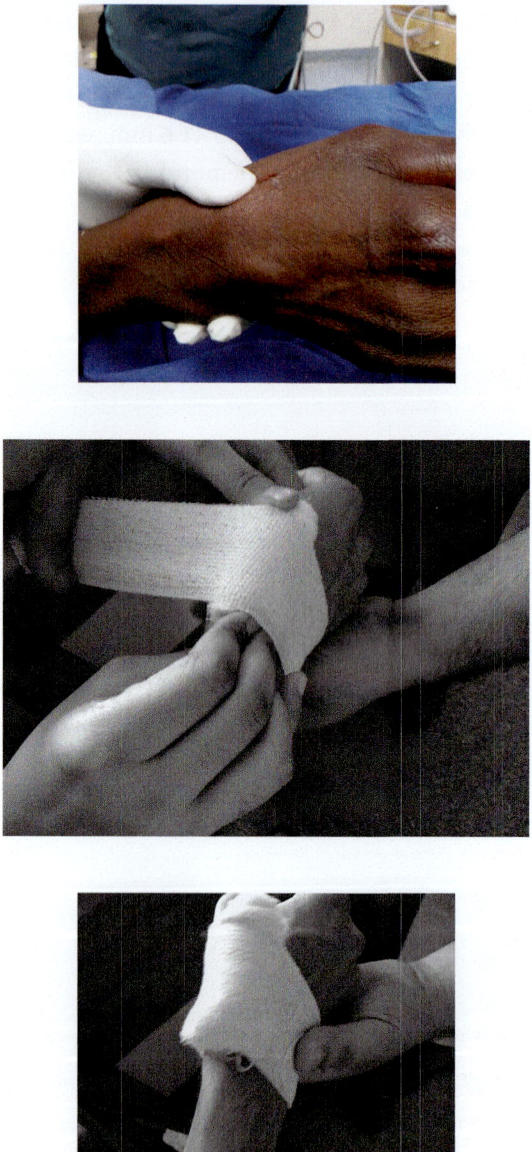

Figure 26.4 f–h Technique of elastic bandage for haemostasis in DRRA cases.

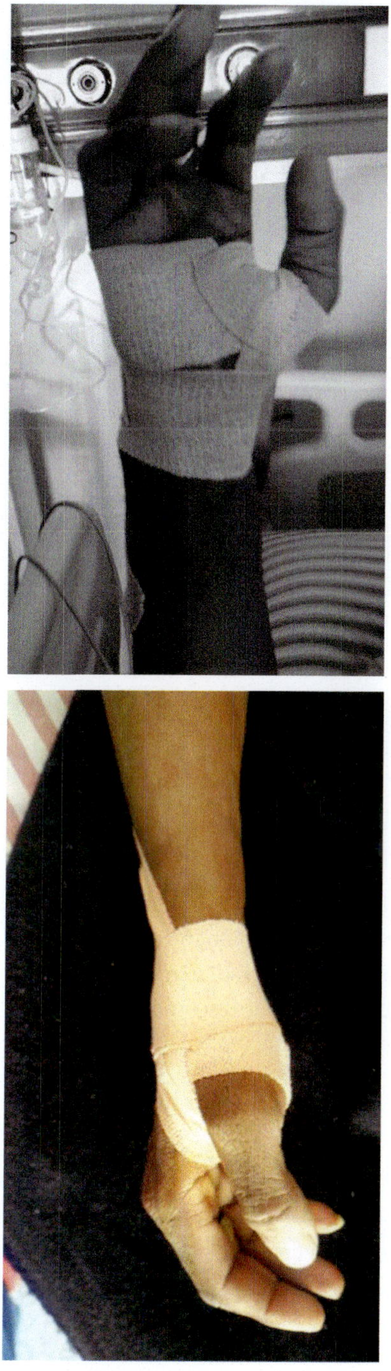

Figure 26.4i–j Final bandage in 2 views

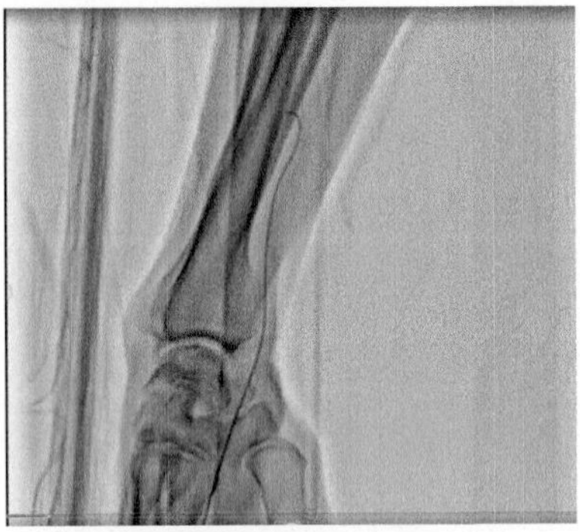

Figure 26.5a Distal transradial access for Angioplasty to RCA in a 67-year-old male. Post successful DRA puncture. The sheath wire could not be advanced.

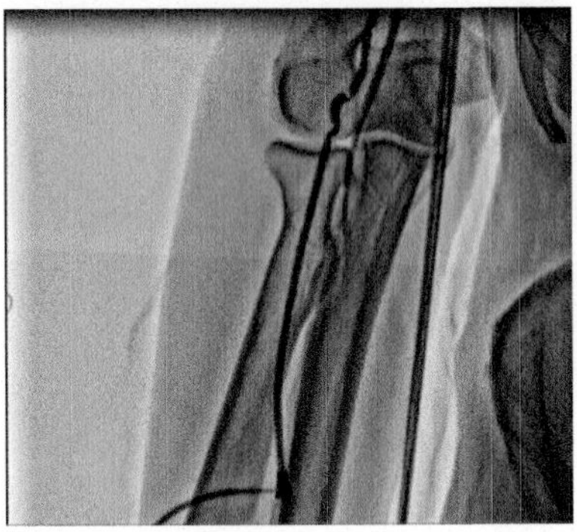

Figure 26.5b After DRA failed puncture of radial artery at the wrist also failed as the sheath wire could not be advanced. This figure shows a successful high puncture of the radial in the forearm shows a diseased tortuous, high bifurcation radial from brachial.

Cubital Loop

Cubital loop with remnant radial (Type 3 bifurcation) was present in 8 (1.46%); bilateral in 1. Of the four cases taken up for 5F angiography via DRA access, the loop was crossed successfully in two cases, while in the remaining two cases, there was *cross-over to alternate access.*

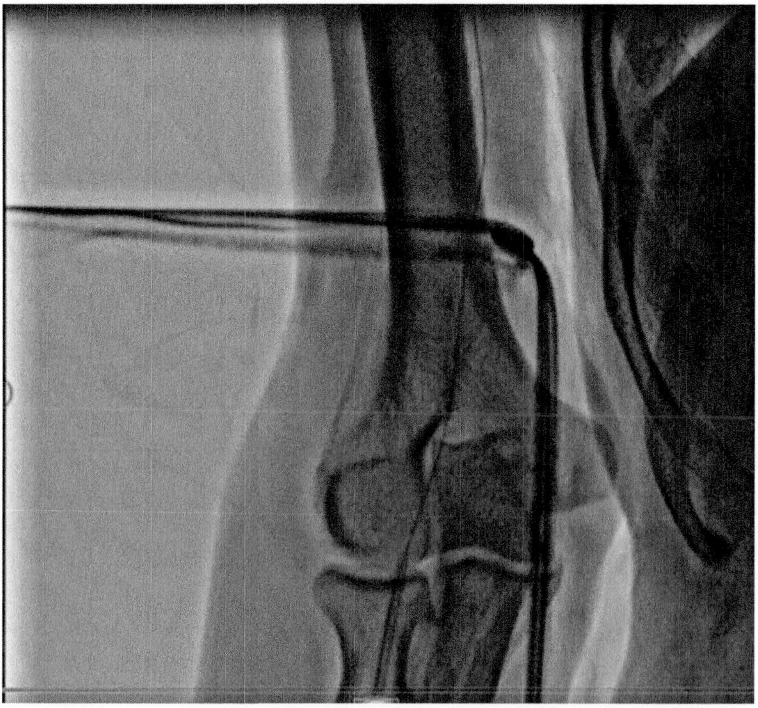

Figure 26.5c An angioplasty wire is used to negotiate the tortuous diseased radial artery.

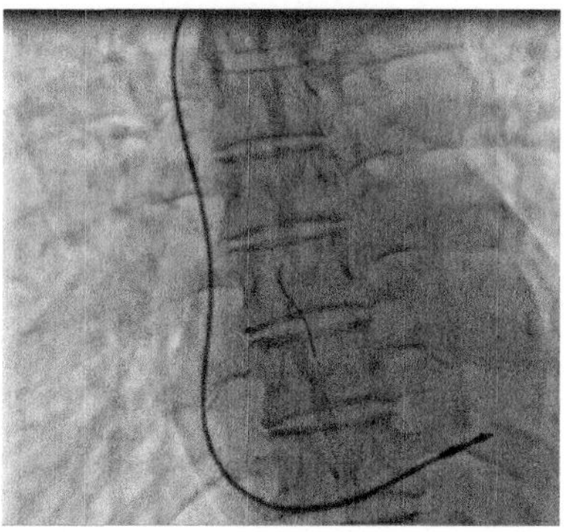

Figure 26.5d Angioplasty wire reaches the ascending aorta. Pacemaker lead is seen in the right ventricle.

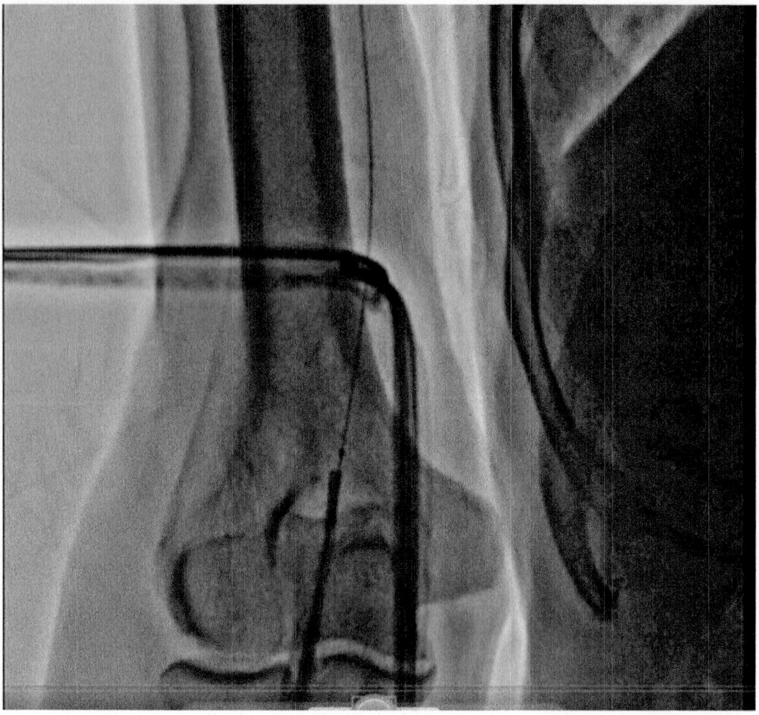

Figure 26.5e A 5 F JR 3.5 is advanced over a deflated balloon on the angioplasty wire.

Complications

By regression analysis, access site complications were found to be similar in both DRA access and RRA groups (1.9% versus 0.35%, $p = 0.12$). A composite end-point of haematoma, non-vascular access site complications and RAO and DRAO was higher in the <1.6 mm DRA access and RRA sub-groups ($p < 0.001$) (Table 26.3).

Radial Artery Spasm (RAS)

Incidence of grade-3 RAS[18] is the same as that with RA access (1.9 versus 2.01% (p = NS) and is managed as for forearm radial access described in chapter 10 on 'Tips and Tricks for Transradial Interventions'.

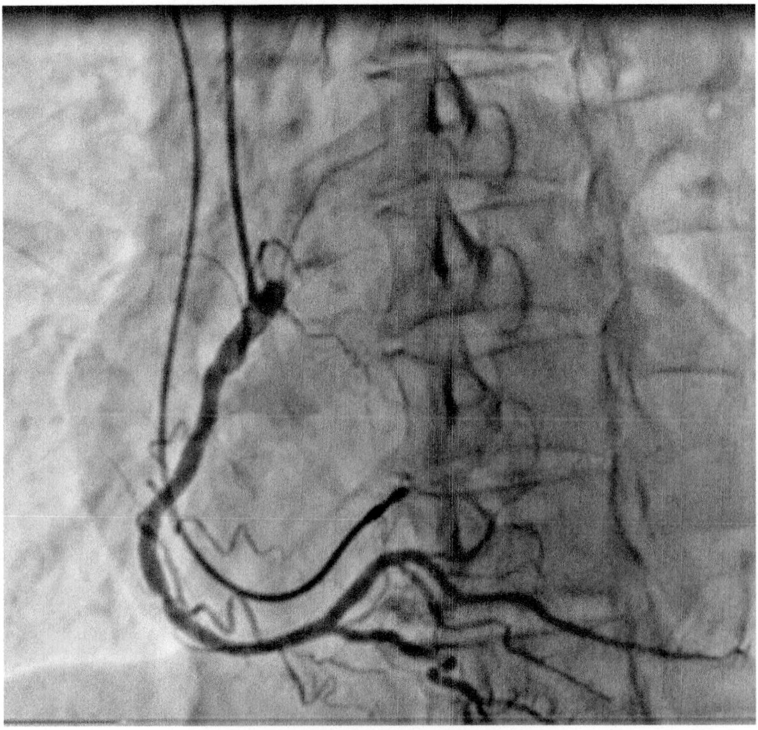

Figure 26.5f A 5F JR 3.5 guiding catheter advanced on the angioplasty wire hooks the right coronary; a 6 F catheter failed to negotiate the type 3 radial bifurcation.

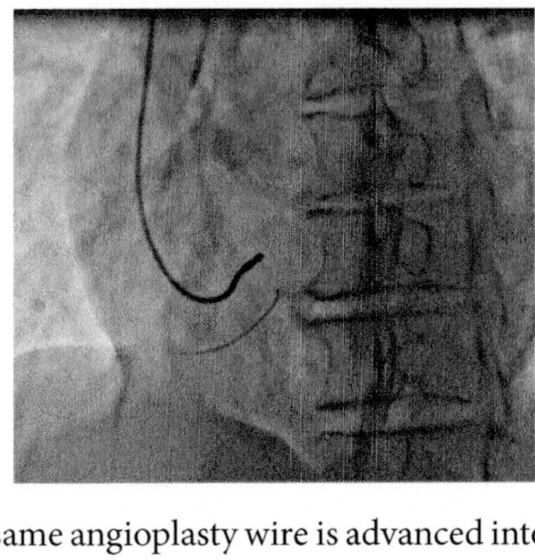

Figure 26.5g The same angioplasty wire is advanced into the RCA across the lesion.

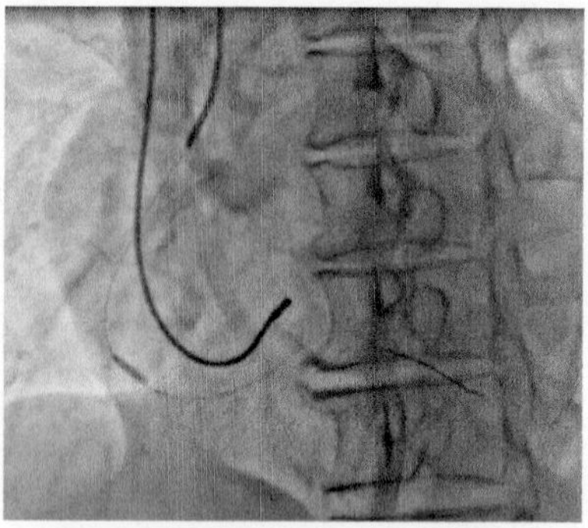

Figure 26.5h Balloon pre-dilatation of the lesion in progress.

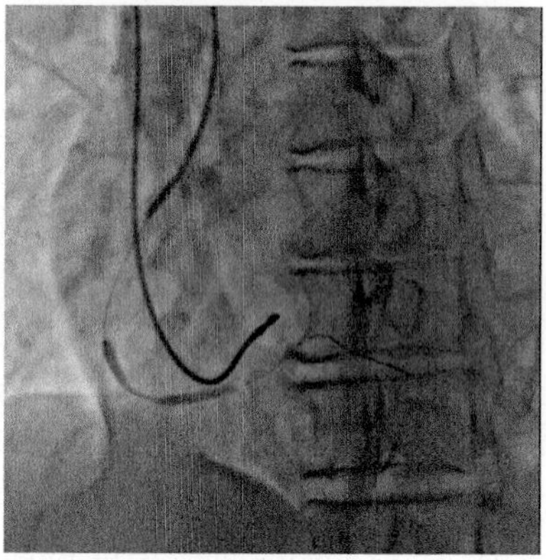

Figure 26.5i Stent deployment in progress.

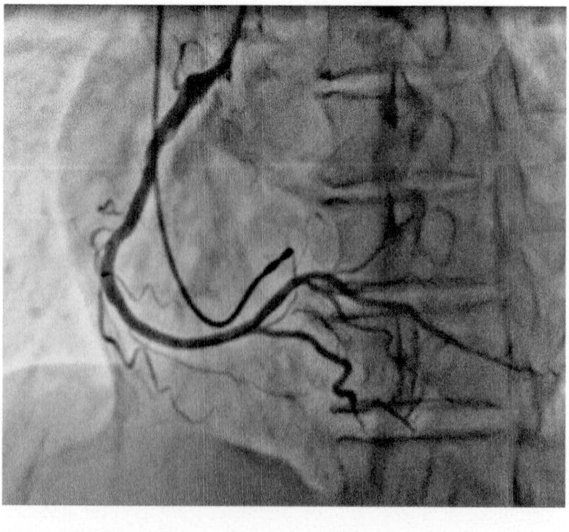

Figure 26.5j Final TIMI 3 flow after post dilatation of stent.

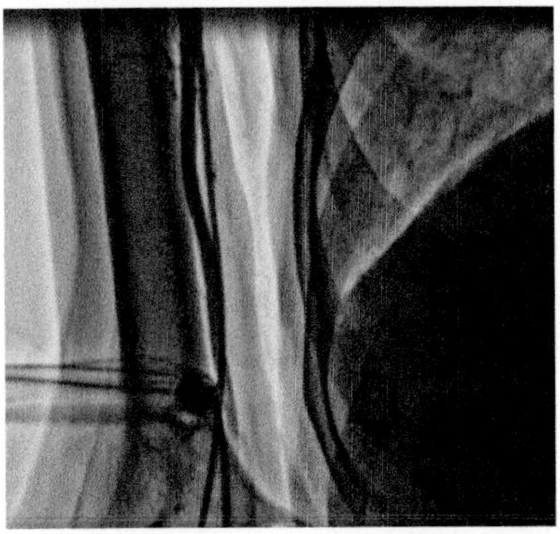

Figure 26.5k Angiogram showing type 3 bifurcation of a narrow radial from brachial.

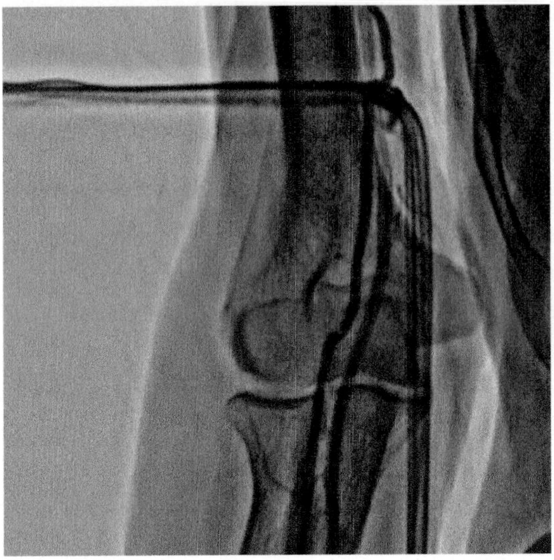

Figure 26.5l High bifurcation of radial from brachial (type 3).

RAO and DRAO

Based on intention-to-treat analysis, the secondary endpoints of RAO and DRAO at Day-30 were 2.9% versus 1.5%, p = 0.12 in RRA group, compared to 2.4% versus 2.5% in DRRA group. Unlike in the PROPHET studies[9,25] which utilized only plethysmography to assess RAO; RAO (and DRAO) were diagnosed with greater accuracy using Doppler ultrasound[17] in the DATA STAR study. In the DRA group, 80% of radial artery occlusions on Day-1 and 100% on Day 30~were found to be associated with RAD ≤1.6 mm; of those developing RAO, 36% developed ≥ grade 3 RAS intra-procedure.

Earlier studies have reported lower rates of RAO,[16,22,23] but they were not powered for conclusion.

Large bore sheaths are associated with higher RAO[26] and patent haemostasis has been shown to reduce RAO.[9,25] Yet, without using patent haemostasis, and with use of bigger sheaths in (6F versus 5F. in 52.4% versus 47.6%), and with PCI in 28% cases, RAO was 2.9% in the standard radial group in DATA STAR study, compared to 3% RAO reported in PROPHET II study[25] which used smaller (5F sheaths in 100%) and did not include any PCI cases in the study.

This real-world data from the DATA STAR study is hypothesis generating and an elastic bandage with gauze ball, using the technique as described, without patent hemostasis, deserves to be compared in a randomized controlled trial, with a compression device and patent hemostasis for assessing RAO with the two different techniques.

RAO was no different from DRAO in the DATA STAR B study because the substrates for occlusion are the same for both and include the following: (i) injury to radial artery endothelium[26,27]; (ii) RA spasm; (iii) mismatch in RA and sheath size[14,17] especially in smaller radial arteries, as is supported by a trend for higher rates of RAO and DRAO observed in subgroups of patients with radial artery diameter <1.6 mm between DRRA and RRA groups.[25] Although it is not clear if RAO would have been different between groups, had patent haemostasis been used; it seems unlikely because our RAO rate without patent haemostasis was comparable to that reported with patent haemostasis in PROPHET 2.

Extravasation

In one case there was perforation of a side branch by the sheath wire; in another instance the artery we cannulated via the snuff box was too small, and test injections (Figure 26.6).

Inability to advance the sheath after successful puncture. This happened in 3 cases: because of the access artery being too small in 1 case

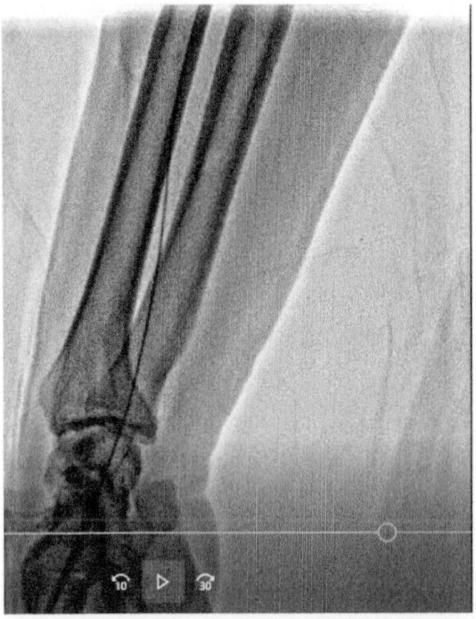

Figure 26.6 Contrast extravasation with check angiogram through partially inserted sheath in DRRA.

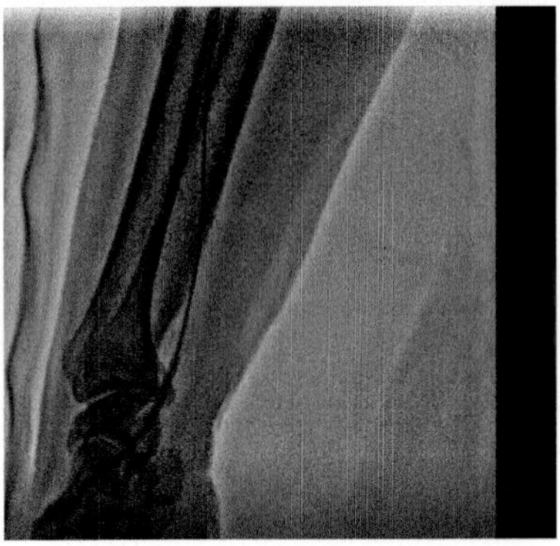

Figure 26.7a Unable to push full length of a 5F Terumo sheath into radial artery after DRA puncture because of small diameter of radial.

(Figure 26.7a); because of a densely calcific narrow RA in another case (Figure 26.7b) and the sheath wire exiting the artery in the third case.

Crossover to Radial or Alternate Access

In 54/282 DRA access failed and of these, 50 were successfully done by RRA. Of the 4 who failed RRA also, 1 was done high right radially, 2 were

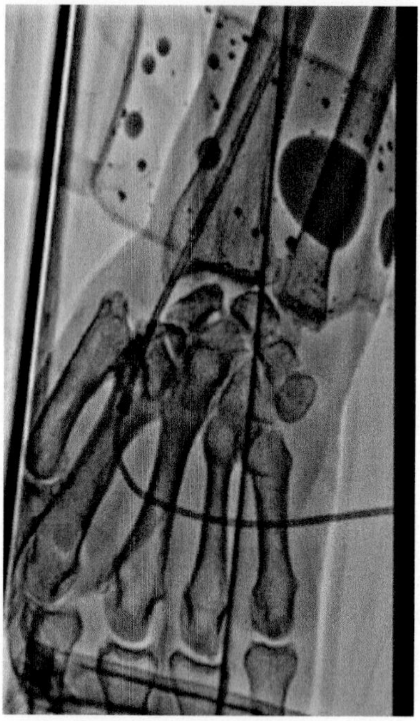

Figure 26.7b Unable to push full length of a 5F Terumo sheath into radial artery after DRA puncture because of calcified radial.

done via left radial and 1 was done transfemorally, because of calcific left radial artery. 4 out of 263 failed RRA and were done transfemorally. All of these patients had RAD <1.6 mm.

Haematoma of Snuffbox

Non-occlusive haemostasis is not required for DRA access though close monitoring for haematoma is still relevant.

- Haematoma post-coronary angiography: In 3 cases (out of n = 282) haematoma developed in the anatomical snuffbox and hand (Figures 26.8a–c) following resumption of heparin infusion 6 hours after procedure.

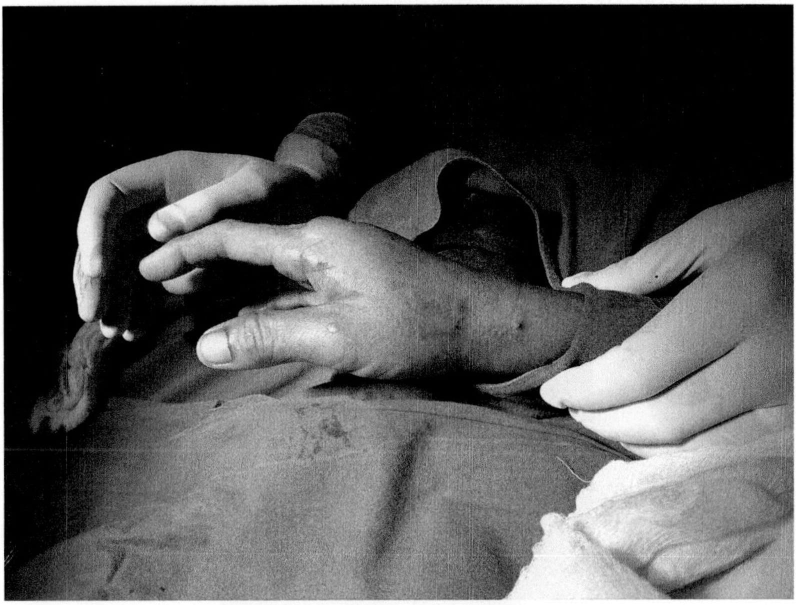

Figure 26.8a Haematoma of snuffbox of hand following DRRA.

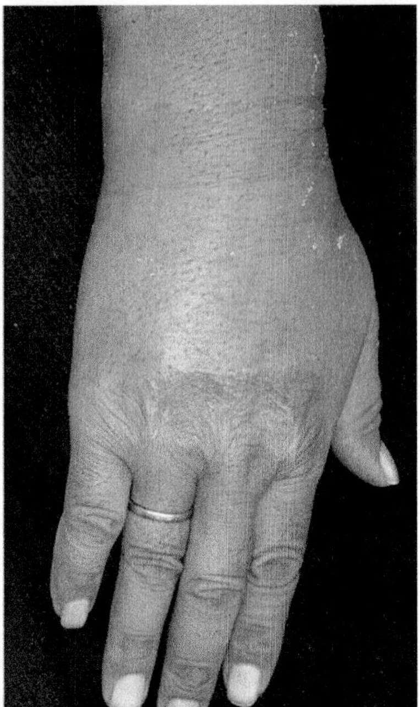

Figure 26.8b Haematoma of hand following DRRA, dorsal aspect.

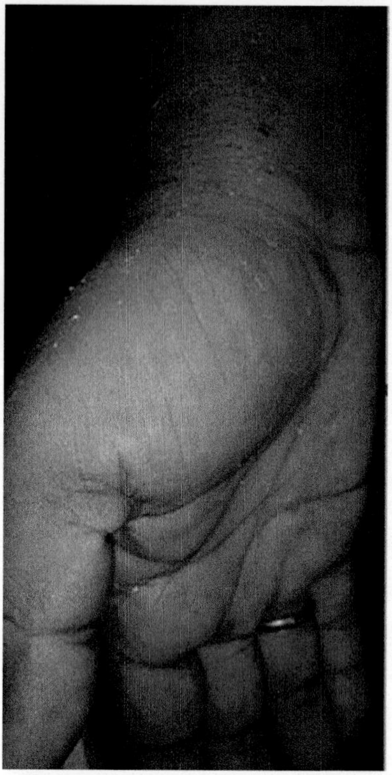

Figure 26.8c Haematoma of hand following DRRA, palmar aspect.

- Haematoma post-angioplasty: Haematoma developed on the dorsum of hand with DRA access 1 hr after angioplasty in one case, on Tirofiban infusion managed by compression bandage (Figures 26.9a and 26.9b). In 2 cases, there was haematoma of the forearm post DRA access angioplasty, managed by compression bandage (Figure 26.10).

Nerve Injury

Numbness on dorsum of hand in distribution of superficial radial nerve was noted in 9/282 cases; which recovered with conservative treatment in all in 4–6 weeks.

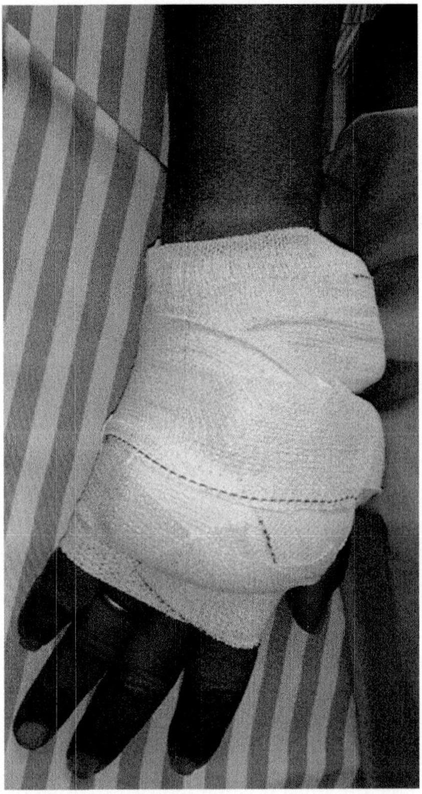

Figure 26.9a Bandage for snuff box haematoma using cotton bandage and elastic bandage for compression showing dorsal aspect of hand.

Learning Curve for DRA Access

While preliminary data shows that there is a steep learning curve; our failure rate dropped from 28% in first 100 cases to 17% in the second 100 and finally to 14% in third 100 cases, hand position and patient cooperation are crucial to successful access.

Distal transradial access has been used for coronary angiography and angioplasty, with 94.9% success in post-CABG patients.[28] A recent meta-analysis which included 6746 patients (dTRA n = 3209 and cTRA n = 3537) from one randomized and four observational studies[29] re-affirmed lower RAO with distal transradial approach (dTRA) (2.30 versus 4.86%, RR = 0.51;

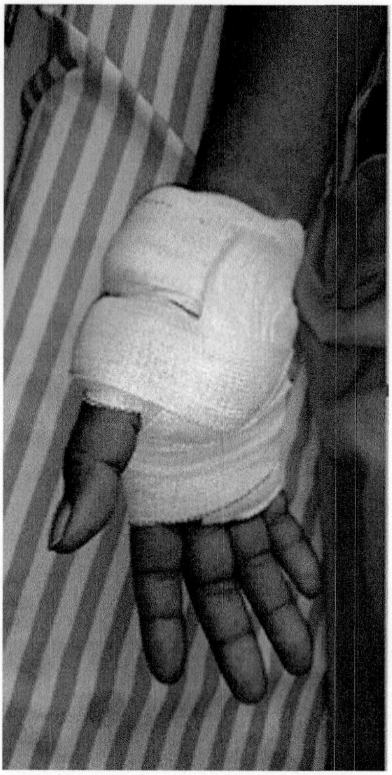

Figure 26.9b Bandage for snuff box haematoma using cotton bandage and elastic bandage for compression showing palmar aspect.

95%CI 0.32–0.81; p = 0.004) compared to conventional TRA (cTRA) with no significant difference in other complications including radial artery spasm (1.42 versus 3.84%, RR = 0.91; 95%CI 0.32–2.62; p = 0.86), and access-site hematomas (1.20% versus 1.24%, RR = 1.01; 95%CI 0.49–2.07; p = 0.99) while the failure rate was similar (5.26% versus 3.75%; RR = 1.36; 95%CI 0.41–4.48; p = 0.62) in dTRA and cTRA groups . However the jury is out and awaits the results of large randomized studies comparing the outcomes with dTRA Vs cTRA. The results of the recently published DIStal Versus COnventional RADIAL Access for Coronary Angiography and Intervention (ClinicalTrials.gov Identifier: NCT04171570)[29] showed that RAO (0.91% vs 0.31%; P = 0.29) and vascular complications were not different between cTRA and dTRA groups; though Crossover was higher with dTRA (3.5% vs 7.4%; P = 0.002), and time to hemostasis was shorter

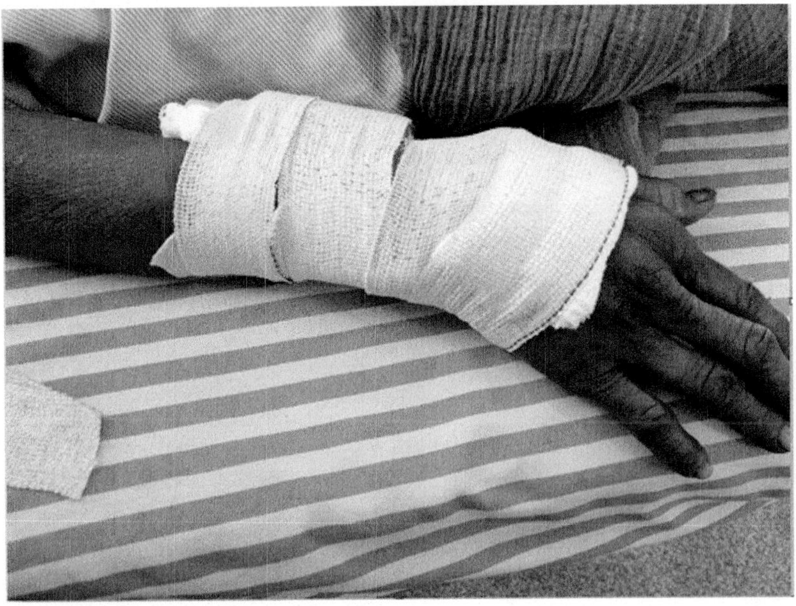

Figure 26.10 Haematoma of the forearm post DRRA angioplasty, managed by compression bandage.

(median 180 vs 153 min; P < 0.001). Also, there was no difference in safety of hand function in cTRA Vs. dTRA in DIPRA study.

Is it Worthwhile Going to All the Trouble with DRA Access Versus RRA?

Despite findings of DATA STAR[20] and DISCO Radial[29] study, even though RAO is similar, it's worthwhile because not only is haemostasis easier and time to hemostasis shorter[29]; using gauze ball and bandage for DRA, no forearm haematoma was reported in the DATA STAR study. Haematoma of hand is easily manageable with cotton bandage roll and elastic bandage compression. Another distinct advantage is that standard radial access is still feasible immediately after completion of first diagnostic or interventional procedure through distal radial artery, even when the gauze-ball bandage is still in place over the anatomical snuffbox (Figure 26.11).

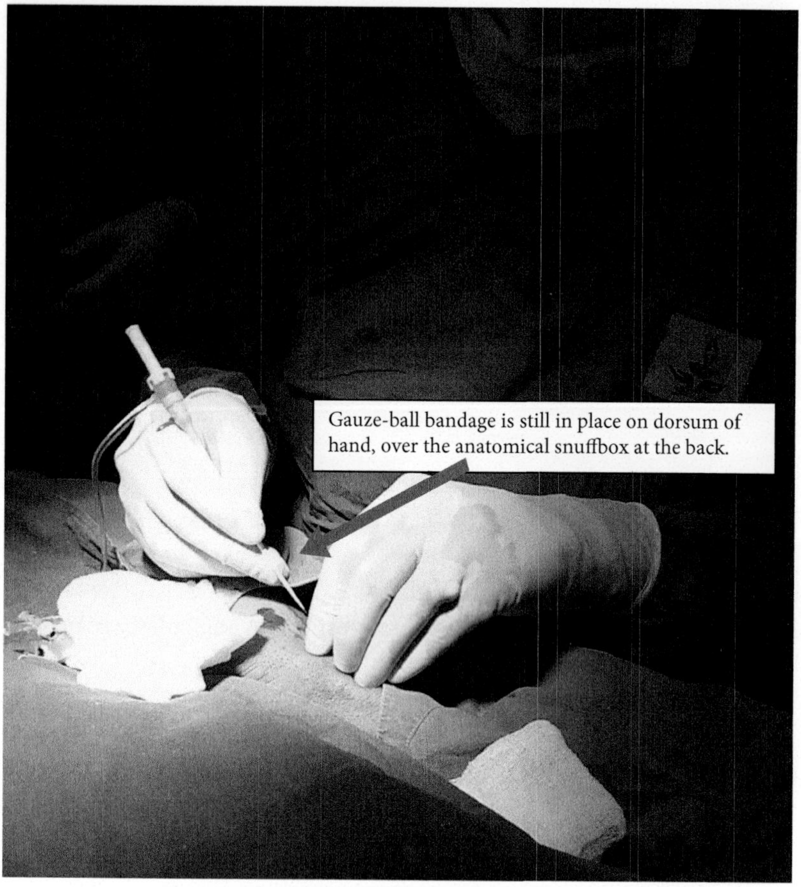

Figure 26.11 Standard radial access is still feasible immediately after completion of first diagnostic or interventional procedure through distal radial artery, even when the gauze-ball bandage is still in place over the anatomical snuffbox.

An update on the subject by the authors, entitled 'DISTAL RADIAL ARTERY ACCESS (DRA) Vs. TRANSRADIAL ACCESS (TRA): CURRENT EVIDENCE' is available as a Chapter in CSI UPDATE, 2022.

For an update on this Chapter, please refer to 'Yashasvi Chugh, Sunita Chugh, Sanjay Kumar Chugh, Distal Radial Artery Access Vs. Transradial Access: Current Evidence. Int J Med Res Rev. 2022; 10(5): 147–153. Available from: https://ijmrr.medresearch.in/index.php/ijmrr/

article/view/1400; Also available by copyright arrangement with IJMRR in: Cardiology Society of India update, 2022.

Conclusion

Based on currently available data, we conclude that distal right radial access at anatomical snuff box is associated with lower puncture success, increased puncture time, and similar rates of RAO and access site complications compared to conventional right radial access at the wrist. DRA access is not associated with less RAO at days 1 and 30 compared to RRA access. However, there were no forearm haematomas, nor any report of compartment syndrome.

References

1. Campeau L. Percutaneous radial artery approach for coronary angiography. *Cathet Cardiovasc Diagn.* 1989;16:3–7.
2. Kiemeneij F, Laarman GJ. Percutaneous transradial artery approach for coronary stent implantation. *Cathet Cardiovasc Diagn.* 1993;30;173–8.
3. Agostoni P, Biondi-Zoccai GG, de Benedictis ML, et al. Radial versus femoral approach for percutaneous coronary diagnostic and interventional procedures: systematic overview and meta-analysis of randomized trials. *J Am Coll Cardiol.* 2004;44:349–56.
4. Biondi-Zoccai G, Sciahbasi A, Bodi V, et al. Right versus left radial artery access for coronary procedures: an international collaborative systematic review and meta-analysis including 5 randomized trials and 3210 patients. *Int J Cardiol.* 2013;166:621–6.
5. Joyal D, Bertrand OF, Rinfret S, et al. Meta-analysis of ten trials on the effectiveness of the radial versus the femoral approach in primary percutaneous coronary intervention. *Am J Cardiol.* 2012;109:813–18.
6. Jolly SS, Amlani S, Hamon M, et al. Radial versus femoral access for coronary angiography or intervention and the impact on major bleeding and ischaemic events: a systematic review and meta-analysis of randomized trials. *Am Heart J.* 2009;157:132–40.
7. Bertrand OF, Belisle P, Joyal D, et al. Comparison of transradial and trans femoral approaches for percutaneous coronary interventions: a systematic review and hierarchial Bayesian meta-analysis. *Am Heart J.* 2012;163:632–48.
8. Deepika K, Palaniappan D, Fuhrman T, et al. Anatomic snuff box radial artery canulation. *Anesth Analg.* 2010;111:1078–9.
9. Pancholy S, Coppola J, Patel T, et al. Prevention of radial artery occlusion-patent hemostasis evaluation trial (PROPHET study): a randomized comparison of

traditional versus patency documented hemostasis after transradial catheterization. *Catheter Cardiovasc Interv*. 2008;72(3):335–40.

10. Bedford RF, Wollman H. Complications of percutaneous radial-artery annulation: an objective prospective study in man. *Anesthesiology*. 1973;38(3):228–36.
11. Davis FM, Stewart JM. Radial artery cannulation: a prospective study in patients undergoing cardiothoracic surgery. *Br J Anaesth*. 1980;52(1):41–7.
12. Slogoff S, Keats AS, Arlund C. On the safety of radial artery cannulation. *Anesthesiology*. 1983;59(1):42–7.
13. Saito S, Ikei H, Hosokawa G, et al. Influence of the ratio between radial artery inner diameter and sheath outer diameter on radial artery flow after transradial coronary intervention. *Catheter Cardiovasc Interv*. 1999;46(2):173–8.
14. Chugh SK, Chugh Y, Chugh S. How to tackle complications in radial procedures: tips and tricks. *Indian Heart J*. 2015;67(3):275–81.
15. Tizon-Marcos H, Barbeau GR. Incidence of compartment syndrome of the arm in a large series of transradial approach for coronary procedures. *J Interv Cardiol*. 2008;21(5):380–4.
16. Kaledin AL, Kochanov IN, Podmetin PS, Seletsky SS, Ardeev VN. Distal radial artery in endovascular interventions. https://www.researchgate.net/publication/319162208 . Research, August 2017. DOI: 10.13140/RG.2.2.13406.33600
17. Kumar Chugh S, Chugh S, Chugh Y, Rao SV. Feasibility and utility of pre-procedural ultrasound imaging of the arm to facilitate transradial coronary diagnostic and interventional procedures (PRIMAFACIE-TRI). *Catheter Cardiovasc Interv*. 2013;82:64–73.
18. Orazio V, Angelina V, Alberto FC, Paolo C, Keisuke S, Luigi F, Giulio G. Early clinical experience with right and left distal transradial access in the anatomical snuffbox in 52 consecutive patients. *J Invasive Cardiol*. 2018;30(6):218–23. Epub 2018 March 15. (Epub Ahead of Print).
19. Kiemeneij F. Left distal transradial access in the anatomical snuffbox for coronary angiography (ldTRA) and interventions (ldTRI). *EuroIntervention*. 2017;13(7):851–7. doi: 10.4244/EIJ-D-17-00079.
20. Chugh Y, Kanaparthy NS, Piplani S, Chugh S, Shroff A, Vidovich M, Nolan J, Mamas M, Chugh SK. Comparison of distal radial access versus standard transradial access in patients with smaller diameter radial Arteries (The distal radial versus transradial access in small transradial ArteriesStudy: D.A.T.A–S.T.A.R study). Indian Heart J. 2021 Jan-Feb;73(1):26–34. doi: 10.1016/j.ihj.2020.11.002. Epub 2020 Nov 11. PMID: 33714406; PMCID: PMC7961259.
21. Lee JW, Park SW, Son JW, Ahn SJ, Lee SH. Real-world experience of the left distal transradial approach for coronary angiography and percutaneous coronary intervention: a prospective observational study (LeDRA). *EuroIntervention*. 2018;14:e995–1003.
22. Flores EA, Todd R. Use of the distal radial artery (DRA) in the anatomical snuffbox as a default access in the cardiac catheterization laboratory. *Catheter Cardiovasc Interv*. 2018;91(Suppl 2):S218.
23. Hull E, Kinsey EN, Bishop WL. Mapping of the snuffbox and cubital vessels for percutaneous arterial venous fistula (pAVF) in dialysis patients. *J Vasc Access*. 2013;14(3):245–51.

24. Pancholy SB, Bernat I, Bertrand OF, Patel TM (2016) Prevention of radial artery occlusion after transradial catheterization: the PROPHET-II randomized trial. *JACC Cardiovasc Interv.* 9(19):1992–9.
25. Rashid M, Kwok CS, Pancholy S, Chugh S, et al. Radial Artery Occlusion After Transradial Interventions: A Systematic Review and Meta-Analysis. J Am Heart Assoc. 2016 Jan 25;5(1):e002686. doi: 10.1161/JAHA.115.002686. PMID: 26811162; PMCID: PMC4859386.
26. Yonetsu T, Kakuta T, Lee T, Takayama K, Kakita K, Iwamoto T, Kawaguchi N, Takahashi K, Yamamoto G, Iesaka Y, Fujiwara H. Assessment of acute injuries and chronic intimal thickening of the radial artery after transradial coronary intervention by optical coherence tomography. *Eur Heart J.* 2010;31(13):1608–15.
27. Marcos Danillo P. Oliveira, Ednelson C. Navarro, Adriano Caixeta, Distal transradial access for post-CABG coronary and surgical grafts angiography and interventions. Indian Heart Journal, Volume 73, Issue 4, 2021, Pages 440–45, ISSN 0019-4832, https://doi.org/10.1016/j.ihj.2021.06.005.
28. Mohanad Hamandi, Marwan Saad, Rimsha Hasan, Michael Megaly, et al. Distal Versus Conventional Transradial Artery Access for Coronary Angiography and Intervention: A Meta-Analysis, Cardiovascular Revascularization Medicine, Volume 21, Issue 10, 2020, Pages 1209–1213, ISSN 1553-8389, https://doi.org/10.1016/j.carrev.2020.03.020.
29. Aminian A, Sgueglia GA, Wiemer M, Kefer J. Distal Versus Conventional Radial Access for Coronary Angiography and Intervention: The DISCO RADIAL Trial. JACC Cardiovasc Interv. 2022 Jun 27; 15(12): 1191–1201. doi: 10.1016/j.jcin.2022.04.032. Epub 2022 May 17. PMID: 35595673.

27

Transradial Coronary Interventions: Research Round-up

Helen Routledge

Since its inception in the late 1980s, transradial coronary intervention has gained global acceptance, and this is indeed the preferred access route in the majority of modern-day cardiac centres across the UK and Europe. The latest European Society of Cardiology (ESC) guidelines, published in 2017, have given a Class IA recommendation to radial access in patients with ST-elevation myocardial infarction (STEMI)[1] and non-STEMI (NSTEMI).[2]

Guidelines are published based on current evidence and for an organization as reputable as the ESC to change its stance on transradial access to be the preferred choice, the said evidence would have been quite convincing. This chapter will take a closer look at the most recent research with regard to transradial access in coronary interventions which may have led to the update mentioned earlier.

As Atul Gawande mentions in his book COMPLICATIONS, 'Medicine is an imperfect science, an enterprise of constantly changing knowledge, uncertain information, fallible individuals, and at the same time lives on the line'. Thus, when ploughing through research and publications, one must be selective in choosing the most reliable of sources. We are hopeful that the information to follow would be accepted by the wider audience as possible reasons why transradial access has gained such prominence.

Patient Safety: Advantages of Transradial Approach (TRA)

Best for ST elevation MI Practices for Transradial Angiography and Intervention: A Consensus Statement from the Society for Cardiovascular Angiography and Intervention's Transradial Working Group

In an era where patient safety has gained global priority especially with regard to invasive procedures, there is a growing body of evidence supporting the transradial approach over transfemoral in better patient outcomes.

The most common complication associated with coronary angiography and angioplasty is bleeding, most often at the access site and also subsequent to peri-procedure anti-thrombotics. Patients at highest risk of bleeding complications are the elderly, those with acute coronary syndromes including STEMI and patients in cardiogenic shock.

Important randomized trials such as RIVAL[3] have demonstrated that the radial approach is associated with a reduction in bleeding and vascular access site complications compared with femoral access, and this is most evident in high bleeding-risk patients. This evidence base was strengthened by a recent systematic review and meta-analysis[4] undertaken by Singh et al. incorporating data from 16 clinical trials and involving over 9,000 patients. The conclusion was that the transradial approach for PCI in STEMI patients significantly reduced all-cause mortality, major and access site bleeding, major adverse cardiovascular events, and length of hospital stay. Interestingly, they report that the greatest reduction in major bleeding was found in the subgroup of trials including only patients undergoing primary percutaneous coronary intervention (PCI) for STEMI.

Clinical trials at times may not provide a pragmatic picture with regard to outcomes as patient selection is dependent on certain exclusion criteria. Would evidence of clinical trials be true in real-world clinical practice? A publication by Mamas and colleagues[12] which analysed data from the British Cardiovascular Interventional Society database, with input from the majority of United Kingdom interventional centres, confirmed that a change to transradial access was indeed associated with lower incidence of mortality, major bleeding and access site complications over a 5-year period.

More recent research also focuses on special circumstances or subgroups of patients where transradial access may be advantageous.

Repeat access is occasionally necessary following the index procedure for a variety of reasons. Recent research from Canada[5] published in the *American Journal of Cardiology* evaluated the safety and feasibility of repeat radial access within 24 hours and 30 days. After evaluating over 500 such patients over two years in this high-volume TRA centre, repeat access within the ipsilateral radial artery within 24 hours and 30 days was found to be safe and feasible with no significant increase in risk of access site complications.

Women have been found to have higher risk from bleeding following PCI than men.[6] The SAFE-PCI trial presented as part of Transcatheter Cardiovascular Therapeutics (TCT) 2013 in San Francisco compared interventional access strategies in women and found distinct advantages with radial access over the femoral route, with a trend towards a reduction of bleeding and vascular complications by about 60% through radial access. Of note though, this advantage was only evident in the whole cohort of women who underwent PCI or diagnostic coronary angiography. There was no distinct advantage in women undergoing PCI alone.

The elderly, being another patient group with a high bleeding risk, almost certainly benefit from a change to transradial intervention with a demonstrated benefit of the radial approach in octogenarians specifically. Patient obesity, defined as a body mass index (BMI) ≥ 40, provides a challenge in performing coronary interventions. Bleeding complications have been found to high in this cohort of patients, during the transfemoral era. The use of transradial approach has been found to have less bleeding and access site complications when compared with a transfemoral approach.[7]

TRA in Difficult Lesions

In the process of performing coronary angioplasty, operators will encounter certain difficult lesions such as chronic total occlusions or heavily calcified lesions. Successful angioplasty in these lesions often involves the use of larger diameter sheaths, multiple balloons and occasionally rotablation. Operators often chose the femoral approach for these lesions assuming that radial access may lead unfavourable outcomes.

A trial by Yin et al.[8] comparing transradial versus transfemoral access for heavily calcified coronary lesions in the contemporary drug eluting stent era had similar procedural success rates (97% versus 99%) but with a significant reduction in access site bleeding in the former (2%) versus the latter approach (16%).

The evidence for using the transradial approach in complex chronic total occlusions though is less encouraging. A recent paper by Tanaka et al.[9] and published in the *Journal of American College of Cardiology* suggests that if cases with J-CTO (Multicenter Chronic Total Occlusion Registry of Japan) scores of ≥3 were examined, the transradial group had a significantly lower success rate than the transfemoral group (35.7% versus 58.2%; $p = 0.04$). However, they did conclude that the transradial approach was indeed feasible in less-complex cases.

The dose of contrast media given to the patient in complex PCI is of particular concern, and this may be a previously less well-recognized benefit of radial artery access. The MATRIX AKI study (9b) demonstrated less AKI in patients undergoing transradial intervention and hypothesized that this may be due to less atherothrombosis or possibly the result of a reduction in bleeding overall.

TRA: Practice Makes Perfect?

Although recent research does prove the worth of transradial access in limiting complications, it remains a challenging procedure and the learning curve maybe prolonged.[10] Gaining adequate competence in the technique through practice would be the logical approach in this regard. Recently, the British Cardiovascular Interventional Society issued guidelines recommending a minimum prerequisite of 50 and 150 radial procedures, respectively, over two years to maintain proficiency to perform PCI.[11] This was further powered by a statement by the European Association of Percutaneous Cardiovascular Intervention, recommending performing >50% of all diagnostic angiography and angioplasty procedures transradially, with a minimum of 80 procedures/annum per operator. A recent review by Nagaraja et al.,[12] published in Cardiac Interventions Today: Radial update, had an excellent summary of data analysed over the years. They suggest that significant survival benefit can be achieved in the hands of high-proportion of radial operators but that the mortality benefit achieved by the transradial approach is not related to total volume or radial volume at the centre level after adjusting for confounding factors.

TRA in Non-coronary Interventions

Although commonly used in coronary interventions, the transradial approach has recently been utilized in a broader range of procedures. A recent single-centre publication from the USA[13] reports excellent short- and long-term outcomes in patients undergoing Alcohol Septal Ablation for HOCM with lower incidence of vascular complications compared to the femoral approach. Transradial access has also been successfully used with less vascular complications in the evaluation of severe aortic stenosis[14] and ventricular septal defect (VSD) closure.[15] The interventional radiologists are beginning to express an interest in the transradial approach in order to improve safety and outcomes for procedures outside of the heart.[(15b)]

TRA: The Cons

With the adaptation of the transradial approach the learning curve described previously will inevitably lead to certain drawbacks. Procedure time would certainly be longer during the early learning phase and common sense would say this may lead to increased radiation exposure to both patient and operator. The question over radiation exposure has been raised a number of times with variable conclusions. This year the RAD-MATRIX analysis reported a higher fluoroscopy time, total dose and operator radiation dose with the radial approach.[16] A recent meta-analysis and systemic review, analysing 24 clinical trials with almost 20,000 patients and published in the Lancet[17] concludes that transradial access for coronary procedures is associated with a small increase in radiation exposure. However, this gap in radiation exposure between transradial and transfemoral access has closed over time, presumably reflecting increased operator experience with transradial access.

Alternative Approaches to TRA

Medicine is a field which is ever evolving and never static. TRA has revolutionized coronary interventions since its inception and is now the preferred choice in most centres around the globe. However, the world of cardiology will always be in flux and thus alternative approaches are being introduced and trialled.

The transulnar route has been used, most often when radial access has been unsuccessful. Most randomized controlled trials have reached mixed conclusions. A recent meta-analysis[19] though raises a more optimistic conclusion: for patients requiring angiography or PCI, transulnar access compared with TRA has similar efficacy and safety except for higher puncture failure rates and access cross-over. More evidence will be needed for ulnar access to be the default choice but a forearm approach as opposed to sole transradial access maybe the norm in the near future.

A more recent innovation is the use of distal left transradial access in the anatomical snuffbox for coronary angiography and intervention. This has been introduced by Ferdinand Kiemeneij,[20] one of the pioneers of TRA and recommended for patients who need or prefer left radial access over right radial access. In addition to operator comfort, the main advantage is postulated to be a reduction in the occurrence of radial artery occlusion post procedure. Further research is needed for this approach to gain more prominence but there is much interest currently in the transradial community.

Conclusion

Quoting Atul Gawande again, 'Medicine is a strange business. The stakes are high, the liberties taken tremendous. We drug people, put needles and tubes in to them, manipulate their chemistry and biology and physics, lay them unconscious and open their bodies to the world. We do so out of an abiding confidence in our know-how as a profession', an interesting perspective from a surgeon. Interventional cardiology is probably no different. With constant publications and data coming through, our own know-how will always remain in a flux. Patients give us their ultimate trust by signing consent forms prior to procedures, accepting risks including death with the hope of better outcomes. In return, it is our duty as a profession to always prioritize their safety and comfort. By analysing the data available thus far and described earlier, at least in coronary interventions, transradial access seems to fulfil these criteria. The introduction of the concept of evidence-based medicine 25 years ago[18] created a paradigm shift in the field of medicine and the way it is taught and practiced. Thus far at least, considering the overall balance of risks and benefits, the evidence most certainly favours the use of transradial access in coronary interventions. However as in life, one must always have a back-up approach and hence to discard the transfemoral approach totally would be foolhardy.

References

1. Ibanez B, James S, Agewall S, et al. 2017 ESC guidelines for the management of acute myocardial infarction in patients presenting with ST-segment elevation. *Eur Heart J*. 2017.
2. Roffi M, et al. ESC Guidelines—Acute Coronary Syndromes Non-ST-Elevation. Presented at: ESC 2015; Aug. 29–Sept. 2, 2015; London.
3. Jolly SS, Yusuf S, Cairns J, Niemelä K, Xavier D, Widimsky P, Budaj A, Niemelä M, Valentin V, Lewis BS, Avezum A, Steg PG, Rao SV, Gao P, Afzal R, Joyner CD, Chrolavicius S, Mehta SR, RIVAL trial group. Radial versus femoral access for coronary angiography and intervention in patients with acute coronary syndromes (RIVAL): a randomised, parallel group, multicentre trial. *Lancet*. 2011 Apr 23; 377(9775):1409–20.
4. Singh, Sukhchain et al. Transradial vs Transfemoral Percutaneous Coronary Intervention in ST-Segment Elevation Myocardial Infarction: A Systemic Review and Meta-analysis. Canadian Journal of Cardiology, Volume 32, Issue 6, 777–90.
5. Am J Cardiol. 2017 Oct 15;120(8):1267–71. doi: 10.1016/j.amjcard.2017.07.009. Epub 2017 Aug 2. Feasibility and Safety of Early Repeat Transradial Access Within 30 Days of Previous Coronary Angiography and Intervention. Barria Perez AE1, Costerousse O1, Cieza T1, Barbeau G1, Déry JP1, Maes F1, Rimac G1, Plourde G1, Poirier Y1, Carrier MA1, Bertrand OF2; Interventional Cardiologists at Quebec Heart-Lung Institute.
6. Duvernoy CS, Smith DE, Manohar P, Schaefer A, Kline-Rogers E, Share D, McNamara R, Gurm HS, Moscucci M. Gender differences in adverse outcomes after contemporary percutaneous coronary intervention: an analysis from the Blue Cross Blue Shield of Michigan Cardiovascular Consortium (BMC2) percutaneous coronary intervention registry. *Am Heart J*. 2010 Apr; 159(4):677–83.

6b. Hoyoun Won, Wang Soo Lee, Sang-Wook Kim, Byung Ryul Cho, et al, for Korea Transradial Coronary Intervention (KOTRI) Prospective Registry Investigators. Safety and efficacy of transradial coronary angiography and intervention in patients older than 80 years: from the Korean Transradial Intervention Prospective Registry J Geriatr Cardiol. 2017 Feb; 14(2): 81–86. doi: 10.11909/j.issn.1671-5411.2017.02.001PMCID: PMC5409348.

7. Hibbert B, Simard T, Wilson KR, Hawken S, Wells GA, et al. Transradial versus transfemoral artery approach for coronary angiography and percutaneous coronary intervention in the extremely obese. JACC Cardiovasc Interv. 2012 Aug;5(8):819–26.

8. Yin W-H, Tseng C-K, Tsao T-P, et al. Transradial versus transfemoral rotablation for heavily calcified coronary lesions in contemporary drug-eluting stent era. *Journal of Geriatric Cardiology: JGC*. 2015;12(5):489–496. doi:10.11909/j.issn.1671–5411.2015.05.004.

9. Yutaka Tanaka, Noriaki Moriyama, Tomoki Ochiai, Takuma Takada, Kazuki Tobita, Koki Shishido, Kazuya Sugitatsu, Futoshi Yamanaka, Shingo Mizuno, Masato Murakami, Junya Matsumi, Saeko Takahashi, Takeshi Akasaka, Shigeru Saito. Transradial Coronary Interventions for Complex Chronic Total Occlusions. JACC: Cardiovascular Interventions Feb 2017, 10 (3) 235–43; DOI:10.1016/j.jcin.2016.11.003

9b. Giuseppe Andò, Bernardo Cortese, Filippo Russo, Martina Rothenbühler, et al. for the MATRIX Investigators. Acute Kidney Injury After Radial or Femoral Access for Invasive Acute Coronary Syndrome Management: AKI-MATRIX. J Am Coll Cardiol. 2017 May, 69 (21) 2592–603.

10. Hess CN, Peterson ED, Neely ML, et al. The learning curve for transradial percutaneous coronary intervention among operators in the United States: a study from the National Cardiovascular Data Registry. Circulation. 2014;129:2277–286.

11. Banning AP, Baumbach A, Blackman D, et al. Percutaneous coronary intervention in the UK: recommendations for good practice 2015. Heart. 2015;101:1–13.

12. Mamas MA, Ratib K, Routledge H, et al. Influence of arterial access site selection on outcomes in primary percutaneous coronary intervention: are the results of randomized trials achievable in clinical practice? JACC Cardiovasc Interv. 2013;6:698–706.

13. Sawaya F, Louvard Y, Spaziano M, et al. Short and long-term outcomes of alcohol septal ablation with the trans-radial versus the trans-femoral approach: a single-center experience. Int J Cardiol. 2016;220:7–13.

14. Sanghvi K, Pancholy S, Patel T. Hemodynamic assessment of severe aortic stenosis via transradial approach is safe. J Invasive Cardiol. 2015;27:E308–E311.

15. Sanghvi K, Selvaraj N, Luft U. Percutaneous closure of a perimembranous ventricular septal defect through arm approach (radial artery and basilic vein). J Interv Cardiol. 2014;27:199–203.

15b. Snelling BM, Sur S, Shah SS, Marlow MM, Cohen MG, Peterson EC. Transradial access: lessons learned from cardiology. J Neurointerv Surg. 2018 May;10(5):487–92. doi: 10.1136/neurintsurg-2017-013295. Epub 2017 Sep 29. PMID: 28963366.

16. Ando, G, Cortese B et al. Rad matrix. JACC 2017 69:21: 2592.

17. Plourde G, Pancholy SB, Nolan J, Jolly S, Rao SV, et al. Radiation exposure in relation to the arterial access site used for diagnostic coronary angiography and percutaneous coronary intervention: a systematic review and meta-analysis. Lancet 2015; 386: 2192–203.
18. Evidence Based Medicine Working Group. Evidence based medicine. A new approach to teaching the practice of medicine. JAMA 1992;268:2420–5.
19. Dahal K, et.al. Transulnar versus transradial access for coronary angiography or percutaneous coronary intervention: A meta-analysis of randomized controlled trials. Catheter Cardiovasc Interv. 2016 Apr;87(5):857–65.
20. Left distal transradial access in the anatomical snuffbox for coronary angiography (ldTRA) and interventions (ldTRI) Kiemeneij F. EuroIntervention. 2017 Sep 20;13(7):851–57.

28

Transradial Peripheral Interventions

N. N. Khanna and Dr. Suparna Rao

Introduction

Transradial access is now the most commonly used approach for coronary interventions in Asia and Europe. Campeau, in 1989, reported the first radial artery access for coronary angiography[1] Kiemeneij and Laarman in 1993 performed the first coronary intervention using radial approach,[2] and now, worldwide, 20% of coronary interventional procedures are performed by radial approach.

The radial approach is now becoming the default approach because of lower rate of complications and bleeding, and immediate ambulation.[3–5]

When to Approach Transradial Approach for Peripheral Interventions

Several studies[6,7] have demonstrated superiority of transradial access for peripheral interventions due to the following reasons:

1. Carotid, subclavian, and vertebral interventions are better approached from the radial artery due to shorter distance to the lesion and better catheter backup support.
2. Superiorly pointed vessels like renal and mesenteric vessels are more easily approached by access from the arm, because of their orientation.
3. In contralateral iliac disease and severe iliac bifurcation disease, the iliac artery and proximal superficial femoral artery are more accessible from the arm.

Patient Selection and Pre-procedural Preparation

The possibility of immediate mobilization post-procedure is comfortable for patients.

Pre-procedure patient evaluation is essential for a successful transradial procedure. Ideal patient characteristics are:

(1) Younger patients (age not more than 70 years),
(2) Haemodynamic stability,
(3) A strong palpable radial artery pulse.

Contraindications to radial access include:

(1) Raynaud disease and other vasospastic conditions,
(2) Radiocephalic fistula for haemodialysis,
(3) No palpable radial artery pulsation.

Assessing Arterial Supply

Arterial supply can be assessed by the following:

- Palmar blush
- Digital pulse oximeter
- Doppler signal
- Doppler of palmar arch

The Allen's test confirms completion of functional palmar arch in the hand. Both radial and ulnar arteries at the wrist level are simultaneously occluded by pressure until the hand blanches. First, pressure is released over the ulnar artery. Normal Allen's test demonstrates reperfusion of the hand within seven seconds. In abnormal Allen's test, reperfusion of the hand takes longer than 15 seconds (Figure 28.1).

Plethysmography with a pulse oximeter placed on the thumb can be alternatively used, and it reduces the number of patients excluded.[8]

Limitations of both the Allen's and plerhysmography tests is well-known. Please see Chapter 23, 'Moving to Forearm Access', for further details.

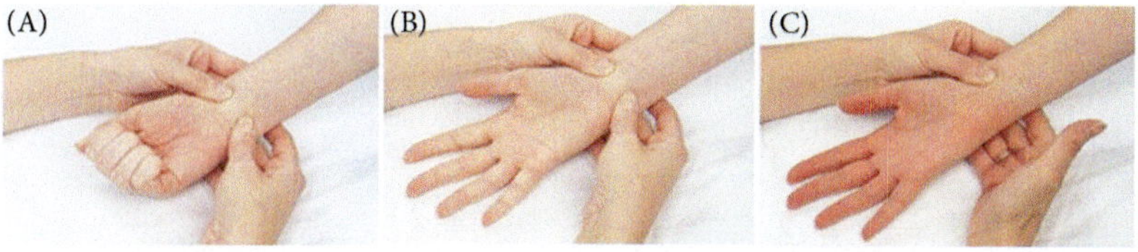

Figure 28.1 Allen's test.

Positioning of the patient for the procedure depends on whether the right or left radial artery is used. A towel is placed underneath the wrist for support. A pulse oximeter is generally placed on the ipsilateral thumb. After gaining arterial access, the arm is placed on side of the body or anteriorly over the belly. This improves the ease of procedure and decreases the radiation hazard to the operator.

Right Versus Left Radial Approach

Although subclavian and vertebral arteries are more easily accessed through ipsilateral radial arteries, left radial artery is usually the preferred access for peripheral interventions.[9]

Left radial approach is preferred for peripheral vascular interventions because of the following reasons:

1. Shorter distance to reach iliac and proximal femoral vessels as there is always a limitation of working length of hardware.
2. More familiar catheter manipulation which mimic those from femoral approach.

Gaining Radial Artery Access and Pharmacological Therapy

The diameter of radial artery is variable. Loh et al.[10] reported a mean diameter of 2.69 ± 0.40 mm in men and 2.43 ± 0.38 mm in women (range 1.15–3.95 mm). However, it depends on ethnicity, body size, and sex.

After giving local anaesthesia (xylocaine/lidocaine), arterial access is gained by a customized radial kit or 21-gauge micropuncture needle

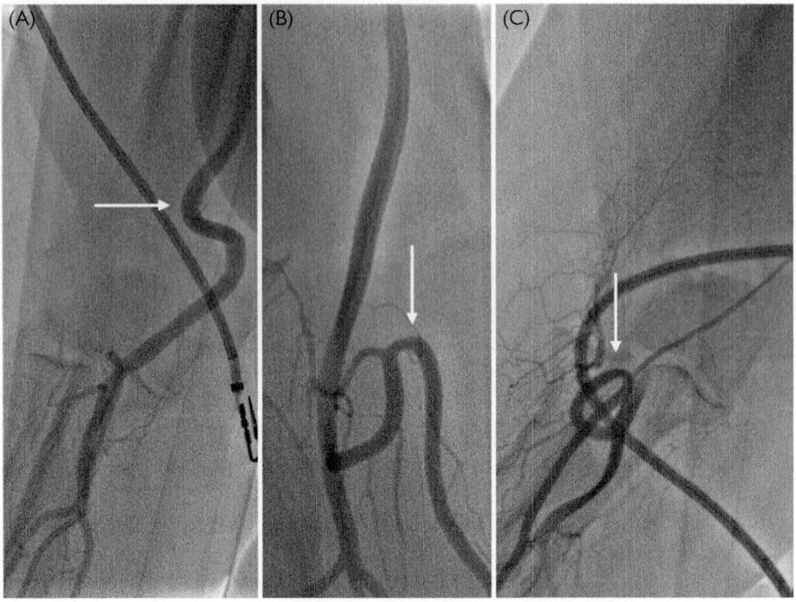

Figure 28.2 Anatomic abnormalities. (A) Tortuosity; (B and C) Loop.

and a 0.018"–0.025" hydrophilic guide wire is passed into the radial artery. A 6-Fr hydrophilic radial sheath is then introduced and 100 U/kg body weight of unfractionated heparin, 100 μg of nitroglycerin and diltiazem or verapamil is given in the radial artery through the side port of the arterial sheath to prevent spasm. A dacron or hydrophilic guidewire is advanced under fluoroscopic guidance. Sometimes resistance is felt because of radial artery loop (2%), spasm or side branch entry (Figure 28.2).

If there is radial artery stenosis, which is seen sometimes in the elderly, it can be first dilated with an appropriate sized balloon.[11–13]

Radial Access for Peripheral Arterial Intervention

Upper Extremity Interventions

Interventions for brachial, axillary, and subclavian arteries are usually performed transradially using long sheaths. The advantage of radial approach is nearness of the lesion and good support and pushability of guide wire for crossing chronic total occlusions. Most of the peripheral stents and balloons are now compatible with 5Fr and 6-Fr sheaths which are used in radial artery approach.

Transradial Access for Carotid Artery Intervention

Carotid artery stenting can be performed through radial approach,[14,15] especially in cases where we have type III aortic arch or bovine aortic arch, and also in cases where there is severe aortoiliac disease, precluding femoral approach. The technique of engaging common carotid artery (CCA) is similar to that of femoral approach. Usually, an Amplatz or Simmons catheter is used to cannulate the CCA. After cannulation, a 0.035" stiff guide wire is passed and parked in the external carotid artery and a 6-Fr braided sheath is passed over it and placed in CCA. After this, a distal embolic protection device is used to cross the lesion in internal carotid artery and the carotid artery stenosis is stented using appropriate sized carotid stent. Post stent dilatation is sometimes required. The embolic protection device is then retrieved and a digital subtraction angiography (DSA) is done for the completeness of the procedure.

Transradial Access for Vertebrobasilar Intervention

It is easier to do vertebrobasilar intervention through ipsilateral radial route because of the ease of cannulation of vertebral artery using a 6-French internal mammary artery catheter. The vertebral artery stenosis is treated in a way similar to coronary artery stenting as the size and lengths of the lesion are similar to coronary artery stenosis. The basilar artery can also be treated in a similar fashion using standard hardware.

Transradial Access for Subclavian and Innominate Artery Intervention

Subclavian artery stenosis or occlusion is commonly seen in atherosclerotic peripheral arterial disease or inflammatory arthritis like Takayasu Arteritis. Usually, they are treated by femoral approach but many a times it is difficult to cross the chronic total occlusion (CTO) of subclavian artery because of poor support of guiding catheter or sheath at the level of aortic arch. Sometimes even the stump of subclavian artery occlusion is not visible and in these situations, radial approach becomes very important as it provides a good delineation of the stenosis/occlusion and provides a very good support for crossing it with hydrophilic or dedicated guide wires. This approach also allows very precise placement of stents

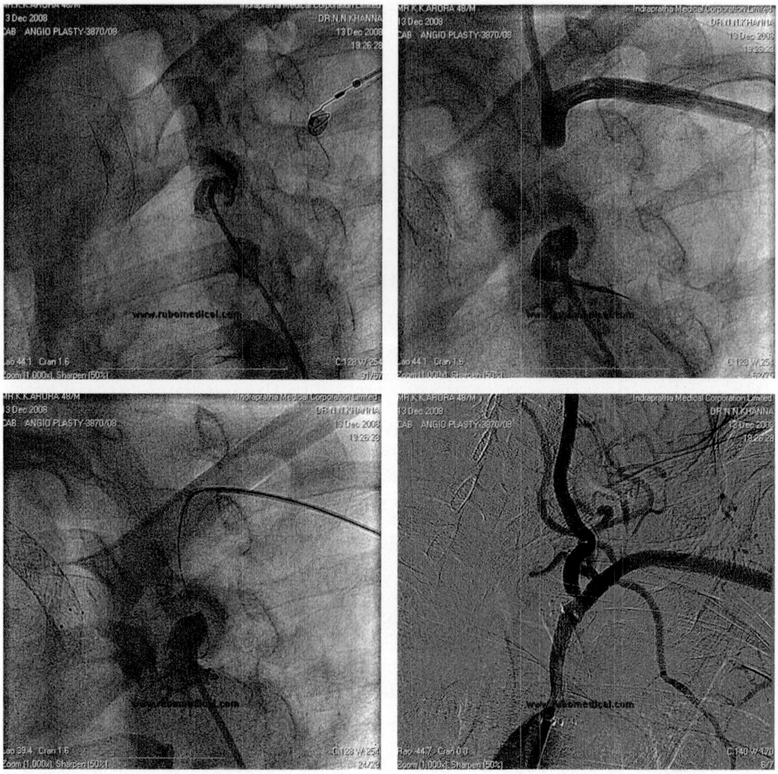

Figure 28.3 Subclavian artery intervention through transradial route.

both at the aorto-ostial level and at the level of take-off of vertebral artery (Figure 28.3).

The procedure of stenting is similar to any peripheral artery stenting.

Transradial Access for Renal Artery Intervention

Many of the renal arteries have superior take off, and they are very difficult to approach from femoral route.[16] It is intuitive to cannulate the renal arteries using multipurpose or JR guiding catheter from the top using radial artery access. The angioplasty is performed without deep intubation using coronary techniques and hardware (Figure 28.4). This technique is also very useful in case of severe aortoiliac disease, especially at the level of juxtarenal and infrarenal aorta and aortic bifurcation. It is also of great importance in case of iliac and femoral disease

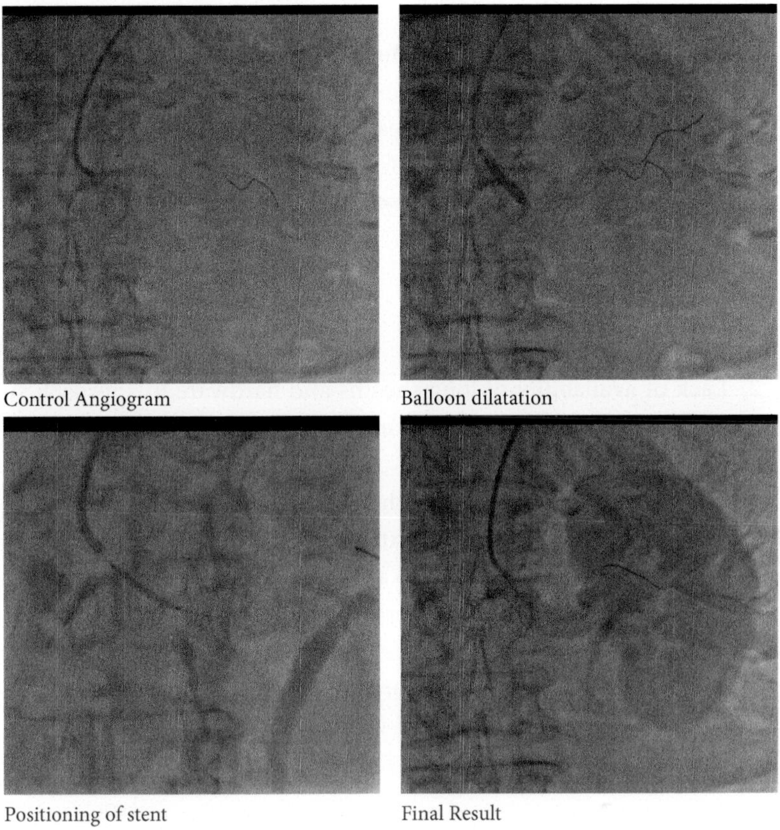

Figure 28.4 Left Radial Approach for Left Renal Artery Stenosis.

and allows the patient to be ambulated immediately after the procedure. The risk of bleeding and access site complications are minimal using left radial artery approach.

Transradial Access for Iliac Artery Intervention

The first transradial stenting of the iliac artery was reported by Flachskampf and colleagues in 2005.[17]

Advantages of transradial access for Iliac Artery Intervention:

1. Patient acceptance
2. No haematoma

3. Immediate mobilization
4. Makes intervention possible in aortic occlusion, severe aortic bifurcation disease, common femoral artery (CFA) and contralateral common iliac artery ostial disease
5. Difficult aortic arch
6. Internal iliac artery coiling

Disadvantages:

1. Restricted sheath size (7 Fr)
2. Lack of availability of long sheaths and hardware to approach superficial femoral artery (SFA) and infrapopliteal lesions

Iliac artery interventions are done through radial access in cases of long iliac artery stenosis or occlusions extending up to the groin where femoral access is not possible. It is also an alternative route in cases of iliac artery occlusions which cannot be crossed retrogradely from femoral artery route. The iliac stent can be placed very precisely at the level of aortic bifurcation just like the femoral approach. Both self-expanding and balloon expandable stents can be used with great precision in treating isolated iliac or aortoiliac lesions using radial route.

Complications

There is increased operator radiation exposure with transradial interventions. The left radial approach is easier to perform because of reasons stated earlier but it is accompanied with higher radiation hazards to the operator as compared to the right radial approach.[18,19] Precisely, 4% of patients lose radial artery pulsations where radial artery is used as an access for peripheral intervention.[20] This incidence can be reduced to 1% with patent haemostasis. Because of completion of palmar arch, these radial artery occlusions are asymptomatic.

Radial artery perforation is rare, about 0.01%,[21] and when it happens, it is caused either by rough manipulation of guide wire or a side branch injury because of guide wire. It can be managed by a prolonged balloon dilatation at the site of perforation after completion of the primary procedure or by external compression using the cuff of sphygmomanometer keeping the pressure to 10 mmHg less than the systolic blood pressure for about 15–20 min.

Compartment syndrome because of bleeding inside the musculofascial compartment of the hand is very rare. Tizon-Marcos et al. reported an incidence as low as 0.004% of patients in the *Journal of Interventional Cardiology*.[22]

Pseudoaneurysms are sometimes seen in cases where the transradial band or the pressure dressing is either not applied properly or removed early. It is also seen in patients with chronic renal failure and patients with multiple punctures or an arteriovenous puncture. They are treated by ultrasound guided compression or thrombin injection. Surgery is rarely required and is indicated when the aforementioned measures fail or there is an associated arteriovenous fistula.

Conclusion

Transradial access for peripheral vascular interventions is being adapted rapidly, because of lower complication rates and early mobility of the patient. In future, longer hardware should be developed for treating more distal lesions in the lower limbs by transradial route.

References

1. Campeau L. Percutaneous radial artery approach for coronary angiography. Cathet Cardiovasc Diagn. 1989;16:3–7.
2. Kiemeneij F, Laarman GJ. Percutaneous transradial artery approach for coronary stent implantation. Cathet Cardiovasc Diagn. 1993;30:173–8.
3. Dehmer GJ, Weaver D, Roe MT, et al. A contemporary view of diagnostic cardiac catheterization and percutaneous coronary intervention in the United States: a report from the CathPCI Registry of the National Cardiovascular Data Registry, 2010 through June 2011. J Am Coll Cardiol 2012;60(20):2017–31.
4. Caputo RP, Tremmel JA, Patel T, et al. Transradial arterial access for coronary and peripheral procedures: executive summary by the transradial committee of the SCAI. Catheter Cardiovasc Interv 2011;78:823–39.

5. Hamon M, Pristipino C, Di Mario C, et al. Consensus document on the radial approach in percutaneous cardiovascular interventions: position paper by the European Association of Percutaneous Cardiovascular Interventions and Working Groups on Acute Cardiac Care and Thrombosis of the European Society of Cardiology. EuroIntervention 2013;8 (11): 1242–51.
6. Sharma GL, Louvard Y, Morice MC, et al. Noncoronary transradial angioplasty with coronary equipment: a less invasive technique. Catheter Cardiovasc Interv. 2002;55:197–205.
7. Yu J, Korabathina R, Coppola J, Staniloae C. Transradial approach to subclavian artery stenting. J Invasive Cardiol. 2010;22:204–6.
8. Barbeau GR, Arsenault F, Dugas L, Simard S, Lariviere MM. Evaluation of the ulnopalmar arterial arches with pulse oximetry and plethysmography: Comparison with the Allen's test in 1010 patients. Am Heart J 2004;147: 489–93.
9. Bertrand OF, Rao SV, Pancholy S, Jolly SS, Rodes-Cabau J, Larose E, Costerousse O, Hamon M, Mann T. Transradial approach for coronary angiography and interventions: Results of the first international transradial practice survey. JACC Cardiovasc Interv 2010;3:1022–31.
10. Loh YJ, Nakao M, Tan WD, Lim CH, Tan YS, Chua YL. Factors influencing radial artery size. Asian Cardiovasc Thorac Ann 2007;15:324–6.
11. Ruzsa Z, Tóth K, Berta B, Koncz I, Szabó Gy, Jambrik Z, et al. Allen's test in patients with peripheral artery disease. Cent Europ. J Med; 2013. pp. 1–6.
12. Pancholy SB, Patel TM. Effect of duration of hemostatic compression on radial artery occlusion after transradial access. Catheter Cardiovasc Interv. 2012;79(1):78–81.
13. Garg R, Pandey R, Darlong V, Punj J. Radial artery cannulation—Prevention of pain and techniques of cannulation: Review of literature. Internet J Anesthesiol 2009;19(1).
14. Folmar J, Sachar R, Mann T. Transradial approach for carotid artery stenting: A feasibility study. Catheter Cardiovasc Interv 2007;69:355–361.
15. Patel T, Shah S, Ranjan A, Malhotra H, Pancholy S, Coppola J. Contralateral transradial approach for carotid artery stenting: A feasibility study. Catheter Cardiovasc Interv 2010;75:268.
16. Trani C, Tommasino A, Burzotta F. Transradial renal stenting: Why and how. Catheter Cardiovasc Interv 2009;74:951–956.
17. Flachskampf FA, Wolf T, Daniel WG, et al. Transradial stenting of the iliac artery: a case report. Catheter Cardiovasc Interv 2005;65:193–5.
18. Neill J, Douglas H, Richardson G, Chew EW, Walsh S, Hanratty C, Herity N. Comparison of radiation dose and the effect of operator experience in femoral and radial arterial access for coronary procedures. Am J Cardiol 2010;106:936–40.
19. Sciahbasi A. The TALENT trial: Transradial approach (left vs. right) and procedural times during percutaneous coronary intervention (oral presentation). May 27, 2010; Paris.

20. John T. Coppola, Cezar Staniloae. Radial Access for Peripheral Vascular Procedures. Endovascular Today. January 2012.
21. Sanmartin M, Cuevas D, Goicolea J, et al. [Vascular complications associated with radial artery access for cardiac catheterization]. Rev Esp Cardiol. 2004;57:581–4.
22. Tizon-Marcos H, Barbeau GR. Incidence of compartment syndrome of the arm in a large series of transradial approach for coronary procedures. J Interv Cardiol. 2008;21:380–4.

29

Transradial Carotid Artery Stenting

Sasko Kedev

Highlights—Pros and Cons of Transradial Carotid Artery Stenting

Pros of transradial access (TRA) carotid artery stenting (CAS):

1. In patients with extensive peripheral vascular disease, TRA maybe a safe alternative.
2. In females, patients with high body mass index and in the elderly, radial access helps reduce the risk of access site bleeding and vascular complications.
3. With complex arch, when cannulation of the common carotid artery is difficult transfemorally,[28] cannulation may be successful transradially.
4. Not only is catheter-induced embolization from the transverse aortic arch reduced with use of TRA in patients with right ICA disease and bovine left ICA disease[37–40]; TRA may be the access of choice in the latter.
5. There may be less hypotension after CAS with use of TRA.
6. TRA allows early mobilization and hence is more comfortable for patients.

Cons of TRA CAS:

1. There is a significant learning curve with TRA procedures.
2. The operator must be facile with transradial interventions and CAS.

3. Proximal protection and larger devices cannot be used freely in all cases.
4. TRA may not be best for patients with type I aortic arch and may take longer than with transfemoral access.
5. Radial artery occlusion is known to occur post-procedure.

Introduction

A proven and viable alternative to carotid endarterectomy for treatment of significant carotid disease is carotid artery stenting (CAS) with embolic protection.[1–7] Though the femoral approach has been used conventionally for carotid stenting, it may be fraught with problems of peripheral vascular disease as well as variations of anatomy of the aortic arch and arch vessels. In fact, most technical failures of transfemoral CAS are related to a complex aortic arch.

TRA may have some distinct advantages, including ease of access to carotid artery in certain types of aortic arch anatomy, reduced strokes from less atheroembolism related to catheter manipulation especially in type III aortic arch with friable atheroma, as well as, reduced need for transfusion for access site bleeding.[8–10]

Since TRA minimizes contact of the catheter with the aortic arch, it may help reduce stroke risk in patients undergoing CAS of bovine left internal carotid artery (ICA) or the right ICA since the distribution of atherosclerosis, with increasing age, is highest in the descending aorta (38.2%), followed by aortic arch (27.6%).[11]

With experience, operators can perform transradial CAS successfully with low risk of complications[12] and is especially advantageous in patients in whom prolonged post-procedure bed rest may be contraindicated, or in those at high risk for bleeding and vascular complications such as the obese and also those with peripheral vascular disease, in whom transfemoral access may be difficult and associated with potential risk of limb ischaemia.[12–28]

The techniques of transradial CAS vary, based on various aortic arch and anatomical carotid variants. The types of carotid variants are: right ICA, bovine left ICA, and non-bovine left ICA.

Transradial CAS

The authors prefer the right radial access as default for CAS, performed using standard procedures. After sheath insertion, injection verapamil or diltiazem (5 mg) is injected intra-arterially through the sheath to reduce radial artery spasm (RAS), along with unfractionated heparin (UH) (50–70 μ/kg, up to 5,000 units) or bivalirudin. Mild anxiolytic such as midazolam in dose of 0.5–1 mg may be given intravenously in the very anxious patients.

The authors prefer to perform a forearm angiography, through the cannula or sheath, with 3 ml of contrast diluted with 7 ml of blood to define the radial artery anatomy from mid forearm to axillary (Figure 29.1).

Though cubital, radial loops, high bifurcation radial, and severe subclavian tortuosities can be negotiated using a soft angioplasty 0.014" wire (Figures 29.2A and 29.2B) and diagnostic carotid arteriography may be feasible; these should be avoided for CAS using large bore devices (Figure 29.2A and 29.2B).

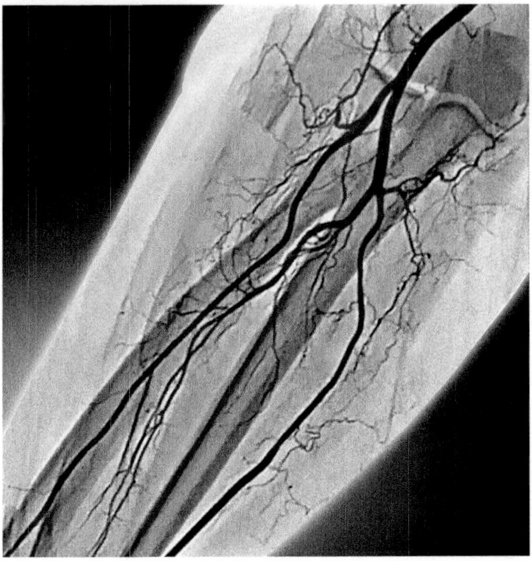

Figure 29.1 Forearm arteriography with normal radial artery diameter.

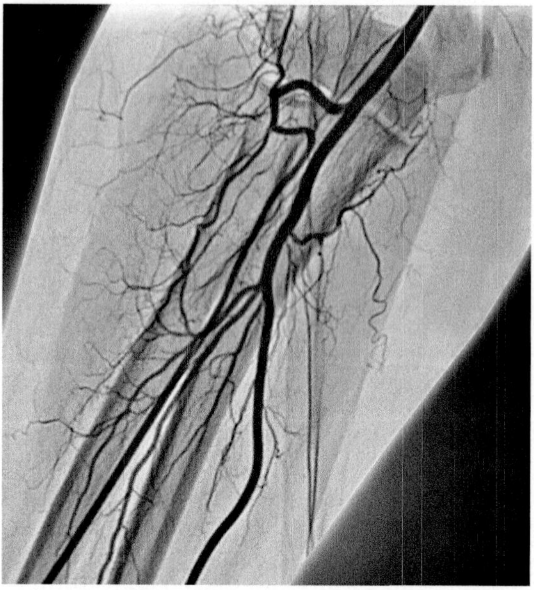

Figure 29.2A RA with 360 degree loop.

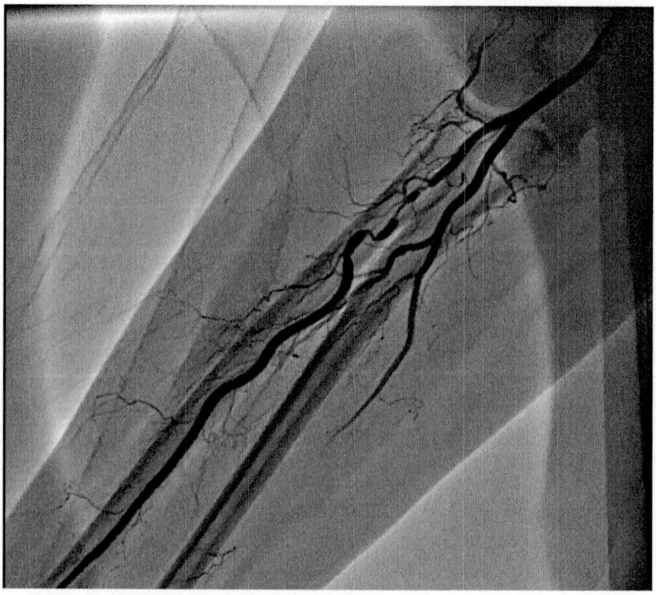

Figure 29.2B Tortuous and spasmatic RA.

Transradial Carotid Angiography (CAG)

The choice of specific diagnostic catheter for CA is based on the type of arch and takeoff of common carotid artery. Hence, different diagnostic catheters are used for right ICA, bovine left ICA, and non-bovine left ICA. For transradial carotid angiography, a 4 French or 5F reversed angle catheter, such as Simmons type 1 or 2, are commonly used. Catheters with a soft reversed angle tip are most easily reformable and least traumatic during CAG and are preferred (Merit Medical, Galway, Ireland).

Prior to CAS, it is desirable to obtain a complete evaluation of the aortic arch as well as bilateral carotid anatomy by CAG, including a right anterior oblique (RAO) angiogram of the innominate bifurcation for right internal CA disease.

A magnetic resonance angiography or computed tomographic angiography should also be performed where necessary.

Methods of Reforming the Natural Reversed Curve of the Simmons Catheters Within the Aortic Arch for CAG

In patients with a very tortuous and dilated aortic arch (Figure 29.3) a Simmons 1 or a Simmons 2 catheter (Terumo, Tokyo, Japan; Merit Medical, Galway, Ireland; Cordis Corporation, Warren NJ, USA) is tracked over a hydrophilic glidewire looped in the ascending aorta; alternatively, a Simmons 2 catheter is negotiated into the descending thoracic aorta over a standard guidewire. By then, withdrawing the guidewire into the primary curve and prolapsing the catheter into the ascending aorta with counterclockwise rotation, sometimes facilitated by a deep breath, the catheter forms a loop on itself which often directly engages the left CA. After angiography of the left carotid, the catheter is pushed, rotated, and withdrawn into the right common CA (Figures 29.4 and 29.5).[29] However, caution needs to be exercised with use of Simmons 2 catheter in the right common CA of women and short patients as the distal limb may reach the bifurcation.

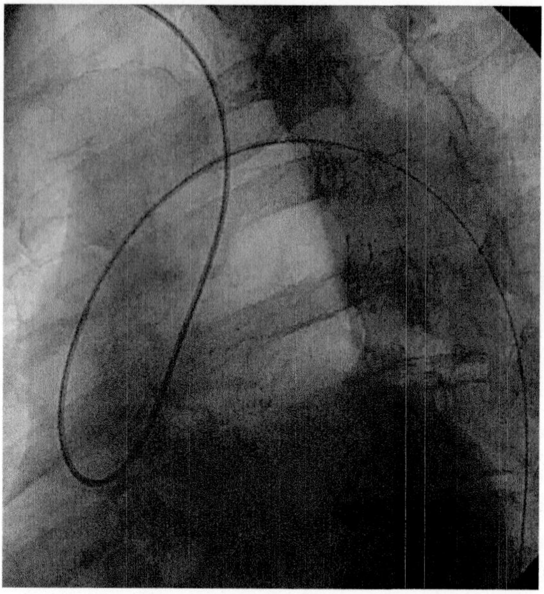

Figure 29.3 Looping technique of a diagnostic Simmons 2 catheter over the hydrophilic wire in the ascending aorta.

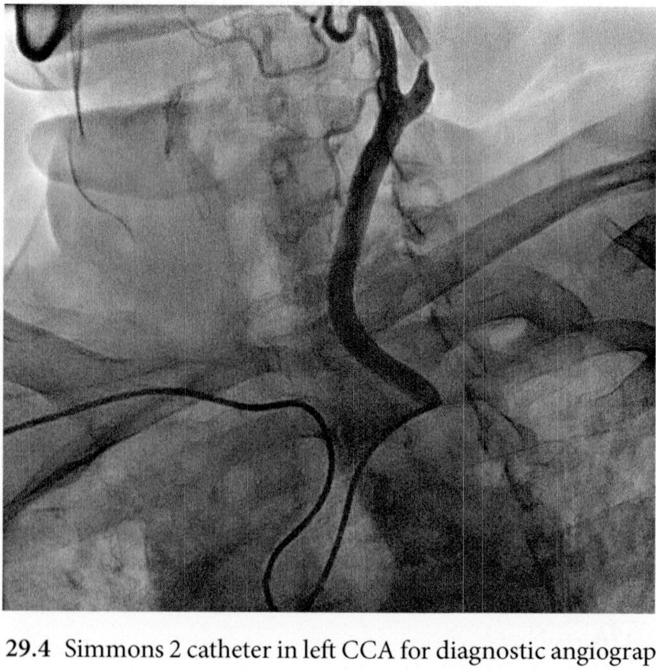

Figure 29.4 Simmons 2 catheter in left CCA for diagnostic angiography.

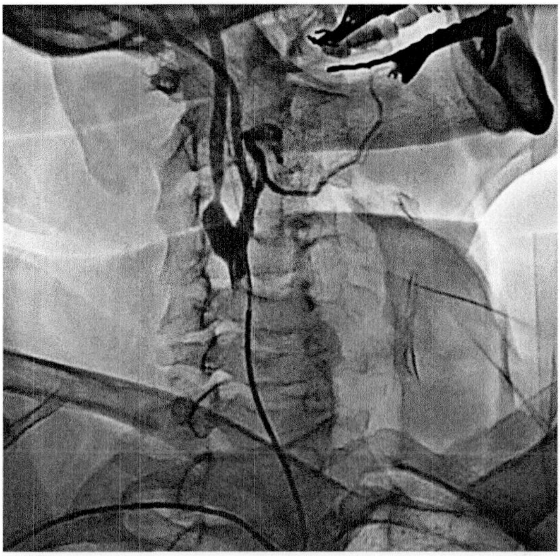

Figure 29.5 Simmons 2 catheter in right CCA for diagnostic angiography.

Techniques of Common Carotid Artery Cannulation

CAS is usually performed through a 5F or 6F long (90 cm) Shuttle Sheath (Cook, Minneapolis, MN, USA), Destination Sheath (Terumo, Tokyo, Japan) or Sheathless PV Guiding System (Asahi Intecc, Aichi, Japan). The same is used for CAS via TRA. Alternatively, conventional (6F–8F) guiding catheters can be used. The pre-procedural radial angiography helps decide on the. Compatibility of the guiding sheath diameter with RA size.

Techniques of Common CA Cannulation

1. Anchoring Technique
2. Telescopic Technique.

Imaging of the aortic arch and takeoff angulation of the arch vessels by computerized tomography angiography, Magnetic resonance angiography and aortography help to choose the technique to be used for cannulation of CA.

Anchoring Technique

A 0.035" glidewire is passed into the external carotid artery; over which a diagnostic Simmon's 1 or 2 catheter tracks. The glidewire is exchanged for an exchange length, superstiff 0.035" J guidewire, over which a guiding sheath is deployed (Figures 29.6B, 29.6C, 29.6D, and 29.6E). Alternatively using same technique, regular guiding catheters (6F–8F) or sheathless catheters (Figures 29.7A, 29.7B, 29.7C, 29.7D, and 29.7E) can be deployed.

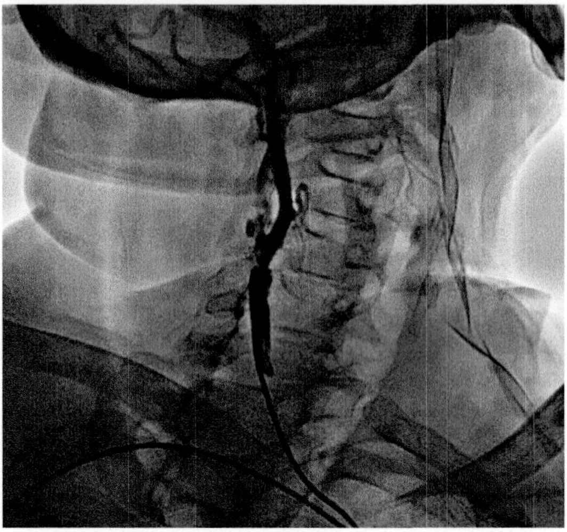

Figure 29.6A Simmons 2 catheter in right CCA.

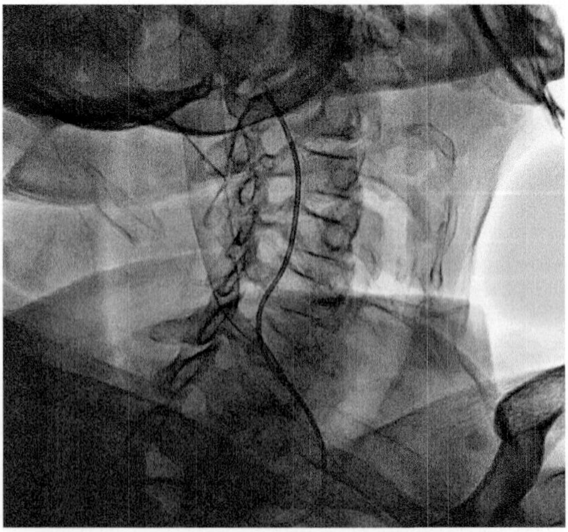

Figure 29.6B Simmons 2 transfer catheter in right ECA.

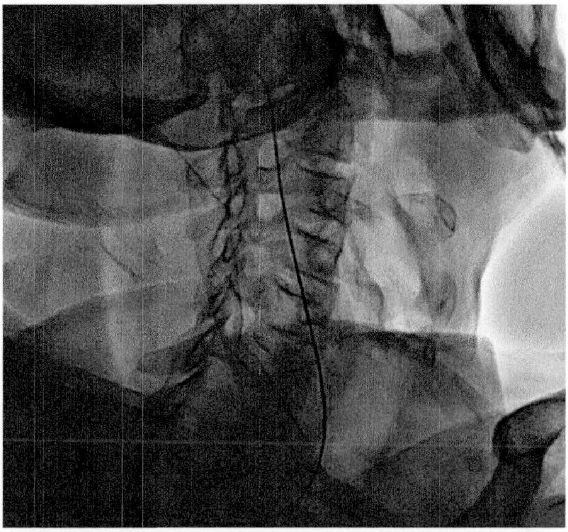

Figure 29.6C Amplatz super stiff guidewire in right ECA.

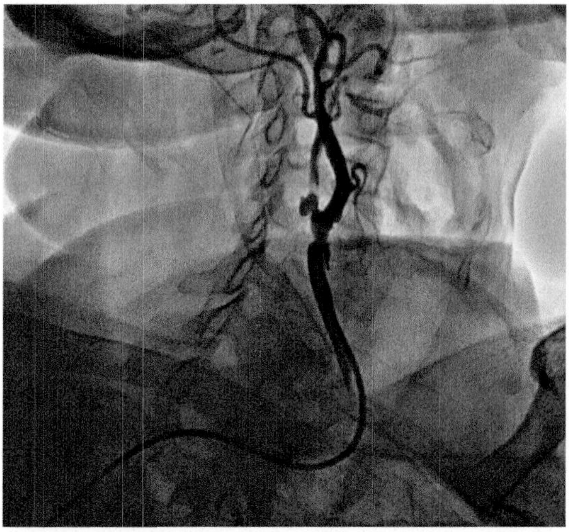

Figure 29.6D Shuttle sheath 6F in right CCA.

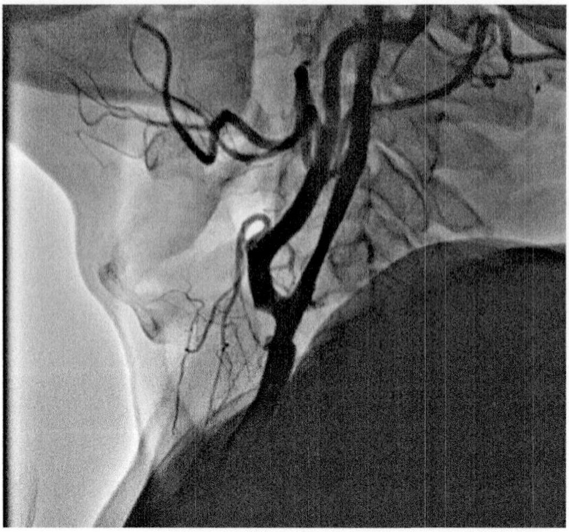

Figure 29.6E Final result after TRA CAS of right ICA (Precise 7.0/40 mm, Cordis).

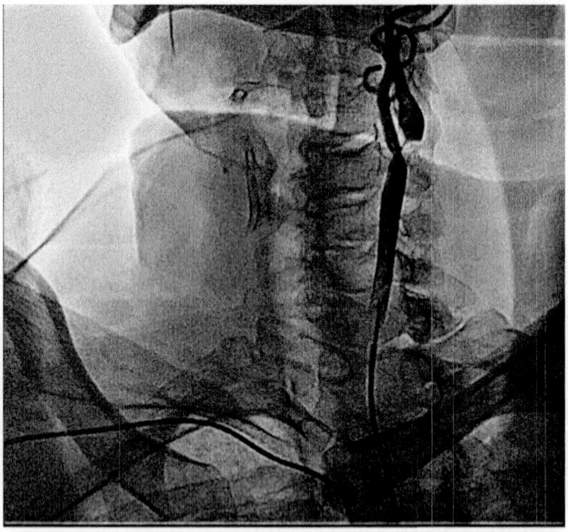

Figure 29.7A Simmons 2 catheter in left CCA.

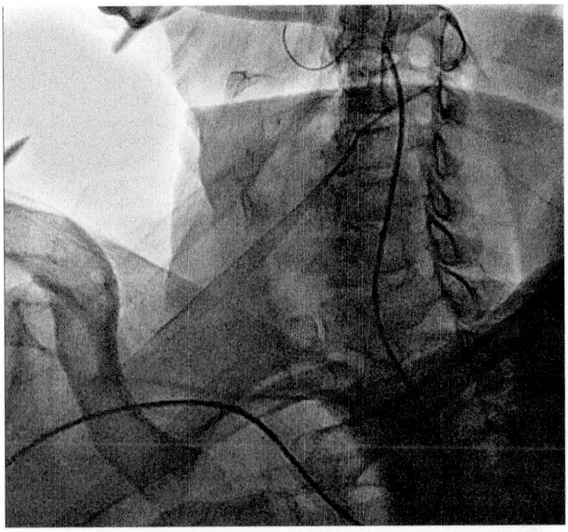

Figure 29.7B Transfer catheter (5F JR guiding catheter) in left ECA.

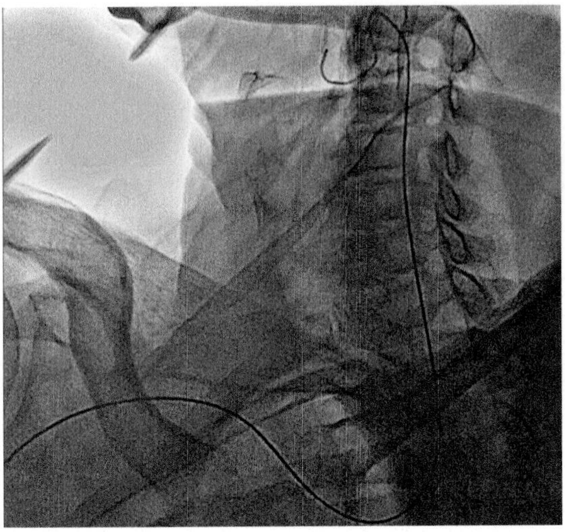

Figure 29.7C Amplatz super stiff guidewire exchange in left ECA.

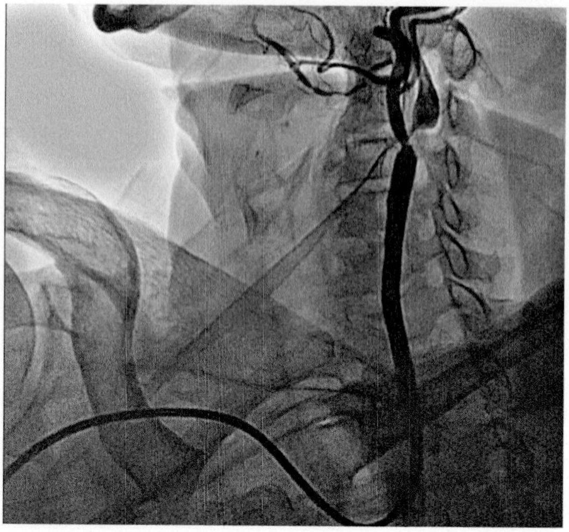

Figure 29.7D Destination 6F guiding sheath in left CCA.

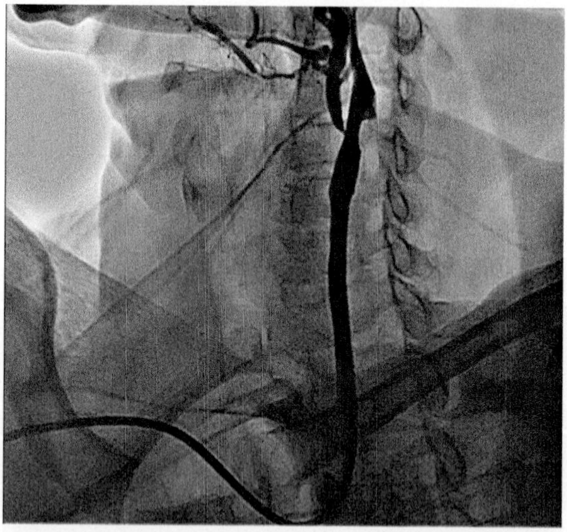

Figure 29.7E Final result after TRA CAS of left ICA (Xact 8-6/40, Abbott Vascular5).

Telescopic Technique

A long (125 cm) wire-braided Simmons 2 catheter (Cook, Minneapolis, MN) is introduced within the shuttle sheath and is used as an introducer. This technique is preferred for sheath deployment for CAS, in which there are extreme angles, like in a sharp takeoff right common CA or a non-bovine left CA (Figures 29.8A, 29.8B, and 29.8C).

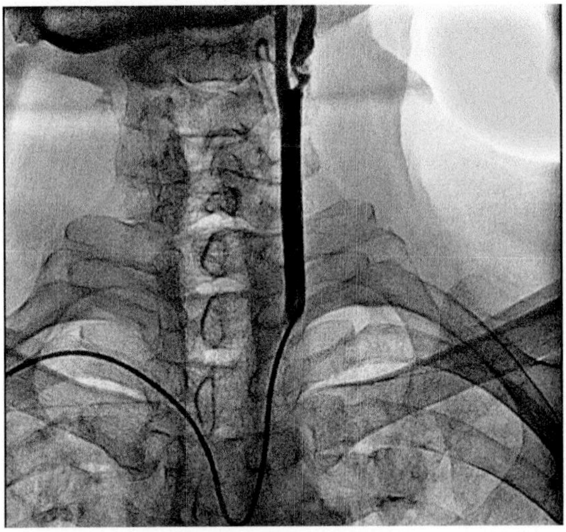

Figure 29.8A Simmons 2 catheter in left CCA.

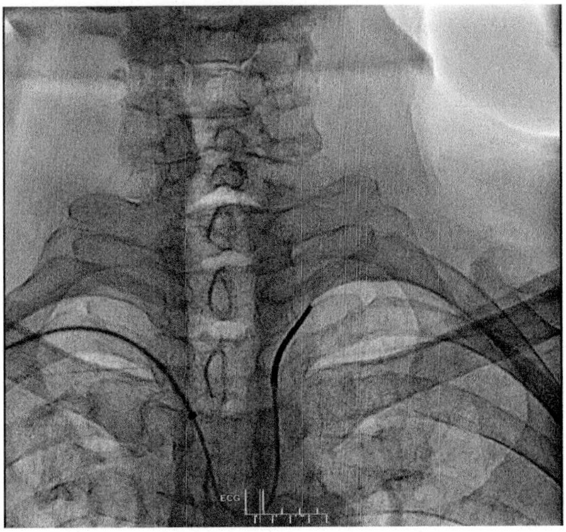

Figure 29.8B 5F braided Simmons 2 (125 cm) catheter into 6F Shuttle sheath.

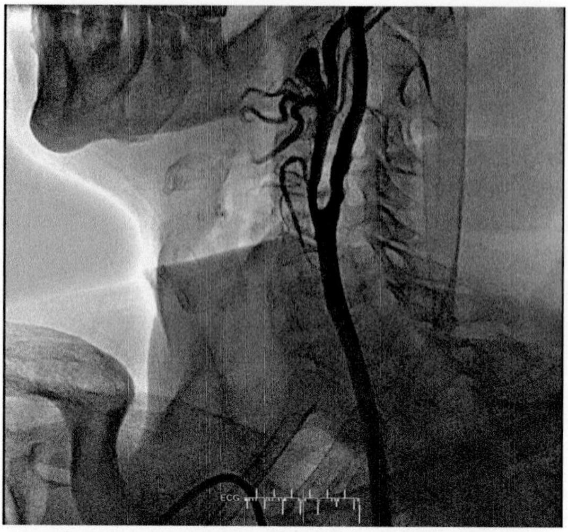

Figure 29.8C Final result after TRA CAS of left ICA (Adapt 4-9/40 mm, Boston Scientific).

With TRA, often, acute angles need to be negotiated. Depending on the severity of the angle between the arm and common carotid artery, different strategies for sheath deployment (direct, simple loop, or deep loop retrograde cannulation) are used based on CA classifications: right, bovine left, and non-bovine left groups.

Direct Cannulation

As discussed earlier, since many procedurally related strokes are because of arch atheroembolization, stroke risk of CAS of right ICA (RICA) and bovine left ICA may be lower with TRA, since TRA reduces contact of catheter with the aortic arch.

RICA CAS

As mentioned earlier, CAG in RAO view shows the innominate (brachiocephalic) artery bifurcation and helps determine the right ICA sheath insertion strategy. A pre-procedure CT also shows the same and helps in decision-making. Direct cannulation of the CA is feasible with right Judkins or internal mammary catheter when angulation is less acute, with presence of a horizontal segment of common CA or subclavian.

Bovine LICA CAS

The right transradial approach is preferred for carotid stenting of left ICA stenosis in a bovine arch,[30] in which the right brachiocephalic and left carotid share a common trunk from the aortic arch, in about 13% of population.[28]

A left anterior oblique view (LAO) the aortic arch is used to visualize the initial takeoff of the bovine carotid. With a horizontal initial segment of the common carotid, a Judkins right or Amplatz R2 diagnostic catheter is successful in engaging the left common CA (Figures 29.9A and 29.9B), usually without much manipulation.

Alternatively, the ECA may be directly cannulated with a hybrid 0.035" Advantage wire (Terumo; Tokyo, Japan) which has a hydrophilic glidewire distal tip, with stiffer nitinol core on the proximal end. This obviates the need of inserting a diagnostic catheter into the external carotid artery.

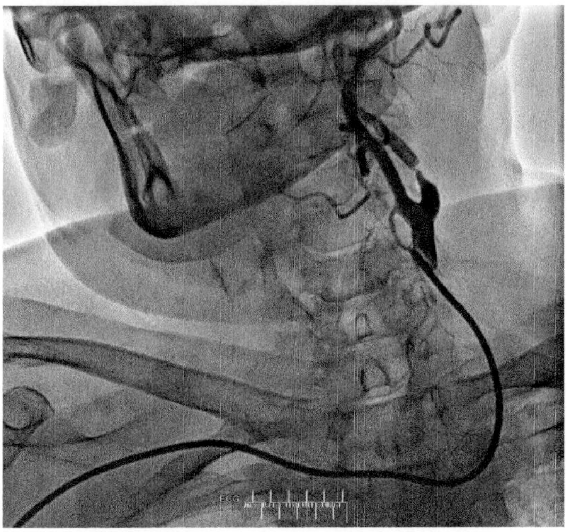

Figure 29.9A 6F Shuttle sheath in left bovine CCA.

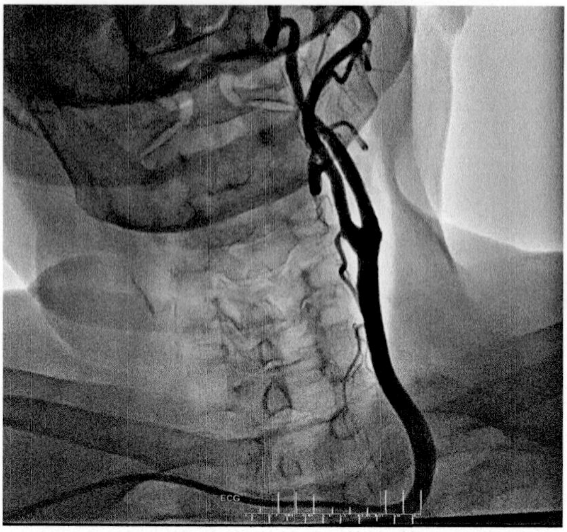

Figure 29.9B Final result after TRA CAS of left bovine ICA (Xact 9-7/40 mm, Abbott Vascular).

Simple Loop Cannulation

With a vertical or acute take-off of CA, a wire braided Simmons 2 catheter is passed into the ECA over a glidewire or extra support angioplasty 0.014" wire and then exchanged for the shuttle sheath over an Amplatz superstiff guidewire. Alternatively, with a very severe angle of takeoff of the right common CA, a telescopic technique, as described earlier, is preferred (Figures 29.10A, 29.10B, 29.10C, and 29.10D). Even with acute angled take off of the common carotid artery from the arch of the aorta right TRA is able to provide adequate support for CAS.

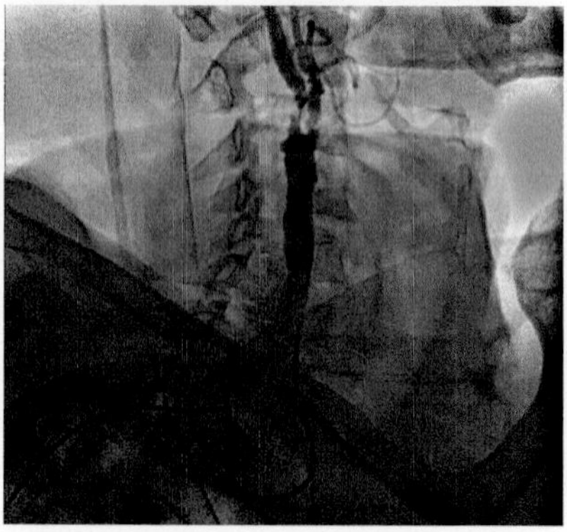

Figure 29.10A Simmons 2 catheter in right CCA.

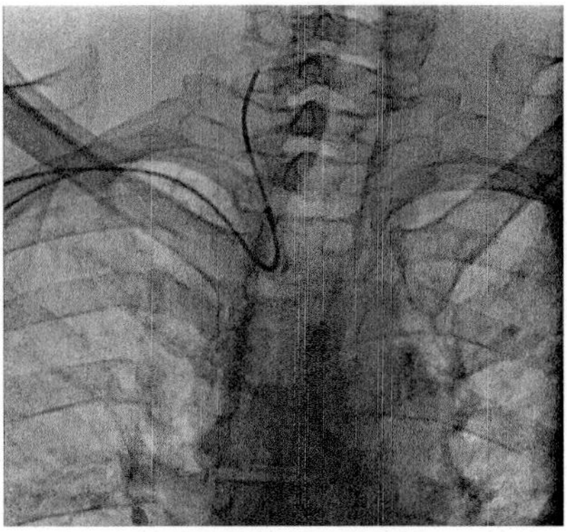

Figure 29.10B 5F braided Simmons 2 (125 cm) catheter into 6F Shuttle sheath.

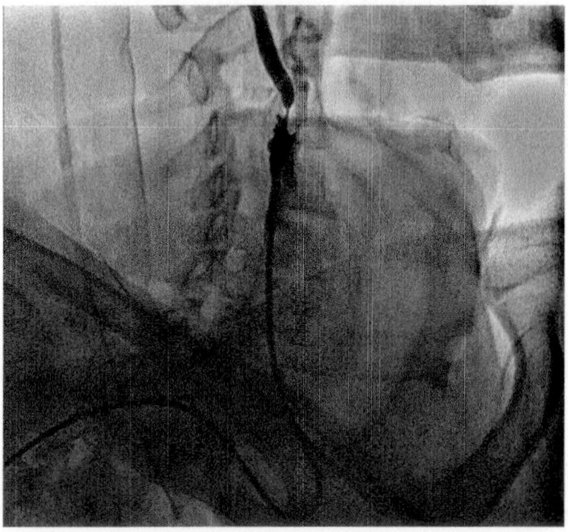

Figure 29.10C 6F Shuttle sheath in right CCA.

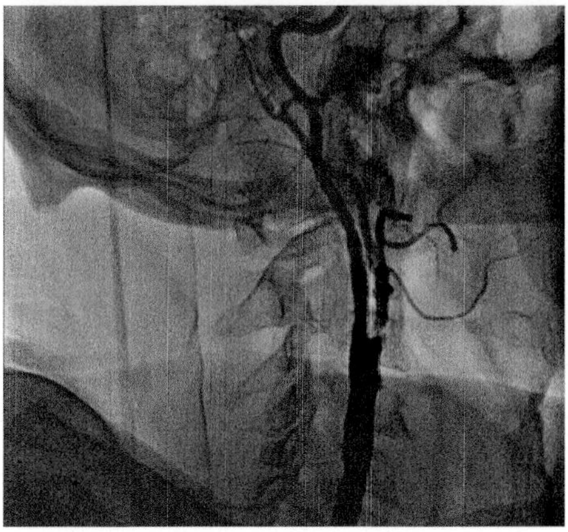

Figure 29.10D Final result after TRA CAS of right ICA (Xact 8-6/40, Abbott Vascular).

Non-bovine LICA CAS

TRA for non-bovine LICA CAS is even more challenging due to the acute angled takeoff of the left common carotid,[12–14] which leads to prolapse of the catheter or sheath into the ascending aorta because of poor inferior support for the catheter or sheath, and can be catastrophic if prolapse occurs during stent delivery.

Generally, a telescopic approach is preferred in cases of non-bovine LICA CAS.

A wire-braided Simmons 2 catheter usually provides adequate support for inserting a guidewire into the ECA. Alternatively, a Simmons 3 catheter can be used in type II and type III arches which are associated with severely acute angled takeoff of the common CA (CCA). The anchoring technique can be used. Though the 'Advantage' and Amplatz superstiff wires provide adequate support for inserting the shuttle sheath, there can be difficulty with extreme angulation. In such situations, a 5 or 6 French multipurpose or Judkins R guide catheter may have to be used as alternative, to facilitate insertion of an Amplatz superstiff guidewire. Again, because the shuttle sheath is liable to kink at the acute angle; a heavily braided, semi-hydrophilic Destination sheath (Terumo, Tokyo, Japan) may have to be used instead (Figure 29.11 and Figure 29.12A, 29.12B, 29.12C, 29.12D, and 29.12E).

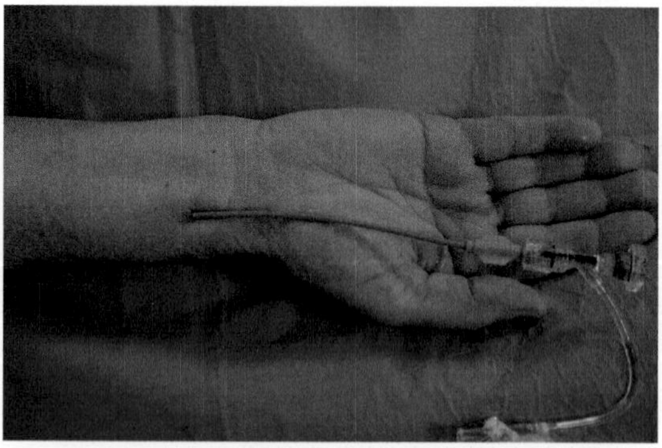

Figure 29.11 6 French Destination guiding sheath (90 cm) through the right radial access.

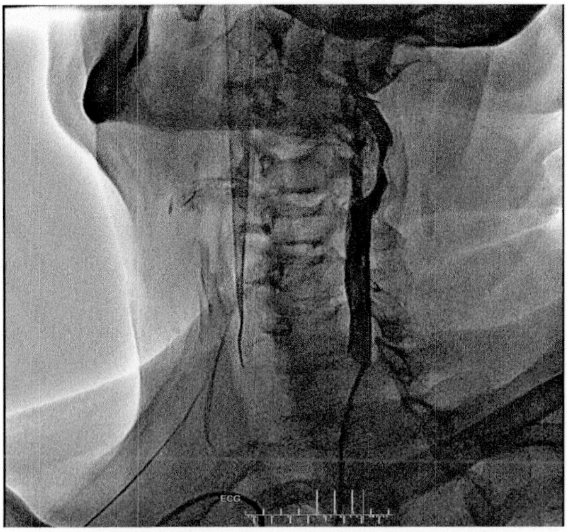

Figure 29.12A Simmons 2 catheter in left CCA.

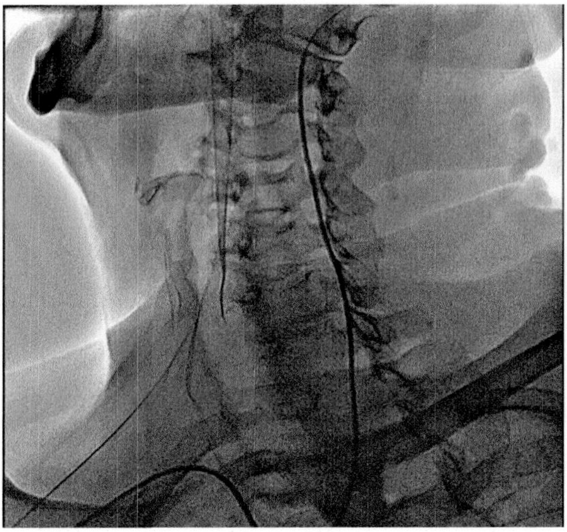

Figure 29.12B Simmons 2 transfer catheter deep in left ECA.

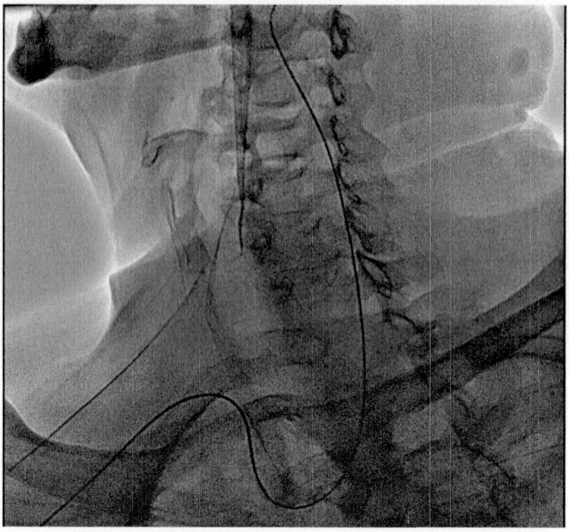

Figure 29.12C Amplatz supersiff guidewire exchange in left ECA.

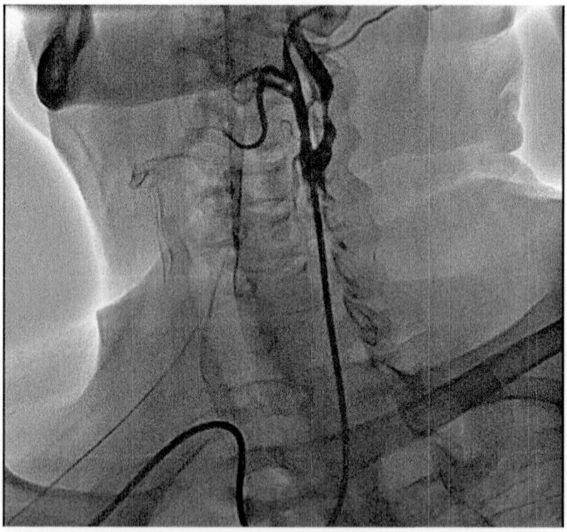

Figure 29.12D 6F Shuttle sheath in left CCA.

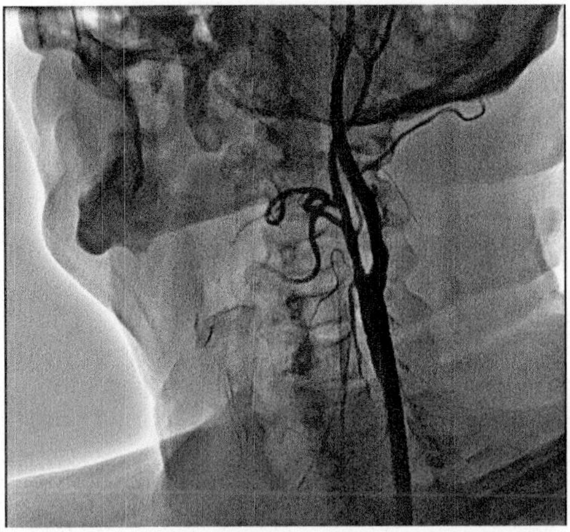

Figure 29.12E Final result after TRA CAS of left ICA (Adapt 4-9/32 mm, Boston Scientific).

RICA CAS

Using left radial access, the right common carotid (RCC) is engaged using a TIG or Simmon's 2 catheter.[14] Using a glidewire, the diagnostic catheter is inserted to ECA, followed by introduction of Shuttle sheath or guiding catheter over a superstiff 0.035" wire and the CAS is then completed using distal embolic protection device (DPD) (Figures 29.13A and 29.13B).

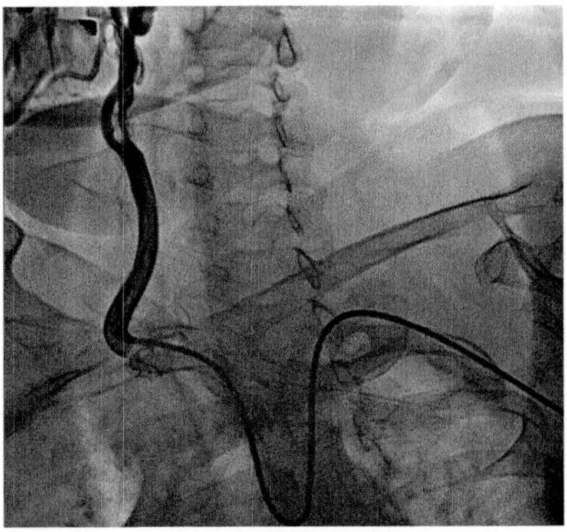

Figure 29.13A 5F Simmons 2 diagnostic catheter in right CCA.

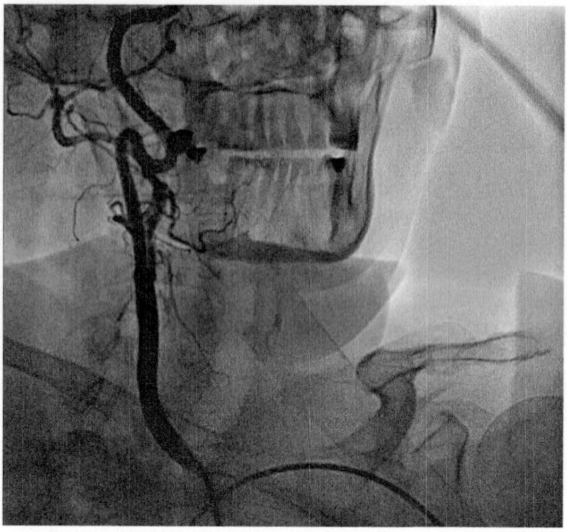

Figure 29.13B Final result after CAS of right ICA from left radial access (Wallstent 7.0/30, Boston Scientific).

Deep Loop Retrograde Cannulation

In unfavourable take-off angulation of the carotids, a Catheter Looping and Retrograde Engagement Technique (CLARET)[15] uses a sheath or a 7 French MP guide catheter for CAS of both right ICA and left ICA with support of the right coronary cusp for inferior support to the catheter or sheath from below (Figures 29.14A, 29.14B, 29.14C, and 29.14D). Of course the catheter system in lacks stability and has the potential to abruptly jump forward in trying to withdraw it.

Transradial CAS with Proximal Protection Device

PPDs have been reported to be better than DPDs for reducing risk of cerebral embolism during CAS.[31,32] A PPD consists of a long sheath. It has a central working lumen, connected to two balloons inflated to occlude the external carotid artery and the common carotid artery.

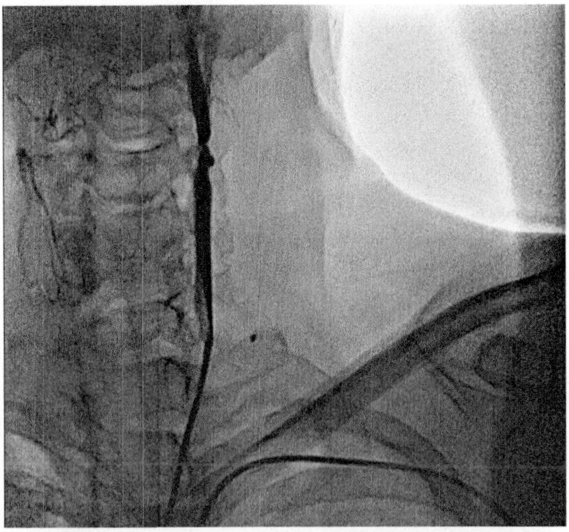

Figure 29.14A Deeply looped 5F MP catheter with retrograde cannulation of in left CCA below bifurcation.

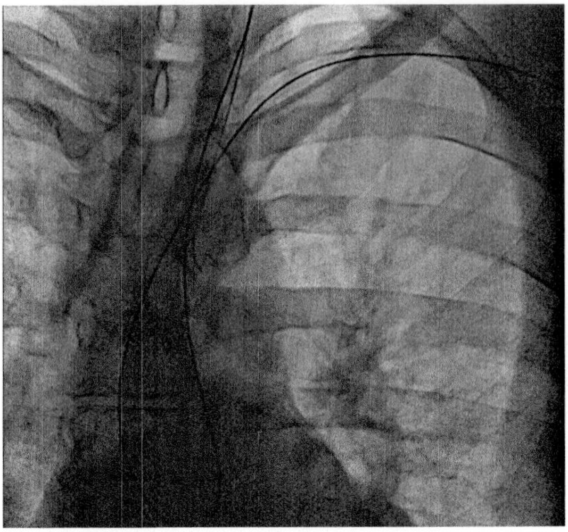

Figure 29.14B Looped Advantage glidewire in left ECA.

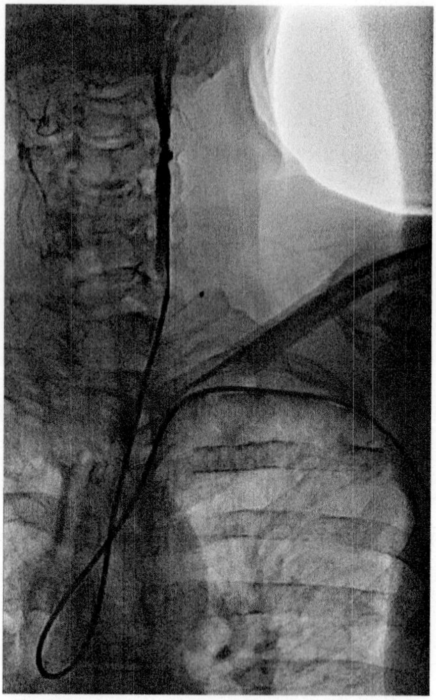

Figure 29.14C Looped 7F MP guiding catheter with retrograde cannulation of left CCA.

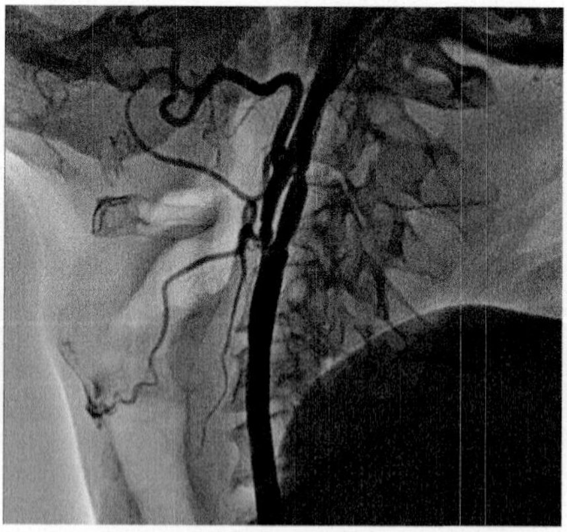

Figure 29.14D Final result after TRA CAS of left non-bovine ICA with deep loop retrograde cannulation technique (Wallstent 7.0/30, Boston Scientific).

Transradial CAS using 8 Fr proximal protection with Mo.Ma device (Medtronic Invatec, Roncadelle, Italy)[17] was first reported by Trani *et al.* Although the feasibility of using 8 Fr sheaths in the radial artery has been reported,[33] a major challenge[34] of transradial CAS is of using the larger and cumbersome (8 or 9 Fr) proximal protection devices (PPDs) transradially, as it may be difficult to insert such bulky devices via smaller radial arteries. Further, transradial CAS with Mo.Ma device can be very challenging and requires the operator to be facile with both radial and carotid interventions.

The authors have used the Mo.Ma device successfully during 21 transradial CAS procedures (Kedev S, MD, personal communication, 2017).

In the anchoring technique, an additional extra support 0.014" angioplasty wire used along with the 0.035" superstiff guidewire inserted in ECA helps to enhance stability of the whole guiding system, in CCAs with angulated take off, facilitating tracking of the stent over the superstiff guidewire (Figures 29.15A and 29.15B).

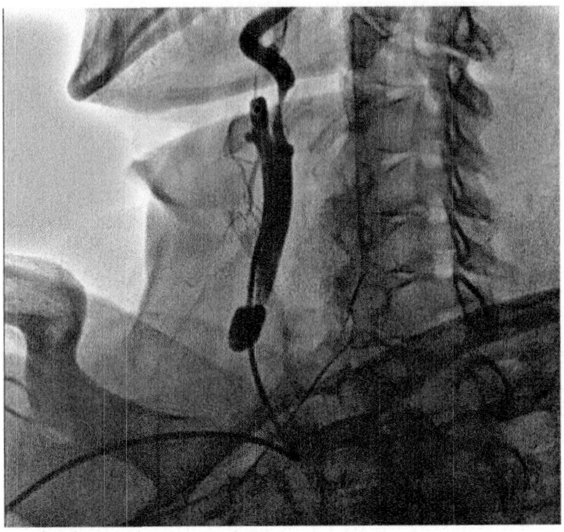

Figure 29.15A 8F Mo.Ma proximal protection device with occlusion of right ECA and right CCA.

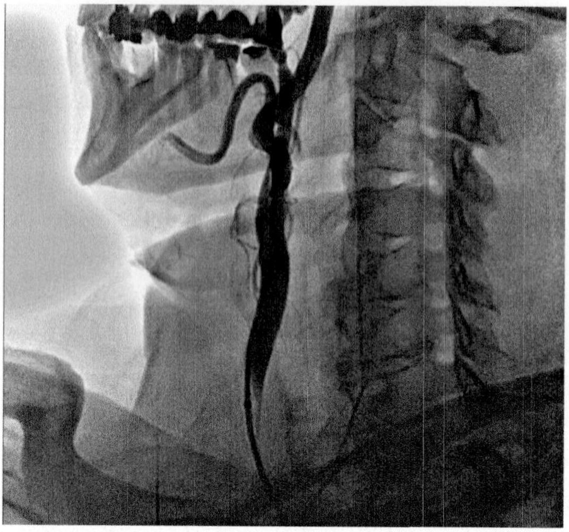

Figure 29.15B Final result after TRA CAS of right ICA under proximal protection with Mo.Ma 8F (Crystalo Ideale 6-9/30 mm, Medtronic, Invatec).

Post-procedure Hemostasis can be Used with a TR Band, Bandage, or Hemostatic Device using Standard Procedures

Patients may be discharged the following day if clinically stable.[35,36]

Limitations

Before embarking on transradial CAS, the operator should first become facile with CAS and with transradial interventions, both of which require significant experience, and have a learning curve,[5,6] because procedural outcomes for both are related to operator experience. It is best to avoid a transradial CAS procedure using bulky devices through severe tortuosity and loops in cubital or subclavian artery.

Contrast injections should be done only after careful bleed-back. Stents should be positioned using roadmap fluoroscopy or bony landmarks. Careful de-airing of small sheaths with bulky stents is important to prevent air-embolization.

Only the carotid Wallstent, Adapt (Boston Scientific, Maple Grove, MN), Precise (Cordis Corporation, Warren NJ, USA), and Crystalo Ideale (Medtronic, Invatec, Roncadelle, Italy) can be delivered through 6F and 7F guiding catheters and 5F shuttle sheaths.

Future Perspectives

Although TRA CAS can be safely performed successfully, improvements in equipment with technological advancement would allow the technique to be widely applicable. Better guiding catheters with dedicated carotid curves could facilitate direct CCA cannulation. Flexible and more supportive sheaths would be useful in patients with angulated origin of the CCA, as lack of inferior support is the cause of most failures. Lower profile, more deliverable stent systems compatible with smaller (5F) catheter systems would not only improve deliverability but also reduce radial artery injury and occlusion.

Conclusions

TRA is an alternative approach for CAS. It is particularly advantageous in patients with extensive peripheral vascular disease and patients with anatomical variations of aortic arch and origin of neck vessels that make cannulation of the common carotid difficult from the femoral approach. Moreover, TRA is associated with reduced risk of bleeding and vascular complications in obese, female, and the elderly patients undergoing CAS.

TRA for CAS in patients with RICA and bovine LICA disease also has the advantage of reducing the risk of possible catheter-induced embolization from the arch since transradial catheters do not traverse this area. Operators must be facile with transradial approach prior to embarking on these advanced techniques of CAS. New operators are encouraged to be comfortable with transradial CAG before undertaking transradial CAS.

Transradial CAS is feasible, and with careful application of appropriate technique, it can be performed safely and successfully with low complication rate by experienced operators.

References

1. Brott TG, Hobson RW, Howard G, et al. Stenting versus endarterectomy for treatment of carotid artery stenosis. *N Engl J Med*. 2010;363:11–23.
2. Silver FL, Mackey A, Clark WM, et al. CREST investigators: safety of stenting and endarterectomy by symptomatic status in the Carotid Revascularization Endarterectomy versus Stenting Trial (CREST). *Stroke*. 2011;42:675–80.
3. Gray WA, Yadav JS, Verta P, et al. CAPTURE trial collaborators the CAPTURE registry: predictors of outcomes in car3.otid artery stenting with embolic protection for high surgical risk patients in the early post-approval setting. *Catheter Cardiovasc Interv*. 2007;70:1025–33.
4. Brott TG, George Howard G, Gary S, et al. for the CREST Investigators. Long-term results of stenting versus endarterectomy for carotid-artery stenosis. *N Engl J Med*. 2016;374(11):1021–31.
5. Rosenfield K, Matsumura JS, Chaturvedi S, et al., for the ACT I Investigators. Randomized trial of stent versus surgery for asymptomatic carotid stenosis. *N Engl J Med*. 2016;374(11):1011–20.
6. Gurm HS, Yadav JS, Fayad P, et al. SAPPHIRE investigators. Long-term results of carotid stenting versus endarterectomy in high-risk patients. *N Engl J Med*. 2008;358:1572–9.
7. White CJ, Iyer SS, Hopkins LN, et al., BEACH Trial Investigators. Carotid stenting with distal protection in 4 high surgical risk patients: the BEACH trial 30 day results. *Catheter Cardiovasc Interv*. 2006;67:503–12.
8. Hill MD, Brooks W, Mackey A, et al., for the CREST Investigators. Stroke after carotid stenting and endarterectomy in the Carotid Revascularization Endarterectomy Versus Stenting Trial (CREST). *Circulation*. 2012;126:3054–61.
9. Macdonald S, Lee R, Williams R, et al. Delphi carotid stenting consensus panel. Towards safer carotid artery stenting: a scoring system for anatomic suitability. *Stroke*. 2009;40:1698–703.
10. Hammer FD, Lacroix V, Duprez T, et al. Cerebral microembolization after protected carotid artery stenting in surgical high-risk patients: results of a 2-year prospective study. *J Vasc Surg*. 2005;42:847–53.
11. Meissner I, Whisnant JP, Khandheria BK, et al. Prevalence of potential risk factors for stroke assessed by transesophageal echocardiography and carotid ultrasonography: the SPARC study: stroke prevention: assessment of risk in a community. *Mayo Clin Proc*. 1999;74:862–9.
12. Etxegoien N, Rhyne D, Kedev S, Sachar R, Mann T. The transradial approach for carotid artery stenting. *Catheter Cardiovasc Interv*. 2012;80:1081–7.
13. Folmar J, Sachar R, Mann T. Transradial approach for carotid artery stenting: a feasibility study. *Catheter Cardiovasc Interv*. 2007;69(3):355–61.

14. Patel T, Shah S, Ranian A, et al. Contralateral transradial approach for carotid artery stenting: a feasibility study. *Catheter Cardiovasc Interv*. 2009;75:268–75.
15. Fang H, Chung S, Sun C, et al. Transradial and transbrachial arterial approach for simultaneous carotid angiographic examination and stenting using catheter looping and retrograde engagement technique. *Ann Vasc Surg*. 2010;24:670–9.
16. Mendiz OA, Sampaolesi AH, Londero HF et al. Initial experience with transradial access for carotid stenting. *Vasc Endovascular Surg*. 2011;45:499–503.
17. Pinter L, Cagiannos C, Ruzsa Z, et al. Report on initial experience with transradial access for carotid artery stenting. *J Vasc Surg*. 2007;45:1136–41.
18. Bakoyiannis C, Economopoulos KP, Georgopoulos S, et al. Transradial access for carotid artery stenting: a single center experience. *Int Angiol*. 2010;29:41–6.
19. Trani C, Burzotta F, Coroleu F. Transradial carotid artery stenting with proximal embolic protection. *Catheter Cardiovasc Interv*. 2009;74:267–72.
20. Coroleu SF, Burzotta F, Fernández-Gómez C, et al. Feasibility of complex coronary and peripheral interventions by trans-radial approach using large sheaths. *Cathet Cardiovasc Diagn*. 2011;79:597–600.
21. Shaw JA, Gravereaux EC, Eisenhauer AC. Carotid stenting in the bovine arch. *Catheter Cardiovasc Interv*. 2003;60:566–9.
22. Gan HW, Bhasin A, Wu CJ. Transradial carotid stenting in a patient with bovine arch anatomy. *Catheter Cardiovasc Interv*. 2006;75:540–3.
23. Levy EL, Kim SH, Bendok BR, et al. Transradial stenting of the cervical internal carotid artery: technical case report. *Neurosurgery*. 2003;53:448–51.
24. Layton KF, Kallmes DF, Cloft HJ. The radial artery access site for interventional neuroradiology procedures. *Am J Neuroradiol*. 2006;27:1151–4.
25. Bendok BR, Przybylo JH, Parkinson R, et al. neuroendovascular interventions for intracranial posterior circulation disease via the transradial approach: technical case report. *Neurosurgery*. 2005;56:626.
26. Eskioglu E, Burry MV, Mericle RA. Transradial approach for neuroendovascular surgery of intracranial vascular lesions. *J Neurosurg*. 2004;101:767–9.
27. Castriota F, Cremonesi A, Manetti R, Lamarra M, Noera G. Carotid stenting using radial artery access. *J Endovasc Surg*. 1999;6:385–6.
28. Yoo B-S, Lee S-H, Kim J-Y, et al. A case of transradial carotid stenting in a patient with total occlusion of distal abdominal aorta. *Catheter Cardiovasc Interv*. 2002;56:243–5.
29. Lee D, Ahn J, Jeong S, et al. Routine transradial access for conventional cerebral angiography: a single operator's experience of its feasibility and safety. *Br J Radiol*. 2004;77:831–8.
30. Layton KF, Kallmes DF, Cloft HJ, et al. Bovine aortic arch variant in humans: clarification of a common misnomer. *Am J Neuroradiol*. 2006;27:1541–2.
31. Montorsi P, Caputi L, Galli S, et al. Microembolization during carotid artery stenting in patients with high-risk, lipid rich plaque: a randomized trial of proximal versus distal cerebral protection. *J Am Coll Cardiol*. 2012;58:1656–63.
32. Bijuklic K, Wandler A, Hazizi F, et al. The PROFI study (prevention of cerebral embolization by proximal balloon occlusion compared to filter protection during carotid artery stenting): a prospective randomized trial. *J Am Coll Cardiol*. 2012;59:1383–91.

33. Wu SS, Galani RJ, Bahro A, et al. 8 French transradial coronary interventions: clinical outcome and late effects on the radial artery and hand function. *J Invasive Cardiol.* 2000;12:605–9.
34. Saito S, Ikei H, Hosokawa G, Tanaka S. Influence of the ratio between radial artery inner diameter and sheath outer diameter on radial artery flow after transradial coronary intervention. *Cathet Cardiovasc Intervent.* 1999;46:173–8.
35. Pancholy S, Coppola J, Patel T, et al. Prevention of radial artery occlusion—patient hemostasis evaluation trial (PROPHET study): a randomized comparison of traditional versus patency documented hemostasis after transradial catheterization. *Cathet Cardiovasc Intervent.* 2008;72:335–40.
36. Pancholy SB, Patel TM. Effect of duration of hemostatic compression on radial artery occlusion after transradial access. *Cathet Cardiovasc Interv.* 2012;79:78–81.
37. Bendszur M, Koltzenburg M, Burger R, et al. Silent embolism in diagnostic cerebral angiography and neurointerventional procedures: a prospective study. *Lancet.* 1999;354:1594–7.
38. El-Koussy M, Schroth G, Do DD, et al. Periprocedural embolic events related to carotid artery stenting detected by diffusion-weighted MRI: comparison between proximal and distal embolus protection devices. *J Endovasc Ther.* 2007;14:293–303.
39. Barbato JE, Dillavou E, Horowitz MB, et al. A randomized trial of carotid artery stenting with and without cerebral protection. *J Vasc Surg.* 2008;47:760–5.
40. Faggioli G, Ferri M, Rapezzi C, et al. Atherosclerotic aortic lesions increase the risk of cerebral embolism during carotid stenting in patients with complex aortic arch anatomy. *J Vasc Surg.* 2009;49:80–5.

30

Complications of Transfemoral Access, Its Prevention, and Management

Saurabh Mehrotra, Pavankumar P. Rasalkar, and Sundeep Mishra

Introduction

Femoral arterial access with the Seldinger technique revolutionized the world of Interventional Cardiology. Over the years, transradial access has replaced transfemoral access as the preferred route, due to the higher rate of complications with the latter. But with the growing number of complex interventions performed these days, transfemoral route continues to be the most frequently used route in catheterization procedures.[1,2] Thus, it is important to have a good knowledge about the proper technique of transfemoral access. This chapter deals in detail about the anatomy of femoral artery, the ideal technique of femoral artery puncture, possible complications, their management, and ways to prevent them.

Applied Anatomy

Common femoral artery (CFA) is the preferred site for puncture for transfemoral access, as its superficial, lies over bony prominence (femoral head), and thus can be compressed against it to achieve adequate haemostasis.[3] CFA is a branch of external iliac artery (EIA). It originates below the inguinal ligament after the inferior epigastric artery branches off the EIA.[4] CFA bifurcates into superficial femoral artery (SFA) and Profunda femoris.

Femoral Puncture Technique

Most ideal site for femoral artery puncture is between inguinal ligament above and bifurcation of CFA below, as shown in Figure 30.1.[5,6] Puncture above the inguinal ligament is termed as high puncture, and puncture at or below the bifurcation is termed as low puncture. Three landmarks can be used to guide puncture of femoral artery, as described later:

1. ***Soft tissue landmark:*** Inguinal crease is the most unreliable of all the landmarks. But, unfortunately, it is the most commonly used, even by experienced operators. In a study, it was found that in

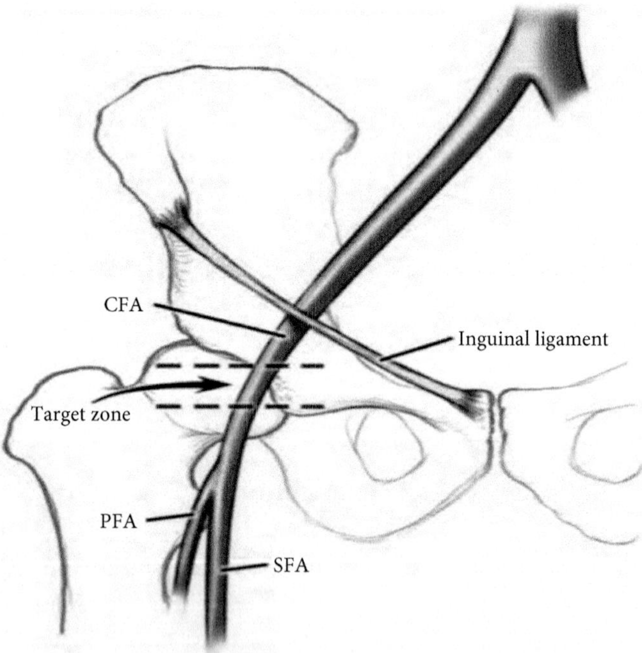

Figure 30.1 The anatomy of the groin and the ideal target zone for arteriotomy of the common femoral artery, which is over the mid third of the femoral head below the inguinal ligament and above the bifurcation of the common femoral into the superficial femoral artery and profound femoral artery. CFA: Common femoral artery; PFA: Profound femoral artery; SFA: Superficial femoral artery

more than 70% of cases the inguinal crease lies below bifurcation of CFA, thus increasing the risk of low puncture and its associated complications.[6,7] We strongly advise against using inguinal crease as a landmark for femoral arterial puncture. Inguinal ligament is a better landmark for femoral artery puncture. It extends from midpoint of pubic symphysis to anterior superior iliac spine. A point 2–3 cm below midpoint of inguinal ligament can be reliably used for femoral artery puncture, as shown in Figure 30.1.[6]

2. ***Area of maximum pulsation of femoral artery:*** Area of maximum pulsation of femoral artery is over the CFA in over 90% of the cases.[6,8] However, this landmark is unreliable when used alone.
3. ***Bony landmark:*** Femoral head is the most reliable landmark. Centre of the femoral head corresponds to CFA. Bifurcation of CFA is consistently found to be below the middle of femoral head.[9] Using fluoroscopic guidance to localize middle of femoral head is the standard recommended technique for femoral puncture.

Complications of Transfemoral Access: Types, Incidence, and Consequences

Types of Complications

Femoral access site complications can be divided into two broad categories clinically: minor and major, as described in Table 30.1 (Figure 30.2). Brief description of each complication is given in the following:

Bleeding: Bleeding is the most common complication of femoral access site. It can manifest clinically as uncontrolled bleed, stable/unstable haematoma, pseudoaneurysm, and retroperitoneal (RP) haemorrhage. Haematomas can lead to haemorrhagic shock in around 10–15% of the cases.[10] Pseudoaneurysm is defined as a communication between femoral artery and the fibromuscular tissue which overlies it, resulting in a blood filled cavity.[11] It is far more common in obese patients. Most common cause for pseudoaneurysm is failure to achieve adequate haemostasis post sheath removal.[12] Haematoma and pseudoaneurysm both present clinically as local site swelling. Difference is that pseudoaneurysm has continuation with lumen of femoral artery whereas haematoma does

Table 30.1 Femoral access site complications are of two types: Minor and Major

Minor Complications	Major Complications
Minor bleed	Pseudo aneurysm
Ecchymosis	AV fistula
Stable hematoma	Hematoma requiring blood transfusion
	RP Hemorrhage
	Arterial dissection
	Thrombo-embolism
	Infection
	Vessel rupture/perforation
	Limb ischemia

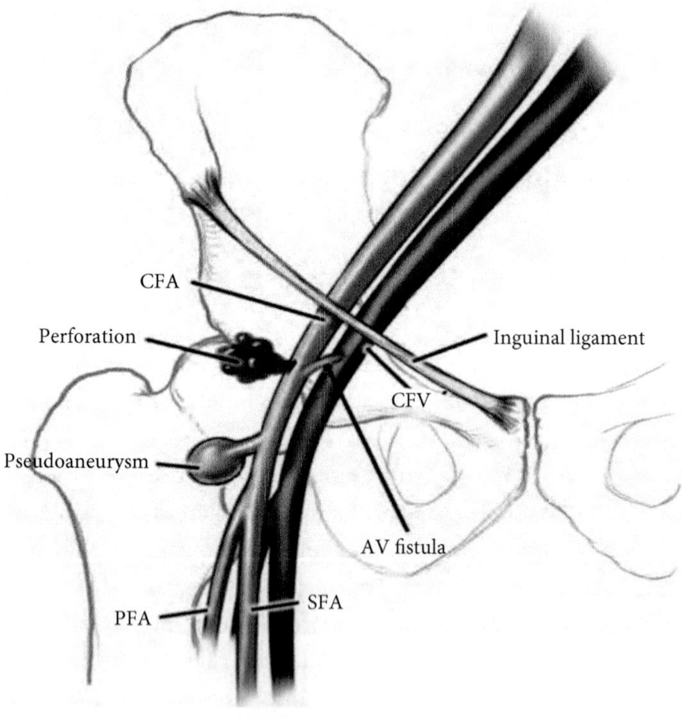

Figure 30.2 Complications of vascular access site in the femoral artery. Pseudo aneurysm (blood-filled cavity communicating with the vessel lumen), arterial perforation and arteriovenous fistula (abnormal communication between the femoral artery and the common femoral vein). AV: Arteriovenous fistula; CFA: Common femoral artery; CFV: Common femoral vein; PFA: Profound femoral artery; SFA: Superficial femoral artery.

not.[10,12] RP haemorrhage is the most catastrophic of all the femoral access site complications. Rather than the bleed per se, it is failure to recognize it in time, which leads to most of the mortalities due to RP haemorrhage. It is commonly missed and thus high degree of suspicion is required to diagnose it in time. RP haemorrhage should always be suspected in patients with unexplained hypotension associated with backache/flank pain, and drop in haemoglobin without an obvious cause.

AV fistula: Defined as a communication between Artery and Vein. In femoral access, it most commonly develops between SFA/profunda femoris and lateral circumflex vein which lies adjacent to the artery.[10] Usually develops after low femoral puncture.

Dissection: Dissection can occur in femoral or the iliac artery. Most commonly, it is in the iliac artery due to associated atherosclerosis and tortuosity.[10]

Thromboembolic complications: These complications are rare but can lead to limb ischaemia.[10,13]

Infection: Infective complications are quite rare, and their frequency is not well defined. However, with increasing use of vascular closure devices, their incidence is on the rise. Infective complications can be local like cellulitis and abscess, or systemic like sepsis. Incidence of local site infection is less than 1%. Most common organisms isolated from infections are *Staphylococcus aureus* and epidermidis.

Neurologic: Neurologic complications include chronic neurogenic pain, paraesthesia, and foot drop. Femoral neuropathy is typically associated with large haematoma and pseudoaneurysm, and rarely with RP haemorrhage. Large haematoma and pseudoaneurysm apply pressure on femoral cutaneous nerve resulting in sensory neuropathy, which is usually reversible once pressure is relieved. Accumulating RP haemorrhage applies pressure on femoral nerve resulting in predominantly motor weakness and pain, which may not be completely reversible even after resolution of accumulated blood.[14]

Incidence: Incidence of femoral access site complications varies widely, depending on the type of complication, population studied, and type of procedure (Diagnostic or Interventional). Incidence is higher for interventional procedures compared to diagnostic, mostly due to larger size of hardware used, prolonged and more intense anticoagulation, and use of powerful antiplatelet agents. Incidence of complications ranges

Table 30.2 Incidences of various femoral access site complications(10,13,18,21,26,43,58–64)

Type of complication	Incidence
Hematoma	2–12%
Pseudo aneurysm	0.5–6.3% (Approximately 1%)
AV fistula	0.2–2.1%
RP hemorrhage	0.15–0.5%
Arterial thrombosis	<0.5%
Arterial dissection	0.01–0.4%
Major bleed after PCI	2–6%

widely from 0% to 17% in diagnostic and interventional procedures.[3] In a study, the incidence of femoral access site complications was 1.8% for diagnostic and 4% for interventional procedures.[15] Incidence of various complications has been given in Table 30.2. It is encouraging that the incidence of complications has decreased over the years, in spite of increasing use of GPIIb/IIIa inhibitors, older age of the patients, and more complex procedures being performed. In Mayo Clinic, the incidence of major bleeding after percutaneous coronary intervention (PCI) decreased from 8.4% in 1994–95 to 3.5% in 2000–05.[16] Reasons for decreasing incidence are: decreased mean sheath size, decreased use of venous sheath, decreased intensity of anticoagulation with unfractionated heparin (UFH) as assessed by peak Activated Clotting Time (ACT), decreased use of post procedural heparin, and decreased procedural time.[17] Incidence is further expected to decrease with more frequent transradial approach, use of better anticoagulation and antiplatelet agents, and better hardware.

Consequences of Femoral Access Site Complications

Femoral access site complications increase morbidity as well as mortality. It increases duration of hospital stay as well as increases the cost. It has been noted that in patients undergoing PCI (Percutaneous Coronary Intervention), who develop femoral access site haematoma, there is fivefold increase in in-hospital mortality and fourfold increase in one-year mortality.[18] In-hospital death and major adverse cardiovascular events (MACE) increases in presence of major or minor bleeding complications.[19] Average hospital stay is 8.9 days for patients with major bleed, compared to 3.1 days for patients without bleeding. Blood transfusion remains an independent predictor of in-hospital and one-year mortality. Patients who develop RP haemorrhage while undergoing PCI have a higher rate of requirement for blood transfusion, increase in duration of hospital stay, and higher mortality.[4] Another issue with access site complications is decision to withhold dual antiplatelet therapy (DAPT). Minor access site complications do not always require discontinuation of DAPT, as stopping DAPT can result in other complications like recurrent ischaemia, stent thrombosis, and myocardial infarction (MI).[17]

Risk Factors

Risk factors for femoral access site complications can be patient related and procedure related, as described in Table 30.3. There are a few

Table 30.3 Risk factors for femoral access site complications[(3,13,65,66)]

Patient related	Procedure related
Female gender	Previous catheterization at same site
Low BMI	Higher dose and longer duration of anticoagulation
Obesity	Use of thrombolytic agents
Low BSA	Use of GPIIb/IIIa inhibitors
Older age	Larger arterial sheath
Peripheral vascular disease	Concomitant use of venous sheath
Renal failure	Prolonged indwelling sheath
Thrombocytopenia	Prolonged procedure duration
Hypertension	Location of arterial puncture
Cardiogenic shock	
Acute MI	

independent predictors of certain complications as described in the following:

1. ***Haematoma requiring blood transfusion:*** Old age, female gender, smaller body surface area (BSA), associated renal failure, emergent procedure in patients with acute MI or cardiogenic shock (CS), and concomitant use of GPIIb/IIIa inhibitors or thrombolytic agents.[18]
2. ***Pseudoaneurysm:*** Old age, female gender, obesity, low puncture, interventional rather than diagnostic procedure, larger devices, and more aggressive anticoagulation.[13,20]
3. ***RP haemorrhage:*** High puncture, especially above the most inferior border of inferior epigastric artery, double/back wall puncture, and use of anticoagulation post procedure.[3,7,13,21]
4. ***AV fistula:*** High/low puncture, multiple puncture attempts, and deranged coagulation parameters.
5. ***Lower limb ischaemia:*** Old age, associated peripheral vascular disease (PVD), associated cardiomyopathy, hypercoagulable state, larger sheath, or catheter size, and vessel dissection.[13]

Management

Diagnosis

Femoral access site complications are suspected based on history (pain, swelling) and physical examination (tenderness, swelling, discolouration, bruit, etc.). Diagnosis is confirmed with imaging. Ultrasonography (USG) is the initial investigation of choice, and in most cases, it is the only investigation that is required to reach accurate diagnosis. USG can reliably and accurately diagnose pseudoaneurysm and AV fistula.[22] It can also accurately diagnose haematoma and arterial thrombosis. For complications like dissection, RP haemorrhage CT angiography is required. Some operators do a check femoral angiogram on table, which can diagnose catastrophic complications like RP haemorrhage in time, and we advise for the same. Table 30.4 enumerates the clinical features, method

Table 30.4 Clinical features, method to diagnose, and possible secondary complications of various femoral access site complications[10–13,26,67,68]

Complication	Clinical finding	Diagnosis	Secondary complications
Hematoma	Pain Swelling Bruising	USG CT	Anemia Neuropathy
Pseudo aneurysm	Pain Swelling Pulsatile mass Systolic bruit	USG	Anemia Neuropathy Rupture Hypovolemic shock Embolization
AV fistula	Pansystolic bruit Thrill Swollen, tender extremity	USG	Steal syndrome High-output cardiac failure Limb claudication Aneurysmal degeneration of the artery
RP hemorrhage	Hypotension Back, flank, hip or abdominal pain Anemia	CT Femoral Angiogram Local Exploration in operating room	Anemia Neuropathy Mortality rate of 6.6%
Thrombo-embolism	5 P's (Pain, Pallor, Parasthesia, Pulselessness, Poikilothermia)	USG	Potential loss of limb
Infection	Sepsis Erythema Abscess	Clinical findings Blood culture	Septic shock Death

of diagnosis, and possible secondary complications of various femoral access site complications.

Treatment

Treatment depends on the type of access site complication, as described in the following:

1. ***Haematoma:*** Treatment approach depends on the size and haemodynamic significance of the haematoma. Small and

haemodynamically insignificant haematomas can be successfully managed by prolonged compression alone in most cases. For larger and haemodynamically significant haematomas, following treatment approach is recommended. Anticoagulation must be reversed to prevent further active bleed. Fluids and blood transfusion (in case of hypotension/fall in haemoglobin) must be given. Initially, prolonged compression (preferably USG guided) can be tried. But, if haematoma does not resolve with compression, immediate femoral angiography must be done from the opposite CFA and puncture site localized. Once localized, balloon tamponade is the initial approach that must be done.[10] In most cases, balloon tamponade successfully seals the puncture site. If not, covered stent can be placed to seal the puncture site. If a large haematoma develops on table, most probably the femoral artery must have been nicked and sheath should be upgraded to a larger one to prevent further perisheath bleed into haematoma.

2. ***Pseudoaneurysm:*** Treatment approach depends on size and associated symptoms. Smaller pseudo aneurysms (less than 3 cm), can just be observed, as most thrombose spontaneously over three to four weeks. For larger pseudo aneurysms, multiple treatment options are available like USG-guided compression, USG-guided thrombin injection, endovascular approaches like coil embolization or placement of stent graft, and surgery. Usual approach is to proceed from a less invasive to more invasive option. USG-guided compression of neck of pseudoaneurysm is the initial approach in most cases. It is sufficient to resolve relatively smaller pseudo aneurysms. If this approach is not successful USG-guided thrombin injection into the pseudoaneurysm sac is the next approach. This option can be directly chosen in relatively larger pseudo aneurysms without trying USG-guided compression as it is more effective. Extreme care must be taken to inject thrombin away from the vessel lumen, as accidental injection into lumen can lead to catastrophic complication of femoral thrombosis. USG-guided para-aneurysmal injection of saline is another option, but it is not as reliable as thrombin injection into aneurysmal sac. Surgery remains the final resort and Gold standard treatment

for pseudoaneurysm. Indications for surgery include failure of a less invasive approach, rapid expansion of pseudoaneurysm, compromised soft tissue viability, associated distal ischaemia or neurodeficit, and presence of mycotic aneurysm. Surgical techniques include direct suturing of the vessel defect after haematoma evacuation or patch angioplasty.[11,12,20,23,24]

3. ***RP haemorrhage:*** Treatment depends on the clinical situation. In most cases, conservative management with fluids, blood transfusion, reversal of anticoagulation, and antiplatelet suffices, as the accumulating RP bleed will tamponade the bleeding site. If conservative approach is unsuccessful or if the patient is in haemodynamic collapse, endovascular approach is recommended. Endovascular techniques include balloon tamponade, coiling, and covered stent. Balloon tamponade is the main method, and it suffices in most cases.[25] Surgery remains the final resort if endovascular approach fails. We recommend check femoral angiogram after completion of procedure, to identify and treat RP haemorrhage in time.
4. ***AV fistula:*** Conservative management suffices in most cases, as most AV fistulas are small, asymptomatic, and close spontaneously. Larger and symptomatic AV fistulas require some kind of treatment. Available treatment options include prolonged pressure bandaging, USG-guided compression, endovascular approach like coil embolization and implantation of covered stents. Surgery is the final resort if a less invasive approach fails.[11,13,26]
5. ***Lower limb ischaemia:*** Treatment depends on etiology. Lower limb angiography confirms the etiology. Most common etiologies are thrombo-embolism and dissection. For thrombo-embolism treatment options include endovascular approach and surgery. Endovascular approaches include balloon angioplasty, catheter directed thrombolysis/thrombectomy, and deployment of stent. If endovascular approaches fails, surgery is the final resort.[13] For dissection, the treatment approaches include removal of hardware like wire and catheter and observation. If unsuccessful or if dissection is flow limiting, endovascular approaches like balloon angioplasty or deployment of stent can be tried. Surgery remains the final resort.[10,13]

Prevention of Femoral Complications

There are various ways of decreasing the incidence of femoral access site complications as described in the following:

1. *Choice of access site:* Access sites most commonly used for diagnostic and interventional procedures in cardiology are radial, brachial, and femoral artery. Brachial access has similar rates of complications as femoral access, except ischaemic complications which are higher in brachial route.[10] Radial route has lower rates of complications than femoral (as low as <0.3%).[27–29] Also, it improves patient comfort level and decreases hospital costs by decreasing incidence of complications.[6,30] Along with the various advantages it offers, radial access has its own disadvantages like increased incidence of arterial spasm, requires better skills, complex procedures requiring larger hardware (≥ 8F) are difficult to perform, increases procedure duration and radiation exposure (in the less-experienced operators), rates of arterial occlusion are higher with lower artery to sheath ratio and prolonged compression time. Incidence of arterial occlusion in earlier studies was as high as 9%[31]; however, in recent studies, the incidence has come down to ≤ 3%. We recommend to use radial access as default strategy whenever feasible, to avoid femoral access site complications.
2. *Imaging-guided femoral puncture:* As described earlier, using fluoroscopic guidance is the best method for a safe femoral arterial puncture. Medial border of femoral head is the most ideal landmark for CFA.[6] Fluoroscopic-guided puncture results in more ideal sheath placement, particularly in obese patients; however, it does not drastically decrease the complication rates.[32] In a study, fluoroscopic-guided puncture decreased the incidence of low punctures, especially in obese and female patients, but did not decrease the complication rates significantly.[33] In another study, it was noted that fluoroscopic guided puncture was associated with significantly lower incidence of arterial injury and pseudoaneurysm, but there was no significant difference in incidence of bleeding complications.[34] Most significant advantage of fluoroscopic guided puncture is decrease in incidence of RP haemorrhage as it avoids high

punctures. Ultrasonography can also be used guiding femoral puncture. In a study, USG-guided puncture vis-à-vis fluoroscopic guided puncture showed lesser number of puncture attempts, lesser time to access artery, lower risk of accidental venipuncture, and lesser incidence of complications like haematoma. However, the better cannulation rates with USG guidance were seen only in patients with high CFA bifurcation.[35]

3. ***Choice of intravenous antiplatelet agent:*** GPIIb/IIIa inhibitors have an influence on incidence of local site complications. Intravenous antiplatelet agents commonly used during interventional procedures are Abciximab, Tirofiban, and Eptifibatide. Various studies have shown that GPIIb/IIIa inhibitors increase the rates of access site complications, especially Abciximab.[36,37] Major reason for increased incidence of complications with Abciximab when compared to Tirofiban and Eptifibatide is that, reversal of antiplatelet activity of Abciximab after stopping is slower compared to other two agents, and Tirofiban and Eptifibatide effect can be reversed effectively with platelet transfusion if bleeding occurs.[38] EPIC trial showed that combination of Abciximab with full dose UFH was associated with increased risk of bleeding. EPILOG trial showed that combination of Abciximab with low dose weight adjusted UFH did not increase rates of bleeding, and also conferred substantial clinical benefit.[39] Rather than routine use, these agents must be used selectively when absolutely essential. In acute coronary syndromes, use of intravenous Cangrelor provides adequate anti-platelet activity for PCI, while the oral loading dose of ticagrelor takes effect; and has the advantage of lower bleeding risk, besides a very short time to onset and offset of action.
4. ***Choice of anticoagulant:*** Most commonly used anticoagulants are UFH and Bivalirudin. Fondaparinux is no longer used as it was found to be associated with significantly higher incidence of catheter thrombosis. Bivalirudin binds to both fibrin bound and unbound thrombin in a reversible manner.[40] Bivalirudin has been compared with UFH with or without GPIIb/IIIa inhibitors in various studies. Bivalirudin when compared with UFH alone was associated with similar rates of ischaemia and lower rates of bleeding.[41] When Bivalirudin alone was compared to UFH and GPIIb/IIIa

inhibitor in patients with STEMI undergoing primary PCI, it was found that 30-day rates of major bleeding and MACE were lower in Bivalirudin group.[42] Another study compared combination of Bivalirudin and GPIIb/IIIa inhibitor with UFH and GPIIb/IIIa inhibitor in patients with moderate or high risk acute coronary syndrome (ACS). Similar rates of ischaemic complications and bleeding were seen in this study.[41] Bivalirudin plus selective GPIIb/IIIa inhibitor was compared with low dose UFH plus GPIIb/IIIa inhibitor in REPLACE-2 trial. Bivalirudin group had lesser major bleed with similar rates of peri-procedural ischaemia.[43] Various trials have compared UFH versus Bivalirudin in ACS (Acute Coronary Syndrome) patients undergoing intervention, with conflicting results.[44–50] Going by the current evidence choice of best anticoagulant during intervention remains unanswered.

5. ***Proper sheath removal:*** Timely and adequate sheath removal goes a long way in preventing complications. Early sheath removal and inadequate compression can lead to complications like bleeding, haematoma, and pseudo aneurysm. Whereas, delayed sheath removal can lead to catastrophic complication like femoral arterial thrombosis. Hence, it is important to remove the sheath at the right time. ACT guided sheath removal is the recommended technique to decrease the complications. An ACT of <150 seconds is taken as standard criteria for sheath removal.
6. ***Use of closure devices:*** Two types of vascular closure devices are available (Table 30.5): Passive and Active. Passive devices enhance manual compression, but some of these devices do not induce immediate haemostasis.[51] Active devices are of three types: Collagen based, Suture based, and Staple based. Advantages of vascular closure devices include: Early mobilization, better patient comfort, early discharge, decreased healthcare cost, and arguably decreased complications.[52] Main advantage of vascular closure devices after diagnostic coronary angiography is shortened time to ambulation. This may become less relevant as more procedures are being performed with radial access.[52] These devices may be of advantage after PCI, where patient is at increased risk of bleeding, although transradial PCI may change this paradigm as well.[52] Complication rates of vascular closure devices versus manual compression

Table 30.5 Enumerates various Vascular closure devices commonly used, their mechanism of action, and important points about each of them[6,69–74]

Closure device	Mechanism of action	Notes
AngioSeal™	Utilizes a collagen plug and anchor mechanism. A suture cinches the anchor and collagen component to form a secure seal	Collagen plug breaks down over months and anchor is absorbed by hydrolysis over months. Similar or lower complications as manual compression
Perclose™	A suture on each side of the arterial puncture site is tied using a preloaded knot tying device. Knot is cinched and suture is cut close to the arterial wall	Suture material is not absorbable
StarClose™	Extravascular clip deployed through peal-away sheath onto the extravascular arterial surface, achieving closure through primary healing	Similar major vascular complications and fewer minor complications as manual compression. The clip is not absorbable
FemoStop™	A belt and air pressure filled bulb is used to compress the artery	Complications result from inadequate compression time or poorly placed compression. Requires significant staff time. Applying device for too long can result in increased risk of arterial and venous thrombosis and injury to femoral nerve
Boomerang™	Percutaneous vascular closure device that promotes hemostasis via intravascular tamponade with complete removal of the system after hemostasis is achieved	Requires significantly shorter staff time than manual compression
Mynx™	Utilizes a water soluble polyethylene glycol sealant that expands inside the tissue tract by absorbing blood and subcutaneous fluids to provide a seal over the arteriotomy site and within the tissue tract	Sealant is fully reabsorbed within 30 days. Avoids cinching or tugging of the artery

(continued)

Table 30.5 Continued

Closure device	Mechanism of action	Notes
ExoSeal™	Visually guided deployment mechanism that delivers a bioabsorbable polyglycolic acid plug atop the femoral artery	Plug is hydrolyzed within 3 months. Avoids cinching or tugging of the artery
Femoral Introducer Sheath and Hemostasis (FISH)™	FISH uses an extracellular matrix closure patch premounted on a 5, 6, or 8 Fr access sheath	Serves as an access and closure device Patch is resorbed within 90 days

remains debatable. Early studies showed higher incidence of access site complications with vascular closure devices.[53] However, newer data suggests that complication rates are similar to manual compression, with earlier time to haemostasis.[54,55] In a study by Arora *et al,* in patients undergoing both diagnostic angiography and PCI, rates of vascular complications were less with vascular closure devices compared to manual compression.[56] With the availability of newer devices, better technique and operator experience, it is likely that use of vascular closure devices will reduce complications and cost, though radial access may still be safer than transfemoral approach with hemostasis via vessel plugs or suture devices and should be considered best practice.[52,57,58]

Summary

The world of interventional cardiology has come a long way since Andreas Gruentzig performed the first angioplasty in 1977. Transradial access is gradually replacing transfemoral access as default route for diagnostic and interventional cardiac procedures. But, with increasing number of complex procedures being performed, transfemoral access remains in picture and is still the most commonly used route for catheterization procedures.[1,2] Transfemoral access is associated with significantly more complications than transradial access. However, the incidence of access site complications can be kept minimum by practicing proper puncture technique, careful choice of anticoagulant and antiplatelet agent, and proper sheath removal. Vascular closure devices have changed the dynamics of femoral access site complications, by decreasing the incidence of complications like bleeding, haematoma, whereas increasing other complications like infection, stenosis, and embolism.[10]

References

1. Louvard I, Lefevre T, Allain A, Morice MC. Coronary angio-graphy trough the radial or the femoral approach. The CARAFE study. Cathet Cardiovasc Interv 2001;52:181–7.
2. Morice MC, Dumas P, Lefevre T, Lougeyre C, Louvard Y, Piechaud J. Systematic use of transradial approach or suture of the femoral artery after angioplasty. Attempt at achieving zero ac- cess site complications. Catheter Cardiovasc Interv 2000;51:417–21.
3. Sherev DA, Shaw RE, Brent BN. Angiographic predictors of femoral access site complications: implication for planned percutaneous coronary intervention. Catheter Cardiovasc. Interv. 65(2), 196–202 (2005).
4. Ellis SG, Bhatt D, Kapadia S, Lee D, Yen M, Whitlow PL. Correlates and outcomes of retroperitoneal hemorrhage complicating percutaneous coronary intervention. Catheter Cardiovasc. Interv. 67(4), 541–545 (2006).
5. Moore KL, Dalley AF. Clinically Oriented Anatomy. 4th Edition. Lippincott Williams & Wilkins, Baltimore, MD, USA, 541–545 (1999).
6. Cox N. Managing the femoral artery in coronary angiography. Heart Lung Circ. 17, S65–S69 (2008).
7. Turi ZG. Optimal femoral access prevents complications. Cardiac Interventions Today 35–38 (2008).
8. Grier D, Hartnell G. Percutaneous femoral artery puncture: practice and anatomy. Br. J. Radiol. 65(752), 602–604 (1990).
9. Garrett PD, Eckart RE, Bauch TD, Thompson CM, Stajduhar KC. Fluoroscopic localization of the femoral head as a landmark for common femoral artery cannulation. Catheter Cardiovasc. Interv. 65(2), 205–207 (2005).
10. Samal AK, White CJ. Percutaneous 19 management of access site complications. Catheter Cardiovasc. Interv. 57(1), 12–23 (2002).
11. Levine GN, Kern MJ, Berger PB et al. Management of patients undergoing percutaneous coronary revascularization. Ann. Intern. Med. 139(2), 123–136 (2003).
12. Tisi PV, Callam MJ. Treatment for femoral pseudoaneurysms (review). Cochrane Database Syst. Rev. 2 (2009).
13. Wiley JM, White CJ, Uretsky BF. Noncoronary complications of coronary intervention. Catheter Cardiovasc. Interv. 57(2), 257–265 (2002).
14. Davis C, VanRiper S, Longstreet J, Moscucci M. Vascular complications of coronary interventions. Heart Lung 26(2), 118–127 (1997).
15. Chandrasekar B, Doucet S, Bilodeau L et al. Complications of cardiac catheterization in the current era: a single-center experience. Catheter Cardiovasc. Interv. 52(3), 289–295 (2001).

16. Sohail MR, Khan AH, Holmes DRJ, Wilson WR, Steckelberg JM, Baddour LM. Infectious complications of percutaneous vascular closure devices. Mayo Clin. Proc. 80(8), 1011–1015 (2005).
17. Doyle BJ, Ting HH, Bell MR et al. Major femoral bleeding complications after percutaneous coronary intervention: incidence, predictors, and impact on long-term survival among 17,901 patients treated at the Mayo Clinic from 1994 to 2005. JACC Cardiovasc. Interv. 1(2), 202–209 (2008).
18. Yatskar L, Selzer F, Feit F et al. Access site hematoma requiring blood transfusion predicts mortality in patients undergoing percutaneous coronary intervention: Data from the National Heart, Lung, and Blood Institute Dynamic Registry. Catheter Cardiovasc. Interv. 69(7), 961–966 (2007).
19. Kinnaird T, Anderson R, Hill J, Thomas M. Bleeding during percutaneous intervention: tailoring the approach to minimise risk. Heart 95(1), 15–19 (2009).
20. Ahmad F, Turner SA, Torrie P, Gibson M. Iatrogenic femoral artery pseudoaneurysms – a review of current methods of diagnosis and treatment. Clin. Radiol. 63(12), 1310–1316 (2008).
21. Sreeram S, Lumsden AB, Miller JS, Salam AA, Dodson TF, Smith RB. Retroperitoneal hematoma following femoral arterial catheterization: a serious and often fatal complication. Am. Surg. 59(2), 94–98 (1993).
22. Azmoon S, Pucillo AL, Aronow WS et al. Vascular complications after percutaneous coronary intervention following hemostasis with the Mynx vascular closure device versus the AngioSeal vascular closure device. J. Invasive Cadiol. 22(4), 175–178 (2010).
23. Lenartova M, Tak T. Iatrogenic pseudoaneurysm of femoral artery: case report and literature review. Clin. Med. Res. 1(13), 243–247 (2003).
24. Chan YC, Morales JP, Reidy JF, Taylor PR. Management of spontaneous and iatrogenic retroperitoneal haemorrhage: conservative management, endovascular intervention, or 69 open surgery? Int. J. Clin. Pract. 62(10), 1604–1613 (2008).
25. Silva JA, Stant J, Ramee SR. Endovascular treatment of a massive retroperitoneal bleeding: successful balloon-catheter delivery of intra-arterial thrombin. Catheter Cardiovasc. Interv. 64(2), 218–222 (2005).
26. Tsetis D. Endovascular treatment of complications of femoral arterial access. Cardiovasc. Intervent. Radiol. 33(3), 457–468 (2010).
27. Jolly SS, Yusuf S, Cairns J et al. Radial versus femoral access for coronary angiography and intervention in patients with acute coronary syndromes (RIVAL): a randomized, parallel group, multicentre trial. Lancet 377(9775), 1409–1420 (2011).
28. Agostoni P, Biondi-Zoccai G.L. Benedictis M. LuisaDe, Rigattieri S, †Turri M, et al. Radial versus femoral approach for percutaneous coronary diagnostic and interventional procedures: Systematic overview and meta-analysis of randomized trials Journal of the American College of Cardiology Volume 44, Issue 2, 21 July 2004, Pages 349–356.
29. Sanmartin M, Cuevas D, Goicolea J, Ruiz-Salmeron R, Gomez M, Argibay V. Vascular complications associated with radial artery access for cardiac catheterization. Rev. Esp. Cardiol. 57(6), 581–584 (2004).
30. Franchi E, Marino P, Biondi-Zoccai GG, De Luca G, Vassanelli C, Agostoni P. Transradial versus transfemoral approach for percutaneous coronary procedures. Curr. Cardiol. Rep. 11(5), 391–397 (2009).

31. Pancholy S, Coppola J, Patel T, Roke-Thomas M. Prevention of radial artery occlusion- patent hemostasis evaluation trial (PROPHET study): a randomized comparison of traditional versus patency documented hemostasis after transradial catheterization. Catheter Cardiovasc. Interv. 72(3), 335–340 (2008).
32. Jacobi JA, Schussler JM, Johnson KB. Routine femoral head fluoroscopy to reduce complications in coronary catheterization. Proc. (Bayl. Univ. Med. Cent.) 22(1), 7–8 (2009).
33. Abu-Fadel MS, Sparling JM, Zacharias SJ et al. Fluoroscopy vs. traditional guided femoral arterial access and the use of closure devices: a randomized controlled trial. Catheter Cardiovasc. Interv. 74(4), 533–539 (2009).
34. Fitts J, Ver Lee P, Hofmaster P, Malenka D. Fluoroscopy-guided femoral artery puncture reduces the risk of PCI-related vascular complications. J. Interv. Cardiol. 21(3), 273–278 (2008).
35. Seto AH, Abu-Fadel MS, Sparling JM et al. Real-time ultrasound guidance facilitates femoral arterial access and reduces vascular complications: FAUST (femoral arterial access with ultrasound trial). JACC Cardiovasc. Interv. 3(7), 751–758 (2010).
36. Lefkovits J, Plow EF, Topol EJ. Platelet glycoprotein IIb/IIIa receptors in cardiovascular medicine. N. Engl. J. Med. 332(23), 1553–1559 (1995).
37. Proimos G. Platelet aggregation inhibition with glycoprotein IIb–IIIa inhibitors. J. Thromb. Thrombolysis 11(2), 99–110 (2001).
38. Mascelli MA, Lance ET, Damaraju L, Wagner CL, Weisman HF, Jordan RE. Pharmacodynamic profile of short-term abciximab treatment demonstrates prolonged platelet inhibition with gradual recovery from GP IIb/IIIa receptor blockade. Circulation 97(17), 1680–1686 (1998).
39. Kereiakes DJ, Lincoff AM, Miller DP et al. Abciximab therapy and unplanned coronary stent deployment: Favorable effects on stent use, clinical outcomes, and bleeding complications. Circulation 97(9), 857–864 (1998).
40. Moen MD, Keating GM, Wellington K. Bivalirudin: a review of its use in patients undergoing percutaneous coronary intervention. Drugs 65(13), 1869–1891 (2005).
41. Stone GW, McLaurin BT, Cox DA et al. Bivalirudin for patients with acute coronary syndromes. N. Engl. J. Med. 355(21), 2203–2216 (2006).
42. Stone GW, Witzenbichler B, Guagliumi G et al. Bivalirudin during primary PCI in acute myocardial infarction. N. Engl. J. Med. 358(21), 2218–2230 (2008).
43. Lincoff AM, Bittl JA, Harrington RA et al. Bivalirudin and provisional glycoprotein IIb/ IIIa blockade compared with heparin and planned glycoprotein IIb/IIIa blockade during percutaneous coronary intervention: REPLACE-2 randomized trial. JAMA 289(7), 853–863 (2003).
44. Navarese EP, Schulze V, Andreotti F, et al. Comprehensive meta-analysis of safety and efficacy of bivalirudin versus heparin with or without routine glycoprotein IIb/IIIa inhibitors in patients with acute coronary syndrome. JACC Cardiovasc Interv 2015;8:201–213.
45. Stone GW, McLaurin BT, Cox DA, et al. Bivalirudin for patients with acute coronary syndromes. N Engl J Med 2006;355:2203–2216.
46. Stone GW, Witzenbichler B, Guagliumi G, et al. Bivalirudin during primary PCI in acute myocardial infarction. N Engl J Med 2008;358:2218–2230.

47. Steg PG, van 't Hof A, Hamm CW, et al. Bivalirudin started during emergency transport for primary PCI. N Engl J Med 2013;369:2207–2217.
48. Shahzad A, Kemp I, Mars C, et al. Unfractionated heparin versus bivalirudin in primary percutaneous coronary intervention (HEAT-PPCI): an open-label, single centre, randomised controlled trial. Lancet 2014;384:1849–1858.
49. Han Y, Guo J, Zheng Y, et al. Bivalirudin vs heparin with or without tirofiban during primary percutaneous coronary intervention in acute myocardial infarction: the BRIGHT randomized clinical trial. JAMA 2015;313:1336–1346.
50. Valgimigli, M., Frigoli, E., Leonardi, S. et al, Bivalirudin or Unfractionated Heparin in Acute Coronary Syndromes. N Engl J Med. 2015;373:997–1009.
51. Dauerman HL, Applegate RJ, Cohen DJ. Vascular closure devices: the second decade. J. Am. Coll. Cardiol. 50(17), 1617–1626 (2007).
52. Bhatty S, Cooke R, Shetty R, Jovin IS. Femoral vascular access-site complications in the cardiac catheterization laboratory: diagnosis and management. Interv Cardiol. 2011;3(4):503–14.
53. Dangas G, Mehran R, Kokolis S et al. Vascular complications after percutaneous coronary interventions following hemostasis with manual compression versus arteriotomy closure devices. J. Am. Coll. Cardiol. 38(3), 638–641 (2001).
54. Koreny M, Riedmüller E, Nikfardjam M, Siostrzonek P, Müllner M: Arterial puncture closing devices compared with standard manual compression after cardiac catheterization: systematic review and meta-analysis. JAMA 291(3), 350–357 (2004).
55. Nikolsky E, Mehran R, Halkin A et al. Vascular complications associated with arteriotomy closure devices in patients undergoing percutaneous coronary procedures. J. Am. Coll. Cardiol. 44(6), 1200–1209 (2004).
56. Arora N, Matheny ME, Sepke C, Resnic FS. A propensity analysis of the risk of vascular complications after cardiac catheterization procedures with the use of vascular closure devices. Am. Heart J. 153(4), 606–611 (2007).
57. Resnic FS, Arora N, Matheny M, Reynolds MR. A cost-minimization analysis of the angio-seal vascular closure device following percutaneous coronary intervention. Am. J. Cardiol. 99(6), 766–770 (2007).
58. Chugh, Yashasvi & Bavishi, Chirag & Mojadidi, Mohammad & Elgendy, Islam & Faillace, Robert & Brilakis, Emmanouil & Tamis-Holland, Jacqueline & Mamas, Mamas & Chugh, Sanjay. (2020). Safety of transradial access compared to transfemoral access with hemostatic devices (vessel plugs and suture devices) after percutaneous coronary interventions: A systematic review and meta-analysis. Catheterization and Cardiovascular Interventions. 96. 10.1002/ccd.29061.

31

STOP PRESS: Transradial Interventions in COVID Times

Yashasvi Chugh, Sunita Chugh, Sanjay Kumar Chugh
On behalf of the COVID working group of Wellness and Radial Intervention Society

Impact of COVID on Healthcare and on Cardiac Patients

The COVID 19 pandemic affected the entire world and overwhelmed the health services world-wide. As a consequence, the non-COVID patients just disappeared from hospitals in these countries, especially in USA, Italy, and Spain; simply because there were no beds left for other patients. While in New York, 911 calls from residents went up, many of which were for cardiac arrests; ST elevation (STE) and non-ST elevation (NSTE) myocardial infarctions (MI) disappeared from emergency rooms, as did strokes. Of course pseudo- MIs or myocarditis masquerading as STEMI and NSTEMI continued to challenge the cardiologists world-wide.

During the COVID- related lockdown period, in India too, it was difficult for patients to reach hospitals. Added to this was their fear of getting infected with COVID 19. As a result non-COVID patients, including ST elevation (STE) and non-ST elevation (NSTE) myocardial infarctions (MI) and strokes disappeared from hospitals in India, between March 22nd and end of April. Thereafter, the emergency patients started trickling in. Meanwhile, departments across the country had had time to think of their management protocols and prepare their standard operating procedures to deal with patients. Catheterization laboratories (CL) devised mechanisms to cope up.

The number of COVID positive cases in India grew from over 3000 per day in March, 2020, to over 9000 per day by end of May, 2020. The directive of the Government, in India, in March 2020 to segregate COVID and non-COVID patients for treatment in separate COVID and non-COVID centers lost clarity by the end of May, 2020 as the number of positive cases climbed and private hospitals had to be roped in. Some private hospitals thus ended-up having both COVID and non-COVID wards, a not very desirable combination, because such a mix increased chances of cross-infection and had the potential to turn hospitals into epicenters of infection, as probably happened at some locations.

In the initial period of the pandemic, the practice at most hospitals in India was that every patient requiring admission in hospital would first be tested for SARS-CoV-2 using reverse transcriptase polymerase chain reaction (RT-PCR). They were then admitted to an isolation ward. Those testing positive were promptly referred to a designated COVID center or ward and the negative ones were then taken up for procedures as appropriate; non-invasive and invasive. Our departmental protocol required us to wear a personal protection equipment (PPE) kit for all procedures in the cath lab (CL), even for patients with a negative RT-PCR report (1), because of concern that a significant proportion of the tests would be false negative, based on reports of false negativity from 100% on day-1 to 38% on day-5, dropping to 21% on day 8, then rising steadily thereafter to 66% on Day 21 (2). Since the turnaround time for the RT-PCR reports was initially 48 hours; until the patient's COVID RT-PCR report was received, the patients had to be treated conservatively, which included thrombolysis for STEMIs, in keeping with the Chinese reports. Only the very sick, such as patients with MI and hemodynamic compromise or those requiring rescue percutaneous coronary intervention (PCI) were taken to CL for procedures at a COVID19 designated facility (1). As the turnaround time for RT-PCR reports dropped to 6 hours at our center, afebrile STEMI or NSTEMI patients without COVID symptoms or breathlessness and normal XRay chest and oxygen saturation, were taken up for interventional procedures as per usual practice and per recommendations of American College of Cardiology, with full or level -1 personal protection (1) for operators.

In the COVID times, since myocarditis caused by SARS-CoV-2 can mimic electrocardiographic changes of both STEMI and NSTEMI and also be associated with raised troponins; cardiologists should be cautious in interpreting electrocardiograms and Troponins, to avoid unnecessary exposure to the CL, cardiologist, and other personnel. Further, in order to keep the risk of contamination of echocardiogram laboratory and exposure of staff and patients to a minimum, an echocardiogram was only advisable for situations where it would favorably alter patient management and outcome. Further guidance on COVID19 is available in our recent publication (1).

Benefits of Transradial Access, Especially for Patient Care During COVID Pandemic

Radial access for coronary diagnostic and interventional procedures is popular worldwide, not only because of enhanced patient comfort, with patients being able to sit up and be able to eat and drink immediately after procedure and ambulate early; but also, more importantly, because of reduced bleeding and vascular complications and enhanced survival in acute coronary syndromes including STEMI (3). Of course training and significant experience is required for operators to become facile to perform complex PCI and primary angioplasty in STEMI. In the latter situation, 'time is muscle' and prompt revascularization is warranted, to achieve the overwhelming survival advantage of transradial PCI over transfemoral PCI in this situation. There is still a huge dearth of experienced radial operators in India, with only a handful facile enough to use radial access as default, or to perform primary PCI for STEMI. As a result, only 30-40% of elective angioplasty and only 2% of all primary angioplasty for STEMI in the country is performed transradially (4). Transradial angioplasty is still a small percentage of total angioplasties in India; even in the National capital region (NCR) of Delhi, which includes Gurgaon, Noida, Ghaziabad and 4zones of Delhi.

Considering the huge number of acute coronary syndrome (ACS) patients including STEMIs requiring PCI; a wide availability of transradial PCI and its easy accessibility to masses would benefit populations worldwide. It is an economical technique which can impact outcomes favorably on a large scale and needs a push for training of cardiologists to make them comfortable in pursuing radial access as default for PCI especially in ACS, including STEMIs per the recent ESC and ACC coronary revascularization guidelines.

In COVID19 times, a shorter hospital stay and lower complication rate with transradial allows a quicker throughput of patients and shortens the contact time between staff and patient, making it a preferred technique compared with transfemoral; because it thus reduces the risk of cross-infection. Contact between staff and patient is further reduced with radial access with the use of a wrist bandage or occlusion band for post-procedure hemostasis (5); unlike manual compression of the groin for an hour after femoral access with femoral access. Hence radial access is better for patients and staff in COVID times.

With radial access, the practice of patent hemostasis or non-occlusive hemostasis post -procedure (6) is labor intensive and requires close monitoring with increased contact between staff and patient. On the other hand, use of gauze ball and bandage (GzBB) (5) has the potential to allow early discharge home, after 3 hours of a transradial angiogram and after 12 hours of transradial angioplasty, based on clinical decision of a consultant. Of course, as per our protocol, the bandage is loosened after 60 minutes. In our practice, the patients remove the GzBB themselves, at home, after 12 hours of procedure. Of course this is only possible with use of a GzBB; not with an occlusion band or device. Further, if the patient requires longer in- hospital stay (5) post-PCI, because of vasopressors or inotropes and /or diuretic infusions for hemodynamic compromise or left ventricular failure, a nurse removes the bandage after 12h in hospital. Radial artery occlusion (RAO) was 2.9% using GzBB, as described, in the standard radial group in DATA STAR study (5), compared to 3% RAO reported in PROPHET II study (6). Further, bleeding complications such as large groin hematomas retroperitoneal bleeds or pseudoaneurysms, which are more common with femoral compared to radial access (3.0 Vs. 0.3%) (7), can lead to prolonged stay, increased cost, more staff-patient interaction, and hence higher risk of cross-infection. Again if surgery is required for vascular or bleeding complications or if there is need for prolonged compression of femoral puncture site to seal off pseudo-aneurysms, then contact between staff and patient is further prolonged with a much higher risk of cross-infection.

Further, pre-procedural ultrasound of arm arteries (8), can be used to select the radial artery with the largest diameter. It is also useful to identify cubital loops or high bifurcation radials in patients. By using the radial artery with larger diameter and straightest course, procedure time and crossover can be minimized, thus reducing the contact time between staff and patient during procedure, as well as concomitant risk of cross-infection.

Again, by performing a pre-procedure ultrasound of arm arteries, one can find at least one suitable artery; radial or ulnar on right or left side (8) and avoid use of femoral access, because, as explained above, femoral access not only requires prolonged groin care with manual compression for hemostasis, it is also associated with higher risk of bleeding and complications. Bleeding complications increase hospital stay and contact between patient and staff and hence risk of cross-infection as well as cost of treatment may increase for these reasons, with development of complications which are more common with femoral access (Femoral Vs. Radial 3% Vs. 0.3%)(7).

A suggestion has been made to perform left distal transradial procedures with the patient prone to reduce the risk of cross- infection in a COVID suspect presenting with electrocardiographic signs of an MI which could be due to SARS-CoV2 myocarditis. In the prone position, there is no option of using the groin for temporary pacing, intra-aortic balloon pump or Impella; or for crossover, should the need arise. Engaging the coronaries with the patient lying prone can be challenging. The technique needs to be tested in large number of patients before its safety and feasibility is established.

In conclusion, in COVID times, it was imperative to minimize contact, and hence exposure, between staff and patients, to prevent cross-infection, Transradial access was advantageous because avoidance of femoral access helped minimize risk of cross- infection and also helped to keep patients safe with reduced bleeding and vascular complications, while also reducing mortality risk in patients with acute coronary syndromes. Early ambulation, and discharge being additional boons for patients.

In COVID times, as in the Pre-COVID era; radial has several advantages over femoral access and is the preferred route for cardiovascular interventions.

I end, with a quote from Charles Darwin-

'It is not the fittest who survive, nor the most intelligent; but those who adapt to change'

References

1. Chugh Y, Chugh S, Chugh SK. Practical guidance for healthcare professionals during the COVID19 pandemic; with special emphasis on care of cardiovascular patients and personal protection. International Journal of Medical Review and Research. June 2020 (In Press).
2. Kucirka LM, Lauer SA, Laeyendecker O, Boon DN and Lessler J. Variation in false-negative rate of reverse transcriptase polymerase chain reaction–based SARS-COV-2 tests by time since exposure. Annals of Internal Medicine doi: 10.7326/M20-1495. Published at Annals.org on 13th May 2020.
3. Hamon M, Pristipino C, Di Mario C, Nolan J, Ludwig J, Tubaro M, Louvard Y., Hammon M. et al. Consensus document on the radial approach in percutaneous cardiovascular interventions: position paper by the European Association of Percutaneous Cardiovascular Interventions and Working Groups on Acute Cardiac Care** and Thrombosis of the European Society of Cardiology. EuroIntervention. 2013;8(11):1242–51.
4. National Intervention Council –Wellness and Radial Intervention Society (NIC WARIS) Data 2016, in Chugh SK, 'Over view of transradial access', in Handbook of transradial interventions. Chugh SK(Ed). Oxford university Press 2020 (In Press).
5. Chugh Y, Kanaparthy NS, Piplani S, Chugh S, Shroff A, Vidovich M, Nolan J, Mamas M, Chugh SK. Comparison of distal radial access versus standard transradial access in patients with smaller diameter radial Arteries(The distal radial versus transradial access in small transradial ArteriesStudy: D.A.T.A - S.T.A.R study). Indian Heart J. 2021 Jan-Feb;73(1):26-34. doi: 10.1016/j.ihj.2020.11.002. Epub 2020 Nov 11. PMID: 33714406; PMCID: PMC7961259
6. Pancholy SB, Bernat I, Bertrand OF, Patel TM (2016) Prevention of radial artery occlusion after transradial catheterization: the PROPHET-II randomized trial. JACC Cardiovasc Interv. 9(19):1992–1999.
7. Agostoni P, Biondi-Zoccai G.L. Benedictis M. LuisaDe, Rigattieri S, †Turri M, et al. Radial versus femoral approach for percutaneous coronary diagnostic and interventional procedures: Systematic overview and meta-analysis of randomized trials Journal of the American College of Cardiology Volume 44, Issue 2, 21 July 2004, Pages 349–356.
8. Chugh SK, Chugh S, Chugh Y, et al. Feasibility and utility of pre-procedure ultrasound imaging of the arm to facilitate trans-radial coronary diagnostic and interventional procedures. (PRIMAFACIE-TRI). Catheter Cardiovasc Interv. 2013;82:64–73

Index

For the benefit of digital users, indexed terms that span two pages (e.g., 52–53) may, on occasion, appear on only one of those pages.

Tables and figures are indicated by *t* and *f* following the page number